U.T.O.P.I.A.

Unified Theory of Oxygen Participation In Aerobiosis:

FIRST EDITION

A Selective World Literature Review

(Hope for Cancer, Heart Disease, HIV/AIDS, Anti-aging and Malaria Patients)

BY

PROF RANDOLPH M. HOWES MD,PHD

(also holding an Honorary Doctorate of Humanities, SLU)
Adjunct Assistant Professor of Plastic Surgery,
The Johns Hopkins Hospital (retired 2013)
Espaldon Professor of Plastic and Reconstructive Surgery,
University of Santo Tomas, Manila
Adjunct Professor of Biological Sciences,
Southeastern Louisiana University

"A mind constrained by misleading doggerel
is difficult to open
and impedes rational consideration
concerning emotional topics.
Ergo, it is necessary to distinguish fact
from manipulated myth,
to dispel generally accepted inaccuracies
and to challenge the power of the uninformed."

R. M. Howes, M.D., Ph.D.

TABLE OF CONTENTS

RONS/excytomers is a term synonymous with "EMODs" electronically modified oxygen derivatives

Necessary edit to shorten the e-book for printer

Throughout this second edition of **UTOPIA**, I left in the original term "**RONS/ excytomers**", which is equivalent to "**EMODs**" (electronically modified oxygen derivatives), which I have used in subsequent versions of my books.

"The cell's intracellular cytoplasmic sea is
an ocean of symphonic motion awash with
incomprehensible complexity."
R. M. Howes, M.D., Ph.D.
1/24/04

Whilst encased in our uterine cocoon,
as the cellular supernova of life begins,
we parasitically tap into Mom's oxygen supply
for perpetuated hits of this gaseous goody.
Thereafter, sleeping for over one third of our lives,
we robotically continuously suck in fresh crucial oxygen,
to feed our lifelong insatiable dioxygen addiction.
Even our thinking organ and our cells for thought,
need a nightly time out; but all the while, under the trusted guidance of
an almighty auto-pilot.
R.M. Howes, M.D., Ph. D.
8/3/04

"Paper by paper, reference by reference, fact by fact,
I am going to paint you a scientific picture,
secure it in the gilded frame of the
Howes Unified Theory
and hang it over the entry door-pore
leading to the stunning
beauty of the intracellular labyrinth.
There, you may behold
the startling and mysterious vistas
of the naked human corpus."
R. M. Howes, M.D., Ph.D.
6/10/04

Great thoughts are a relative rarity;

whereas,

great mistakes are commonplace.

R. M. Howes, M.D., Ph.D.

8/19/04

"Some findings of greatness, occur by accident,

others by serendipity, whilst others require nigh pathological levels

of progressive persistence from conception, to birth,

through growth and development.

Over two decades have passed since the seed of

the Howes Singlet Oxygen Delivery system germinated

in my frontal lobes, and now,

as muscular momentum of contractions build, my idea is birthing.

I feel it,

and excitedly await its arrival,

so I can hear baby discovery's first joyous cry,

"Eureka."

R. M. Howes, M.D., Ph.D.

6/08/04

"Lascivious oxygen carries on curt, torrid affairs

with throngs of willing electrons,

whilst maintaining a most meaningful relationship

with its photon mate."

R. M. Howes, M.D., Ph.D.

5/23/04

"Excytology, the study of excited states, will thread the scientific needle of truth,

which we will use to pierce the toughened hide

of the bloated, corpulent body

of medical ignorance,

in our quest for cures."

R. M. Howes, M.D., Ph.D.

5/27/04

"It would require Occam's bush-hog to cut away the fluff and gratuitous academic verbosity in today's scientific publications."
R. M. Howes, M.D., Ph.D.
5/25/04

"Within the matrix of the virtual nano-world of cellular signaling, oxygen's multiple personalities go about
their intricate peripatetic tasks, with an arrogant assurance
earned over eons of time."
R. M. Howes, M.D., Ph.D.
5/26/04

"Singlet oxygen is spawned from the erotic mating ritual
between stately hydrogen peroxide and perky hypochlorite.
From this molecular true romance, is born the excited singlet love-child, which,
within micro-seconds, rises to be a great leader
of electrons."
R. M. Howes, M.D., Ph.D.
5/26/04

"Obfuscation of scientific truth
by the deceptive smoke of meaningless associations
and the arcane mirrors of manipulated data
must be eschewed.
We must demand scientific exactitude."
R. M. Howes, M.D., Ph.D.

"The verity of the nature of oxygen radicals
can only be realized by acknowledgement of the condition
resultant to their absence: death and rigor mortis.
The way of the radical
is the way of life."
R. M. Howes, M.D., Ph.D.
6/11/04

"The electromagnetic puppeteer dictates the
cadence and thoughts of the aerobiotic legions."
R. M. Howes, M.D., Ph.D.
5/2/04

"Scare tactics of the oxy-morons have spawned a generation of oxy-phobes, who
believe that ground state oxygen, itself,
is a diabolical "toxin," which only acts as a
catabolic cellular assassin."
R. M. Howes, M.D., Ph. D.
5/9/04

"The electron never rests.
Nonetheless, oxygen occasionally naps,
until enlivened by an
electron volt jolt."
R. M. Howes, M.D., Ph.D.
7/11/04

"In searching for the road of truth, for the Free Radical Theory of Aging and
Oxidative stress, I found that it was riddled with gaping paradoxical potholes of
contradiction,
which rendered it impassable.
In fact, I found that this avenue to enlightenment
had been completely blockaded by bricks of biochemistry.
The theory had been distributed and taught from
a passage in the Great Book of
Medical Mythology, along with phlogistin,
spontaneous generation, thymic hypertrophy
and hormone replacement therapy."
R. M. Howes, M.D., Ph.D.
7/18/04

"Paper by paper, reference by reference, fact by fact,

I am going to paint you a scientific picture,

secure it in the gilded frame of the

Howes Unified Theory

and hang it over the entry door-pore

leading to the stunning

beauty of the intracellular labyrinth.

There, you may behold

the startling and mysterious vistas

of the naked human corpus."

R. M. Howes, M.D., Ph.D.

6/10/04

"Lascivious oxygen carries on curt, torrid affairs

with throngs of willing electrons,

whilst maintaining a most meaningful relationship

with its photon mate."

R. M. Howes, M.D., Ph.D.

5/23/04

"Persistence transforms the weakling acorn

into the mighty oak of the informed, which can withstand

the wicked winds of ignorance

throughout a storm of discovery

and a vortex of controversy."

R. M. Howes, M.D., Ph.D.

5/3/04

I PREFACE

"Oxygen: aerobic life's lone elixir."

R.M. Howes, M.D., Ph.D.

8/04/04

By careful intent, I have subtitled my book "A selective review of the world literature."

I did not call it "definitive," "complete," "comprehensive," "unabridged," or "all that you can ever hope to know about oxygen." The subject of oxygen and reactive oxygen species or active oxygen is expansive enough to give Google a megabyte migraine, let alone, a mere mortal, such as myself. Add to that, discussions of cancer, arterio-sclerosis, diabetes, HIV/AIDS, malaria, immunosuppression, etc. and the subject matter reaches critical mass. Ergo, I have presented a "selective review" which both supports and negates my Unified Theory and the rationale for my singlet oxygen delivery system. I present my take on the issues and then you can decide if you feel that it has any profound meaning but, please approach it open mindedly.

As was pointed out by medical historian, Albert S. Lyons, in his book, Medicine: An Illustrated History, "All of us in any century are just as encased in the beliefs and practices of our times as were our progenitors in theirs. The tradition-shattering anatomist Andreas Vesalius still subscribed to the ancient doctrine of the four humors; Ambrose Pare while pioneering in the management of wounds also believed in witches; the revolutionary experi-mentalist William Harvey proved the circulation of the blood, yet accepted "vital spirits" as a contribution to the heart." Medical history illustrates a long and difficult trek in overcoming ignorance and there are no guarantees that we are presently near the end to that arduous journey or that we are about to collect the pot of golden truth at the end of the medical rainbow.

The role of RONS/excytomers (free radical oxidative and nitrative species/electronic excitation states) was ad-vanced nearly a half a century ago and has served as an endless and gargantuan source of speculation, conjecture and controversy. **Countless attempts using antioxidants to remedy problems associated with over 100 disease states and to stall aging have failed. They have failed because the theory is obviously wrong.** Had the theory been correct, we would be living disease-free for life spans approaching that of Methuselah (969 years); but, none of this has come to pass. The conundrum of aging and disease will not be solved by trying to pin the blame for all-things-bad on oxygen. In fact, attempts to do so have terribly complicated this scope of scientific investigation.

**"With freshmanic amazement and
sophomoric curiosity,
I study the hidden wonders and arcane
secrets of the aerobic cell.
What my peers see as a metabolic
melee and free radical fracas,
I view as a molecular marvel
of unparalleled design.**

**Yet, it is emblazoned with an
unmistakable and splendid imprint,
that is common throughout our cosmos:
the signature of the electromagnetic field. "**

R. M. Howes, M.D., Ph.D.

7/11/04

**"The electron never rests.
Nonetheless, oxygen occasionally naps,
until enlivened by an
electron-volt jolt."**

R. M. Howes, M.D., Ph.D.
7/11/04

Oxygen made a good target because of its crucial role in the metabolism of all aerobic cells. Thus, it could be linked to almost anything the cell was doing but the proposal that happenstance associations were "cause and effect" was the main factor which led so many down the "corridor of confusion." Complete deficiencies or mega-doses of countless other natural substances in the body, could also be similarly demonized by the worry-mongers and given the moniker of "deadly." The nearly unbelievable role of oxygen in sustaining aerobic life is illustrated by the frequently overlooked fact that a constant and invariant supply of O_2 is essential to maintain the life force. **Blood, if oxygenated, carries the life force within its bio-fluid; whereas, un-oxygenated blood is just bio-fluid.** In man, this requires that the body circulate its entire volume of blood every minute of our lives, or 1,440 times/day, or 525,600 times/year or 36,792,000 times for a 70 year old man...at rest! The human heart beats over 2.5 billion times and pumps 5 million gallons of blood in the average lifetime. This illustrates the amazing capability of **"specialized flesh"**, all the while on auto pilot. All of this work and energy is expended primarily to remove O_2 from the air and to transport it to all of our cells, for the perpetuation of life as we know it. **To me, it is incomprehensible that nature would work so very hard to actively bring an alleged "killer substance, a toxin, a poison, e.g., (O_2)" into its midst but it would logically do so to sustain itself with the life rendering energy potential possessed by oxygen. With billions of years to perfect aerobic metabolism, I remain highly circumspect that the generation of superoxide or hydrogen peroxide from one of every 20 processed oxygen molecules, which passes through the electron transport chain en route to oxidative phosphorylation, is the result of a "leak" or a colossal design flaw. A glaring mistake of this magnitude is implausible, since it had billions upon billions of years to get it right. Obviously, we have been looking at the situation from the wrong perspective. Any evolving system, possessing the ingenuity to create beautifully complex molecules, such as the O_2-binding heme proteins, surely would have corrected a "lethal leak" occurring directly in the midst of its most vital chemical pathway. There is a general failure to appreciate the imposing biochemical grandeur encased within the living/breathing cell and its inter-connectedness to the whole organism.**

Basic energy-producing metabolism for aerobic organisms starts with $^3\sum gO_2$ (ground state oxygen) and ends with H_2O (water). At first glance, that appears ever so simple but that is far from the actual case.

O_2 plus direct divalent electron reduction and 4 hydrogen abstractions leads to **$2H_2O$.**

In between, there are **only a couple of intermediate oxygen derivatives,** which are $O_2^{.-}$ (superoxide anion radical), H_2O_2 (hydrogen peroxide) and the hydroxyl radical **(.OH).** Both $O_2^{.-}$ and H_2O_2 are essential steps in the mitochondrial electron transport chain and its coupling to oxidative phosphorylation for ATP (adenosine triphosphate) production. All other reactive oxidative and nitrative species **(RONS)** are formed by secondary mechanisms, of which there may be hundreds or even thousands of intermediates or complexes. **In many reactions, intermediates are involved, e.g., exciplexes, diradicals, excytomers and/or zwitterions.**

Studies are further complicated by combining all of the RONS under one incorrect "radical" heading and by not recognizing their individual reactivities or chemical properties. It is inexcusable that these known inaccuracies are perpetuated. The situation only worsens when one reviews the literature on "antioxidants and antioxidant enzymes." **Sweeping erroneous generalities are everywhere and appear to be readily accepted** but the true biochemical facts must be applied to make interpretation of the data as accurate as possible. For example:

- It is rarely pointed out that many of the standard antioxidants can serve equally well as reductants or that pro-oxidants can also serve as antioxidants.
- The idea that any free radical or oxidant is merely present to kill us or to make us ill, is a blatant distortion of biochemical facts. Tragically, the erroneous concept that RONS/excytomers are only agents of destruction and harm has been indelibly etched into the medical, scientific and lay psyche.
- It is rarely pointed out that free radicals and oxidants play an ever-increasing role in indispensable and crucial cellular signaling functions and they are operative at many metabolic levels.
- It is rarely mentioned that either standard or large doses of antioxidants can be harmful or even deadly.
- It is even more rarely mentioned that normal steady state levels of RONS/excytomers are necessary to maintain cellular homeostasis and to fend off infections and cancer via their **bactericidal, fungicidal, parasiticidal, virucidal and tumoricidal activity**.
- Antioxidant enzymes can also generate free radicals and oxidants, further confusing the unknowing reader of the literature, and antioxidant enzymes are frequently inhibited or inactivated by various RONS/excytomers.
- Rarely mentioned is the possible reaction of hydrogen peroxide with transition metals which produces the superoxide anion, not the hydroxyl radical.
- RONS and singlet oxygen did not come on the scene for just the past 100 years, when cancer, heart disease and CNS disease rates started to soar or for just the past ½ century, since the free radical theory was introduced. They have been around since aerobic life evolved on Earth, which was approximately 2.3-2.5 billion years before these diseases became causes celebres. Actually, they have been around since light (photons) first reacted to excite a pigment, in the presence of oxygen. During the intervening eon, these alleged killers of aerobic life (RONS/excytomers) should surely have destroyed aerobic life, according to the predictions of the free radical theory, but they did not. In fact, it sustained aerobic life and accompanied the evolutionary process. Consequently, **Dr. Harman, and the oxy-moronic sycophants**, did not release RONS and excited states upon helpless and vulnerable aerobic life forms. They just mistakenly attributed all disease states and aging to them.
- Evolutionary history has proven the predictors of doom and gloom to be wrong, as it relates to RONS/excytomers and aerobic cellular interactions.
- The probable interaction of RONS with themselves or feed back/self-control of RONS/excytomers is rarely mentioned. Control of RONS levels does not necessarily require antioxidants, either endogenous or exogenous, once one understands the myriad of inter-actions possible with RONS. I believe that complex RONS/RONS interactions may be, in a large part, self-regulating.

U.T.O.P.I.A. (Unified Theory of Oxygen Participation In Aerobiosis) is the compelling theory of the fall of **O_2**, its **RONS** and its primary electronic excitation state, $^1\Delta_g O_2$ (metastable singlet delta oxygen), as a crucial, stately component of all aerobic life, to its present lowly status as the primary agent of all human diseases and aging. I consider the many factors involved in getting adequate amounts of these RONS to the cellular level. I consider the many consequences of reactions with O_2 and RONS. In particular, I discuss some of the data which discounts the Free Radical theory of aging and oxidative stress. I present clinical study models to illustrate my points. Even though there is a plethora of persuasive data, which is claimed to support the free radical theory of aging and oxidative stress, I do not and can not subscribe to its basic premise.

Medical and scientific literature concerning oxidative metabolism is loaded with confusing, conflicting, contradictory and controversial data. Nothing is more disturbing than the claims by thousands of researchers that **O_2 is a toxic killer**, contrasted with the claims of thousands of alternative practitioners that **O_2 therapy is a cure**. On the one hand, O_2 and its products are blamed for causing over 100 human diseases; whereas, on the other hand, O_2 therapy is touted as the cure for these very same diseases. This makes one wonder if all of the authors are right, if half are right/wrong, or if none of them are right, such that the variables under investigation really make no difference at all. Thus, we must continue to look for "patterns of predictability" to lead to a greater understanding of the unbelievable complexities of the living/breathing cell.

I have become increasingly skeptical and weary of overly exaggerated interpretations of in vitro studies and at epidemiological associations which are presented and touted as cause and effect relationships. Remember, by definition, a cause invariably leads to its effect. The introduction of biometry, which is the application of statistics to biology and medicine, has been a double edged microtome. Causality may be unrelated to correlations.

I have been involved with studies in oxidative metabolism and electronic excitation states since the mid 1960s, when I had the privilege of working with the enthusiastic Dr. Richard H. Steele in the Department of Biochemistry at Tulane School of Medicine. Dr. Steele was a role model who truly personified a true gentleman and a scholar. Even though my diversified career(s) have taken me through general and plastic surgery at the great Johns Hopkins Hospital, an owner of radio stations, rancher, country/singer/performer and writer, inventor of the Arrow-Howes multi-lumen venous catheter, Bourbon Street night club owner and an owner of oil and gas wells, I have never lost sight of my love for the study of O_2 and its biochemical involvement in the cell. In fact, I have rededicated my life to these fascinating studies.

> **"The raw materials needed to construct
> a man are worth less than
> five dollars of basic chemical components.
> Yet, when properly oxygenated, hydrated,
> nourished and assembled,
> they form entities of value beyond estimation,
> which we love and call
> 'self and our fellow man'."**
>
> R. M. Howes, M.D., Ph.D.
>
> 7/11/04

My laboratory and clinical studies are presently backing up my **Unified Theory**. **One good clinical study is worth countless expert opinions.** Once the simplicity of my singlet oxygen delivery system is understood and its potential bactericidal, virucidal, fungicidal, parasiticidal and tumoricidal properties are appreciated, we should have the ability to successfully treat a vast variety of bacterial, fungal, viral and neoplastic diseases. With an optimistic slant, for the real cures to these diseases, we will have to wait, like Macbeth, for tomorrow, tomorrow and tomorrow.

Because of the enormity of the subject matter, I have had to perform a selective review of the world literature. In particular, I have especially taken a close look at the agents used in my $^1O_2$ delivery system, e.g., H_2O_2 and $NaOCl$, and delta singlet oxygen, which is produced from their reactivity. Undoubtedly, my book will spark controversy, but I sincerely hope that it may, in some way, stimulate discoveries in this most exciting area of medical science and thus, bring cures to the patient's bedside and lessen pain and suffering for mankind. I fully realize that I am swimming upstream, against a downward tide of established articles and authors. I have kept in mind the fact that the same O_2 and H_2O_2 which can propel a rocket into and through interplanetary space, can also serve as the power source to drive the biochemistry inside intracellular space for all aerobic cells.

I offer gratitude and thanks to my beautiful wife, Robin, for whom I coined the phrase, "typing and griping" and for her overall superb assistance in the preparation of this manuscript. I also wish to thank my fine parents for their DNA contribution, ethics and morality and to the pantheistic God, who gave me the energy for this undertaking.

I have presented **highlights** of each section, preceding that section for quick review and further, I have emphasized highlights which I consider most relevant by putting them in dark red color. For those readers who wish more details, they can readily proceed to the main text for detailed discussions and references. References have been kept within the text for ease of photocopying.

Randolph M. Howes M.D., Ph.D.

II HOWES BLANK VERSE PARODY AND AUTOBIOGRAPHICAL SKETCH

"A long, long time ago, on a tiny, insignificant
planet called Earth,
its primordial broth, bathed a biochemical gumbo,
irradiated it with sunlight and lightning bolts, brought it to a boil,
let it cool and TAH-DAH!
A replicative molecule was spawned. Being educable,
over millennia it overcame narcosis and became aware
that it was aware....aware of itself.
Narcissism rapidly ensued and it became obsessed with self-replication.
The hardy helix hastily scaled the phylogenetic tree,
crawling through you and slithering over me.
Willing to make all sacrifices, it now offers up its human host,
to the god of immortality to feed its mania and
to secure the dubious title of
"cancer."

R. M. Howes, M.D., Ph.D.

6/18/04

"God said, 'Let there be light .'
and singlet oxygen emitted its photon
into the chemical nightscape,
illuminating the cell's dark reactions.
And the light was good.
Now excited carbonyls and oxygen impart their photon energy
bringing about the perpetual resurrection of the electron;
thus, empowering the momentous cycle of light
and the great circle of life."

R. M. Howes, M.D., Ph.D.

6/11/04

"The living/breathing cell is a cornucopia
of exciting electron affinities,
a thermodynamic treasure trove of
biochemical perplexities and
a temple of uncertainty for medical and scientific curiosity.
The cellular conundrum is a deliciously clever concoction
cooked up by an all-knowing Riddler."

R. M. Howes, M.D., Ph.D.

6/18/04

II.1 "THE R. M. HOWES, M.D., PH.D. TRIBUTE TO THE LIVING/BREATHING CELL."

The living /breathing cell is a heterogeneous isothermal conglomerate, containing a dynamic commingled biochemical infrastructure, held rather precariously, yet intentionally, in a most meaningful spatial conformation by lipid interlinks utilizing weak non-covalent and covalent forces, and capable of assimilating nutrients and processing data during energy production. Stretching the laws of thermodynamics, it maintains steady states of oxygen free radicals and electronic excitation states far from equilibrium.

With an uncanny degree of self awareness, the living/breathing cell is :

Self-sustaining
Self-contained
Self-adjusting
Self-assembling
Self-medicating
Self-healing
Self-replicating
Self-mutilating
Self-mutating
Self-terminating

It is an anti-chaotic/anti-entropic living unit, one hundred trillionth of the whole man, which carries on light speed to-and-fro cross talk within itself and throughout the whole, all for the sake of self-survival. As I grapple with its spiritual overtones, I am awe-struck by its biochemical beauty, mystified by its ability to pass on the self-replication dictum and inspired by its will to live and thus, to win.

The living /breathing cell is home to the savant of living matter and to the pundit of protoplasm. (R.M. Howes, 2004)

> "Medicine's history and its practice teaches us that physicians and scientists alike, can be blinded by obviousness and entrapped by ignorance."

R. M. Howes, M.D., Ph.D.

5/2/04

**"Future's shape is sculpted by the
persistent kneading hands of
the impossible dreamer."**

R. M. Howes, M.D., Ph.D.

5/2/04

**"To be possessed with the gift to see the unseen or
to know the unknown, even for a fleeting second,
can be an unparalleled blessing,
rife with reward or
a daunting flash of peril,
the immediate result of which
will be determined, not by ultimate
truth, but by the amplitude of reactionaries."**

R. M. Howes, M.D., Ph.D.

5/25/04

**"Remember, I am the one who wishes to be studious,
when others do not want to study,
to be diligent, when others do not want to work
and the one who remains curious for discovery,
whilst others remain pacified.
I am the doer.
I can. I will. I must."**

R. M. Howes, M.D., Ph.D.

5/25/04

**"The achievers drink
from the endless stream of opportunity
and bathe in the waters of wisdom
to heal
their wounds of criticism."**

R. M. Howes, M.D., Ph.D.

5/3/04

**"Even though our oro-gastrointestinal tract is teeming
with microbial life, we maintain healthy homeostasis.
Self-cure overcomes nature's insults,**

along with man's nostrums
and levels the playing field for crystal therapy, urine drinking,
cupping, magnets, acupuncture, hexing,
Western medicine and the
like. Medicine's recorded history teaches that,
in spite of man's meddlesome tendencies,
we are bolstered and sustained by self-cure
and its best buddy,
placebo."

R. M. Howes, M.D., Ph.D.
8/12/04

In our living state,
we are bounded by space and time.
Death extricates us from the confines of our skins,
thus, coalescing our essence with the spirit of endless space.
Our quietus frees us from the stressful restraints of time,
allowing us to frolic in infinity.

R.M. Howes, M.D., Ph.D.
8/21/04

II.2 HOWES PRESENTS THE SOPHISTRY AND UNWRITTEN RULES OF THE PSEUDO-SCIENTIST

1. Publish or perish is a fact of life and is more than adequate justification for submitting any contrived pretext of fact or drivel.

2. Any publication counts, as long as you can get it into print .

3. Extensive use of "may", "can", "could", "might be" , "may be", "perhaps", is encouraged.

4. Each successive interpretation of the data should increase by one order of magnitude, in verbal certainty.

   Thus, the progression would be:

   > May
   > Could be
   > Is thought to be
   > Is likely
   > Is now believed to be
   > Is convincingly
   > Has been shown to be
   > Vast amounts of data have proven beyond doubt (all cleverly based on the same original data).

5. Perform only in vitro experiments because you can basically control your results and make wild extrapolations to in vivo models.

6. Rely heavily on opinions and support of fellow pseudo-scientists. They can help you sell almost any cockamamie theory.

7. Use statistical slight of hand and mathematical mirror tricks to get a straight line association between 2 unrelated variables.

8. Resort to logarithms of logarithms, if necessary, for this technique will produce a false linearity between darn near anything.

9. Assert cause and effect relations between variables which are clearly circumstantial, especially epidemiological data and the more preposterous, the better.

10. Cause and effect relations will garner big grant money and guarantee publication.

11. Apply for federal funding because so few applications are read with scrutiny and even fewer are understood.   Besides, the government has tons of tax payers' money.

12. History has proven, with certainty, that funds and fame are there for the taking; so, belly on up to the trough, good buddy. Ain't life beautiful.

III HOWES' JOCULAR MALAPROPISMS FOR SCIENTIFIC/MEDICAL INVESTIGATORS

"Alarmageddon" - refers to every dooms day theory such as:

    Earlobe creases related to heart attacks
    Thigh length and diabetes
    Death by free radicals
    Being eaten alive by chain reactions of lipid peroxidations

"Free Radi-Crap" theory - refers to Drs. Harman and Ames theory of aging and oxidative stress

"Oxy-morons" - refers to followers of the Free Radi-Crap theory

"Oxy-phobes" - refers to those who live in constant fear of free radicals

PART I - INTRODUCTION

1.0 PREHISTORIC AND PRIMITIVE MEDICINE

Materials for this section were excerpted from: Lyons, A.S. and Petrucelli, II, R.J. Medicine: An Illustrated History, H.N. Abrams, Inc., Publishers, 1978.

Little is known about prehistoric and primitive medicine, other than that which can be gleaned from bony artifacts and cave drawings. Most authors refer to magic, voodoo, good and bad spirits and gods, sorcery, and shamanism. Interestingly, the North American Indians who recovered from serious illness were looked upon with awe as possessed of unusual powers. I believe that this was a recognition of those with a strong constitution or a highly developed system of **"self-cure."** Throughout recorded history, most healers have been accorded positions of high respect and were believed to possess great knowledge in tribal lore and tradition. Healers have always been required to **"practice the state of the art"** but in the African Congo and with the American Indian, their wealth could be confiscated, if they practiced "bad medicine," which was not in accord with tradition. Obviously, this situation is currently instituted by ambulance chasers and medical malpractice trial lawyers. During these times, the "healer," dressed in ceremonial garb, would attempt to suck out the cause of the disease. He would then regurgitate, with lots of fanfare, arrowheads, small frogs or other strange objects thought to be the cause of the illness. Specialization has also been around for centuries, as with the Amerindians who had specialists to treat sickness, injuries, snakebites or to address the weather. The North American medicine man carried his medicine bag, which was sometimes a human scrotum, containing artifacts symbolic of good luck and representing his spiritual force for healing. Even this is somewhat reminiscent of a modern physician receiving his first black bag. **How quickly I learned that it was the contents of one's head, and not the content of the black bag, which contained the true elements for successful healing.**

Treatment for illnesses varies immensely from culture to culture. Some "doctors" may ensnare an offending evil spirit in a cockroach, which was enticed to eat of food crumbs or blood; whereas, others may suck out evil by passing an egg or a black hen over the head of the patient. Nonetheless, the American Indian had a keen knowledge of the medicinal properties of plants, using laxatives, emetics, diuretics, local analgesics, sedatives and anti-febrile plant concoctions. Surgery was rather symbolic, as in the removal of arrows, or remindful of Galen's doctrine of laudable pus, in that the Dakota tribe would place a strip of bark between the edges of a healing wound to allow for drainage and promote healing. Obstetrics was practiced by the women and following delivery of a baby, some cultures practiced expulsion of the placental remnants by massage, which is analogous to the Crede maneuver seen in modern hospitals. On Marco Polo's travels he described the practice of couvades, in which the father took to bed as if he had been bearing the child and he performed rituals to draw away evil spirits from the mother and child. Meanwhile, the mother returned immediately to work in the fields.

Communicable diseases had been recognized. In Asia, smallpox scabs were pricked into the skin since ancient times and the Chinese had been known to blow powdered scabs into the nostrils. Isolation of the sick had been practiced by the ancients but was discontinued in medieval hospitals and during the American Civil War and resulted in terrible contagions. As Dr. Lyons states, "Many of primitive man's most favored techniques had no rational or pharmacological basis, but he certainly recognized the psychological benefits to the sick of a healer's even appearing to do something effective and that **under certain conditions the body seems better able to cure itself." I believe that this is a lesson that we should be mindful of today.**

Mesopotamians, who were located in Asia between the Tigris and the Euphrates rivers, believed that many diseases were a result of punishment of the gods and relied on divination to uncover the sins of their patients. They had a taboo against touching the sick and this tradition was carried over into the Hebrew culture and later became a significant factor in public hygiene. Hepatoscopy, which was the examination of the liver with other organs of sacrificial animals, was used in diagnosis. Medications were administered according to rituals and were given by mouth, applied as salves, blown into orifices, inhaled as vapors and inserted as suppositories and enemas. Additionally, the time of day and the position of constellations influenced the administration of medicines. The Code of Hammurabi (c. 1700 B.C.) indicated a knowledge of surgery and at that time, there were references to the snake as a symbol of healing. In the Sumerian epic of Gilgamesh, the search for the secret of immortality was ended when a snake stole and ate the plant of everlasting life. Immediately, **the snake shed its skin and appeared rejuvenated, which garnered it the symbol of regeneration and the cure of illness**. Proudly, we wear the staff and the snake as a modern symbol of the healing art. The Code of Hammurabi also described the cautions and the punishment for performing "bad surgery" when it stated that, "If a doctor has treated a man with a metal knife for a severe wound, and has caused the man to die, or has opened a man's tumor with a metal knife and destroyed the man's eye, his hands shall be cut off." I believe that this would have served as a formidable deterrent to unnecessary surgery.

 Mesopotamian characteristics passed down to orthodox Jews and their hygienic laws influenced isolation of the sick, time and location of burial, frequency of sexual intercourse, washing before meals, bathing after coitus and menstruation and restriction of activities on the seventh day. With the severe Assyrian restrictions placed on the seventh day, the king engaged in no official business and **physicians were not even permitted to treat the sick.**

Biblical passages attest to the esteem given to physicians with statements such as, "When thou feelest sick call upon God and bring the physician, for the prudent man scorneth not the remedies of the earth." The Jewish Talmud indicates that they relied upon the Greek humoral theories which attributed disease to the imbalance of **the four humors of the body: phlegm, blood, yellow bile and black bile.** The Jews also followed the Greek philosophers in specifying **the four elements of the universe as air, fire, earth and water.** Circumcision, the seal of the covenant, was the most common form of surgery. The Edwin Smith Papyrus (about the 17th century B.C.) concerned itself with surgical matters from the head down but stopped abruptly at the mid-chest.

Egyptian history reveals that the evil Seth, who together with his sister and consort, Nephthys, was a prime agent for bringing diseases to humans and he destroyed the eye of Horus. **Thoth, physician to the gods and the source of all knowledge**, healed the eye. The influence of these stories led to the custom of sibling marriages and it was estimated that by the 2nd century A.D., two-thirds of the citizens of Arsinoe were offspring of sibling unions. **Sir William Osler referred to Imhotep as "the first figure of a physician to stand out clearly from the mists of antiquity."** Thus, the two important Egyptian healing divinities were Toth and Imhotep.

In the medical history of ancient India, Sushruta wrote, "Only the union of medicine and surgery constitutes the complete doctor. The doctor who lacks knowledge of one of these branches is like a bird with only one wing." Surprisingly, the students of medicine, in India, make commitments, which closely resemble the Hippocratic Oath of Greece.

According to ancient Chinese cosmology, the universe was created not by divinities but self-generated from the interplay of **nature's basic duality**: the active, light, dry, warm, positive, masculine *yang* and the passive dark, cold, moist, negative *yin*. All things were a combination of these basics. **The driving principle of the universe was the *tao*, "the way"** and disregard of the tao led to illness in Confucianism. Chang Chung-ching was the equivalent of Hippocrates. Examination of the radial pulse was of prime importance to Chinese doctors and each pulse had three distinct divisions, which led to hundreds of possible characteristics and a ten-volume treatise, *Muo-Ching*. Thus, **a physician could determine the symptoms, diagnosis, prognosis and proper treatment by an intensive palpation of the pulse**. Since it was considered improper for a physician to intimately examine a female, special ceramic, ivory and wooden dolls were pointed to by the invalid to indicate where discomfort was felt.

Acupuncture is a well-known form of Chinese medical therapy, designed to drain off excess *yang* or *yin*, and has been around since before recorded history. Long needles are inserted into the skin into any of **365 points along the 12 meridians** that traverse the body and transmit an active life force called *ch'i*. Each of these points is related to a specific organ and **virtually every illness, weakness and symptom is thought to be amenable to correction by acupuncture.** Later, the Japanese adopted 660 points for acupuncture and moxibustion. The Chinese developed moxibustion along with acupuncture and it follows the same points and meridians for placement of the moxa. **Moxibustion involves the burning of a small mound of a powdered plant, usually mugwort, on the patient's skin to produce a blister.** I believe that these inflicted discomforts could be a considerable inducement to get well and not return for follow up visits. The Chinese felt that it was proper to show no emotion to pain and they recount the story of the general treated by Hua T'o, who played chess while Hua T'o incised his flesh and scraped the bone.

Not only did the Chinese attempt to prevent smallpox by placing scabs from smallpox pustules into the nostrils but they also ingested powdered fleas from cattle infected with cowpox. **Medical knowledge was thought of as a secret power** that belonged to each physician and he kept his secrets closely guarded.

A study of Greek medical history reveals that **virtually any of the Greek gods could cause disease.** Apollo and his sister, Artemis, could shoot certain "arrows" which would bring on illness or widespread pestilence and/or others which would produce the deterioration and death of old age. Also, **they believed that the life force, *thymos*, was in all parts of the living organism** and that it was maintained by factors which came from outside the body (food, drink and air) as well as actions of internal body functions (movement of bodily fluids, including blood) and that **_thymos_ could escape from wounds and by exhalation, leaving the body at death. I could interpret this to mean that, at least in part, they were referring to oxygen as _thymos_.** For the Greeks, the *psyche* referred to the soul, individual personality or spirit, which went to the underworld after death. By the 4th century B.C. at the time of Aristotle, the heart was believed to be the site of consciousness. *Pharmaka*, the name widely used for drugs, applied to wound coverings used for magic, poison, curing, soothing, analgesia, drying and healing.

1.0.0 Roman Times

After 146 B.C., Rome wielded hegemony over Greece and the Hippocratic method greatly influenced Roman medicine. The Etruscan inheritance on medicine relied on religious healing, as was seen at the College of Augurs, which had a special divinity for each disease or symptom or even epidemics. By legend, **the Greek medical deity, Asclepios (Aesculapius in Latin)** was introduced in Rome in 295 B.C. in the form of snakes sent from the temple of Epidaurus. Eventually, **patients wanted more than treatment by gods and snakes and insisted on drugs.** Does this sound familiar in the 21st century? The Roman upper class detested manual work as did the Greeks and thought that practicing medicine was unworthy of cultured men. The early respect given by the Romans to the Greek physician, Archagathos was the appellation *vulnerarius* (wound healer) but who later became known as *carnifex* (butcher). Most Roman practitioners were mainly freedmen and slaves and upper class Romans frequently had a private slave-physician for his private use and who was occasionally hired out.

Cornelius Celsus (fl. 14-37), who was not a physician, composed the eight books, *De Medicina*, which recorded much of the information on Alexandrian and Roman medicine. **Celsus is best known for his description of inflammation: redness and swelling with heat and pain (*rubor et tumor cum calor et dolor*), and which is still used today.** Next was Caius Pliny (23-79), who was a brilliant outspoken atheist and did not believe in an afterlife, also believed in one-footed people who used their giant foot to protect them from the rain. Pliny also expressed belief "in rains of milk, blood, flesh, iron, sponges, wool, and baked bricks." Rufus of Ephesus (c. 110-180), made great contributions on the eye, the pulse and also **he believed in the *pneuma* (the Stoic's idea of a vital force borne in the air).** Obviously, I would have liked Rufus a lot.

The Greek physician, **Galen (c. 129-c. 200), dramatically influenced medicine for the next 1,500 years with his dogmatic approach and original thinking.** Galen openly mocked those who disagreed with him and he gained great knowledge as the physician of the gladiators. **Aristotle has said, "Nature does nothing without a purpose."** and Galen insisted that he could perceive what that purpose was in such things as organs and tissue. He accepted the four fundamental humors as sources of health and illness and classified personalities into corresponding types: phlegmatic, sanguine, choleric and melancholic, which we also still use today. Teachers of subsequent years, accepted Galen's works, without question, even though Galen had always believed in "discovery by experiment." Galen introduced pharmaceutical "Galenical" concoctions called "theriacs" (Greek for wild beast), which were at times composed of over 100 ingredients and were listed in European pharmacies through the last quarter of the 19th century. His most notable contribution was his "doctrine of laudable pus," which lasted until the time of Pare and the Napoleonic wars.

Jesus Christ of Nazareth maintained a type of **divine supernatural healing, which later medieval philosophers would call *praeter naturam* (beyond nature - where all rules covering the here and now were suspended).** Luke, one of the authors of the Bible, was a physician and "touching" was an important aspect of Christ's healing, even touching the hem of His garment.

The fall of Rome to the Goths in 476 and the Fall of Constantinople in 1453 to the Turks is frequently used to mark the beginning and the end of **the Middle Ages.** This period was also known as the **"Age of Faith."** Many types of medical practices followed, such as the Celtics under Druid leadership, the Russians led by *volkhava* (wolf men) and the Teutonic women were useful healers as bloodsuckers during war. Throughout the Dark Ages, the Church and the papacy grew to become a controlling influence over medicine and law. **The Christian belief in the meditation of the Holy Ghost as the only possibility for cure led to the gradual abandonment of all but the simplest surgical procedures**, such as bloodletting, amputation and tooth extraction. St. Benedict forbade the study of medicine and the Healing Mission of Christ was institutionalized in a manner that was to control medical care for the next 500 years. Also, the Church maintained control over universities throughout the Middle Ages. The wrath of God was expressed in disease, famine, pestilence and civil strife and was later morphed into a kinder image of the Gentle Shepard looking after his flock. Basically, the Middle Ages was an unusual combination of old science and mysticism.

Miracle cures and the intercession of saints grew in frequency. From about 500-1000, the intercession of saints and the divine peaked with the belief in the intercessory powers of the Virgin (so-called Mariolarity), which was pushed by the French troubadours' cult of chivalry. After 1300, magical cures, chants, superstitions and dung-filled amulets were used to influence healing of illness and diseases. St. Thomas Aquinas (1225-74) believed so strongly in the Aristotelian thought that it led to the pronouncement of William of Occam **(Occam's razor): the simplest explanation should be applied to observed natural phenomena**. This led to the doctrine of efficient causation, which was known as Thomism or Scholasticism.

The period known as the **Renaissance sprang forth in the mid-fifteenth century**. The arrival of a "Renaissance man" such as Copernicus was a physician, with a strong knowledge of physics and astronomy. This was the time for abandonment of the pseudo-Hippocratic doctrine that "wounds which were not curable by iron were curable by fire."

Finally, **the 17th century arrived and was known as the "Age of the Scientific Revolution."** This was a time for new directions in medical thought, application of mathematics, the rise of atomism and scientific experimentation. Robert Boyle (1627-91) was a proponent of atomism and he devised a pump, with **which he demonstrated the necessity of air for life. Three cheers for Boyle**, who later formulated Boyles' Law and who was knowledgeable on a variety of subjects, such as respiration, magnetism and blood chemistry, even though he was not a physician. However, this great scientist, when dealing with therapeutics (A Collection of Choice Remedies, 1692) was satisfied to recommend a hodgepodge of messes with ingredients such as worms, horse dung, human urine and moss from a dead man's skull.

This thumbnail historical sketch, of man's mistakes and advances, brings us up to modern methods of data collection and theories of disease causation.

1.0.1 Modern Data and Disease Causation

Greater variability of causation is associated with the more complex human diseases. Diseases, such as cancer, have multi-factorial causes, which must be considered when interpreting the plethora of today's data. Increasingly, genetics seems to play more of a role in disease causation. We know of many factors, which are linked to cancer causation such as viruses, chemical pollutants, irradiation, etc. but they are usually associated with "something else" which facilitates cancer development. That "something else" **may be as basic as oxygen consumption rates, oxygen tissue utilization or the ultimate production of oxygen free radicals and electronic excitation states**. As difficult as it is, the data must be considered on a case-by-case basis, a cell-by-cell basis, a tissue-by-tissue basis and so on, until we can identify unifying characteristics of causation. That is precisely what I have attempted to do in this selective world review. I have looked for "the canary in the coal mine" and have utilized an overview approach of relevant published data and considered known genetic anomalies as study models, where available.

Others, such as Dr. Tim Key of the University of Oxford, states that "Tobacco is linked to 30% of cancer cases, diet is involved in and estimated 25%, alcohol in about 6% and obesity in 5%." They have utilized the unifying concept in their analysis. However, this does not guarantee that the concluding concepts are correct and I believe that this is the case with Dr. Harman's (and Ames) free radical theory of aging and oxidative stress.

In an interview with Franklin Cameron, Dr. Harman stated that, "I knew when Mother Nature finds something that works, she uses it over and over, like variations of a theme. **I approached the problem with the idea that there is a single cause of aging.** This cause would be responsible for the aging and death of everything, modified by genetics and environment." **He concluded that free radicals of oxygen were the source of basically all human disease and aging**. I submit that he so biased his initial approach, that it forever forced him to try to knowingly manipulate the data to fit the biased concept. The acceptance of this apocryphal concept has led generations of oxy-morons to follow in lock step. Based on decades of evaluation, **I believe that his conclusion that there is a singular cause for all human disease and aging is, at best, naive and at worst, just plain wrong.**

After a selective review of the world's literature, I have found that others are also beginning to **seriously question and reject the hallowed free radical theory**. Research by University College of London, published in Nature in February 2004, states that the theory may be incorrect and flawed. Dr. Tony Segal said, **"Many patients might be using expensive antioxidant drugs based upon completely invalid theories."** Since the 1970s, pharmaceutical companies have developed and flooded the market with drugs, including vitamins and dietary supplements, designed to mop up or inactivate the production of damaging free radicals, which are produced during normal metabolism of oxygen. Tons of vitamins A, C and E are consumed on a daily basis and are regarded as healthy because they attack free radicals. This is being done and perpetuated, even though **the data relating to it is contradictory and at times indicates considerable potential harm or even death from many of these antioxidants**. The power of the lay press, the media and the pharmaceutical industry is enormous. Unfortunately, their bottom line is profit and not the well being of our citizenry.

Dr. Segal further states, **"Our work shows that the basic theory underlying the toxicity of oxygen radicals is flawed."** Segal's group discovered that production of lytic enzymes, which are triggered by potassium flow, are responsible for digestion of foreign invaders and that free radicals are by no means the toxic particles they had been accused of being. Segal said, **"Pharmaceutical companies have spent millions on what effectively amounted to a red herring. All the theories relating to the free radical causation of disease and the therapeutic value of antioxidants, at the very least, must be re-evaluated."**

I feel that an entire multi-billion dollar industry, including lecturers, publishers, health gurus, antiaging clinics, drug manufacturers, etc., is likely based on the extremely shaky ground of speculation and not the terra firma of scientific experimentation.

After cataloging numerous DNA mutations that are associated with cellular progression from normalcy to malignancy, it is becoming obvious **that events in the tissues surrounding cancer cells play a major formative role**. Some researchers have shown that a cancer cell's so-called microenvironment can determine its tumorigenic potential. Lisa Coussens, Ph. D. of the University of California, San Francisco, says, "You can't proliferate as a cancer cell all by yourself unless you can orchestrate that microenvironment to allow you to proliferate." It is becoming increasingly clear that **only certain tissues permit cancer growth with particular DNA mutations. Mutations in the BRCA1 gene can go on to cause breast cancer and ovarian cancers but not cancers in the skin or gut.** There must be something in the tissue in the breast and ovary that allows cells with

BRCA1 mutations to proliferate. Additionally, **cancer cells are able to settle down and start proliferating only in certain regions of the body.** Mina Bissell, Ph.D. of the Lawrence Berkeley National Lab, has shown that the abnormal behavior of cancer cells is due not only to mutations from within but also to influences from without (JAMA 2003; 290: 1977-1979). **I believe that the micro-oxygen environment is a major player in the "allowance" of either primary, secondary or metastatic tumor growth. I am referring to the RONS/excytomer micro-environment and not to just ground state oxygen, as was proposed by Otto Warburg.** The microenvironment of RONS/excytomers is a key factor in my Unified Theory, especially as it relates to the non-linearity and tri-phasic nature of RONS/excytomer and/or RONS/excytomer complexes. Throughout my writings I have argued against the use of the term "inducer" (when applied to hypoxia) and have insisted on the use of the term "allowed." I believe that, in many instances, **it is the absence of RONS/excytomers which "allows" cancer to develop; whereas, in other circumstances, RONS/excytomer levels either hold cancer cells in abeyance or if RONS/excytomer levels are high enough, they cause death of the cancer cells by induction of apoptosis.**

I am reminded of the words of the Irish author, Elizabeth Bowen, who said, "One can live in the shadow of an idea without grasping it."

Studies show that the microenvironment influences include the extracellular matrix, a network of macromolecules that provides structural scaffolding, and the stroma, a connective tissue framework consisting of fibroblasts, immune cells and fat cells. Please remember that many of these cells are capable of generating RONS/excytomers (fibroblasts, immune cells and even fat cells) and fat cells are capable of trapping RONS/excytomers, due to the presence of high concentrations of polyunsaturated lipids. Reportedly, **normal cells respond to the presence of cancer cells much like they would to injury.** Signals are sent to step up the production of various enzymes and inflammatory factors, which are dumped into the matrix. A state of cell proliferation and extracellular matrix degradation ensues. Dr. Coussens said, "The difference is that in wounding, the signals are turned on and then turned off; in the context of a tumor, the signals are turned on and not turned off."

Major factors associated with:

1. **obesity** - heart disease, post menopausal breast cancer, endometrial and colon cancer, diabetes.
2. **low fruit and vegetable intake** - lung cancer, heart disease, esophageal, gastric and colorectal cancer
3. **physical inactivity** - breast cancer, heart disease, prostate, colon and rectal cancer, diabetes
4. **unsafe sex** - cervical cancer
5. **tobacco** - lung and aerodigestive cancer and all other cancers
6. **alcohol** - heart disease, diabetes, liver and esophageal cancer and selective other cancers
7. **pollution** - lung cancer and mesothelioma

A recent report from Vanderbilt University showed that **transgenic mice with defective stroma fibroblasts develop aggressive epithelial tumors.** The tumors developed because the fibroblasts were unable to respond to transforming growth factor B (TGF-B), a cytokine involved in processes such as differentiation, development and wound healing (Science 2004; 303: 848-851). **I believe that the tumor cells developed because the microenvironment "allowed" them to do so because of a deficiency of RONS/excytomer production.** Research by Mary Helen Barcellos-Hoff, Ph.D., of the Lawrence Berkeley National Laboratory has demonstrated that TGF-B expression has a great impact on cell death and proliferation following tissue exposure to radiation, a known carcinogen (Cancer Res. 2002; 62: 5627-5631). Barcellos-Hoff also said, "We all have pre-neoplastic disease, but it stays in situ. And as long as it stays in situ, we're good." **These statements are consistent with my Unified Theory in regards to the "held in abeyance stage" of cancer by adequate levels of RONS/excytomers.**

A number of studies have shown that modifying the interactions between tumor and stroma cells can hinder cancer progression and even revert tumor cells to a normal phenotype (Int J Cancer 2003; 107: 688-695). I suspect that this is beginning to sound a lot like **spontaneous regression**, which I have covered in detail in this book. Dr. Coussens has found that clinical trials with drugs that inhibit tumor-associated **matrix metalloproteinase**

(enzymes that degrade the extracellular matrix) have been disappointing (Nat Rev Cancer 2002; 2: 657-672). Interestingly enough, there is little discussion of oxygen's role in any of the above study models and I believe that is a serious oversight.

1.1 FIRST, DO NO HARM ("PRIMUM NON NOCERE")

The basis of the creed of the physician is to, "First, do no harm." Patient safety and care has been and should continue to be the objective of all medical endeavors. The history of medicine has had a circuitous and checkered past. Any student of medical history quickly learns that the "standard of care" is a fleeting entity, as its concepts and embodiments can drastically change within single generations, let alone over the course of recorded history. Yet, looking at the history of medicine reveals that the **"dogma de jour"** (**dogma of the day), can hold medical advances at a virtual standstill for many centuries at a time.

Examples taken from the days of Galen's laudable pus, through today's dilemma regarding hormone replacement therapy, are illustrative of the frequent absence of free thinking and open minds prevailing to determine the course of patient care. At times, one can only thank divine providence or nature's wondrous healing powers for the perpetuation of mankind, in spite of man's erroneous intervention in what has been called **"the practice of medicine."**

1.1.1 The Hippocratic Method

The Hippocratic method has had a profound influence on Western medicine.

The principles of the Hippocratic method are outlined as follows:

1. Observe all.
2. Study the patient rather than the disease.
3. Evaluate honestly.
4. **Assist nature**.

During the Renaissance, **Paracelsus** burned the works of Avicenna and Galen to illustrate his **need to rely on his own observations**, rather than those of the authorities. Hippocrates also relied on his own observations but based them upon the past works of others, realizing that knowledge did not start with him. Similarly, **our present view of medical and scientific truth will likely be viewed as primitive and foolhardy by generations of the future.**

The mere fact that a procedure is called a "therapy" or that a drug is called a "medicine" does not guarantee you that it is good for you, that it will not cause you serious harm or that it may not be lethal. Past centuries have seen the powerful roles of the church and the state influencing medical practices but these pale in comparison with the **gold-plated-iron-fist with which the pharmaceutical industry** controls the attitude and acceptance of pharmaceutically friendly regulations governing the entirety of the medical enterprise.

RMH Note: Modern medicine has focused on synthetic drugs for therapy and we have seen an alarming rise in resistant bacteria, mutated viruses and adverse chemical pharmacological reactions.

In that regard, **Big Pharma certainly follows the Golden Rule, in that "He, who has the gold, makes the rules."** They market and promote **"pharmaceuticide."**

2.5 billion prescriptions are written annually (1998), about nine for every man, woman and child and about 700 on a lifetime basis. On the basis of these considerations, a leading national authority has concluded that prescription drugs may pose the single most important class of unrecognized and avoidable cancer risks for the entire U.S. population (Moore, T.J. Prescription for Disaster. Simon & Schuster, New York, 1998).

An additional concern is that there is such a flood of daily scientific data pouring onto the pages of countless journals and publications, that the singular practicing physician is relying more and more on the advice of the commissioned pharmaceutical detail man to instruct him on advisability of administration of drugs to his patients. Simply put, the doctor barely has the time to take care of his patients, let alone keep up with the information avalanche of publications. Continuing medical education programs are a needed and an under-utilized method of physician education.

Traditionally, physicians have been viewed with great respect by their fellow man and it will be a continuing challenge to maintain that lofty position. The mantra of Big Pharma seems to be **"profit, profit and more profit"** but maintaining this monetary approach will erode the moral foundations of ethical medical practice. Physicians must find a way to maintain their own identity, continue to put the patient first and be the independent caregivers that they took an oath to be.

The Institute of Medicine and the National research Council have concluded that the **government should ban suspect dietary supplements, even in the absence of direct evidence of harm to humans** and recommended changes to the Dietary Supplement Health and Education Act. **A decade ago, there were about 4,000 supplements on the market; today there are about 29,000, with another 1,000 new products introduced each year** (Dietary supplements: A Framework for Evaluating Safety. http://www.edu/books/0309091101/html/). Today's regulations only guarantee that the contents of the supplement must be accurate and that the supplement will dissolve when taken; otherwise, this is an unregulated pharmaceutical industry which generates $19 billion annually. Pharmaceutical companies continue to with hold negative data and medical products continue to be pushed by physicians who have a proprietary interest in the products they promote or write about.

"Caveat emptor."

1.2 THE SCIENTIFIC METHOD

1.2.1 It is Elementary, Watson.

The bedrock for the interpretation of medical and scientific research data is the **scientific method**. Unfortunately, it frequently appears that the scientific method has either been ignored or has been manipulated for selfish purposes. **For scientific work to maintain quality and reliability, it must adhere to the principles of the scientific method.** It can only ascribe probabilities to differences with observed events and it can not "prove" a hypothesis, such as can be done with a geometrical theorem. By disproving the null hypothesis (the hypothesis that the experimental treatment had no effect), we can say that the observed difference is "significant."

As research scientists, we must be open-minded, yet remain skeptical. We must be more critical of our work than any of our peers and readily be willing to point out its weaknesses. As humbling as this can be, it provides for a method of self correction, honesty and integrity. As basic and applied research scientists, we must strive to bolster these honorable professions. We must be unafraid to question conventional interpretations of scientific data, and if the re-interpretation yields more accurate concepts, we must be open-minded regarding its acceptance.

To quote H. L. Mencken, "The value the world sets upon motives is often grossly unjust and inaccurate. Consider, for example, two of them: mere insatiable curiosity and the desire to do good. The latter is put high above the former, and yet it is the former that moves one of the most useful men the human race has yet produced: the scientific investigator. What actually urges him on is not some brummagem idea of Service, but a boundless, almost **pathological thirst to penetrate the unknown**, to uncover the secret, to find out what has not been found out before. His prototype is not the liberator releasing slaves, the good Samaritan lifting up the fallen, but a dog sniffing tremendously at an infinite series of rat-holes." Indeed, intellectual curiosity is a great motivator, but I believe that the desire to do good is equally important.

Recently, following the death of Francis Crick, Herbert Boyer, who co-founded Genentech, Inc., said, "When I was a student, he was one of my heroes. He was an iconoclast. **He challenged established thinking. It's what all the great scientists do."** Crick, who was the co-discoverer of DNA with James Watson, reportedly walked into a pub in Cambridge, England, in 1953 and announced that they had, "found the secret of life." Crick didn't have a "wet lab" where he could conduct experiments at the San Diego-based Salk Institute where he worked. Instead, he sat in his office and thought. Then, he went home and thought. He said he didn't like to socialize - and he declined just about every invitation for public appearances because it cut into his thinking time.

Ironically, **the DNA cellular dictatorship described by Watson and Crick, is now undergoing serious challenges.** A 2004, cloning experiment published in the August issue of Genes and Development, indicates that the body itself, has the ability to reverse cancer. Lynda Chin of the Dana-Farber Cancer Institute and Harvard Medical School said, "Drugs that target the cancer epigenome may prove to be a key therapeutic opportunity for diverse cancers." In other words, it might be possible to silence a cancer gene. Nucleic acids consist of : purine and pyrimidine bases, a sugar backbone and phosphodiesterase linkages (double stranded by base pairing).

Cancer begins when certain genes mutate, or when a certain, inherited version of a gene somehow gets turned on. This can happen through various so-called epigenetic processes - when other molecules in a cell affect genes without actually altering the sequence of DNA. In the experiment, Konrad Hochedlinger and Robert Blelloch, both researchers in Jaenisch's lab, took the nucleus from a melanoma cell and injected it into a hollowed-out mouse egg cell. This started the egg growing as if it had been fertilized by sperm. They did not allow this embryonic mouse to develop, but harvested from it embryonic stem cells - immature cells that have the potential to become any cell in the body at all. They put these stem cells into healthy mouse blastocysts - very early embryos only a few days old. Some of these developed into healthy, normal mice. **"It's important to note that the stem cells from the cloned melanoma were incorporated into most, if not all, tissues of adult mice, showing that they can develop into normal, healthy cells,"** Blelloch said. They included skin pigmentation cells, immune cells and connective tissue. **This could only have happened if the cancer cells had lost their malignant qualities**, at least temporarily, the researchers said. But when certain cancer related genes in these mice were activated, they developed malignant tumors at a much faster rate than normal mice, the researcher added. Many researchers want to try similar experiments with human cancer cells. I believe that this type of data points out the importance of cellular and DNA redox status and the significance of RONS steady state levels and their signaling capabilities. Nonetheless, it shows that cancer cells, encoded with malignant DNA, can be influenced or reprogrammed to become or appear to be benign, even though the DNA is encoded with a malignant sequence.

1.2.2 Nonsense and Non-science

A hypothesis is an attempted explanation for why the observed facts are as they are. Obviously, the conclusions reached from the interpretation of data can change as the collection of the data base changes. When I worked as a technician with **Nobel Laureate, Dr. Andrew V. Schally, co-isolator of thyrotropin releasing factor,** he told me that it was better to work on the isolation and identification of compounds rather than on mechanisms, because the identity of compounds will not change; whereas, explanations with mechanisms are more likely to change as more data is collected, allowing for different and changing mechanistic interpretations. Fortunately, over my lifetime I have been influenced by stimulating conversations with many great minds. At Tulane, I had the privilege of meeting and speaking with **Nobel Laureate, Dr Linus Pauling**. While completing my general surgery and plastic surgery training at the Johns Hopkins Hospital, I had the opportunity to work with the late **Dr. Albert L. Lehninger**, who contributed so much to the study of the mitochondrion. Some of my work there, which was unpublished, demonstrated that the WBCs of patients coming off of the cardiac by-pass pump were emitting huge amounts of chemiluminescence. I attributed this to the exposure of the WBCs to the foreign substances which make up the by-pass pump system. And in later years, I had many fascinating conversations with **Nobel Laureate, Dr. Fritz Lipmann**, discoverer of co-enzyme-A and its importance in intermediary metabolism. Also, in the Potpourri section of this book, I will share with you a poem, which I especially prepared and presented to **Nobel Laureate, Dr. Louis Ignarro. I feel that exposure to these great minds has been a privilege and I keep their images as guide lines in formulating my research.**

Above all, a good hypothesis should be able to predict future observations and support past collected data. Unfortunately, this is not the case in many areas of science today. Far too often, it appears that the data has been skewed, doctored or tampered with, such as to garner support for further funding or to feed the "publish or perish" voracious appetites of academia or feed the funding hunger of basic science research. Just this type of nonsense and non-science leads directly to research papers of today that are filled with inconsistencies, contradictions and **"paradoxes."**

Statistical concepts go from numerical measures to probability and sampling, to principles of testing with univariate tests and bivariate relationships. Statistics are a useful method for finding patterns in data and inferring important connections between measured events. However, **statistics can be manipulated to support outrageous claims. In scientific and medical investigative studies, we gather data, organize data and analyze data, all of which are subject to errors.** Chan et al. found that the reporting of trial outcomes is not only frequently incomplete but also biased and inconsistent with protocols. Published articles, as well as reviews that incorporate them, may therefore be unreliable and overestimate the benefits of an intervention (Chan, A.,

Hrobjartsson, A., Haahr, A., Gotzsche, P. and Altman, D. Empirical evidence for selective reporting of outcomes in randomized trials. Comparison of protocols to published articles. JAMA 2004; 291: 2457-2465).

The American Cancer Society released articles, in Jan. 2004, stating that, "Cancer Deaths to Decline in 2004," and "Cancer Deaths Falling in U. S., Annual Report Shows." However, the first page of the 2004 statistics states that the incidence and mortality data in this report will be age-adjusted to the 2000 U. S. population standard. They point out that this change will affect the comparability of these reports and **will produce some "apparent" dramatic changes** in the rates of cancer incidence and mortality, rates at different ages, magnitude of improvement in cancer, and racial and ethnic differences. Thus, the obvious question is, "How can you trust their conclusions?"

Hippocrates of Cos (c. 460-377 B.C.) was believed to be **the greatest physician of his time**; even so, a few scholars still question if he ever lived at all.. The Hippocratic books are thought to be **the starting point for careful observation and experimental work.** In the 5th century B.C., **Socrates** the Athenian (c. 470-399 B.C.) constructed a rational system of ethics which questioned conventional prejudices and beliefs. He was accused of subverting all that Athenians had always, and rightly, taken for granted, which likely led to his having to commit suicide by being required to drink hemlock. **Plato** (c. 427-347 B.C.), a contemporary of Hippocrates, a student of Socrates and the teacher of Aristotle, was the heir to Socrates and became interested in cosmology and human physiology. Next, it was **Aristotle,** son of a physician and pupil of Plato, who honed his skills as a lecturer and helped shape many of the techniques and methods used in science in the Middle Ages and the Renaissance and was considered the father of comparative anatomy. And in the 17th century, it was **Galileo Galilei** (1564-1642) who pointed out that Aristotle's conclusions, relative to physics and astronomy, were wrong. Additionally, Aristotle erroneously placed the seat of intelligence in the heart, confused nerves, ligaments and tendons and linked veins from the liver to the right arm and veins from the spleen to the left arm.

Tenents of the various sects of medicine (Dogmatism, Empiricism, Methodism, Pneumatism and Eclecticism) extended from the 4th century far into the Christian era. Interestingly, the doctrine of the *pneuma*, which was the all-pervading cosmic principle of the Stoics, (*pneuma* referred to the breathing in of the spirit, which went first to the heart and then through the arteries to all parts of the body) extended up to the practices of Aretaeus of Cappadocia (c. A.D. 120-180). **One could interpret *pneuma* as being oxygen.** These belief systems had strong influence on scientific thinking and the development of the scientific method.

In general, **scientists follow the course of 1) making observations, 2) developing a hypothesis, 3) formulating a theory and 4) debate and collection of data to either validate or invalidate the theory.**

Hypotheses are deduced from analysis of observed data and are validated by the accuracy of predictability and reproducibility. Hypotheses that are supported by a wide array of predictable observations come to be known as **theories**. If your collected data is not capable of being analyzed by deductive reasoning, then it is not going to allow itself to be evaluated by the Western scientific paradigm. At times, it seems as though our scientific community has temporarily over looked these basic tenents and rely totally on p-values (probability values) or figures of significance, while simultaneously ignoring common sense.

Additionally, we must realize that many phenomena are not amenable to being investigated utilizing the scientific method. **The complexities perpetually existing within a living entity are far removed from the simplicity of the test tube.** It is invalid to assume that complex mind-body relationship studies are worthless, merely because the scientific method cannot be readily applied to them.

1.2.3 Junk Dealers

Occasionally, falsified data gets into publications. Fortunately, it is ferreted out and exposed rapidly. In the scientific arena, we stand upon the shoulders of those investigators who have labored before us. We are linked into an **intellectual cumulative continuum** for our knowledge base. We must strive to maintain its purity.

In the JAMA, April 14, 2004 edition, pages 1776-1777, Dr. Michael Kalichman reviewed the book, <u>Science in the Private Interest: Has the Lure of Profits Corrupted Biomedical Research?</u> by Sheldon Krimsky. Rowman & Littlefield Publishers, 2003. Dr. Kalichman states the following:

"Dr. Sheldon Krimsky's new publication adds voice to two other recent books that examine the commercialization of academia (Bok, D. Universities in the marketplace: the commercialization of higher education. Princeton, NJ, Princeton University Press, 2003) (Etkowitz, H. MIT and the rise of entrepreneurial science. New York, NY, Routledge, 2002). Krimsky's premise is that **academia is fundamentally altered by increasing partnerships with the private sector.** With the compilation of case histories, data and analyses, Krimsky has clarified what is at stake in a way that warrants our attention.

" By looking closely at how research topics are chosen, how research is funded, and how policy decisions are made, Krimsky demonstrates that certain hypothetical fears are now realities. **The definition of successful research programs has been narrowed to those most likely to yield a marketable product, rather than to those that generate new knowledge.** Decreases in communication and sharing are inevitable consequence of protecting personal interest. **The work that is being done, and that is ultimately published, tends to favor the interest of those who fund the research.** The obvious risk is flawed results, whether due to unconscious or conscious biases. Finally, and most importantly, the independence and perceived integrity of academic researchers is eroding. This is also likely reflected in the fact that over 30% of today's patients seek out help though alternative medicine. With an increased emphasis on opportunities for accumulating personal financial wealth, it is to be expected that researchers, the funders of the research and the public will become increasingly cynical about the motives driving academic science. Ironically, **the ultimate outcome could be that the original credibility afforded by partnerships with academic researchers will be lost.** If Krimsky is right about these directions, then academia will have sold out a valuable mission in exchange for short-term profits.

"The message of this book is relevant to most of us. Teachers of the responsible conduct of research will find ample material for an entire course on the subject of conflicts of interest. **Educators and basic researchers should be concerned about the shifting of the academic mission toward profit and away from knowledge creation and student instruction.**

"Unfortunately, the problems enumerated by Krimsky clearly outweigh those few documented instances in which academia chose the principles of openness and free publication over the risk of a loss of external funding."

We live in a scientific world in which collection of data may be flawed, observations may be misinterpreted and conclusions may change as quickly as the results of the next experiment's data exits the computer's printer. Hypotheses can be modified and theories can be altered. As science gets closer to applying quantum mechanics and particle physics to our inner molecular workings, of the already present multitudes of biochemical and enzymatic nanomachines, we seemingly get ever closer to what I term the **"cellular uncertainty principle."** Unfortunately, with today's degree of rapid and world wide communications, junk science can be dispersed faster than tabloid headlines of aliens landing in Washington D. C. All too often, **associations are sold as truth and epidemiological trends are preached with gospel-like zeal,** which is usually directly tied to a profit motive. Clearly, many shaky hypotheses and erroneous associations have been converted into perceived **virtual dogma** by clever marketers.

Many areas related to the pharmaceutical industry, weight loss methods, hair growth aids, dietary supplements, antioxidants, vitamins, antiaging schemes, fat burners, cancer cures, miracle drugs, etc. are reportedly based on scientific and medical data. **These areas are rife with quackery, fraud and outright lies, all at the expense of legitimate science and** are examples of "pharmaceuticide."

Dr. James Le Fanu's book, "<u>The Rise & Fall of Modern Medicine</u>" (Abacus, 1999), is a must-read for all scientists, medical investigators and physicians. Even many lay people would understand and follow its logic, even though I believe that its basic title implying the fall of modern medicine is arguable.

1.2.4 Quick to Judge, Slow to Change

Scientific advances seemingly move at glacial speed or, at times, not to move at all. On other occasions, if and when it does move, it may even move in the wrong direction. I believe that I will show that such is the case with today's **"free radical phobia".** Rarely do we see true quantum leaps in scientific discovery. Dr. James Le Fanu cites many interesting examples of **medical and scientific intellectual impaction** and asserts that frequently the most important discoveries are made by novices or by accident.

On 1/23/04, syndicated columnist, William Rusher, was discussing alleged global warming and the response to Bjorn Lomborg's book, "The Skeptical Environmentalist: Measuring the Real State of the World" (Cambridge University Press, 2001), Rusher says:

> "On the specific subject of global warming, Lomborg demonstrates that the scientific evidence is dubious, the warnings of doom are vastly exaggerated and the cost of efforts to reduce the human contribution to the growth of greenhouse gases (as under the Kyoto Protocol) would be in the neighborhood of hundreds of trillions of dollars.

> Well, needless to say, the roof fell in on Lomborg. Scientific American ran an 11-page spread of articles by various certified "experts" denouncing him and his findings.

> What we are seeing in operation here is herd mentality of a large segment of the scientific community. Some alleged scientific "certainty," almost always with leftist policy implications, is fastened upon and endowed with the force of unarguable gospel. The media take up the cry, and the public--always nervously on guard against the latest supposed scientific threat to our survival, from acid rain to the ozone hole—is flogged to a fever pitch of anxiety. Scientists who agree are marginalized and dismissed. Eventually the hysteria dies down, until some new peril is identified and publicized.

> Fortunately, there are always a few scientists, such as Lomborg, who refuse to be silenced. We owe them a tremendous debt of gratitude."

Another current example of the sloth speed of scientific discovery relates to studies on AIDS. On 1/21/04, USA Today ran a story entitled, "Biggest-ever AIDS vaccine trial draws stinging criticism." Excerpts from the article were as follows:

> "When the world of AIDS vaccine research erupts into controversy, as it did last week, the source is often pent-up frustration over the snail's pace of progress and the best use of research money. **More than 20 years into the epidemic, only one vaccine has completed two large-scale clinical trials. It failed both.**

> If the vaccines fail as expected, however, scientists face major challenges. They still haven't figured out what kind of immune response they need to provide protection, much less how to obtain it. What's more, evidence suggests that researchers may have focused much too narrowly on potential vaccines that activate just one part of the body's immune system."

> At times, it seems to me as though we, in the USA, have regulated ourselves into "a body at rest" and that **we have to balance patient safety with the progressive momentum to overcome the inertia of being overly cautious.**

2 OXYGEN OVERVIEW

The effects of free radicals on biological materials were proposed about 50 years ago and **Denham Harman described free radicals as " Pandora's box of evils,"** which accounted for diseases, aging and cancer. This set the tone of the role of free radicals for decades. In 1969, McCord and Fridovich discovered superoxide dismutase (SOD) and investigators were more encouraged than ever to find and identify the damage inflicted by radicals upon all cellular components (McCord J.M. and Fridovich, I. Superoxide dismutase: an enzyme function for Erythrocuprein (hemocuprein). J. Biol Chem 244: 6049-6055, 1969). It was not until the late 1970s that a slight change in attitude toward free radicals in biological systems was to emerge, with the 1977 work of Mittal and Murad showing that the O_2^- anion effected the formation of the "second messenger" cGMP. Subsequent work with nitric oxide and hydrogen peroxide has demonstrated regulatory control of smooth muscle relaxation and in the inhibition of platelet adhesion and T-cell production of IL-2. In 1991, hydrogen peroxide was shown to produce activation of transcription nuclear factors in mammalian cells and indications for the positive effects of free radicals were beginning to be recognized.

2.1 THOUGHTS ON THE LIFE FORCE

It appears to me that, just as a computer has to have a constant supply of electrons to function, so does the human brain. The brain does so by utilizing atmospheric air with its 21% O_2 levels, which acts as a "vaporized wire" passing through the nostrils and going into the lungs, from which the O_2 is extracted and carried by the blood stream to the brain. In the brain, and elsewhere throughout the body, it serves as a source for the electron flow in the electron transport chain and for NADPH oxidase, thus providing an energy supply (an internal flow of electricity or electrons, actually a circuit) to the brain and because of its connection to oxidative phosphorylation, it provides energy for the entire organism.

In countless studies, cells have been fragmented, fractured, broken, homogenized, passed through osmotic gradients, and centrifuged at 100,000 rpms to end up with a "pellet", which is then subjected to a wide array of artifactual in vitro conditions, in attempts to discover the workings of the living/breathing cell. Not only have these artificial conditions critically deviated from normalcy, but they also lack the vital "life force." It is little wonder that we have such difficulty in utilizing this type of data for predictive purposes.

I will discuss the role of oxygen and its **"chemical cousins" (RONS)** in great detail, as regards health and disease.

2.2 "TO BEAT OR NOT TO BEAT ?" THAT IS THE QUESTION...AND OXYGEN IS THE ANSWER

The human brain and heart can survive for only brief intervals of O_2 deprivation without sustaining irreversible damage or cell death.

If one looks at **levels of consciousness**, decreasing levels of O_2 results directly in decreased levels of consciousness. Pilots or those exploring high altitudes, experience confusion, and dizziness up to the point of total loss of consciousness, with progressively decreasing levels of O_2. Conditions such as ischemic encephalopathy, present with decreased brain oxygen levels and with the attendant mental confusion pattern. **If the O_2 levels are stopped for just a few minutes, one can experience death of brain neurons**, in an irreversible fashion and brain function ceases. Again, this is analogous to pulling the plug on a computer, thereby stopping or interrupting its power supply.

One can see that a situation can exist whereby the brain still has an O_2 supply but does not function properly, such as in traumatic unconsciousness or coma. This would be analogous to traumatizing a computer, whereby it is still plugged into a power supply but does not function. Thus, it appears to me that at least one fundamental requirement for consciousness is the presence and flow of a constant supply of electrons via oxygen. Furthermore, **I believe, as do others, that the reactivity of ground state oxygen is far too slow to participate in usual brain function (thinking, thought storage and retrieval) and that speeds of electromagnetic phenomena can be achieved primarily by oxygen radicals and electronic excitation states.**

In individuals who expire calmly, the life force leaves them concurrent or simultaneous with the cessation of breathing. **In other words, when the constant and invariant supply of oxygen is gone, so is life, as we know it**. Not only is oxygen directly tied or linked to consciousness but it is also directly linked to the life process itself. At times, it appears that some scientists have overlooked these most basic of observations. There is a plethora of comments condemning O_2 and its modifications, which tend to overlook its beneficence.

I can only feel that conditions such as dementia and Alzheimer's disease are related at least in part, to lowering of oxygen levels and RONS in the brain. Investigators utilizing hyperbaric oxygen treatments have made interesting contributing studies to these areas but **it has received little attention or mention. Studies show that, although the brain is only 2% of the total body weight, it requires 20-25% of the body's consumed oxygen.** Additionally, **brains shrink at the rate of 20-30 grams per decade until the age of 60, and 30-40 grams thereafter**. The average male brain weighs 1,350 grams, that of females 1,200grams; but females have a slightly higher proportion of brain to body. Brain size is roughly proportional to body size. The heart and the brain have the highest requirements for oxygen than any other organ or tissue in the body. Additionally, heart and brain cells have low levels of superoxide dismutase and catalase, again indicating that these tissues have a need for higher levels of reactive oxygen products and peroxide and excited states.

Just as with the living/breathing cell, the complexities of the human brain should not be underestimated. By way of illustration, **the National Academy of Sciences estimates that, "a single human brain has a greater number of possible connections among its nerve cells than the total number of atomic particles in the universe."**

Studies on the toxicity of massive doses of hydrogen peroxide, given intravenously to laboratory animals, show that it selectively injures the lungs, thymus, liver and kidneys. I believe that **this indicates that both the heart and the brain can "handle or tolerate" excessively high levels of peroxide and oxygen**. In fact, it appears that these two tissues require higher levels of peroxides and oxygen. Also, I feel that non-polar oxygen species such as hydrogen peroxide, singlet oxygen or hypochlorite, may be the way to treat certain ischemia or O_2 deficiency conditions, since these species can readily cross cell membranes. Additionally, peroxide would be more stable but it could be rapidly decomposed by catalase, while in the blood stream.

Further, if one were to attempt to administer $^1O_2$ or $^1O_2$ generating reagents, one would have to consider the short

life time of singlet oxygen as 3-4 μs and short diffusion distance, such that it would have to be generated at or near the target site. This would, however, give concerns for air embolism in the small arterioles of the brain, which could be lethal but this could theoretically be overcome by decreasing concentrations of reagents or decreasing the flow rates of reagents, as was done using H_2O_2 in the 1960s by Urschal's group at Baylor. Hypochlorite could break down to chlorides or chloramines and be harmful in that form. Thus, perhaps a better route would be to try to increase levels of ground state triplet oxygen. This can be done by either increasing the concentration of inspired O_2, increasing the O_2 carrying capacity of hemoglobin, by a hyperbaric oxygen chamber or by a combination of all of these modes. Of interest is the fact that the Baylor group found that intra-arterial administration of H_2O_2 had the same physiological effect on O_2 saturation as did hyperbaric O_2 administration.

The main effect of stroke or heart attack is that they interrupt or stop the flow of oxygen to either the heart or the brain. **Nearly 90% of all strokes result from clots that block the brain's arteries, cutting off circulation and starving the brain cells of oxygen**. In surgery, we can tourniquet off the blood supply to the arm or hand for up to 2 hours before irreversible damage occurs. Yet, the heart or the brain can only tolerate oxygen stoppage for a few minutes, as is evidenced with angina, myocardial infarction or stroke. Oxygen is, indeed, magical or an essential to these vital organs in sustaining life as we know it.

Many investigators have shown that **calcium is essential for production of RONS** and believe that elevated calcium levels are responsible for activation of RONS-generating enzymes and formation of free radicals by the mitochondrial respiratory chain. Conversely, **an increase in intracellular calcium concentration may be stimulated by RONS** and H_2O_2 has been recently shown to accelerate the overall channel opening process in voltage-dependent calcium channels in plant and animal cells. Data support the speculation that **Ca^{2+} and RONS are two cross-talking messengers in various cellular processes** (Gordeeva, A.V., Zvyagilskaya, R.A. and Labas, Y.A. Cross-talk between reactive oxygen species and calcium in living cells. Biochemistry (Moscow), Oct. 2003, vol. 68, no. 10, pp. 1077-1080.). Please keep in mind that many investigators believe that Ca^{2+} overload is considered to be the final pathway leading to cell death under pathological conditions. I believe that this is related to RONS induced apoptosis.

2.3 RONS, ALZHEIMER'S DISEASE AND METALS

Nearly all mammals accumulate toxic deposits of a protein called beta-amyloid in the brain as they age. It forms distinctive plaques and tangles. University of Melbourne researcher Professor Colin Masters, an international authority on brain disorders that cause dementia, says that Alzheimer's causes massive damage to neurons but even in late stages much of the damage may reversible.

Beta-amyloid production varies between individuals. As the plaques clog neural tissue, they kill off nerve cells en masse. The gradual build up of amyloid accelerates with age, hastening the descent into dementia.

Remove the amyloid, or slow its build up, and you could cure or prevent Alzheimer's disease. But that is literally an insoluable problem. **Amyloid deposits stubbornly resist dissolving by enzymes or chemicals, even in laboratory tests on brain tissue**, so the chances of developing amyloid-busting drugs for living brains is remote.

Alzheimer's disease selectively erodes the area of the brain rich in neurons responsive to the neurotransmitter acetylcholine, a key player in higher brain function and memory. New drugs keep healthy neurons firing in the brains of Alzheimer patients, but may only retard their symptoms by less than a year.

One of Masters' former PhD students, Dr. Ashley Bush, may have found an even more potent therapy for Alzheimer's disease: a genuine amyloid-busting drug that may halt the disease in its tracks. A decade ago, Bush began to suspect heavy metals played a central role in forming the amyloid deposits that kill off brain cells. His interest was in zinc and copper - not aluminum, whose folkloric reputation as the culprit in Alzheimer's was debunked in the early 1990's.

In 1999, Bush and his colleagues tested the world's first amyloid plaque-dissolving drug in mice, with remarkable results. It's **an old antibiotic, clioquinol**, which was used to treat travelers' diarrhea until it was withdrawn in the 1970's because it induced vitamin B12 deficiency.

Bush became interested in clioquinol because of its ability to trap and remove copper and zinc, two metals with essential roles in cell metabolism, especially in the brain.

A psychiatrist by training, Bush left Masters' group in 1992 to join Professor Rudi Tanzy's team at Harvard Medical School in Boston, Massachusetts. Soon after, he made a crucial discovery: copper levels in the mammalian brain increase with age in concert with the build-up of amyloid deposits. Moreover, the metals - and amyloid deposits - concentrate in the areas damaged most by Alzheimer's disease: the neocortex, focus of higher brain functions and memory, and the hippocampus, which regulates memory storage.

The next step was to find out how beta-amyloid deposits poison neurons. Bush suspected the answer lay in the highly reactive nature of **copper, which catalyses formation of a natural bleach, hydrogen peroxide**. In living tissue, hydrogen peroxide rapidly breaks down into harmless water, but the reaction also spawns one of the most dangerously reactive molecules in nature: the hydroxyl radical, the active bleaching agent in hydrogen peroxide.

Bush believes the brains of Alzheimer's patients literally fizz with hydrogen peroxide, overwhelming the enzymes that normally defuse toxic radicals. **Of course, I think that his belief is wrong and that additional H_2O_2 may be needed by the demented brain.** The 1999 experiment was the acid test of his hypothesis. As of mid-2004, there has been no positive follow-up the this theory, that I have been able to find.

He administered clioquinol to aging, transgenic mice expressing a particularly malignant form of the human APP gene. Uniquely among mammals, rats and mice don't develop plaque deposits with age; their form of APP has no equivalent copper-binding site.

Bush hoped to see signs of a reduction in plaque aggregation and hydrogen peroxide production - the latter causes symptoms similar to drunkenness: confusion and clouding of higher mental functions like reasoning and memory, but definitive results are still pending.

Alzheimer's disease continues today with little hope in sight and there have been no major breakthroughs based on the blocking peroxide or hydroxyl radical.

The **two hallmarks of Alzheimer's disease (AD) victims are neurofibrillary tangles and amyloid plaques in the brain.** The latter constitutes mainly of an aggregated protein called beta-amyloid. The plaques are dense deposits of a protein fragment called *amyloid*, mixed with inflammatory cells (a type of glial cell and invading white blood cells), and detritus. The beta-amyloid originates from a membrane protein called amyloid-precursor protein (APP) and is present in healthy brains in a soluble form. Since the amyloid plaques occur only in AD patients (**RMH Note: Presently, this is a point of dispute**), the aggregation process from beta-amyloid to the plaques is a key event. This is supported by the fact that factors promoting this aggregation are risk factors for the AD (e.g., the allele e4 of the apolipoprotein E). Thus, conditions influencing this aggregation are of high interest. Studies in vitro, in cell cultures and AD model mice all indicate an important role for metals and RONS in this context. Alois Alzheimer described tangles, which were twisted fibrils of a *tau* protein and remnants of the extensive network of tubules that normally maintains the structure and integrity of the neuron.

Complicating the picture is the fact that some Alzheimer's patients never develop amyloid plaques and it appears that tangles are usually formed before plaques. Also, it appears that **the onset of dementia corresponds to the loss of neurons and not to the quantity of amyloid in the brain.** Further, injections of amyloid into young monkeys does not produce dementia as it does in old monkeys and not all human patients with mutations in APP or the presently genes produce only amyloid plaques but only form tangles in old age. **It appears that Alzheimer's disease can not be produced by amyloid alone.** Also, people with no genetic susceptibility to amyloid formation still deposit amyloid in their brains and if oxidation is prevented by antioxidants, *tau* will not coagulate. An important observation may be the fact that tau becomes abnormally phosphorylated in Alzheimer's disease but it appears that this is not necessary for tau deposition. And tau fibrils can form even in the absence of phosphate.

Some investigators believe that inflammation plays a crucial role in Alzheimer's and even refer to it as **"arthritis of the brain."** Actually, I believe that the chances are very good that both arthritis and Alzheimer's disease are due to the presence of presently undetectable pathogens (pathonanogens); so, in that sense, I agree with them, but only in that sense. It has been shown that patients taking NSAIDs have about half the risk of developing dementia and it appears that people with sources of brain inflammation, such as stroke, traumatic brain injury and viral infections, have several times the risk of dementia.

It was shown that Zn, Cu and Fe are found in the amyloid plaques and in vitro studies revealed that these same metals promote the aggregation of beta-amyloid. The ligands of the metal are most likely histidine and perhaps an oxygen (from water or amino-acid). Moreover, beta-amyloid with bound Cu/Fe are able to produce H_2O_2, an RONS, probably by reducing O_2. Reportedly, this can be blocked by TNF-α and β. However, **close scrutiny of the data as it relates to plaques, tangles, amyloid and dementia, is filled with confusing inconsistencies and presently, there are no cause and effect relationships established.**

Certain heavy metal compounds are important environmental allergens, such as mercury dichloride ($HgCl_2$) and it may contribute to the development of allergies.

Preliminary experiments that I have conducted have revealed that when nearly totally blocked human coronary arteries are bathed in my singlet oxygen system, the arteriosclerotic plaques were dissolved within 3 minutes. However, the concentrations used in my in vitro experiment would require considerable modifications to be used on in situ plaques but solubility is a function of infusion rate and concentration of reagents. **The bottom line is the fact that my singlet oxygen system did dissolve plaque in human arteries (unpublished study by me). I truly believe that it has great potential for future clinical use and begs for investigation.**

3 PATHONANOGENS

Cancer is reaching pandemic proportions on a world wide basis. Additionally, many investigators have postulated that "stealth pathogens" are causing wide spread increases in autoimmune diseases. There has been no success in finding these stealth pathogens. For a number of years now, I have had the idea that many of these run-away unexplained diseases is being caused by agents which exist below the level and size of viruses and I call these nanobugs (or pathological chemicals), **"pathonanogens."** Furthermore, I feel and theorize that these pathonanogens are present in many disease conditions and act as nanomachines or nanomolecules, especially for the autoimmune diseases. **These pathonanogens alter metabolism of the normal cell in such a way as to produce disease symptomatology, similar to that seen with prions.** I predict that we will isolate and identify many of these pathonanogens.

3.1 DENHAM HARMAN: THE FIRST "OXY-MORON"

Past investigators have referred to a group of compounds called Reactive Oxygen Nitrogen Species (RONS). Unfortunately, free radicals of oxygen have been demonized and referred to as "biochemical bad boys," "chemical terrorists," "killers," and "rats in hiding" that run wild and wreak havoc, chaos and annihilation throughout the cell. These are also referred to by at least a dozen other demonic notations.

I believe that it is just these kinds of inaccurate characterizations (B.S.) that lead to statements such as those uttered by "an herb doctor" on National Public Radio on the morning of 8/22/04, when he said, "The human body produces over 17 tons (34,000 pounds) of free radicals during a lifetime." Of course, he immediately hawked a dietary herbal supplement, which one could **purchase**, to not only compensate for these dangerous free radicals but also to improve one's self esteem, correct bowel habits and overall, lead to a wonderful and wholesome life.

We must recognize that with oxygen modifications (RONS/excytomers), each has their own specific properties, reactivities, solubilities, rates of reaction, half-lives, diffusion distances, etc. It is time that we avoid the garbage-can term "reactive oxygen nitrogen species and oxygen free radicals" and refer to each individual oxygen/electron modification by its true name, such as, superoxide ion, hydrogen peroxide, singlet oxygen, hypochlorous acid, peroxynitrite, hydroxyl radical, etc. **This aspect of recent terminology was recently addressed by Nathan as follows:**

> Some scientists write as if the terms ROI and RNI lack precise definitions, or conversely, as if all members of each class fit one definition. ROI and RNI are sets of related molecules with individually distinct chemical and biological properties. ROI refers to all oxidation and excitation states of O_2, from superoxide ($O_2\cdot-$) up to but excluding water, that arise in physiological environments, including singlet oxygen ($^1O_2^*$), ozone (O_3), hydrogen peroxide (H_2O_2), hypohalites and the hydroxyl radical ($OH\cdot$). RNI refers to all oxidation states and reactive adducts of nitrogenous NOS products, from NO up to but excluding nitrate (NO_3-), that arise in physiological settings, including nitroxyl ($NO-$), nitrosonium ($NO+$), higher oxides of nitrogen, S-nitroslthiols (RSNOs), peroxynitrite ($OONO-$), and denitrify iron complexes. **No two ROI have identical biological properties, nor do any two RNI**. Their distinctive properties arise from differences in such features as reactivity, half-life and lipid solubility.

> Some discussions of ROI and RNI assume that RNI cause only nitrosative reactions, whereas only ROI cause oxidative reactions. Oxidative reactions includecarbonylations, hydroxylations, peroxidations, or oxidation of sulfhydryl to disulfides or sulfenic, sulfinic, or sulfonic acids. Nitrosative reactions include nitrosylation of sulfhydryl or metals and nitrations of tyrosine residues. Actually, various ROI can oxidize or reduce, and RNI can lead to both nitrosative and redox reactions. It is critical that many of these reactions are reversible, such as formation of methionine sulfoxides and cysteinyl nitrosyls, disulfides and sulfenic acids.

> With respect to biologic actions of ROI and RNI, some authors use the terms oxidative stress or nitrosative stress in a neutral sense indistinguishable from perturbation. However, most use it to mean reactions that threaten or cause harm. The frame of reference of the present discussion is that ROI and RNI are routinely produced throughout the aerobic biome. Evolution has capitalized on their properties to put them to use as signaling molecules, including in the special case of host defense. From this perspective, the molecules usually

referred to as antioxidant and antinitrosative defenses spend most of their time acting as integral parts of homeostatic signaling systems. As with any aspect of physiology, production of ROI and RNI can become excessive to the point that it is maladaptive, if not for the producing cell, then for a target cell. In those circumstances, the systems that catabolism ROI and RNI, or reverse their effects, act as defenses.

Since **oxygen reacts with basically all other elements**, except the noble gases, I feel that all molecular combinations with oxygen should be termed **oxygen modifications**, if they are bonded to, complexed with or have reacted with oxygen. In short, what I am saying is that oxygen is much more basic to chemical reactions on planet earth than has been previously appreciated by many. Its uniqueness, such as its ground state triplet multiplicity, indicates its special role in all aerobic chemistry and most life processes from plants through primates, from bacteria through mammals and perhaps even the chemistry of viruses and/or minerals.

In inorganic chemistry (not involving carbon based molecules) there are basically only 2 types of chemical reactions: **oxidation** (which removes negative charged electrons) and **reduction** (which adds a negative charged electron).

Humans consume about 250 grams of oxygen every day, and of this, approximately 3-5% is converted to superoxide anion (O_2^{-}) and other modifications of oxygen (Rice-Evans, C A and Burdon, R H. Free radical damage and its control. Amsterdam: Elsevier, 1994; p. 25-27). **That calculates out to 12.5 grams of superoxide per person per day.**

These are overwhelming quantities of **superoxide, which are likely rapidly converted to hydrogen peroxide.** Thus, **it seems ludicrous to believe that these effects can be overcome with milligram quantities of antioxidants per day.** Even more important is the issue as to whether or not these oxygen modifications, such as superoxide anion, should be decreased, trapped, or quenched. Only recently have we found organisms in the abyss of the oceans, whose life cycles is not tied to light and oxygen but these are, by far, the extremely rare exceptions on planet Earth.

Different energy levels within a compound result in different physical characteristics and chemical reactivities. For instance, water can exist as a vapor, a liquid or a solid, depending upon whether or not it is steam, fluid or ice and this is with the same chemical formula of H_2O. Unquestionably, this should be regarded as dihydrogen oxygen, since 8/9ths of its mass is oxygen and as such, **water is merely another form of oxygen. I believe that this is, at least in part, responsible for water's healing and life sustaining properties.** Perhaps, this can best be illustrated by the fact that the jellyfish is composed of nearly 90-95% water.

Likewise, carbonates, phosphates, nitrates, etc. should be looked upon primarily as oxygen with another chemical moiety attached to it, yet, keeping **oxygen as the prime mover.** Indeed, **oxygen, along with its electronic and molecular modifications, is the prime mover.** Another example of changing characteristics and reactivities is within the RONS family, whereby, **simply moving an electron to higher energy orbitals or the addition or subtraction of a single electron, results in remarkably different chemical characteristics and reactivities.** Figures vary but it is said that humans are 2/3 oxygen and the earth's crust is 50% oxygen. In fact, it is said that oxygen is more plentiful, in the body, than all of the other elements combined. That fact alone, should make oxygen's unique role readily apparent.

Thus, **water is just another form of oxygen; yet, water is rarely discussed in biochemical experiments, other than being used as a solvent medium.** In fact, it is the primary solvent medium within human beings and its participation in all of the body's biochemical mechanisms could be of paramount importance. We may have simply overlooked the significance of the water-form or the dihydrogen modification of oxygen. Also, please remember that H_2O_2 is oxygenated water.

Of utmost interest is the fact that **everything in us, on us and around us is made up of about 92 naturally occurring elements and about 115 natural and synthesized elements** and/or combinations thereof. Everything in our known world is made up of this handful of elements. It is their combinations, which give rise to new products with seemingly totally new properties. It is with this theme in mind that I have come to the concept of oxygen and its many combinations, as being of utmost importance to all living things. **Oxygen is the "prime**

mover" and is numero uno in living/breathing biological systems. All aerobic cells must constantly breathe, just as collectively for an individual, we must constantly breathe.

We must have a constant, invariant and never ending supply of oxygen, with its unique reaction qualities, to supply the energy for all aerobic activity and to maintain a state of cellular and organismal homeostasis. Even the component enzymes of the glycolytic biochemical pathways (anaerobic), are made of oxygen combinations. Furthermore, the phosphate groups of ATP are, themselves, made of oxygen combinations.

American physiologist, Walter Cannon (1871-1945), coined the term **"homeostasis"** and pointed out that strenuous exercise generates sufficient heat to curdle or "cook" body proteins unless rapidly dispersed and that the lactic acid produced by the muscles, during exercise, would destroy cells if it were not removed or inactivated.

It gets particularly interesting when oxygen's electron configuration is altered from the triplet multiplicity ground state, to electron rich states or electronically excited states. In that regard, the electron ranks next in order of prime importance, when it comes to oxygen's reactivities and properties. Therefore, **the electron is the "secondary mover."**

4 LIFE FORCES

4.0 ILLNESS AND THE LIFE FORCE

Practitioners at the time of Hippocrates no longer considered illness as a punishment. The Stoics, in the 4th and 3rd centuries B.C. considered illness as an evil to be avoided at all costs and they preached virtue rather than health as the highest good. Actually, suicide was justified for illness under their code. The Greeks key principle was that all body fluids were composed of varying proportions of blood (warm and moist), phlegm (cold and moist), yellow bile (warm and dry), and black bile (cold and dry). When these humors were in balance, the body was in good health and the life force was strong. This represented the hypothesis that the Greeks used to organize their concept of health and disease. Nobel Laureate, Peter Medawar was quoted as saying, "Science without the underpinning of hypothesis is just kitchen arts."

4.1 OXIDATIVE AND NON-OXIDATIVE KILLING MECHANISMS

The major role of the neutrophil is to protect the body against infectious organisms and, in my opinion and that of many others, against cancer. The killing event is thought to occur with the participation of both oxidative and non-oxidative mechanisms. Metchnikoff described the process of phagocytosis, in which the neutrophil engulfs the foreign agent and forms a phagosome, wherein fusion of intracellular azurophilic granules and specific granules occur. Specific granules activate the complement cascade and contain collagenase and gelatinase.

Oxidative mechanisms, producing bacterial cell death, usually follow a massive increase in the consumption of oxygen by the neutrophil and is referred to as the **respiratory burst**. The respiratory burst is a sequence of four metabolic events which consists of (1) a massive, **10-15% increase in oxygen consumption**, (2) formation of the superoxide anion by a one electron reduction, (3) formation of hydrogen peroxide by another one electron reduction and (4) activation of the hexose monophosphate shunt, which is used to regenerate NADPH. NADPH is nicotinamide adenine dinucleotide phosphate, and NADP+ is the oxidized form of NADPH.

Molecular ground state dioxygen is converted to superoxide by NADPH oxidase and NADH oxidase. Superoxide is converted to hydrogen peroxide by **superoxide dismutate at a rate that is 100 times faster than spontaneous non-enzymatic conversion**. Oxidative mechanisms can be mediated by myeloperoxidase (MPO) or may be independent from MPO.

4.1.1 Bacteria, Viruses, Fungi, Parasites and Tumors/Cancer

Hydrogen peroxide is utilized in myeloperoxidase-dependent bacterial killing, where it combines with chloride (Cl-) to form hypochlorous acid or with bromide (Br-) to form hypobromous acid. These oxidized halogens are potent antimicrobial agents. These reactive oxygen species can recombine or be converted to other species such as **singlet oxygen (which is bactericidal, fungicidal, virucidal, parasiticidal and tumoricidal)** or the hydroxyl radical.

Oxygen-independent mechanisms also play a part in bacterial killing in anaerobic conditions. Some of these non-oxidative agents are acids, lysozyme, lactoferrin, defensins, BPI, azurocidin, serine proteinases, elastase, cathepsin G, and proteinase 3.

There are many forms of active oxygen, they have different half lives and reactivities. **RMH Note: I refer to these RONS as the "chemical cousins" of ground state oxygen.** They can chemically alter cells via lipid peroxidation, protein oxidation, carbohydrate and protein cleavage and DNA base alterations. They can alter cellular redox states and gene expression (O_2 Paradox, page 328).

4.2 NEUTROPHILIA

Neutrophilia, an over production of neutrophils, can be associated with infections, where the total blood **granulocyte pool is increased 5-6 times normal**. Established infections maintain elevated neutrophil counts. Similarly, **exercise** or an epinephrine injection **can increase the circulating granulocyte pool by up to 50% for brief time periods of up to 20-30 minutes.**

Neutrophilia can also accompany a rapidly growing neoplasm, when the tumor outgrows its blood supply. This is thought to be due to tumor necrosis factor-alpha (TNF-α). However, **I feel that this is the body's attempt to kill the tumor by mobilizing more neutrophils to produce more oxidative killing species, and as a matter of fact, if the body could mount a large enough neutrophil response, we would see a course identical to that which occurs in spontaneous tumor regression or following a successful course of Coley's toxin. This is also analogous to the formation of large quantities of singlet oxygen during PDT, which are tumoricidal.**

5 EPIPHANY OF 12/31/03: HOW TO RECONCILE THE MANY CONFLICTS OF THE DATA

My use of the word "epiphany" does not refer to the January 6th church festival or to its Greek origins referring to the manifestation of a god, but rather refers to the nigh "intellectual high" described by Bertrand Russell. However, it may not be unlike the rapture described with spiritual or emotional ecstasy.

It has occurred to me (and apparently to others), that if the figures regarding the number of oxidative hits per day to each aerobic cell in the human body are true, then **we all have (potential or pro-neoplasia) cancer in us at all times.** There is an enormous amount of data supporting this rather disconcerting hypothesis. So much so, that I am forced to accept it as being correct. Ergo, we must be correcting and/or removing oxidatively damaged nuclear and mitochondrial DNA at all times. The important factor is whether or not we can use our natural defenses to remove or **eliminate these uncorrected intracellular cancerous events**, which I think we do by our steady state levels of RONS and excited states, because of their tumoricidal properties and capability.

If the level of these reactive oxygen species and excited states are reduced below normal levels, there is the probability of developing or "allowing" tumors and cancer or an infection to occur. Conversely, in times of need, such as the overt manifestation of cancerous cells or the onset of an infection, the body is called upon to generate even more of these important tumoricidal and bactericidal oxygen species.

In other words, **RONS and excited states serve in at least a biphasic or triphasic manner as both the cause and the cure of cancer, just as with many chemotherapeutic agents and radiation.** Similarly, we all have bacteria constantly in us (i.e., in our gut, lungs, mouth, the air we breathe, the food we eat, esophagus, wounds and even our blood stream, particularly following each bowel movement) but we do not have constant infections. However, we constantly have the potential for an infection or for cancer to manifest itself in every aerobic cell at all times. **Oxygen is constantly being metabolized**, from the moment of conception until the moment of death, in every aerobic cell in our body. Consequently, reactive oxygen species and oxygen excited states are constantly being generated in every aerobic cell in our body and they are causing potentially mutagenic events on a constant basis. **Steady state levels for hydrogen peroxide, hypochlorous acid and superoxide anion have been measured by investigators.** Plus, common sense tells us that steady states must be produced at all times or we would die of an imminent infection, since germs are present outside and inside the body at all times.

5.1 RONS STEADY STATES

Healthy tissue maintains a steady state of $[H_2O_2]$ of 10^{-9} to 10^{-7} (Physiological Reviews 1979, 59: 564).

In 1999, Juan and Buettner calculated the steady state levels to be as follows:

    $[H_2O_2]$ss in red cells is 10^{-10} M
    $[H_2O_2]$ss in mitochondrial membrane is 10^{-8} M
    $[H_2O_2]$ss in liver cells is 10^{-8} M
    $[O_2]$ss is $10-5$ M, much higher than $[H_2O_2]$
    $[O_2^{\cdot-}]$ss in cells is 10^{-10} M

Physiologic ratios of $[O_2]/[H_2O_2]$ is $> 10^3$ and thus, O_2 is much higher than H_2O_2 levels.

Michael Thun M. D., vice president of epidemiology and surveillance research for the American Cancer society, stated that, "Cancer is not an inescapable fact of life." (ACS Statistics for 2004, www.cancer.org/docroot/stt/stt_0.asp). This double negative statement does not recognize the fact that cancers are perpetually being constantly created and constantly destroyed in all of our aerobic cells, due to some of the products of oxidative metabolism, such as reactive oxygen species and electronic excitation states. Thus, **cancer formation is inescapable** but it is usually stopped before it can move to stages of progressive growth. As a matter of fact, **as a developing, dividing and growing embryo and fetus, all of our lives started as cancers**; yet, we are usually not terminated in utero.

RONS in neutrophils are stimulated by phorbol esters or phormyl peptides proceed via protein kinase C (PKC), which is affected by weak magnetic fields. Thus, **RONS generation by neutrophils can be substantially modulated by weak magnetic fields.**

We derive our energy from oxidation, which requires at least slightly prooxidant conditions. (Halliwell)

5.2 EXCYTOLOGY, EXCYTOMERS AND EXCYTOMER PATHWAYS

In 1977, I introduced some new terms into the excited state literature. **"Excytology" refers to the study of interactions of electronic excitation states of atoms, molecules and/or complexes with cells.** Therefore, any biological pathway involving cellular generation or reaction with excited states would be, by definition, proceeding through an "excytomer pathway" such as the Howes Excytomer Pathway. Likewise, atoms, molecules and/or complexes which are in an electronically excited state are referred to as "excytomers." (Howes, R.M., Steele, R.H. and Hoopes, J.E. The role of electronic excitation states in collagen biosynthesis. Perspect Biol and Med 1977; 20(4): 539-544).

Oxygen, in its varying electronic configurations and states, is the primary reason that we do not have an infection or a tumor to appear at any and all times, even from conception and birth. This is due to the WBC's ability to deal with these bacteria, fungi or viruses by their generation of free radicals and excited states of oxygen with the oxidative or respiratory burst. Again, similarly, if the level of these oxygen species is reduced below normal levels, then there is the likelihood of developing ("allowing") an infection, repeated infections or prolonged infections. My approach explains the many **"paradoxes"** associated with oxygen metabolism.

5.3 UNIFIED THEORY LEVELS OF RONS

Levels of RONS and excited states according to my Unified Theory:

Apoptosis of neoplastic cells	➜	**Highest levels of RONS and $^1O_2$ (PDT, Howes System)**
Abeyance of neoplasms and Infections	➜	**Homeostatic levels of RONS and $^1O_2$ (normal levels)**
Allowance for pro-neoplasia	➜	**Deficient levels of RONS and $^1O_2$ (immunosuppression)**

Basically, cancer is in part related to white blood cell levels, which is related to their ability to produce the oxidative burst and produce reactive oxygen species and electronic excitation states. My approach also implies that any factor affecting oxygen's availability to the mitochondrion, can and will affect whether or not an individual will be in a homeostatic state of health or develop illness.

It is also related to oxygen levels of the blood and the oxygen carrying capacity of the blood and specifically to the WBC's ability to produce an oxidative burst. This is further related to such variables as hemoglobin, iron deficiency, chronic granulomatous disease, ethnicity, immunosuppression etc. In fact, it is related to and complicated by **any factor which affects a normal amount of oxygen** from reaching the white blood cell. Additionally, it can further be affected by any white blood cell **intracellular** defect or problem with normal oxidative metabolism. This, in turn, is also related to levels of antioxidants and antioxidant enzymes. My approach makes it readily apparent **that we now may be working against ourselves by the routine administration of antioxidants, antibiotics, chemotherapy and irradiation.** At this juncture of our scientific ignorance, I would bet the ranch on it.

5.3.1 Antibiotics and Cancer

It has been known for many years that certain antibiotics can cause immunosuppression. It is also well known that prior to surgical resection of most cancers, most patients are routinely placed on prophylactic antibiotics. This may be the beginning of reducing our natural self-cure ability. The February 18 issue of JAMA, 2004, reported that all levels of antibiotic use were associated with increased risk of breast cancer and death from breast cancer. This report was met with an avalanche of criticism, even though the data was persuasive.

The report showed that antibiotic use for 1-50 cumulative days reportedly was associated with a 50% increase in breast cancer risk. Antibiotic use for more than 1,000 cumulative days was associated with a 100% increase risk. The primary objection to this startling data was that there is no plausible biological link between antibiotic use and breast cancer. However, **since antibiotic use can suppress the immune system, this is, indeed, a plausible link between antibiotic use and cancer formation.** Additionally, antibiotics may help block the effect of Coley's toxin-types of treatment. This effect could be augmented when combined with chemotherapy and irradiation.

5.4 EPIPHANY OF 3/26/04: DNA IS THE MOST SELFISH MOLECULE

I have been impressed that in complex living ecosystems that each species or specific DNA template tries to perpetuate itself at the peril of most others. Selfish is defined as, "taking care of one's own interest, comfort or pleasure excessively or without regard for others." Animals and/or plants of an intertwined ecosystem consume the others to perpetuate themselves. It is as though the cell or the individual organism is a means for that specific DNA to make more of itself. It is like the old saying that, "a chicken is an egg's way of producing more eggs." Similarly, the cell, all of its organelles, and the collective known as the organism is DNA's way for making more of itself. That is selfish. It can only make one speculate as to why or how this occurs and to question if it is at the pleasure of DNA. In a world in which Arabs kill Jews and Jews kill Arabs and the Irish kill Englishmen and vice versa , (all over ideology) one can only wonder what motivates the pleasure of the DNA. This extrapolates down to the rivalry of football and soccer teams, etc., whereby specific DNA, desires to perpetuate DNA only of its own likeness. In humans, we have developed techniques whereby we can clone desirable DNA that serves our purposes of food or shelter (trees, corn, soy beans, etc.) and in doing so, we perpetuate ourselves (our own specific DNA). DNA, in its many forms, is anything but altruistic.

6 SPONTANEOUS REGRESSION

6.1 NOT SEEING THE OBVIOUS

Frequently, **cancer patients suffer from immunonological deficiencies due to a tumor load and aggressive cytotoxic therapies such as, chemotherapy and irradiation. Cytotoxic therapies often leave patients with a considerable risk of secondary malignancies** (Bokemeyer, C., Kuczyk, M.A., Kohne, C.H., Haupt, A. and Schmoll, H.J. Risk of secondary neoplastic after treatment of malignant germ cell tumors of the testis (in German) Med Clin 1996; 91: 703-710), (Malpas, J.S. Long-term effects of treatment of childhood malignancy. Clin Radiol 1996; 51: 466-474), (Shapiro, C.L. and Recht, A. Late effects of adjuvant therapy for breast cancer. J Natl Cancer Inst Monogr 1994; (16):101-112), (Forbes, J.F. Long-term effects of adjuvant chemotherapy in breast cancer. Acta Oncol 1992; 31: 243-250). Before the onset of cancer, most patients state that they were never ill and as one acquaintance told me, "I thought I was the healthiest person in St. Helena Parish, until I developed this breast cancer." To paraphrase an old aphorism, "If doesn't kill you, it probably makes you tougher."

With the example of spontaneous regression (SR) of cancer, it is obvious that we have the capacity to kill cancer and that we do it by the activity of oxygen and the white blood cell (WBC). In general, **regression** connotes that the clinical presentation of the cancer cells are decreasing in overall number and effect; whereas, **remission** means that the cancer cell number is not overall increasing and the clinical picture is stable. Also, **with the spontaneous recovery from infections, we routinely and frequently demonstrate the innate ability to generate more than normal levels of oxygen species to produce bactericidal, fungicidal or virucidal events**, without causing untoward effects or harming adjacent normal cells or their constituents. In fact, it is only through the generation of augmented levels of reactive oxygen species and excited states that we are able to maintain the normal health of the body.

The body normally contains antioxidant compounds and enzymes to deal with excesses, if and when they occur. **These few spontaneous regression patients unquestionably prove that we have the innate ability within us to kill cancer, just as we can kill bacteria, fungi, parasites and viruses, on a daily ongoing basis.**

I have analyzed the essentials of the body's method and mimicked the mechanism which the white blood cell uses for the self-cure of cancer and the foreign invader killing event. That mechanism is duplicated in my singlet oxygen delivery system by the use of hydrogen peroxide and sodium hypochlorite to produce singlet oxygen and which has been responsible for the astounding clinical results of my studies. I am more encouraged than ever with the direction of my work.

My work and theoretical approach of the **Howes Singlet Oxygen Delivery System turns the possibility of a self cure into a probability of a self cure.**

I whole heartedly concur that the limited effectiveness of conventional complex tumor killing mechanisms (chemotherapy and radiation) necessitates new therapeutic strategies based on tumor biological (and biochemical) knowledge (Gilde, K. Magy Onkol 2003; 47(1): 3-11. Epub 2003 Apr 24).

Likely, spontaneous regression has been around for millennia and even though it was observed, its full ramifications were either not appreciated or not able to be duplicated. Medical literature indicates that spontaneous regression was recorded as early as 1742. It has been referred to as "a hidden treasure buried in time" (Hoption Cann, S.A., van Netten, J.P., van Netten, C. and Glover, D.W. Med Hypotheses 2002 Feb; 58(2): 115-119).

Spontaneous regression is probably even rarer than previously believed and the incidence may be **one in every 140,000 cases** of cancer rather than the one per 60,000 to 100,000 cancer cases as earlier thought (Chang, W.Y. Hawaii Med J 2002 Oct; 59(10): 379-387). Reportedly, **in recent years the incidence of spontaneous regression has been becoming even more of a rarity.** This is theoretically due to the frequent use of chemotherapy, irradiation and antibiotics, all of which to one degree or another, suppress the immune response.

Some authors state that the term spontaneous regression implies "without apparent cause" but I tend to think of it more **as "having been triggered but happening on its own,"** without the intervention of the medical profession. Clearly, it has a reason or a cause.

Primarily, only two texts and one monograph have been devoted to spontaneous regression of cancer. Both texts were published in 1966: Tilden Everson and Warren Cole's book, "Spontaneous Regression of Cancer" and William Boyd's, "The Spontaneous Regression of Cancer." The only monograph written was the proceedings of an international conference on spontaneous regression of cancer held in 1974 at the Johns Hopkins School of Medicine and it was published in 1976 by the National Cancer Institute.

Dr. Tilden Everson and Dr. Warren Cole established the standard for the definition of spontaneous regression as **"the partial or complete disappearance of a malignant tumor in the absence of all treatment or in the presence of therapy considered inadequate to exert a significant influence on [the] disease** (Everson, T. and Cole, W. Spontaneous regression of cancer. Prog Clin Cancer 1967; 3: 79-95). Some investigators require that the original presence of cancer had to be proven by microscopic tissue examination. Such rigorous standards, in an evaluation of the medical literature between 1900 and 1965, found 176 cases of spontaneous regression of cancer (Everson, T. and Cole, W. Spontaneous regression of cancer. Philadelphia, PA W.B. Saunders, 1966).

All considered, **spontaneous regression has been reported about 10,000 times, but only about 1000 cases meet the definition of Everson and Cole** (Challis, G.B. and Stam, H.J. The spontaneous regression of cancer: A review of cases from 1900 to 1987. Acta Oncol 1990; 29(5): 545-550). Spontaneous regression or remission of clinical malignancies (SR) is a rare event (Nagorsen, D., Marincola, F.M. and Kaiser, H.E. In Vivo 2002; 16(6): 551-556).

6.2 COLEY'S TOXIN

I am fascinated by the work of Dr. William Coley, (active career 1890-1936), a prominent New York surgeon. Dr. Coley's daughter, **Helen Coley Nauts**, is primarily responsible for reviewing and analyzing her father's life work, after his death in 1936. She deserves the credit for keeping his work alive and bringing it to a new generation of enthusiasts.

Additionally, Donald H. MacAdam has written an interesting book on spontaneous regression which has provided some of the references in this text (MacAdam, D.H. Spontaneous regression: cancer and the immune system, 2003; Xlibris Corp). MacAdam's book is well referenced, concise and clear. Other important references for spontaneous regression include: (Kleef, R., Jonas, W.B., Knogler, W. and Stenzinger, W. Fever, cancer incidence and spontaneous remissions. Neuroimmunomodulation 2001; 9: 55-64). The literature reveals that **fever associated infections are linked to spontaneous regression in over 22% of leukemia cases, over 15% of cancers of the bone and connective tissue, over 11% of melanoma cases and over 7% of lymphoma cases** (O'Regan, B. and Hirshberg, C. Spontaneous remission: an annotated bibliography. Sausalito, Institute of Noetic Sciences, 1993).

Dr. Coley's story has been researched, written and posted by Vera Bradova on the web at www.geocities.com/HotSprings/Villa/5443/alts/coley.html. and is the basis of the scenario which follows:

Reportedly, **Dr. Coley developed his toxin treatment regime for SR in the 1890's and continued to use it until he retired in the 1930's**. Dr. Coley had studied medicine at Harvard and eventually became the head of the Bone Tumor Service at Memorial Hospital, which is commonly known today as Memorial Sloan Kettering Cancer Center. During his practice, he had a young patient and friend of John D. Rockefeller, Jr., by the name of Bessie Dashiell, who required a below the elbow arm amputation due to a particularly virulent bone sarcoma of the hand. Although the operation was successful, she died painfully several months later from widespread metastasis.

Discouraged, and determined to do better, Coley reviewed the sarcoma records of the previous 15 years. He found the records of a sarcoma patient, who had developed erysipelas skin infections on two occasions. Miraculously, upon recovery from the infections and fevers his sarcomas had spontaneously regressed and he was discharged in good health, and remained so for many years. Dr. Coley set out to intentionally artificially induce erysipelas infections in inoperable cases. After a rocky course of trial and error, **he later discovered that he could get the desired effect by mixing attenuated strains of Streptococcus pyogenes (the cause of erysipelas) (exotoxin-containing gram-positive organisms) with Serratia marcescens (which contained a lipopolysaccharide, LPS) (endotoxin-containing gram-negative organisms),** which would produce fever, rash, chills, shakes and other symptoms, which are today referred to as the "cytokine flu."

Dr. Coley's first success with his toxin was with a young boy with a huge abdominal tumor, who after many toxin injections and bouts of fever and chills, did successfully have regression of his tumor. He died of a heart attack 26 years after the successful regression of his tumor. In some cases, **Coley's toxin was administered from just a few months on up to several years, helping 40% of his patients, and perhaps curing 10%.** Other medical observers had noticed that infectious diseases such as, erysipelas, tuberculosis, syphilis, malaria, gangrene, mumps and measles resulted in tumor regression.

Although there was considerable skepticism throughout the medical community, it was tried by physicians, including the Mayo Clinic, up until World War II. One of the reasons that Coley's toxin was not more successful is reportedly due to the fact that the medical community became infatuated with x-rays and radium, and the entire thrust of cancer treatment was turned in that direction. It is mind boggling to read of the extent that this "magical" radioactive substance came to be viewed as a panacea -- people drank "radium water", rubbed radium creams and lotions into their skins, and expected radium to cure dreaded diseases like cancer. In particular, the new head of Memorial Hospital, Dr. James Ewing, had little interest in Coley's toxin but had enthusiasm for radiation.

At a 1934 symposium on Ewing's sarcoma, Dr. Coley presented 22 toxin treated patients and had 12 survive for five years, whereas, 22 radiation treatment patients had no survivors (3 were too early to evaluate). Curiously, even faced with this data, Dr. Ewing urged his colleagues to use radiation for bone cancer and all cases of unexplained bone pain, even though, he knew that radiation markedly harms bone marrow.

The toxins were continued until the 1950's when the American Cancer Society put it on the infamous blacklist, although it was later removed in the 1970's. Coley's toxin remains a controversial alternative cancer therapy, even though it is a cheap and easily made but it is a non-patentable substance.

Dr. William Coley studied spontaneous regression and found that it was linked to an occurrence following a severe infection, with accompanying hyperthermia. He developed a bacterial vaccine which, when properly administered, could and did induce complete cancer regression, on occasions and which included regression of metastatic lesions. The work "fell into obscurity" until recently. **Researchers have concluded that 'the connection of febrile infection and tumor regression is the most frequent association found in the literature.'** (Maurer, S. and Kolmel, K. Spontaneous regression of melanoma, monography No. 19. New York, Cancer Research Institute, 1997). In general, this follows the "hygiene hypothesis," which basically says that too much cleanliness in childhood, leads to decreased resistance to diseases later in life. I believe that there is merit in this approach.

Others had also arrived at the concept that a bout with an infectious disease could result in a reduced risk of developing cancer. In 1899, a medical practitioner, D'arcy Power, stated that, "**Where malaria is common, cancer is rare**." (Power, D. The local distribution of cancer and cancer houses. Practitioner 1899; 62: 418-429; quoted in Graner J. History of infectious disease oncology, from Galen to Rous. Infectious causes of cancer. Goedert, James J., ed. Totowa, New Jersey: Humana Press, 2000, p. 6). Additionally, **it had been observed that the survival outcome of lung operations was favorably influenced if the patient had experienced a postoperative infection.** Fifty percent of such patients with post op infections survived five years after surgery, whereas, only 18% of patients without infections had the same survival time. (Ruckdeschel, J.C., Codish, S.D. and Stranahan, A. et al. Postoperative empyema improves survival in lung cancer: documentation of a natural experiment. N Engl J Med 1972; 287(20): 1013-1017). In a study on 194 patients with bronchiogenic carcinoma, it was found that 54% of patients with post op empyema infections survived 5 years in comparison to 27% of patients without post op infections. (Takita, H. Effect of postoperative empyema on survival of patients with bronchiogenic carcinoma. J Thorac Cardiovasc Surg 1970; 59: 642-644).

Apparently, Nietzsche was correct when he said, "What doesn't kill us, makes us stronger," (of course, within limits).

Today, sterility of aseptic surgical techniques and wide spread use of antibiotics stifle the body's natural response to infection. Additionally, chemotherapeutic agents and irradiation further suppress the body's natural abilities to deal with cancer. We have and are suppressing the very systems that have evolved over millennia, to protect us by surveillance and killing of cancer cells and foreign invaders. **Immune system cells can be taught to seek out and kill cancer cells** (Hall, Stephen S.A. A commotion in the blood. London: Little, Brown and Company, 1997; p. 351-352). **Immunocompromized patients develop cancer at a rate that is 10-100 times that of healthy individuals** (Jenson, H. Leiomyoma and leiomyosarcoma. Infectious causes of cancer. Goedert, James J., ed. Towota, New Jersey: Humana Press, 2000, p. 145).

Our immune systems have the ability and duty to keep the ever-present cancer within us at bay, to kill it if it tries to grow and to reverse it if it has developed. Immunosuppressed patients, such as AIDS patients or organ recipients, who subsequently develop cancer, can have a reversal or spontaneous

regression of the cancer, once the immunosuppressing drugs have been terminated (Seachrist, L. Spontaneous cancer remissions spark questions. J Nat Cancer Inst 1993; 85: 1892-1895).

Studies now indicate that **cases of spontaneous regression are likely effectuated by the immune system,** thus, producing a **self-cure of cancer.** In what would now be an unethical and illegal human study, **healthy young men and terminally ill cancer patients had viable human cancer cells injected into them during the 1950's, in hopes of getting a better understanding of the human immune system.** Interestingly, in **all the healthy young men, all of the new cancerous nodules disappeared but in some of the cancer patients, histologically positive cancerous nodules continued to grow up until the time of their deaths** (Southam, C.M., Moore A. and Rhoads, C. P. Homotransplantation of human cell lines. Science 1957; 125: 158) (Southam, C. M. Tumor immunity in man. Clin Bull Mem Sloan Kettering Cancer Center 1971; 1: 40). I believe this to be a very important study. Unbelievably, **today's standard of care, which utilizes chemotherapy and irradiation, essentially wipes out our natural ability to deal with mutagenesis.** And even more unbelievably, these principles of Dr. Coley have been around for 100 years.

Recently, Wake Forest University **researchers have developed a tumor resistant breed of mice** from their usual study animals. These mice apparently have a genetic mutation that protects them by the cytologic **destruction of cancer cells by innate leukocytes, without apparent damage to normal cells. (This is analogous to my singlet oxygen system and to PDT).** Also, **these same white cells, when transplanted to another animal, can protect it from cancer and it appears that they have resistance to a wide array of cancer cells.** The proposed immunological attack on the cancer does not involve the T lymphocytes, as other immunological responses tend to do. Mainly, leukocytes of the innate system, which includes neutrophils, macrophages and natural killer cells, are responsible for killing of the cancer cells (Cui Z., Willingham, M.C., Hicks, A.M., Alexander-Miller, M.A., Howard, T.D., Hawkins, G.A., Miller, M.S., Weir, H.M., Du, W. and DeLong, C.J. PNAS 2003; 100(11): 6682-6687).

Hormones, especially estrogens and androgens, can have an impact on cancer progression or regression (Jensen, E.V. and Jacobson, H. I. Basic guides to the mechanism of estrogen action. Recent Prog Horm Res 1962; 18: 387-414) (Oliver, S. Trends in prostate cancer mortality in England, Wales and the USA. The Lancet Oncology 2000; 1: 136). **Many factors have been implicated in eliciting spontaneous regression of cancers including various etiological sources of infection, hyperthermia, blood transfusions, biopsies, partial surgical resection, hormonal factors, termination of immunosuppression drugs and elimination of a carcinogen.**

6.3 THE POWER OF THE MIND

Psychoneuroimmunological factors such as prayer, religion, love, meditation, a positive attitude, a do or die mind set, hypnosis or placebo effect have also been implicated as possible causative agents prompting spontaneous cancer regression. The power of the mind, over biological and biochemical bodily processes, including the immune response, is unquestionably an important parameter to be reckoned with, even though it is frequently difficult to measure or quantitate with the scientific method.

In fact, a study of alternative medical practices revealed that over 80% of cancer patients use religious practices as an adjunctive form of therapy (Cohen, L., Gerner, J. and Baile, W. Forum: complementary and alternative medicines. The Lancet Oncology 2000; 1: 55-56).

6.4 INFECTIOUS AGENTS

Spontaneous regression has been associated with almost all common infectious agents (Hoption Cann, S.A., van Netten, J. P., van Netten, C. and Glover D.W. Spontaneous regression: a hidden treasure buried in time. Med Hypotheses 2002; 58: 115-119). This includes links of spontaneous regression with malaria, erysipelas, diphtheria, gonorrhea, measles, gangrene, hepatitis, smallpox, influenza, syphilis, tuberculosis and anti-rabies treatment (Stephensen, H. E., Delmez, J. A. and Renden, D. I., et al. Host immunity and spontaneous regression of cancer. Surg Gynecol Obstet 1971; 133: 649).

However, as to the underlying mechanism, irrespective of spontaneous regressions varied etiological factors, **Warren Cole wrote, "I am convinced that an increase in immunologic resistance, temporary or permanent, is the best explanation of spontaneous regression."** (Cole, W. H. Spontaneous regression of cancer and the importance of finding its cause. Natl Cancer Inst Monogr 1976; 44: 5-9). A complex mathematical analysis by Stephensen et. al. of 224 spontaneous regression cases concluded that **all 224 cases were due to the same underlying mechanism** (Stephensen, H. E., Delmez, J. A. and Renden D. I., et al. Host immunity and spontaneous regression of cancer. Surg Gynecol Obstet 1971; 133: 649). That mechanism is felt, by most investigators, to be a potent immunological response.

However, the real question is, **"Is there a most basic, singular and essential biochemical step, reaction or mechanism that is the product of this immune response, and which can explain other forms of cancer cell kill, such as photodynamic therapy, radiation and chemotherapy?"** I firmly believe that there is such a biochemical explanation that will unify the vast array of data relating to cancer causation and tumoricidal activity. Furthermore, I believe that I have found the specific agent responsible for both photodynamic therapy and spontaneous regression of cancer. **I believe that the Howes Singlet Oxygen Delivery System produces and delivers that agent to cancer cells. That agent and that step concerns the transformation of ground state triplet oxygen to its more reactive counterparts, such as singlet metastable delta oxygen, hydrogen peroxide, hypochlorous and hypobromous acid, superoxide, nitric oxide, peroxynitrite and the hydroxyl radical.**

6.5   IS THE FETUS A CANCER?

Investigators have observed that trophoblastic chorionic villi appear during normal pregnancy 80% of the time. In the postpartum period these cells return to normalcy. My interpretation of this observation is that the fetus is being treated as cancerous tissue and consequently, a pregnant individual has the same systemic response to cancer as it does to the fetus. It has also been observed that following the pregnancy, the breast tissue returns to normal.

In many cases, an autoimmune disease may flare up during pregnancy, only to subside after the birth. This argues strongly for a concomitant reaction towards the fetus or for the hormonal changes associated with pregnancy.

If my interpretation of these observations are correct, and if my observations regarding severe infections effect on spontaneous regression of cancer are also correct, then predictably, pregnant females that experience severe infections during fetal development, should have an increased or elevated rate of stillborns, fetal deaths and miscarriages. **Consistent with my Unified Theory, abruption of the placenta, some infectious disorders, fetal chromosomal aberration/malformation and internal disease such as diabetes are some of the conditions that are associated with stillbirth.** (Petersson, K. and Hulthen-Varli, I. Researchers show growing interest in antenatal mortality. Increased understanding of intrauterine fetal death may reduce the number of cases in the long run. Lakartidningen 2003; 100(32-33): 2512-2516).

In fact, **infection is the most common cause of intrauterine fetal death.** The most common factors associated with intrauterine fetal death could be identified **as infections (24%),** placental insufficiency/intrauterine growth restriction (22%), placental abruption (19%), intercurrent maternal conditions (12%), congenital malformations (10%), and umbilical cord complications (9%) (Petersson, K., Bremune, K., Bottinga, R., Horsjo, A, Hulthen-Varli, I., Kublickas, M., Norman, M., Papadogiannakis, N., Wanggren, K. and Woff, K. Diagnostic evaluation of intrauterine fetal deaths in Stockholm 1998-9. Acta Obstet Gynecol Scand 2002; 81(4): 284-292).

Spontaneous regression of leukemia has been associated mainly with bacterial infections (Wiernik, P. H. Spontaneous regression of hematologic cancers. Natl Cancer Inst Monogr 1976; 44: 35-38). However, **lymphoma regression has been associated with viral infections** (Stephenson, H.E., Delmez, J. A. and Renden, D. I., et al. Host immunity and spontaneous regression of cancer. Surg Gynecol Obstet 1971; 133: 649). In fact, lymphoma and adult T-cell leukemia are both thought to be partially caused by human T-cell lymphotropic virus type I (HTLV-I) infection (Matsuoka, M. Adult T-cell leukemia/lymphoma. Infectious causes of cancer Goedert J. J., ed. Towata, New Jersey; Humana Press, 2000, p. 211-229).

A review of twenty years with worldwide cancer research indicates a viral, bacterial and parasite etiology for fifteen to twenty percent of all cancers (Barsch, H. Studies on biomarkers in cancer etiology and prevention: a summary and challenge of 20 years of interdisciplinary research. Mutat Res 2000; 462(2-3): 255-279).

The association between some infectious disorders and fetal morbidity and mortality is well documented. The thesis focuses mainly on two agents: toxoplasma gondii and provirus B19. Disseminated toxoplasma infection may cause fetal death. Several reports have shown that provirus B19 can cause fetal death in the second trimester, mainly in combination with hydrops fetalis. Some authors have reported that **the infection might also be an important cause of stillbirth in late pregnancy in non-hydropic cases** (Petersson, K. Diagnostic evaluation of fetal death with special reference to intrauterine infections. Fredagen den 31 maj 2002, kl. 9.15).

The earlier infections occur in intrauterine life the more severe they are. When the infection develops during embryogenesis, the lesions are much more serious. Infections acquired in utero may result in resorption of the embryo, abortion, stillbirth, neonatal death, intrauterine growth retardation (IUGR), or prematurely (Bittencourt, A.L. and Garcia, A.G. Pathogenesis and pathology of hematogenous infections of the fetus and newborn. Pediatr Pathol Mol Med 2002; 21(4): 353-399).

6.6 MALARIA, PREGNANCY AND FETAL DEATH

Cancer researcher, D'arcy Power, had observed in 1899 that, **"Where malaria is common, cancer is rare."** (Power, D. The local distribution of cancer and cancer houses. Practitioner 1899; 62: 418-429; quoted in Graner J. History of infectious disease oncology, from Galen to Rous. Infectious causes of cancer. Goedert, James J., ed Totowa, New Jersey: Humana Press, 2000, p. 16). Brian Greenwood observed in 1968 the fact that areas of high incidence of malarial infections had low rates of autoimmune diseases, such as multiple sclerosis, rheumatoid arthritis and lupus and further, he related it to malarial tolerance. It also appears that dementia is low in these same areas.

Increase malaria is associated with: decreased cancer

decreased autoimmune diseases (multiple sclerosis, arthritis, lupus)
decreased dementia (Alzheimer's disease)

Whereas, AIDS is associated with increased Alzheimer's disease.

In 2000, D. Taramelli published a paper in *Laboratory Investigation* in which he found that feeding malarial pigment to the immune cells produced a rise in oxidative stress and a 5 fold increase in the activity of the stress protein heme oxygenase.

If my Unified Theory is correct, then I would anticipate that females with malaria would also have an increased rate of fetal deaths and stillbirths. Since their immunologic system, which has been bolstered by their infection, is set up to detect and destroy cancer, it should attempt to treat the developing fetus in the same manner as it would a developing cancer. The analogy of a developing fetus to a cancer has been put forth by many authors for many years. Such is the case, with pregnant malaria patients.

Approximately 4 million fetal deaths occur each year, 98% of them in developing countries. **Known risk factors for fetal deaths include demographic and social correlates such as advanced maternal age; chronic maternal conditions such as anemia and sickle cell disease; maternal infections such as syphilis, HIV and malaria**; inadequate maternal nutrition; and maternal complications (both antepartum and intrapartum). (Improving Birth Outcomes: Meeting the Challenge in the Developing World (2003). http://www.nap.edu/openbook/0309086140/html/134.html).

Pregnant women are a high risk group, and should be targeted for specific malaria protection. **Malaria infections and disease can increase the risk of complications and death for both the mother and child.** (Malaria: Case Management Update. Malaria in Pregnancy. WHO SAMC Information for action leaflet).

Actually, **hydrogen peroxide is an effective agent in killing malaria.** Both nonlethal Plasmodium yoelii and lethal Plasmodium berghei were **killed in vitro by hydrogen peroxide** at concentrations as low as 10(-5) M. Higher concentrations were required in the presence of added normal erythrocytes. Injection of hydrogen peroxide in vivo significantly reduced P. Yoelii parasitemia but had less effect on P. berghei (Dockrell, H.M. and Playfair, J.H.L. Killing of blood-state murine malaria parasites by hydrogen peroxide. Infection and Immunity 1983; 39(1): 456-459).

After considering the fact that "where malaria is common, cancer is rare" it occurred to me that this could be due to the fact that malaria patients had taken antimalarial medications or hydrogen peroxide, which could have generated ROS or excytomers, and these agents could have been responsible for the reduced levels of cancer in malaria patients. This approach led me to the following fascinating paper by Dr. Rowen.

7 ARTEMISININ (ANTIMALARIAL) AND REACTIVE OXYGEN SPECIES

7.1 MALARIA INTRODUCTION

Annually, 100 million people suffer a malarial illness and over 1 million people (primarily African children) die, according to the World Health Organization (WHO, Malaria unit. 1993. Global malaria control. Bull. W.H.O. 71: 281-294). Other estimates go as high as 1.5-2.7 million people being killed by this parasite every year and another 300-500 million people are reported to have the disease (Cristina Valencia, U., Lemp, E. and Anaocco, A.L., Quantum yields of singlet oxygen, O_2 ($^1\Delta_g$), production by antimalaric drugs in organic solvents. J. Chil. Soc. Soc. V. 48, N 4(2003) ISSN 0717-9324.). Over 40% of the world's population is at risk of malaria infection and patients with severe and complicated disease, the mortality rate is between 20-50%.

For many years, quinine was the only drug used for the treatment of malaria. Later, the **appearance of resistant strains and the occurrence of undesirable side effects**, led to the development of synthetic antimalarials, of which quinicrine was the first. Subsequently, chloroquine, primaquine, mefloquine and amodiaquine have also been used and most of these synthetics have pharmacological activity in the treatment of other diseases, such as lupus erythematosus, polymorphous light eruption, cutaneous lymphoma, **rheumatoid arthritis**, etc. (Tonnesen, H.H., Kristensen, S., and Nord, K., (19196(In *The Phostability of drugs and drug formulations*, H.H. Tonnesen Ed., Taylor & Francis, Washington D.C.). Synthetic antimalarials derived from quinoline caused photosensitized side effects undesirable for the skin and the eye.

Skin pigmentation, corneal opacity, cataract formation and other irreversible forms of retinal damage (retinopathy) could lead to blindness. Malaria is a disease found in regions of high light intensity; thus, protective measures (clothing, sun blockers, sunglasses or eye wraps) are recommended for patients receiving antimalarial drugs. The accurate mechanisms for these reactions in humans is unknown, although singlet molecular oxygen, $O_2(^1\Delta_g)$ and free radicals including superoxide/hydroperoxyl or peroxyl adduct, carbon-centered and nitrogen-centered radicals have been invoked as responsible for these phototoxic effects. Singlet molecular oxygen reactions are important in biological systems, where it can play deleterious (damaging valuable biomolecules) and/or beneficial roles (Briviba, K., Klotz, L.-O. and Sies, H. Biol Chem 1997; 378: 1259) (Hulten, L.M., Holmstrom, M. and Soussi, B. Free Radical Biol Med 1999; 27: 1203). Then, **the relevance of the singlet oxygen-mediated photosensitizing effects of the antimalarials will be related to the efficiency of the drug to produce $O_2(^1\Delta_g)$.**

Investigators have irradiated a number of antimalarials (amodiaquine, chloroquine, hydroxy-chloroquine, mefloquine, primaquine and quinicrine) and have shown that all antimalarial drugs sensitize the formation of $^1O_2$ in organic media (ethanol) and show significant quantum yields, with the sole exception of primaquine, which was the only one to effectively quench $^1O_2$. All drugs investigated absorbed light in the UVA region of the spectrum (320-400nm), and these wavelengths will penetrate Caucasian skin. It has also been shown that several antimalarials for complexes with melanine in vitro (Kristensen, S., Orsteen, A.L., Sande, S.A. and Tonnesen, H.H., (1994) Free Radical Biol. Med., 27, 1203.).

A main feature of biological systems is their microheterogeneity, resulting in several coexisting microphase, form the very polar aqueous microenvironment to the highly hydrophobic lipidic regions.

Artemisinin derivatives, such as Arteether products, are the fastest acting schizontocides for rapid parasite clearance, acting as a blood schizontocide and the presence of **the endoperoxide bridge is believed to generate $^1O_2$.**

The parasite responsible for the vast majority of fatal malarial infections, Plasmodium falciparum, can kill people in a matter of hours. Sadly, most P. falciparum have become resistant to chloroquine, and some, in Southeast Asia, have also developed resistance to mefloquine and halofantrine and multi drug resistance is expected to develop in Africa soon. **Endoperoxide** antimalarials may be effective in warding off the resistant strains.

The endoperoxide bridge (C-O-O-C) is unique among the other antimalarial drugs. The first-generation Artemisinin drugs are being widely used in Thailand, Myanmar, Vietnam and China, where multidrug resistant parasites are common (Meshnick, S.R., Taylor, T.E. and Kamchonwongpaisan, S. Artemisinin and the antimalarial endoperoxides: from herbal remedy to targeted chemotherapy. Microbiol Rev 1996; 60(2): 301-315).

The following material was excepted or modified, in part, from an article by Robert Jay Rowen, M.D. entitled, "Artemisinin: From Malaria to Cancer Treatment," which appeared in the Dec. 2002 edition of the Townsend Letter for Doctors & Patients.

7.2 HISTORY OF ARTEMISININ

Artemisinin, the key ingredient obtained from Artemisia annua, has a long history of use as an antimalarial remedy. Artemisia annua, or "sweet wormwood," is mentioned in the Recipes For 52 Kinds Of Disease found in the Mawangdui Han Dynasty tomb, dating from 168 B.C. In that work, the herb is recommended for use for hemorrhoids. It is also mentioned in the Zhou Hou Bei Ji Fang (Handbook of Prescriptions for Emergency Treatments) written in 340 A.D. The major active principal was first isolated in 1972, and investigators at the Walter Reed Army Institute of Research located and crystallized the active component in 1984 (Klayman, D. Qinghaosu (Artemisinin): Antimalarial drug from China. Science 1985; 238: 1049).

Artemisinin and two synthetic derivatives, artemether and sodium artesunate, were evaluated in the 1970's. **Recent studies indicate that the opening of the peroxide ring of the molecule, which generates singlet oxygen, is responsible for the fast cytotoxic action of artemether.** A number of the tropical countries have conducted trials. In China in 1979, wherein 2,099 patients infected with P. viva and P. falciparum, Artemisinin had good therapeutic effects and **improved or cured all patients**. Furthermore, the treatment with Artemisinin was **without any obvious side effects**. Artemisinin is also effective in cerebral malaria. Body temperature of patients normalized within 72 hours and asexual parasites were eliminated within 72 hours. However, there was a relapse rate of 21% (China Cooperative Research Group on Qinghaosu and its Derivatives as Antimalarials. J Trad Chin Med 1982; 2: 17).

7.3 HUMAN CLINICAL STUDIES

In clinical trials in Vietnam, children ages 1 to 15 years were randomly selected to receive Artemisinin suppositories or oral quinine. The results indicated that the suppositories rapidly cleared asexual P. Falciparum parasitemia in children and confirmed the problem reoccurrence rates (Arnold, K., Hien, T.T. and Chin, N.T., et al. A randomized comparative study of Artemisinin suppositories and oral quinine in acute falciparum malaria).

Artemisinin has been extensively researched for malaria and has been used on over a million patients, mostly in China and Vietnam. It is very helpful for drug resistant malaria. Extensive review articles are available documenting the extensive testing that has been done (Transactions of the Royal Society of Tropical Medicine and Hygiene. 1990; 84: 499-502) (Bharel, S., Gulati, M., Abdin, P. and Srivastava, S. Structure biosynthesis and functions of Artemisinin. Fitoterapia 1996; Vol. LXVII No. 5) (Gulati, a., Bharel, S., Srivastava, M. and Abdin, M.Z. Experimental studies on Artemisinin, an herbal remedy for malaria. Fitoterapia 1996; Vol. LXVII No. 5).

Various oral dosage regimens have been adopted in treating over one million patients. **Early studies suggested that an optimum total dosage of 3 grams (about 50 mg/kg) was administered over a 3 to 5 day period**. In most cases, parasite and fever clearance times were in less than two days. Recurrence were much more common with tablets than with parenteral formulations. Because of the very rapid clearance time of fever and parasites, the use of Artemisinin was favored, and recurrences, which were common, were treated with Artemisinin again or with another drug (Hein, T. and White, N. The Lancet 1993; 341: 603-651).

About twelve years ago, Dr. Leo Galland and Dr. Herman Bueno worked together in New York City and began using Artemisinin as a broad spectrum antiparasitic agent.

"Artemisinin is a powerful oxidant. I have used it orally to treat small bowel bacterial overgrowth and for Clostridia overgrowth and (along with other herbal extracts, such as berberine, grapefruit seed extract and oregano oil) as a treatment for intestinal parasites." Leo Galland, M.D.

Very recently, news reports have trumpeted Artemisinin as a leading treatment for malaria. Affected nations are calling for it to be accepted as the number one first line treatment, but **the USA has blocked its acceptance as the primary treatment, alleging yet more studies are needed**.

For the past ten years, the Hoang medical family, with three generations of sophisticated physicians, have used Artemisinin in combination with several other herbs to treat cancer and eliminate necrotic material from the body; for example, from wounds; from intestines of people who have ulcerative colitis, and from Crohn's disease. The efficacy of **Artemisinin compound is very impressive for the treatment of breast cancer and possibly to prevent it**. It is not only because of direct anticancer activity, but also due to hormonal balancing properties of the Artemisinin. Herein, doses of 300 mg twice per day were adequate with other herbs (Personal communication from Dr. Hoang, M.D., 2002).

"The herb itself, Artemisia annua, is one of the best things for PMS, cramping, excessive bleeding and all symptoms of hyper-estrogenemia and hyperprolactinemia." Dr. Hoang, M.D.

7.4 RONS AND $^1O_2$

Considerable evidence has accrued that the killing of parasites is mediated by free radicals. One piece of evidence is the observation that **Artemisinin derivatives lacking the endoperoxide bridge, a known source of oxygen free radicals, are devoid of antimalarial activity**. Further evidence included observations that the in vitro antimalarial activities of **Artemisinin and artesunate are enhanced by high oxygen tension and by the addition of other free radical generating compounds, such as doxorubicin, miconazole, castecin and artemitin**. Similarly, **antioxidants (free radical scavengers) such as *a*-tocopherol, catalase, dithiothreitol, ascorbate and reduced glutathione block antimalarial activity**. Conversely, ***a*-tocopherol deficiency enhances the antimalarial action of Artemisinin against P. yoelii in mice and inhibitors of endogenous antioxidants promote Artemisinin action**. In aggregate, the observed potentiation of the Artemisinins by other oxidant agents and the inhibition of Artemisinin action by antioxidants provides strong indirect evidence for the importance of free radicals, especially oxygen free radicals.

Most free radical generating drugs are thought to cause "oxidant damage" by producing oxygen free radicals, such as superoxide, which then cause indiscriminate damage to the cell. Artemisinin derivatives were at first thought to act in this manner. Artesunate was shown to induce lipid peroxidation in both infected and uninfected erythrocytes, as well as membrane protein thiol oxidation in isolated erythrocyte membranes. These Artemisinin-induced membrane effects could underlie other observed effects of artemisinin derivatives, such as hemolysis, decreased erythrocyte deformability and premature lysis of infected erythrocytes. However, lipid peroxidation, membrane thiol oxidation, and most of the other effects could be observed only at very high drug concentrations (>100 uM), suggesting that these nonspecific oxidant reactions may not be mediating Artemisinin killing of parasites.

According to Meshnick et al, artemisinin derivatives have now been shown to affect parasites very differently from other oxidant drugs. Instead of reacting with oxygen and producing large quantities of oxygen-containing free radicals such as superoxide and OH., Artemisinin itself becomes a free radical in a reaction catalyzed by iron (Meshnick, S.R. Free radical and antioxidants. Lancet 1994; 344: 1441-1442). A large body of data has now accumulated to support this mechanism. **Before you discount the oxidative killing mechanism, I caution you to remember that H_2O_2 and RONS are known to have antimalarial properties** (Free oxygen radical generators as antimalarial drugs, the Lancet, 25 Dec 1982, pp. 1431-1433). Currently, there is evidence to the contrary and singlet oxygen is likely involved. Also, endoperoxides are well known producers of $^1O_2$.

High doses of the artemisinins appear to have specific neurotoxic effects, when given in laboratories in massive doses, both in vitro and in vivo. However, since the drug has been used safely in millions of people, this neurotoxin effect is unlikely to be clinically relevant and this observation is invalid as to its safety.

Artemisinin contains an internal peroxide group. Due to this group, reactive oxygen is already present in the molecule. This belief is in agreement with the observations that derivatives of Artemisinin lacking the peroxide moiety, are devoid of antimalarial activity (Ames, J.R., Ryan, M.D. and Klayman, D.L. Charge transfer and oxy radicals in antimalarial action. J Free Rad Biol Med 1985; 1: 353-361). **Artesunate drugs open the endoperoxide group and release $^1O_2$ and form RONS and carbon radicals.** The definitive action is still unknown but the peroxide bridge plays an essential role. After being opened in the plasmodium, it liberates $^1O_2$ and forms RONS and the carbon radicals.

Additional support for oxygen-mediated toxicity of Artemisinin is generated from other studies. **The antimalarial activity of Artemisinin in vitro, against P. Falciparum, could be enhanced by increased oxygen tension. Drugs such as miconazole and doxorubicin, which are known to work via oxygen radical effects, enhance the activity of artesunate, a derivative of Artemisinin. The effectiveness of Artemisinin is reduced by catalase, dithiothreitol and alpha tocopherol** (Krugkrai, S.R. and Thavong, Y. The antimalarial action of Plasmodium falciparum of ginghams and artesunate in combination with agents, which modulate oxidant stress. Transr Soc Trop Med Hyg 1987; 81: 710-714).

Furthermore, Levander, et al. found that manipulation of the host antioxidant defense status could provide prophylactic or therapeutic enhancement for the control of malaria. In this study, **mice were fed with diets deficient in vitamin E or a diet supplemented with cod liver oil, which would deplete antioxidants. Vitamin E deficiency enhanced the antimalarial action of Artemisinin against P. yoelii, but selenium deficiency did not. A diet containing 5% cod liver oil had a very strong antimalarial action** (Levander, O., Ager, A. and Morris, V.C. Qinghaosu, dietary vitamin E, selenium and cod liver oil: effect on susceptibility of mice to the malarial parasite Plasmodium yoelii. Am J Clin Nutr 1989; 5: 346-352).

Artemisinin has been shown to work through oxygen and carbon based free radical mechanisms. Its structure includes an endoperoxide bridge. **Peroxides can generate free radicals in a Fenton type reaction when exposed to unbound ferrous iron. Malaria, which grows in the erythrocytes, has the opportunity to accumulate much excess iron, which can spill into the unbound form.** Electron microscopy has confirmed destruction of plasmodium membranes with morphology typical of free radical mechanisms.

With the knowledge of **a high accumulation of iron in cancer cells**, researcher Henry Lai and Narenda Singh of the University of Washington became interested in possible Artemisinin activity against malignant cells. In 1995, they published a paper in Cancer Letters concerning the use of Artemisinin against numerous cancer cells lines in vitro. This article has mobilized interest in Artemisinin as an addition to anticancer treatment (Lai, H. and Singh, N. Cancer Letters, 1995; 91: 41-46).

There are a number of properties shared by cancer cells, which favor the selective toxicity of Artemisinin against cancer cell lines, and against cancer in vivo. In addition to higher rates of iron flux via transferrin receptors than normal cells, **cancers are particularly sensitive to oxygen radicals** (May, W.S. J Membr Biol 1985; 88: 205-215).

A subsequent article appeared in Life Science in 2001 by Singh and Lai on the selective toxicity of Artemisinin and holotransferrin towards human breast cancer cells (Singh, N.P. and Lai, H. Life Sci 2001; 70(1): 49-56). In this article, rapid and complete destruction of a radiation-resistant breast cancer cell line was achieved when the in vitro cell system was supported in iron uptake with holotransferrin. The cancer cell line was completely nonviable within 8 hours of combined incubation with minimal effect on the normal cells.

Artemisinin becomes cytotoxic in the presence of ferrous iron. **Since iron influx is naturally high in cancer cells,** Artemisinin and its analogs selectively kill cancer cells under conditions in vivo. Further, it is possible to increase or enhance iron flux in cancer cells using the conditions that increase intracellular iron concentrations. However, **intact in vivo systems do not need holotransferrin, the living body provides all the necessary iron transport proteins.**

A third paper, by Efferth et al., published in Oncology in 2001, stated that the antimalarial artesunate is also active against cancer (Efferth, T., Dunstan, H., Sauerbrey, A., Miyachi, H. and Chitambar, C.R. Antimalarial artesunate is also active against cancer. Oncol 2001; 18(4): 767-773). This article described dramatic cytotoxic activity against a wide variety of cancers including drug resistant cell lines. **Artesunate (ART)** is a semi-synthetic derivative of Artemisinin, and has been analyzed for its anticancer activity against 55 cell lines by the Developmental Therapeutics program of the National Cancer Institute, USA. **ART was most active against leukemia and colon cancer cell lines**. Mean growth inhibition 50% (GI 50) 1.11 microM and 2.13 microM respectively. Non-small cell lung cancer cell lines showed the highest mean (GI 50 26.62 microM) indicating the lowest sensitivity towards ART. Intermediate GI 50 values were obtained for melanomas, breast, ovarian, prostate, CNS and renal cancer cell lines. Most important, a comparison of ART's cytotoxicity with those standard cytostatic drugs showed **that ART was**

active in molar ranges comparable to those of established antitumor drugs. Leukemia lines resistant to either doxorubicin, vincristine, methotrexate or hydroxyurea were tested. Remarkably, none of these drug resistant lines showed resistance to ART. The theorized reason for this is the absence of a tertiary amine in ART, present in virtually all other chemotherapy agents, which is required for cellular transport systems to usher the drug outside the cell.

7.5 CANCER CELLS ARE DEFICIENT IN ANTIOXIDANT ENZYMES

Cancer cells are notoriously deficient in antioxidant enzymes - both forms of superoxide dismutase, the manganese form in mitochondria and the copper zinc form in the cell cytoplasm are generally low in cancer cells. Cancer cells are grossly deficient in catalase and glutathione peroxidase, both of which degrade hydrogen peroxide. It is these deficiencies in antioxidant enzymes, which lead to the use of many of the **common chemotherapeutics which are superoxide generators** (Levine, S.A. and Kidd, P.M. Antioxidant adaptation: its role in free radical pathology. Allergy Research Group, San Leandro, CA 1985).

The higher iron fluxes, especially associated with the reproductive phase of tumor cells, should render these cells even more susceptible to oxidative damage via hydrogen peroxide and superoxides. Normally, the profound catalase deficiency in cancer cells is credited with creating vulnerability to oxidants, in relationship to IV vitamin C or intravenous (IV) hydrogen peroxide. However, **since all of these protective antioxidant enzymes are most often deficient in transformed cells, the oxidant vulnerability should be enhanced dramatically, and further so, due to enhanced unbound iron during cell division.**

Dr. Hugh Riordan has suggested that very high doses of intravenous (IV) vitamin C can kill cancer cells via conversion of vitamin C to hydrogen peroxide and due to deficiency of catalase. For this procedure to work, very high levels of IV vitamin C are required to reach "kill concentrations." Intravenous (IV) vitamin C may be one of the best-documented alternative cancer treatments (Journal of Orthomolecular Medicine, Special Edition, 1999).

Artemisinin may be a most effective method, and certainly one of the easiest, of delivering a knock-out oxidative stress to cancer cells.

Artemisinin is appealing for oral use in that the pharmacodynamics, dosage and toxicity have been well studied for use in relationship to the treatment of malaria. Artemisinin is relatively safe with little side effects even at high dosages (70 mg/kg per day) in short term malaria use.

Artemisinin has two semi-synthetic derivatives. Artesunate is a water derivative with no reported toxicity at usual levels. However, its serum half-life is relatively short. **Artemether is a lipid soluable derivative, effective in cerebral malaria and therefore may be more effective in brain cancers by better penetration of the blood-brain barrier (BBB). Dorland's Medical Dictionary, 27th ed.,** defines the BBB as the barrier separating the blood from the parenchyma of the central nervous system (CNS) consisting of the walls of the capillaries of the CNS and the surrounding glial membranes. Artemether, however, has been reported to cause some neural toxicity in laboratory models in rather high doses. Artemisinin has an intermediate half life and can cross the blood-brain barrier. The two semi synthetic derivatives are available overseas in both oral and injectable for artesuante and artemether. Artemisinin derivatives have immunosuppressive activity. Also Artemisinin's anticancer activity was potentiated if the cancer cells were first loaded with iron by exposure to transferrin.

As mentioned, Lai used holotransferrin, which is iron-loaded transferrin, to further sensitize tumor cell lines to the oxidizing properties of dihydroartemisinin, which is derived from the parent compound metabolically in vivo. A human leukemia cell culture, Molt-4-lymphblastoid cells, and normal human lymphocytes were used in this experiment.

U.T.O.P.I.A.

A significant decrease in cell count was noted with Artemisinin alone, with p<.035. Greater effects were noted when transferrin and dihydroartemesinin were used together. In combined treatment, considerable tumor cell death was observed at a concentration of dihydroartemisinin of 1 μM after 8 hours of incubation. Furthermore, there is reason to believe that Artemisinin can work at lower concentrations in vivo than in vitro, due to destruction of the Artemisinin molecule in vitro.

Lai suggests that this procedure would be most effective for the treatment of aggressive cancers, in which large numbers of transferrin receptors are expressed on the cell surface. It may not be effective for T cell leukemias, which have defective internalization of transferrin receptors and therefore may not be susceptible to this treatment.

Some investigators say that antimalarial endoperoxides are not likely to be useful for therapeutic purposes, such as anticancer drugs, but that directed-synthesis programs might lead to endoperoxides with useful anti-infective and/ or anticancer activities (Woerdenbag, H.J., Moskal, T.A., Pras, N., Malingre, T.M., El-Feraly, F.S., Kampinga, H.H. and Konings, A.W. Cytotoxicity of Artemisinin-related endoperoxides to Ehrlich tumor cells. J Nat Prod 1993; 56: 849-856). **I interpret this to basically mean that only when pharmaceutical companies develop patentable (profitable) endoperoxide drugs, will they be of great utility in treating many human diseases**.

7.6 CONCLUSION

Artemisinin has been used for about 30 years in Vietnam and China for cancer treatment. And the experience with Artemisinin for this purpose is increasing. This history probably led to the recent cited cancer research with Artemisinin.

The fact that Artemisinin's direct antineoplastic effects closely resemble that of high-dose intravenous vitamin C is intriguing. **The potential benefit of Artemisinin in cancer treatment should be further explored because it is simple, safe, well-understood and capitalizes on the multifold weakness in cancer cells to defend themselves against oxygen radicals.** Enhancing the oxidant activity with other oxidation agents (such as carnivora, ultraviolet blood irradiation, H_2O_2 or high oxygen tension itself) may add significant synergism. Adding Artemisinin to low dose chemotherapeutic regimens inducing cytotoxicity via free radical mechanisms (such as doxorubicin), may safely add to the effectiveness of such treatment.

8 HOMESPUN PHILOSOPHY 101

**"I must resuscitate oxygen's embattled image
and effectuate the renaissance of its
aristocratic attributes."**

R. M. Howes, M.D., Ph.D.

5/4/04

Today's **data deluge** puts one onto the hopeless and hapless downward path leading to the abyss of scientific arrogance and hubris. Reportedly, **there are more than 25,000 scientific publications, which produce in excess of one million articles annually**.

One must be able to appreciate the panorama of the life process, in hopes of getting one's mind around its imaginary margins. This, "let's back up and take a look" approach may provide the point of prospective to see a glimpse of the miraculous and overwhelming forest of life. **I believe that the thread that runs so true is directly through the center of the orbitals of the oxygen molecule.   Furthermore, it has been right before our eyes all along, but we just haven't seen it.**

I was mentored by Dr. Steele, who was mentored by Dr. Albert Szent Gyorgii, who said that if a scientific principle was true and significant, that " **it would stick up out of the grass**, easy to see, kind of like a sore thumb." Today's investigators rely totally on manipulations of statistical methods to ascertain "the significance" of their observations; frequently, in apparent denial of common sense. However, our concept of common sense and the state of the art of medicine (or state of ignorance) does change over the course of time. Thus, we must try to continually update our thinking, which will require a constant updating of our knowledge data base.

With spontaneous regression of cancer having been verified in over 1,000 cases world wide, this proves, that **under the proper circumstances, the human body is capable of monitoring and killing cancer**. We do not have to run that experiment. Nature has done it for us. All we have to do is to find and duplicate the agents responsible for this event. **My singlet oxygen delivery system has done precisely that**.

The Howes Singlet Oxygen Delivery System produces rapid cancer cell kill, with minimal damage, if any, to normal cells because they have the requirements to deal with a steady state of singlet oxygen and reactive oxygen nitrative species (RONS) on an on-going basis. The reagents of hydrogen peroxide and sodium hypochlorite are broken down into sodium chloride and water (saline) and ground state oxygen, all of which are essential products needed by the human body.

8.1 HERE IS THE SHOCKER

We tend to see spontaneous regression only as it relates to cancer, however, we know that the same system of protection utilizes the same immune system, the same mechanisms of oxidation, the same oxidative metabolism and the same reactive oxygen species and electronic excitation states to control or to keep bacteria, viruses, fungi and parasites at bay in our bodies all of the time. In fact, I believe that this rare, mysterious, strange sounding phenomenon (spontaneous regression) is one of the most common occurrences in the body. Perhaps, I can best illustrate this as follows:

Bacteria always present on humans:

Bacteria on skin of adult: 300 million
Bacteria in human mouth: 100 million
Bacteria breathed in daily: 100,000
Bacteria in large intestine: 70 trillion*
    (aids in digestion)
    (Source: World Features Syndicate)

Theoretically, each of these bacteria should result in an infection or they should rapidly over-run the body but, they do not. They are killed off or undergo spontaneous regression at an alarmingly high rate, otherwise each of these "infections-waiting-to-happen" could or would manifest itself as such. This is truly a "woulda', coulda', shoulda'" scenario. **Our immune cells, hence our white blood cells, hence our oxidative metabolism, hence reactive oxygen species and electronic excitation states, are constantly performing spontaneous regressions of bacteria. Just as with ever-present cancer, we keep these ever-present infections at bay with our innate abilities to effectuate a spontaneous regression.**

To illustrate this point, I refer to the 1998 work of Carl Nathan, who states that **there are only two antimicrobial mechanisms of macrophages which have been specifically identified and genetically established: production of reactive oxygen intermediates (ROI) by phagocyte oxidase (phox) and reactive nitrogen intermediates (RNI) by inducible nitric oxide synthase (iNOS).** To determine whether additional mechanisms exist, he generated mice doubly deficient in each pathway (phoxNOS-/-). Even when reared under SPF conditions with antibiotics, phoxNOS-/- mice were markedly susceptible to spontaneous infections with indigenous flora. **This means that in animals that cannot generate reactive oxygen species or reactive nitrogen species, they will experience lethal infections from bacteria that are normally present in their bodies and kept under control by these oxygen modifications.** Nathan demonstrated that bactericidal assays with wild type, phox-/-, iNOS-/- and phoxNOS-/- macrophages showed that ROI and RNI are the predominant antimicrobial products of mouse macrophages with respect to the organisms tested, although a weaker antibacterial mechanism exists that is independent of phox and iNOS.

Nathan further states that **these findings predict a corresponding importance of RNI- and ROI-resistance mechanisms in pathogens.** Peroxiredoxins are a recently identified, widely distributed family of proteins with the unusual ability to catabolize peroxides without intrinsic metal, heme, or flavin prosthetic groups. The canonical peroxiredoxin ahpC, already known to participate in resistance to ROI, was found to be essential for resistance of Salmonella typhinurium to RNI as well. Salmonella disrupted in ahpC became hyper-susceptible to RNI. ahpC from either Mycobacterium tuberculosis or S. typhimurium fully complemented the defect. ahpC and its homologs are the most widely distributed gene family known some of whose members protect cells from RNI, and provide the first known enzymatic defense against an element of antitubercular immunity.

ROI and RNI have powerful anti-tumor potential, whether generated by the innate immune system, drugs or x-rays. Interference with the glutathione redox cycle markedly enhanced the therapeutic potential of ROI against mouse tumor cells in vitro and also in vivo without host toxicity (Nathan, C.F., Arrick, B.A., Murray, H.W., DeSantis, N.M. and Cohn, Z.A. Tumor cell antioxidant defenses: Inhibition of the glutathione redox cycle enhances macrophage-mediated cytolysis. J Exp Med 153: 766-782, 1981). However, human tumor cells were markedly more resistant than mouse tumor cells to ROI, and the biochemical basis of this resistance was not attributable to known pathways. RNI resistance among tumors has yet to be systematically studied. Novel pathways - perhaps peroxiredoxins - may help account for the resistance of human tumors to ROI and may confer resistance to RNI as well. Inhibition of such pathways is predicted to render tumors more susceptible to immunotherapy, both through apoptosis and necrosis of malignant cells and through interference with angiogenesis (Nathan, C. and Cohn, Z.A. Antitumor effects of hydrogen peroxide in vivo. J Exp Med 1981; 154: 1539-1553) (O'Donnell-Tormey, J., DeBoer, C. and Nathan, C.E. Resistance of human tumor cells to oxidative cytolysis. J Clin Invest 1985; 76: 80-86).

Accumulation of polymorphonuclear leukocytes (PMN) in lungs is a central event in the pathogenesis of inflammatory lung injury associated with Gram-negative sepsis (Malik, A.B. and Lo, S.K. Vascular endothelial adhesion molecules and tissue inflammation. Pharmacol Rev 1996; 48: 213). **Generation of superoxide anions (O_2^{-}) by NADPH oxidase complex of PMN is indispensable to the host defense response, as it is essential for killing of invading microorganisms.** NADPH oxidase is a multisubunit complex that generates O_2^{-} in one-electron reduction of O_2 using electrons supplied by NADPH (Dodd, O.J. and Pearse, D.B. Effect of the NADPH oxidase inhibitor apocynin on ischemia-reperfusion lung injury. Am J Physiol 2000; 279: 11303). NADPH oxidase subunits, gp91phox and p47phox, are essential components of this complex (Jackson, S.H., Gallin, J.I. and Holland, S.M. The p47phox mouse knock-out model of chronic granulomatous disease. J Exp Med 1995; 182:751). Mutations in these subunits in **chronic granulomatous disease** (CGD) patients (Segal, B.H., Doherty, T.M., Wynn, T.A., Cheever, A.W., Sher, A. and Holland, S.M. The p4phox-/- mouse model of chronic granulomatous disease has normal granuloma formation and cytokine responses to Mycobacterium avium and Schistosoma mansoni eggs. Infect Immun 1999; 67: 1659) **or targeted deletions of these genes in mice resulted in PMN incapable of the respiratory burst and failure of PMN bactericidal function.** gp91phox knockout mice also had increased the susceptibility to Staphylococcus aureus and Aspergillus fumigatus, two important causes of infection in patients with CGD, and a high mortality compared with wild-type mice (Morgenstern, D.E., Gifford, M.A., Li, L.L., Doerschuk, C.M. and Dinauer, M.C. Absence of respiratory burst in X-linked chronic granulomatous disease mice leads to abnormalities in both host defense and inflammatory response to Aspergillus fumigatus. J Exp Med 1997; 185: 207).

The superoxide anions generated by the NADPH oxidase complex of phagocytic cells serve the primary function of killing invading microorganisms (Hiraoka, W., Vazquez, N., Nieves-Neira, W., Chanock, S.J. and Pommier, Y. Role of oxygen radicals generated by NADPH oxidase in apoptosis induced in human leukemia cells. J Clin Invest 1998; 102: 1961) (Gallin, J.I., Buescher, E.S., Seligmann, B.E., Nath, J., Gaither, T. and Katz, P. National Institutes of Health Conference: recent advances in chronic granulomatous disease. Am Intern Med 1983; 99: 657) (Ward, P.A., Till, G.O., Kunkel, R. and Beauchamp, C. Evidence for role of hydroxyl radical in complement and neutrophil-dependent tissue injury. J Clin Invest 1983; 72: 789).

No viral infection is more common than the common cold and it is common knowledge that we do not, presently, have any medical agents to combat the cold virus. We are told that antibiotics are useless against viruses, so, our best bet is to get plenty of rest, drink lots of fluids and take antipyretics, if the fever gets too high. We are told this because, "It has to run its course" and it does. It does so because our bodies immune system, hence our white cells, hence our oxidative metabolism, hence reactive oxygen species and electronic excitation states (excytomers), are killing off the cold virus and producing spontaneous regressions for each bout of the common cold. Vaccines do not work because there are too many species of viruses to prepare a vaccine for each and still be able to timely administer it to the patient, such that they can build up immunity. Every time we recover from a cold, we have experienced a spontaneous regression or self-cure.

Even more intriguing is the possibility of being able to willfully turn on our innate self-cure system for spontaneous regression. We get glimpses of this ability in cases of herpes simplex (warts) and herpes genitalis (genital herpes). **There are many reliable accounts of warts disappearing or spontaneously regressing secondary to the powers of suggestion (the mind).** It is not uncommon for warts to recede following a post hypnotic suggestion or following "treatment by a gifted member of the community" who has the ability to remove warts. I feel that this is another example of stimulating (turning on and turning up) our immune system, hence our white blood cells, hence our oxidative metabolism, hence reactive oxygen species and electron excitation states, to effectuate these "healings." The possibilities of this **mind-over-immune-system** are enormous. We know that **we have the ability to willfully generate reactive oxygen species because of the body's responses to sexual arousal, i.e., nitric oxide generation produces vasodilation and penile erection willfully.**

Both, herpes simplex and herpes genitalis symptoms and lesions are believed to appear under conditions of stress or "when your body is run down." Stress is one of the best and most common known causes of immunosuppression. Suppressing the immune system allows these ever-present viruses to manifest themselves. In other words, during periods of immunosuppression, these viruses are no longer held at bay. However, recovery is based on the reestablishment of homeostasis by the intervention of our immune system and our innate ability for self-cure. This is another example of turning on our immune system, hence our white blood cells, hence oxidative metabolism, hence reactive oxygen species, and effectuating more spontaneous regression or self-cure.

Even in his daily syndicated newspaper columns, Princeton and Tulane Medical School graduate, Dr. Peter Gott frequently refers to, "......our bodies phenomenal abilities to cure themselves."

8.2 NOW FOR THE REAL KICKER

To get an appreciation of exponential notation, the Molecular Expressions web site, compares the size of the Earth to the size to the size of a plant cell, which is a trillion times smaller:

Earth = 12.76 X 10^{+6} = 12,760,000 meters wide (12.76 million meters)

Plant cell = 12.76 X 10^{-6} = 0.00001276 meters wide (12.76 millionths of a meter)

Vast amounts of data accumulated by many different investigators have established that every cell in our body has over 100,000 mutagenic oxidative events occurring in our DNA every day. This means that:

  100,000 mutations times (estimates go as low as 10,000 in humans)
  75 trillion cells times (estimates go as high as 100 trillion cells in the human body)
  365 days per year times

Years (age of individual) equals the number of spontaneous regressions that have occurred in that individual. That makes it very common! By my calculations, that totals about 1.12×10^{20} . That is the number of times that spontaneous regression of cancer has occurred in a 60 year old human. In other words, **the cancer was there but it was removed, corrected or eliminated gazillions of times**. **Potential cancer or pro-neoplasia**, as we commonly know it, continually undergoes spontaneous regression. Similarly, we have warded off exponential numbers of **potential infections** over our life spans by continual spontaneous regressions or self-cure, via this same mechanistic process involving oxidative metabolism. This is another solid component in my **Unified Theory**.

Another example of the utility of exponential notation is as follows: a factor of 10^{25} stands between the longest and the shortest known forms of electromagnetic waves. Denton said a pile of 10^{25} playing cards would reach half way across the observable universe.   Our sun's light and heat between near-ultraviolet and near-infrared is the width of just one card in the cosmic stack.

8.2.1 DNA Repair

DNA photolyase is a DNA repair enzyme which recognizes and removes dimers that have formed between pyrimidine nitrogenous bases, such as T<>T, on the same strand as each other, as a result of too much ultraviolet radiation. The enzyme can only do this in the presence of visible light, which is usually in the blue/UV-A region for catalysis.

Thus, I ask, **could the photolyase that repairs DNA be activated by decay or photon emission from singlet oxygen?** If so, this explains the fact that DNA repair increases with exercise. There are other dark reactions which produce chemiluminescence such as the chlorination of tryptophan by HOCl, myeloperoxidase-H_2O_2-HOCl, and taurine chloramines and could also serve to activate photolyase. This pathway would also provide for another useful task for electronic excitation states, especially since we are now finding that they are much more frequently present and involved in cellular metabolism than had previously been known or postulated. If such a pathway is found, I would call it **"the $^1O_2$ nano-lightning pathway for DNA repair."**   This could also serve as the same source of light for activation of the many intracellular photosensitive compounds, in an environment which was previously thought to be only an arena of "dark reactions." Natural photoexcitable sensitizers are: tetrapyroles (bilirubin), flavins, chlorophyll, hemeproteins, NADH (reduced pyridine nucleotide). Remember that UVA (320-400 nm) plus a sensitizer reacts with O_2 to produce $^1O_2$.

Also, while I am speculating wildly, it is conceivable that the brain's "heavy breathing" and O_2 utilization is the result of the innate need for excited states and photons necessary to carry on the electromagnetic aspects of thinking and memory.

8.3 POINTS OF CONVERGENCE

Throughout this book and its associated discussions, I have aimed for points of convergence to emerge from the near chaotic state of the data. My scope of inquiry has considered the following:

Points of convergence: **Cancer, spontaneous regression, arteriosclerosis, PDT, HIV/AIDS, malaria, pregnancy, smoking, hydrogen peroxide, sodium hypochlorite, singlet oxygen, respiratory burst, inflammation, oxygen consumption, cellular oxygen levels, RONS levels, exercise, immuno-suppression, antioxidants, hypoxia, aging, hypericin, obesity, chronic granulomatous disease, Down's syndrome, diabetes, etc.**

UTOPIA CONNECTIONS AND CONVERGENCE

My studies of the biochemical intricacies connecting reactive oxygen radicals and excited states has led me to the following unifying concepts:

- RONS and excited states have levels or ranges, which I prefer to call zones, which determine certain biological outcomes, relative to the appearance of cancer and infection. Zones of RONS and excited states appear to be multi-phasic and at least triphasic. In general, these zones refer to the whole organism but due to the heterogeneity of tissue and/or organs necessitates that they be considered on an individual basis at times.

- **Howes' TRIPHASIC ZONES OF RONS & EXCITED STATES**

- **Apoptosis Zone** - the **highest zone (hyper-zone)** of RONS and excited states. Based on the results of thousands and thousands of papers, it is well established that very high levels of RONS and excited states which can be produced by PDT, many chemotherapeutic drugs, radiation and the Howes Singlet Oxygen delivery system, **will kill cancer**. Also, a hyper-stimulated immune system, such as is seen in spontaneous regression of cancer, **kills cancer**.

- **Abeyance Zone** - the **middle zone (mid-zone)** of RONS and excited states. Based on the fact that millions and millions of people go through life without the manifestation of cancer is evidence, par excellence, for the existence of this mid zone of ROS and excited states, which **holds cancer cell development in abeyance**. It is an accepted scientific fact that all aerobic cells undergo exponential numbers of potentially mutagenic oxidative damaging events on a continual basis yet, **millions do not manifest or develop continual infections or tumors in a life time**. This is the zone of **homeostasis**.

- **Allowance Zone** - the **lowest zone (hypo-zone)** of RONS and excited states. This zone is based on the millions of cases of patients with immunosuppression (acquired or innate) and on genetic diseases such as chronic granulomatous disease, obesity and diabetes. We know that low levels of ROS and excited states **allow the development of cancer**.

"Aerobic life is choreographed by its oxygen instructor to perform the dance of the electron."

R. M. Howes, M.D., Ph.D.

2/25/04

PART II - OXYGEN AND FREE RADICALS (RONS)

9 OXYGEN

9.1 DISCOVERY OF OXYGEN

Prokaryotic-like cells date back 3.5 billion years and eukaryotic cells go back 2.7- 2.1 billion years ago.

Oxygen supports all life on this planet and is essential to combustion as well as respiration, and yet its very existence was not known until the 1770's, when scientists began to concern themselves with air and how it affects combustion. **The ancient Greeks considered air to be an element composed of a single substance, and this view persisted through the centuries.** It took major scientific breakthroughs to discover oxygen.

In 1770, G.E. Stahl, a German physician, proposed a theory that received widespread acceptance. He claimed that all inflammable objects contained a material substance that he called **"phlogiston,"** from a Greek word meaning **"to set on fire."** When an object burned, it poured its content of phlogiston into the air, and when all its phlogiston was gone, it stopped burning. Wood lost its phlogiston very rapidly, so that its passage into air was visible as flames. Stahl suggested that the rusting of metals also depended on the loss of phlogiston to surrounding air, except that metals lost their phlogiston so slowly that rusting was a gradual process.

Experiments to learn more about the principles of combustion were made in 1772 by a Scottish chemist, Joseph Black, and his student, Daniel Rutherford. They tried burning candles in closed containers of air and found that the candles eventually went out even though the containers still held a large amount of air. Mice put into these containers promptly died. Holding to the phlogiston theory, Rutherford, came to the conclusion that the burning candles emitted phlogiston but a given volume of air could hold only a certain amount of phlogiston. When the saturation point was reached in the closed container, the air would not accept any more phlogiston and the candle would go out because it could not continue to emit phlogiston. Rutherford believed that, in like manner, a living creature gives up phlogiston while breathing and when placed in air that is already saturated with phlogiston, can no longer breathe and must die.

The **demolition of the phlogiston theory** began with experiments carried on in 1774 by Joseph Priestly, an English clergyman who was interested in science. His experiments involved the heating of mercury by exposing it to sunlight concentrated through a magnifying glass. The heated mercury became coated with a reddish powder, which Priestly reheated at a higher temperature. The powder evaporated and turned into two gases, one of which was mercury vapor. The mercury vapor condensed into drops of mercury in the test vessel as it cooled. The other gas was invisible, but priestly knew it existed because when he placed a smoldering splint of wood into it, the wood burst into flame, and mice put into this invisible gas became hyperactive. **Priestly stuck to the phlogiston theory** to explain these results. He thought that heated mercury lost some of its phlogiston and turned into mercury rust. When this rust was heated, it absorbed phlogiston from air and turned back into mercury. The invisible gas had also lost its phlogiston, and it drew phlogiston rapidly from the smoldering wood splint, causing the splint to burst into flame.

Priestly later traveled to Paris, where he discussed his experiments with a brilliant French chemist, Antoine Lavoisier, who had been carrying on his own experiments in combustion. Lavoisier's experiments had convinced him that **phlogiston did not exist** and combustion was caused by the combination of fuel with air. However, he was unable to prove his theory until Priestly described his experiments with heated mercury. Lavoisier had burned candles in closed containers and he had observed that only one-fifth of the air was consumed during burning and the remaining four-fifths would not support combustion. After his discussions with Priestly, one with phlogiston and one without - was really only one kind of air that contained two substances. **Lavoisier called** the one-fifth of the air that supported combustion "oxygen" (from the Greek words meaning "acid-producing," because he thought (wrongly), that oxygen was a necessary component of all acids). The four-fifths of the air that does not support respiration or combustion he called "azote" (from the Greek words meaning "no life"). Azote today is known as "nitrogen."

Lavoisier made many contributions to the advancement of chemistry. One of the most significant was his belief in the importance of accurate measurements during experimentation. He arrived at his conclusion on the non-existence of phlogiston because of his accurate measurement of weight gains and losses during combustion. He demonstrated that there is no change in total weight during any chemical reaction in a closed system. Therefore, he concluded that air cannot change its properties by gaining or losing phlogiston and consequently phlogiston did not exist.

In succeeding years, methods for isolating oxygen and other gases were developed and improved. The next problem that researchers faced as how to measure the oxygen content in a gaseous atmosphere. Michael Faraday, an English chemist and physicist, is noted for discoveries in electricity and magnetism. In 1848, while he was investigating the magnetic susceptibility of matter, he discovered that oxygen could be drawn into a magnetic field, and in fact was far more susceptible to a magnetic field than most other gases. Faraday developed a simple measurement method by suspending a test sample in a non-uniform magnetic field and observing the difference in magnetic susceptibility between the sample and the surrounding medium. Later, researchers found that the magnetic susceptibility (paramagnetism) of oxygen decreased markedly when it was heated. In the following decades, Faraday's principle of the paramagnetism of oxygen led to the design of a large number of instruments based on Faraday's discovery - the magnetodynamic, the thermomagnetic and the magnetopneumatic oxygen analyzers - are used for oxygen measurements and analysis.

'Give me the power to induce fever and I will cure all diseases.'
Parmenides (ca 540-480 BC)

(Some of the materials in this section have been excerpted or modified from http://teaching.ust.hk/~bisc376/chapter1.doc

9.2 BRIEF HISTORY OF OXYGEN

The element oxygen (chemical symbol O) exists in air as a 'double' molecule, two atoms being joined together to give O_2 **(dioxygen).** Oxygen was first isolated and characterized between 1772 and 1774 by the individual skills of three great European scientists - Scheele, Priestley and Lavoisier. Oxygen appeared in significant amounts in the Earth's atmosphere some 2.5×10^9 years ago, and geological evidence suggests that this was due to the photosynthetic activity of certain microorganisms, the blue-green algae. As they split water to obtain their essential requirement for hydrogen atoms, blue-greens released tons of oxygen into the atmosphere, creating perhaps the worst case of environmental pollution ever recorded on this planet. The slow and steady rise in atmospheric oxygen concentrations was accompanied by the formation of the ozone layer in the stratosphere. Both oxygen and the ozone layer acted as critical filters against the intense solar ultraviolet light striking the surface of the Earth. Ascending in altitude from the Earth's atmosphere into outer space, we see a change from relatively heavy molecules such as O_2, N_2 and H_2O to lighter molecules, atoms and ions (such as hydrogen atoms and H^+) and electrons, which are dominant above 800 km. The universe contains vast amounts of hydrogen (H) and Helium (He). **Perhaps the Earth may be regarded as a unique center of potential oxidation capacity in an otherwise reducing universe.**

The percentage of oxygen in air is now approximately **21 per cent**. This makes oxygen the second most abundant element in the atmosphere. The first is nitrogen, N_2, at approximately 78 per cent. **However, the actual mass of oxygen in the atmosphere is negligible when compared with that present as part of the water (H_2O) molecule in oceans, lakes, and rivers and that present as part of mineral ores (e.g., metal oxides such as the aluminum ore bauxite, Al_2O_3) in the Earth's crust, where oxygen is by far the most abundant element.**

When the Earth's atmosphere changed from a highly reducing state of the oxygen-rich state that we know today, the anaerobic life forms existing at that time either adapted, died or retreated to places with little or no oxygen. Present-day anaerobic bacteria (which are killed by O_2 or cease growing when O_2 is present) are presumably the evolutionary descendants of organisms that followed this avoidance strategy. They are found in the mammalian colon, rotten foods, infected wounds, dental plaque, deep in soil and similar places. However, these are not a salubrious environment: in retrospect, organisms that evolved the capacity to cope with oxygen (by evolving antioxidant defense mechanisms) did best, because they could simultaneously evolve to use oxygen for efficient energy production and for other oxidation reactions. Thus, every textbook of biochemistry explains how **anaerobic metabolism** of one molecule of the sugar glucose gives only two molecules of ATP (adenosine triphosphate, the energy currency of the cell), whereas **aerobic (oxidative) metabolism gives 36 or 38 ATPs per glucose** (depending on textbook source quoted). The evolution of efficient aerobic respiration allowed the development of complex multicellular organisms. However, since Earth's organisms consist mainly of water, and O_2 is poorly soluble in water (it is much more soluble in organic solvents), transport of necessary O_2 to all the cells in a large organism required the evolution of high-capacity O_2 transporter molecules, of which the red-brown protein **hemoglobin** (Hb) in our red blood cells is the prime example.

Aerobic life forms use oxygen to oxidize ('burn') fuels rich in carbon and hydrogen (foods) to obtain the heat and other forms of energy essential for life. **The carbon becomes carbon dioxide (CO_2) and the hydrogen becomes water (H_2O).** Thus, the burning of glucose to provide energy in the body can be written as

$$C_6H_{12}O_6 + 6O_2 \rightarrow 6CO_2 + 6H_2O$$

The carbon in glucose is oxidized to CO_2; the O_2 is reduced to water. Fats can also be burned: they yield more energy per gram than carbohydrates and so they are our major body food stores. **Amino acids can also be burned: the nitrogen is first removed from them and eventually excreted in the urine as urea.** The burning of dietary fuels in the cells **produces ATP**, a central energy source which is used to drive movement and building up of cell components.

9.3 OXYGEN PROPERTIES

Oxygen is a stable, odorless, tasteless and colorless gas. I have already pointed out its limited solubility in water. However, this limited solubility is vital to the survival of fish and other aquatic organisms, and essential for normal respiratory functions in many. **Oxygen has to dissolve in water to cross the alveoli of the lungs and reach the transport protein hemoglobin.** Oxygen solubility in water (like that of most gases) decreases with increases in temperature - if the oceans and rivers get warmer, some fish and other aquatic organisms may not receive sufficient oxygen.

The air dissolved in water contains a higher percentage of oxygen (34 per cent) than does dry air (21 per cent), because O_2, although poorly soluble, is more soluble than is nitrogen. As already mentioned, oxygen is considerably more soluble in organic solvents than it is in water. For example, **the fat solvent chloroform ($CHCl_3$) at 10°C can dissolve up to 219.5 ml of oxygen per liter at one atmosphere pressure, whereas under the same conditions water dissolves only 38.2 ml of oxygen.** These differences in solubility are important when considering the availability of oxygen for chemical reactions inside living systems: **organic regions may contain more oxygen than aqueous regions.** The membranes that separate cells from the environment and separate the different compartments within **cells contain an interior organic phase**, in which oxygen may tend to concentrate.

9.4 OXYGEN TOXICITY AND ANTIOXIDANTS

It is stated that a problem with oxygen can be that it oxidizes organic molecules, including foods, plastics, paints, hydrocarbon fuels (petroleum, gasoline, natural gas, etc.), rubber and human tissues. Fortunately, the rates of these oxidations are very slow at normal temperatures. **They can be increased by enzymes (such as those that catalyze oxidations of foodstuffs in aerobic cells) or by heat,** as in combustion of hydrocarbon fuels. **Theoretically, defenses may prevent these oxidations by removing catalysts, by being preferentially oxidized (thus, protecting key cell components), or by repairing the damage caused by oxygen.**

Biological oxidation has been metaphorically compared to "the rusting of a car" or to "the browning of a cut apple." However, **this naïve analogy is woefully lacking in the complexities occurring continuously inside aerobic, living/breathing cells and only projects harmful and negative views of oxidation.** This is wrong. This is like comparing the flame of a cup cake candle to the burning surface of the sun. Even more pathetic is the fact that some of these lame analogies have presented by trained biochemists. This has led, either directly or indirectly, to a steadfast religious zealot-like belief in the theory of oxidative stress and the free radical theory of aging. **Biased scientific experimentation in the area of oxidative stress is reaching levels of prejudice whereby experiments are being manipulated to support this flawed theory and this is occurring on a daily basis.** Further, **if the data does not fit the oxidative stress theory, whereby the theory should be discarded, they ascribe the true data to an anomaly or a "paradox."** That is supposed to solve everything but it only further prejudices the experimental data, and, in essence, **throws good data at a bad theory.**

A previous author has stated that, "One of the results of the ceaseless investigation which characterizes the medical world of the present, is the retesting of many of the theories, which, on account of their age, or their apparent rationality, have almost assumed the finality of facts. If ever a theory seemed rational and well grounded, that which regarded wind-instrument players and glass blowers as particularly prone to emphysema would seem to have been one. The examination of two hundred and eighteen glass blowers by the authors mentioned showed only five cases of emphysema, a result which is decidedly destructive to the current belief on this point. Fischer's article of two years ago showed almost identical results so far as wind-instrument players were concerned, as he found that in five hundred military musicians there was no case of emphysema, even in individuals over fifty. **Thus, another idol is shattered."** I feel that this is woefully analogous to the fall of the flawed free radical/oxidation theory and **this above case was presented 100 years ago.** (Munchener Med Woch., Feb. 9, 1904).

Many of today's investigators are setting up experiments with such bias, that their data is destructively tainted before the experiments have even begun. This was unheard of prior to the1970's but it is readily accepted in the 21st century. This can only weaken and obscure the validity of the scientific method and fill countless journals with junk science. **It will only serve to perpetuate the demonization of oxygen, the phobia of free radicals, feed the hunger of 21st century snake oil salesmen and put off the realization of the wonders of oxygen in sustaining all aerobic life forms.**

Guilt, by epidemiological association, must not be allowed to cloud our ability to see true cause and effect relationships. **Please remember that a cause, by definition, invariably leads to its effect.**

10 OXYGEN MODIFICATIONS (DERIVATIVES)

Here is the standard nonsense/non-science erroneous description used to describe the "oxygen paradox."

Oxidative damage is the foremost theory as to what causes the deterioration that comes with age. The concept is known as the "oxygen paradox': we require oxygen to turn the food we eat into cellular fuel, but the side effects of this oxygen metabolism are detrimental to our health. The process takes place in the mitochondria, where electrons are striped from energy-rich substances--in particular, glucose--while converting them to the kind of fuel that cells can use. In the process, electrons go astray, resulting in the formation of highly reactive molecules known as free radicals. Roy L. Walford, a gerontologist and a pioneer of calorie restriction research, refers to free radicals as "great white sharks in the biochemical sea--short-lived but voracious agents that oxidize and damage tissues." This analogy to a great white shark is laughable…..inaccurate, but laughable.

Oxygen modifications (including reactive oxygen species and/or excitation states; derivatives; RONS/excytomers) have been viewed as an all encompassing class. This erroneous fundamental premise tends to suggest that a free radical is a free radical is a free radical or that the non-radical forms of oxygen all react the same. **This orthodox view is misleading, erroneous, confusing and just plain wrong, wrong, and wrong.   The take home message is simple: we must arrive at a point of adequate chemical and biochemical sophistication where we treat each of these entities in a manner which reflects its specific individual characteristics and reactivities.** Anything less is unacceptable with today's understanding of free radical and electronic excitation state chemistry. Nonetheless, I feel that I have to still use the RONS designation, such that those indoctrinated in this clumsy nomenclature can easily follow along with my text.

10.1 THE "FREE RADI-CRAP" THEORY OF AGING AND OXIDATIVE STRESS

Hensley and Floyd have described the historical course of oxygen modification chemistry as follows:

"The existence of free radicals, as chemical entities, was inferred 100 years ago but not universally accepted for some 30-40 years. The existence and importance of free radicals in biological systems was not recognized until the mid 1950's, by a small number of visionary scientists who can be credited with founding the field of reactive oxygen biochemistry. For most of the remaining 20th century, reactive oxygen species (ROS) were considered a type of biochemical "rusting chemical" that caused stochastic tissue damage and disease. As we enter the 21st century, reactive oxygen biochemistry is maturing as a discipline and establishing its importance among the biomedical sciences. **It is now recognized that virtually every disease state involves some degree of oxidative stress.** Moreover, we are now beginning to recognize that ROS are produced in a well-regulated manner to help maintain homeostasis on the cellular level in normal, healthy tissue."

(Hensley, K. and Floyd, R.A. Reactive oxygen species and protein oxidation in aging: a look back, a look ahead. Arch of Biochem and Biophy 2002; 397(2): 377-383).

Respectfully, I vehemently disagree with their implication of oxidative stress being causal in virtually every disease state but I do agree with the increasing recognition that RONS and excited states are normal metabolic products which are intimately involved with maintaining homeostasis. Erroneous interpretations of this variety, I now refer to as "The Free Radi-Crap Theory of aging and oxidative stress."

In *Science*, in 1954, Rebecca Gerschman published a paper entitled, "Oxygen poisoning and X-irradiation: a mechanism in common." This paper led to the supposed link between oxygen free radicals and cellular damage, which was later used as the basis for the free radical theory of aging and oxidative stress.

Recent studies in a variety of cell types have suggested that cancer chemotherapy drugs induce tumor cell apoptosis in part by inducing formation of reactive oxygen species (RONS). Investigators demonstrated that, at least in B lymphoma cells, chemotherapy-induced apoptosis occur using a mechanism that does not involve oxidants. Hydrogen peroxide, which reportedly kills cells by a non-apoptotic pathway, caused increases in both protein and lipid oxidation (Senturker, S., Tschirret-Guth, R., Morrow, J., Levine, R. and Shacter, E. Induction of apoptosis by chemotherapeutic drugs without generation of reactive oxygen species. Arch of Biochem and Biophy 2002; 397(2): 262-272). Free radicals and reactive oxygen species (RONS) have been thought to be associated with the etiology and/or progression of a number of diseases and in aging. **Many of the proteins oxidatively modified by free radicals contain side-chain carbonyl derivatives**, which can be used as markers for protein oxidation. The protein carbonyl content has been quantitated as a function of age for human cultured dermal fibroblasts, lens, and brain tissue. The carbonylated proteins and peptides are highly susceptible to proteolytic degradation (Moskovitz, J., Yim, M.B. and Chock, P.B. Free radicals and disease. Arch of Biochem and Biophy 2002; 397(2): 354-359).

10.2 FREE RADICALS (RONS)

The concept of free radicals requires a brief review of some elementary chemistry. An atom consists of a central nucleus (containing positively charged protons and neutral neutrons), with electrons orbiting around it. The electrons associate in pairs, and each pair moves in its own region of space around the nucleus. A **free radical is defined as any species capable of independent existence (hence the term 'free') that contains one or more unpaired electrons.** The free radical nature of an atom or molecule is usually denoted by a superscript dot (e.g., H ., O_2^- , .OH). Molecules can be free radicals if one or more of the atoms present have unpaired electrons. Indeed, **the diatomic oxygen molecule (O_2) qualifies as a free radical because it contains two unpaired electrons. Other gaseous free radicals include nitric oxide (.NO) and nitrogen dioxide (.NO$_2$).** Thus, ground state oxygen is a diradical. By contrast, the gas ozone (O_3) is not a free radical - there are no unpaired electrons in its molecules. Free radicals of different types vary widely in their chemical reactivity, but in general they are more reactive than nonradicals. Fortunately, however, **oxygen is an exception to this rule: it is not a particularly reactive free radical because of peculiarities in its arrangement of electrons.** Also, not all free radicals react violently and in the termination of a free radical, by reaction with an antioxidant, another free radical is created. Thus, **every time a free radical reacts with a non-radical, another free radical is created.**

When two free radicals meet, their unpaired electrons can join to form a pair, and both radicals are lost. Thus, **it takes a radical to kill a radical.** However, **since most molecules present in living organisms do not have unpaired electrons, any free radicals that are produced will most likely react with nonradicals, generating new free radicals.** Hence, free radical reactions tend to proceed as **chain reactions.** Webster's New Lexicon dictionary defines a chain reaction as, "a process of change in which a product of the change initiates further change." This is a basic principle of free radical chemistry but I believe that it can also be applied to most intracellular chemical events because it is unlikely that any event occurs alone, without inducing further changes in the living/breathing cell. Just because further events occur does not mean that these events are destructive; to the contrary, they are overwhelmingly beneficial or the cell would rapidly die. **It has been stated that only one lipid radical is necessary to start a chain reaction of lipid peroxidation, but obviously, in nature this is not a problem since lipid radicals are constantly present.**

**"Relative to oxygen metabolism,
the most damaging chain reaction that occurs,
is the uncontrolled dispersal of misinformation and
the perpetuation of erroneous conclusions."**

R. M. Howes, M.D., Ph.D.

8/21/04

The take-home message is that free radical chain reactions within the cell do not occur in the same manner as atomic fission, in that they appear to be self-limiting or the outcome of such intracellular chain reactions would also be self-annihilation.

Unpaired electrons can be associated with many different atoms and molecules. Hence **many different free radicals exist**. For example, the structure of many proteins is stabilized by joining sulphur atoms together by covalent bonds to form disulphide bridges. These disulphide bridges can be broken to give **sulphur radicals**, if one of the two electrons from the covalent bond remains on each sulphur atom

S - S → S. + S.

Among the mechanisms by which these and other radicals can be generated is the grinding of proteins (e.g., during the processing of food material). The protein keratin present in human fingernails is rich is disulphide bridges, and sulphur radicals can be detected in fingernail clippings. However, **in biological systems, most attention has been focused on the oxygen radicals and unfortunately, in a negative way**. Reduction of oxygen can produce a number of free radicals such as superoxide, peroxyl and hydroxyl.

"Within the matrix of the virtual nano-world of cellular signaling, oxygen's multiple personalities go about their intricate peripatetic tasks, with an arrogant assurance earned over eons of time."

R. M. Howes, M.D., Ph.D.
5/26/04

10.3 SUPEROXIDE RADICAL

The superoxide anion is thought to be the most widely produced free radical in the body. It is a mono-radical resulting from the monovalent reduction of ground state molecular oxygen. In the presence of protons, its dismutation leads to O_2 and H_2O_2.

Many investigators believe that O_2^- is nearly immediately converted to H_2O_2 within the cell.

One out of every 20 of the O_2 molecules or 5% of the O_2 passing along the electron transport chain is converted into O_2^- and this occurs when one of the electron carriers, called Coenzyme Q, passes the electron to O_2 instead of the next electron carrier. Superoxide is not very reactive and is primarily converted to H_2O_2 which is also not very reactive. The O_2^- is much more reactive when protonated and becomes the HO_2. species. Yet, there is considerable hoopla constantly in the literature accusing both of these RONS as being "chemical killers." Even more shocking is the fact that both O_2^- and H_2O_2 are needed to help protect and regulate the body and not to harm it. **Please keep in mind that O_2^-, in aqueous solutions, is a reductant, not an oxidant.** In fact, an ideal place for O_2^- to give up its spare electron is to lose it to iron.

White cells deliberately generate O_2^- to kill invading pathogens. An enzyme, NADPH oxidase, is found on the surfaces of macrophages and neutrophils and is stimulated by invading pathogens to produce O_2^-. The neutrophil also contains myeloperoxidase which reacts with H_2O_2 and salt (chloride ions) to produce $^1O_2$. **Myeloperoxidase** is in such high concentrations in neutrophils that it gives a **greenish color** to phlegm during times in which our bodies are fighting respiratory infections.

In biological tissues, **superoxide can be nonenzymatically converted into H_2O_2 and $^1O_2$** (Steinbeck, M.J., Khan, A.U. and Karnovsky, M.J. Extracellular production of singlet oxygen by stimulated macrophages quantified using 9, 10-diphenylanthracene and perylene in a polystyrene film. J Biol Chem 268: 15649-15654).

Superoxide is produced enzymatically by:

- NADPH oxidases (phagocytosis)
- Mitochondrial cytochrome c oxidase (cell respiration)
- Liver Cytochrome P 450 (oxidation of xenobiotics)
- Xanthine oxidase (ischemic reperfusion)
- Prostaglandin synthetase
- Lipoxygenase
- Aldehyde oxidase
- Amino acid oxidase
- Myeloperoxidase
- NADPH-cytochrome P-450 reductase
- flavoprotein dehydrogenases

A major source of O_2^- is cytochrome$_{b5}$ and the autoxidation of ubisemiquinone.

Autoxidation produces superoxide anion (O_2^-):

Catecholamines

Hemoglobin
Myoglobin
Reduced cytochrome c
Thiol
Fe++

70-90% of O$_2$ uptake during the respiratory burst goes to O$_2^-$ formation but this goes to produce singlet oxygen. Shift of oxygen to this system reduces electron transport and lactic acid accumulates and is transported to the lysosome. **Acid pH aids in the production of singlet oxygen.** It also allows hydrolytic enzymes, like lysozyme and proteases, that have acidic pH optima, to act more effectively. Ingested bacterial cells are killed.

Bacteria (e.g., Streptococcus pyogenes) which contain carotenoid pigments are resistant to singlet oxygen toxicity because the carotenoids quench its action. This fact argues against the administration of large doses of beta-carotene during a Strep infection. Keep in mind that capsulated bacteria are often very resistant to phagocytosis and that in the case of Streptococcus pneumoniae, strains with capsules (smooth) are enormously more virulent than non-capsulated strains.

Mycobacterium tuberculosis can survive and grow inside macrophages, likely due to production of cell wall glycolysis that remove ROS (**some bacteria have catalase to break down hydrogen peroxide**) and these types of organisms that survive inside phagocytes produce persistent diseases.

Cell membrane NADPH-oxidase is activated to produce O$_2^-$ by:

Immunologic-coated bacteria
Immune complexes
Complement 5a
Leukotrienes

Organelles that can produce O$_2^-$ are:

Mitochondria, which are the main source of O$_2^-$
Microsomes, which produce 80% H$_2$O$_2$ at 100% O$_2$
Peroxisomes
Nuclei
Chloroplasts

Superoxide anion is generated at the ubiquinone site in complex III and approximately 3-5% of all electrons passing through the electron transport chain are directed this way.

Ubiquitination - protein modification by the conjugation of ubiquitin moieties.

Superoxide anion and hydrogen peroxide are constantly being produced by:

Mitochondrial respiratory chain
Electron transport chain
Endoplasmic reticulum
Nuclear membranes

Superoxide is formed upon one-electron reduction of oxygen mediated by enzymes such as NADPH oxidase or xanthine oxidase or from the respiratory chain. The half-life of O$_2^-$ in tissues is dependent on the presence of the enzyme superoxide dismutase in different cellular compartments. Some believe that **most superoxide is rapidly converted to hydrogen peroxide and that very little superoxide anion, per se, actually exists.** In my opinion, this is a most important consideration and it provides for high steady states of hydrogen peroxide. Reactive oxygen species are also produced in the organism as a part of the primary immune defense.

Superoxide is made by adding one electron on to an oxygen molecule. The added electron pairs with one of the two unpaired electrons already present in O_2, leaving one unpaired electron.

(1) O_2 + e- O_2^- (superoxide radical)
(2) O_2^- +2H+ +e- H_2O_2 (hydrogen peroxide)
(3) H_2O_2+e-   OH-+.OH (hydroxyl radical)
(4) .OH.+e-   OH- (hydroxyl ion)
2OH-+2H+ H_2O
    Overall O_2 + 4H + 4e- H_2O

The chemical behavior of O_2^- differs greatly depending on what it is dissolved in. **In water, O_2^- is not very reactive. It can sometimes act as a weak oxidizing agent, by accepting one more electron.** For example, it can oxidize **ascorbic acid (vitamin C).**

Ascorbic acid + O_2^- + H+$\rightarrow$ ascorbic acid radical + H_2O_2

hydrogen peroxide

Superoxide in aqueous solution more often acts as a reducing agent.

(e.g., it reduces ferric (Fe3+) iron salts):

Fe3+ + O_2^- $\rightarrow$ Fe2+ + O_2

Upon donating its electron, O_2^- is oxidized and reforms dioxygen. **However, in organic solvents, O_2^- is far more reactive and dangerous. Thus any O_2^- generated in the interior of biological membranes might do considerable damage or it may participate in chemical reactions or be rapidly converted to hydrogen peroxide.**

Many tissue effects of superoxide appear to be produced from the secondary formation of other oxygen radicals in addition to direct reactions of superoxide for its conjugate acid with biological targets, such **as lipids** (Dix, T.A. and Aikens, J. Mechanisms and biological significance of lipid peroxidation initiation. Chem Res Toxicol 1993; 6: 2-18), **catecholamines** (Macarthur, H., Westfall, T.C., Riley, D.P., Misko, T.P. and Salvenini, D. Inactivation of catecholamines by superoxide gives new insights on the pathogenesis of septic shock. Pros Natl Acad Sci 2000; 97: 9753-9758**), and DNA** (Dix, T.A., Hess, K.M., Medina, M.A., Sullivan, R.W., Tilly, S.L. and Webb, L.L. Mechanism of site selective DNA nicking by the hydrodioxyl (perhydroxyl) radical. Biochemistry 1996; 35: 4578-4583).

Superoxide in aqueous media undergoes a spontaneous second order reaction with itself, a dismutation reaction that yields one molecule each of H_2O_2 and oxygen in a relatively slow reaction at pH 7.4 (the second order rate constant is of the order of 10 to the 4.5th power), when compared with the rate at which superoxide or HO_2^- can abstract an H-atom from such key biological targets as catecholamines or the allylic CH in lipid where the second order rate constant exceeds 10^7 .

Although the dismutation would be spontaneous at physiological pH at high superoxide concentrations, the concentration of superoxide approaches 10 μM (physiological) as the self reaction slows down considerably and its lifetime becomes extended by many seconds. Consequently, nature has evolved a class of superoxide dismutase (SOD2), enzymes to remove this potentially deleterious free radical byproduct of oxygen metabolism. **These enzymes can react rapidly with superoxide (rates approaching or exceeding 10^9 power) and dismutate the radical to the nonradical products, O_2 and H_2O_2, faster than superoxide can react with other potential biological targets.** The short half-life should not be misinterpreted as mitigating the potential reactivity of O_2^- because the half-life is actually quite long in relation to the **phenomenal diffusion coefficient of the radical.** Given that superoxide can interact with a variety of biological target molecules, the reaction with the enzyme literally can shunt the superoxide production into H_2O_2 and oxygen. Thus, theoretically, in vivo, the presence of highly active **SOD enzymes will lead to an increase in the local concentration of H_2O_2.**

The foregoing collection of data presents an overwhelming number of ways in which O_2^- is produced in the cell. Surely, not all of these are the result of evolutionary mistakes and it seems plausible to me that even enzymes, such as superoxide dismutase, may have evolved to more efficiently produce H_2O_2. **Basically, all cells continuously form O_2^- and submitochondrial particles generate O_2^- at a rate of 4-7 nmol/min^{-1}/mg protein^{-1}** (Chance, B., Sies, H. and Boveris, A. Hydroperoxide metabolism in mammalian organs. Physiol Rev 59: 527-605, 1979).

Again, I feel that this is a most important aspect of superoxide chemistry, in that it provides an adequate and continual supply of life-sustaining hydrogen peroxide. I feel that my take on this position is bolstered by the fact that nature has developed the peroxisome expressly for the purpose of hydrogen peroxide production (during fatty acid oxidation). Hydrogen peroxide is a non-radical and is readily diffusible throughout the cell. In fact, I look at the production of **superoxide anion as an innate pathway for hydrogen peroxide production,** which allows for an adequate source of **singlet oxygen** production following reaction with hypochlorous acid or otherwise. Likely, this is the basis for the low level chemiluminescence which has been known to be produced by cells and the human body for decades and may be the source of **biophotons,** primarily described by Russian investigators. **This constant supply of singlet oxygen can then serve the body in its many capacities as an anti-inflammatory, anti-bacterial, anti-fungal, anti-virucidal and anti-cancer agent. Thus, I believe that H_2O_2 and $^1O_2$ may be two of the most beautifully designed molecular structures in the aerobic cell and in the human body.**

In theory, tissue toxicity from extracellular superoxide generation seems to be based on its direct reactivity with numerous types of biological molecules (lipids, DNA, RNA, catecholamines, steroids, etc.) and from its dismutation to form H_2O_2 and the concomitant reduction of ferric ion to ferrous ion (Fenton reaction); reaction of these two products can yield the highly **toxic hydroxyl radical that may cleave covalent bonds in proteins and carbohydrates, cause lipid peroxidation, and destroy cell membranes.** There are **three strategies available to "detoxify"** or prevent formation of locally produced oxygen radicals: 1) **deliver SOD** or an SODm to the area; 2) **deliver catalase** or a relative peroxide scavenger, or 3) **chelate (and thereby inactivate) the trace iron** that catalyzes the reaction (Cuzzocrea, S., Riley, D.P., Caputi, A.P. and Salvemini, D. Antioxidant therapy: A new pharmacological approach in shock, inflammation and ischemia/reperfusion injury. Pharmacol Rev 2001; 53: 135-159).

10.3.1 RONS, ADP Availability and Sleep

More O_2 is reduced to O_2^- rather than water, if the proton gradient at the mitochondrial matrix is high, then the proper flux of electrons through the ETC is energetically less favored. Thus, since the proton gradient is coupled to the conversion of ADP to ATP, **mitochondrial ROS production is especially strong if the availability of ADP is low.** It has been proposed that, since ATP consumption and ADP availability is particularly low during **sleep** periods, when muscular activity is low, the mitochondrial oxidative stress may be particularly high at night. **I believe that, if this is true, it is because sleep is a time of rejuvenation and it requires high levels of RONS/excytomers to do so, according to my Unified Theory. Perhaps, this is the reason that rest is recommended to recover from many forms of illness. In fact, if it is true that RONS generation is increased during rest, perhaps this is the reason that humans sleep for 1/3 of their lifetimes. More importantly, the mystery of the need for sleep has eluded us up to now and this may represent the biochemical basis for the need for sleep.**

RONS production reportedly increases in skeletal muscle tissue after immobilization and

is this is consistent with what I would expect during healing of wounds, injuries or fractures. Obviously, prolonged immobilization leads to muscular atrophy and would not be expected to occur in nature. I feel that this is also consistent with my view on the reperfusion "paradox", which increases levels of RONS/excytomers, in that, in nature, decreased perfusion was likely due to injury and/or having sustained a contaminated wound (a biting-tearing type of injury) . It would be logical for the contaminated tissues to produce high levels of RONS/excytomers to ward off infections, kill pathogens and promote healing.

10.4 HYDROXYL RADICAL

The hydroxyl radical is the most reactive oxygen species. X-rays or gamma rays can split water molecules and form the .OH radical. It is so reactive that it only exists for **1 billionth of a second** and must react with other molecular constituents at the site of its generation. It is formed in vivo upon high energy irradiation (e.g., x-rays) by homolytic cleavage of water or from hydrogen peroxide in a metal-catalyzed process. **UV light energy is insufficient to split water, but it can cleave hydrogen peroxide to yield the hydroxyl radical.** Due to its high reactivity, this radical immediately reacts with surrounding target molecules at the site where it is generated. It is considerably more reactive than superoxide.

The **hydroxyl radical is the most reactive oxygen radical** known to chemistry. It has tremendous potential for causing biological damage, since it attacks all biological molecules as soon as it comes into contact with them, which may set off free radical **chain reactions**. This event must be quite rare or the cell would be destroyed by uncontrolled free radical chain reactions. DNA contains a backbone of the sugar deoxyribose linked by phosphate groups. Attached to deoxyribose are the purine bases adenine and guanine and the pyramiding bases cytosine and thiamine. **Adenine pairs with thiamine and guanine with cytosine (A-T, C-G).** This pairing is essential in allowing DNA to copy itself when cells divide, and in reading the genetic information contained in DNA. Hydroxyl radicals can attack all constituents of DNA. For example, if it adds to guanine and makes a hydroxyguanine radical, it can then form 8-hydroxyguanine. 8-Hydroxyguanine can be misread when DNA is copied, introducing a mutation. **RMH Note: Some describe this as DNA damage and that it is repairable and not transmissible.** Some say that free radical damage to DNA is one of the main causes of genetic mutation and accounts for the high rates of cancer suffered by radiation victims. This may be true with high levels of exposure, such as an atomic blast, but please keep in mind the interesting results of the studies involving the exposure of hundreds of thousands of people to low level radiation and the resulting increase in longevity attributed to radiation hormesis, which is presented later in this book. Also, keep in mind that the energetics occurring within the cell are magnitudes of differences away from those associated with atomic explosions.

Most of our knowledge about the chemistry of .OH has been provided by radiation chemists, since exposing water to x-rays or gamma-rays generates .OH. Indeed, **most of the damage done to living organisms exposed to excess ionizing radiation is caused by the consequences of .OH radical attack on biological molecules. However, this may not be an exact corollary to what happens in non-ionizing intracellular events.**

Hydroxyl radicals can add on to biological molecules, as illustrated by their reaction with guanine. **They can also convert themselves back into water by pulling off hydrogen atoms (hydrogen atom abstraction) from a biological molecule, as happens in lipid peroxidation.** Since .OH reacts so fast with everything, any .OH generated combines with whatever is in the human body next to it: it doesn't last long enough to migrate anywhere else.

It is accepted that the most reactive oxy radical is HO. It was proposed erroneously many years ago that it could be produced from the interaction of O_2^- and H_2O_2 by a chemical process known as the Haber-Weiss reaction. However, **detailed studies of the rate of this reaction have shown that the Haber-Weiss reaction could not take place under physiological conditions**, even though it is still referred to in the literature. An alternative explanation, which is now widely accepted, is that trace amounts of metal ions, primarily **ferrous ion,**

react with H_2O_2 in what is known as the **iron-catalyzed Fenton reaction to produce the hydroxyl radical. Under normal cellular conditions ferrous ion is not present in vivo,** but it may be produced by the action of superoxide on ferric ion present in iron storage proteins, thus, liberating soluble ferrous ion. **There is considerable debate** as to whether protein-bound metal ions (e.g., lactoferrin, hemoglobin, etc.) catalyze this reaction to any great degree.

Recent attention has been drawn to what is called "site-specific," hydroxyl radical formation, wherein an iron ion bound to a macromolecule catalyzes HO. generation at the actual site on the substrate where cleavage eventually ensues.

Thus, in the body, the .OH radical is produced exclusively by the iron-catalyzed Fenton reaction. Also, it must be produced in small quantities or the integrity of the cell would be rapidly destroyed. Additionally, **it seems likely that harmful hydroxyl radicals which are produced at a finite or specific cellular locus would have a tendency to react with other hydroxyl radicals (since they are being generated from the same locus), to produce beneficial hydrogen peroxide.** Thus, the mere formation of the hydroxyl radical may not spell instant disaster since it may be converted to H_2O_2, which is less reactive and can readily diffuse throughout the cell.

Some authors say that since all three RONS (e.g., O_2^{-}, H_2O_2 and .OH), can interact and be formed from each other, they can be considered to be equally dangerous. Thus, they could work together and create **"an insidious catalytic system."** I believe that this is more scare tactics of the oxy-morons. If this is true, let's all gather hands and go and jump off of the nearest high bridge because life is going to be "a living Hell." This is more Free Radi-Crap nonsense. It takes enormous volumes of O_2 and RONS to keep us going. Shockingly, a 70 kilogram/154 lb. adult with a 1% "leak" would produce annually 1.7 kilograms of O_2^{-} (presumably and/or H_2O_2 or .OH) and a 5% leak would generate an astonishing 8.5 kilograms of O_2^{-} in a year. In other words, **at a 5% leak of O_2^{-}, an average adult would produce more than his entire body weight in O_2^{-} in 6 years.** If he lived to be a healthy 83 years, he would have produced over 10 times his body weight in oxygen free radicals (705 kg of O_2^{-}) and many individuals appear to do this and are just fine. So, my question is "How toxic are RONS?" They do not sound very toxic to me.

Nick Lane states that it is likely that both iron and H_2O_2 are present at steady-state concentrations of about 10^{-6} gm/kg body weight. He then uses Avogadro's number (6.023×10^{23} molecules in one mole of any substance) and calculates that **we produce about 50 .OH radicals in each cell every second or that in a day, each cell generates 4 million .OH radicals. Thus, in the average body of 100 trillion cells (figures vary), we would produce 4×10^{17} .OH radicals per day.** Again, I ask "How toxic are RONS?" (Oxygen: The molecule that made the world. Nick Lane, Oxford University Press, 2002). Lane goes on to refer to James Lovelock who estimated that **"the damage done by breathing for 1 year is equal to** a whole-body radiation dose of 1 sievert (or 1 joule energy per kilogram) and would be 10,000 times more dangerous than a chest x-ray (50 micro-sieverts of radiation) and **50 times as dangerous as all the radiation that we normally receive from all sources in the course of an entire lifetime."** I believe that "something is drastically wrong with this picture." It does not make sense.

10.4.1 Peroxyl Radicals

Peroxyl radicals (ROO.) can be generated in the process of abstraction of a hydrogen atom from polyunsaturated fatty acids (PUFA). **ROO. are relatively long-lived species with a considerable diffusion path length in biological systems.**

Further products generated in lipid peroxidation are aldehydes. The reaction of aldehydes with amine groups of peptides and proteins has been suggested as a mechanism involved in the modification of lipoproteins.

Peroxyl (ROO.) and alkoxyl (RO.) free radicals are also synthesized essentially from polyunsaturated fatty acids either in a direct and controlled way or in an indirect and uncontrolled way. Peroxyl (ROO.) free radicals result from the action of oxygenases (COX or LOX i.e., cycloxoygenase and lipoxygenases) and lead to the eicosanoid pathway and in case of alkoxyl (RO.) result from the action of .OH leading to the formation of an oxygen free radical ROO. This constitutes the initial phase of lipid peroxidation.

10.5 HYDROGEN PEROXIDE

H_2O_2 is an incredible compound which has been called "a gangland thug" and it turns violent upon meeting a rival gang member, such as an iron-containing protein and produces the all-feared .OH radical. The .OH will attack DNA, producing mutations and results in CANCER formation....Oh, No. **Probably no single substance has been applied to open wounds with greater frequency than H_2O_2.** For decades upon decades, wounds have been and continue to be washed, bathed, scrubbed and cleaned with 3% H_2O_2. In short, wounds have been flooded with peroxide. Ergo, we have an excellent clinical study model and, according to the free radical phobics, all of these open wounds, with iron containing hemoglobin (blood), dripping from them, should be producing .OH, DNA mutations and cancer, cancer and more cancer, at these wound sites.....but that has not happened! That's right..... **millions upon millions of wounds have been directly and repeatedly exposed to H_2O_2 and instead of becoming cancerous, the wounds have healed.** Surely, the oxy-morons will attribute this undisputable fact to **just another "paradox."**

If two hydroxyl radicals ever meet, they can join their unpaired electrons and make an oxygen-oxygen covalent bond, giving H_2O_2 (hydrogen peroxide), a product with no unpaired electrons. I believe that this reaction saves the cell from rapid destruction by .OH and allows for the beneficial effects of hydrogen peroxide and electronic excitation states. In my opinion, this is another ingenious pathway for hydrogen peroxide formation, which, although it has been known for many years, has basically gone unrecognized by most investigators.

.OH + .OH →H-O-O-H

Another ingenious way for the **body to produce H_2O_2** is by the **deactivation of $^1O_2$** by NADPH as follows:

NADPH + $^1O_2$ + H^+ → $NADP^+$ + H_2O_2

(Bodaness, R.S. and Chan, P.C. *FEBS Lett.* 1979; 105: 195-196).

Superoxide radicals generated in aqueous solution also make H_2O_2. One O_2^- gives up its electron to another one. The first is oxidized to O_2, and the second is reduced to H_2O_2. The overall reaction is called the **dismutation of O_2^- ,**

2 O_2^- 2H+→ H_2O_2 + O_2

A few enzymes exist in the body that make H_2O_2 directly. For example, **the amino acids incorporated into proteins by the human body are all L-type (this term describes the three-dimensional arrangement of their atoms in space).** The alternate D-type amino acids are not used. However, they can be produced by bacteria in the gut and enter the body. These 'unnatural' D-amino acids are destroyed by a **D-amino acid oxidase** enzyme. The unwanted D-amino acids are oxidized, and the electrons removed from them are **used to reduce O_2 to H_2O_2.** Proteolysis (protein breakdown) is enhanced by 20-400 μM H_2O_2, whereas mill molar concentrations inhibit proteolysis and may lead to the intracellular accumulation of oxidized proteins. It is important to remember that oxidized proteins and amino acids are always present in the cell and that the living/breathing cell has homeostatic mechanisms for maintaining the redox potential of the cell.

Several human tissues (especially gut), contain the enzyme **xanthine oxidase** which oxidizes the complex molecule hypoxanthine to xanthine, and then oxidizes the xanthine further to uric acid. Uric acid is excreted in human urine: we do not have an enzyme to break it down further. **When xanthine oxidase acts upon xanthine and hypoxanthine both O_2^- and H_2O_2 are generated**. The amounts of xanthine oxidase can increase as a result of tissue injury in certain human diseases, generating extra O_2^- and H_2O_2. These products are thought to be involved in lipid peroxidation.

Most H_2O_2 is broken down to H_2O and O_2 by catalase in aqueous solutions. In fats and oils of the body, H_2O_2 is broken down by glutathione peroxidase. They are called glutathione peroxidases because they transfer the energy of the reactive peroxides to a very small sulphur containing protein called glutathione, whose reactive center contains selenium to carry reactive electrons from the peroxide to the glutathione. It is the glutathione that is the antioxidant in the reaction , not the selenium, as many health food companies would have you believe. **Selenium, by itself, is a potent oxidant**, which can be very toxic if taken in high doses.

H_2O_2 is a pale blue liquid, which mixes readily with water, diffusing easily in the body and crossing membranes. It has been used for many years as a bleach and to disinfect wounds. Since it does not have unpaired electrons, it is not a free radical. **However, if one extra electron is added to H_2O_2, it makes .OH. Hence, some believe that H_2O_2 is a mobile time bomb**: it is **poorly reactive itself**, yet it can make .OH at any time if an electron is supplied to it. Where can this electron come from? One source is certain metal ions - those whose valencies differ by one. Iron is the prime example:

Fe2+ → Fe3+ + e-
Ferrous → Ferric
H_2O_2 + e- → .OH + OH-

The net reaction is the **Fenton reaction**

H_2O_2 + Fe2+ → .OH + OH- + Fe3+

For many years, chemists have mixed iron (II) sulphate (ferrous sulphate, $FeSO_4$) and H_2O_2 to make .OH. Indeed, the Fenton reagent was first described in the 1890's by the Cambridge chemist, H.J.H. Fenton, who showed that mixtures of ferrous salts and H_2O_2 could oxidize most organic molecules. **Some titanium, copper, cobalt and chromium salts also convert H_2O_2 into .OH.**

It is frequently pointed out that H_2O_2 will react with iron to produce the .OH radical but curiously, it does not react with the iron contained in the heme proteins such as catalase.

Superoxide can react with hydrogen peroxide to produce the hydroxyl radical as follows:

O_2^- + H_2O_2 → .OH + OH- + O_2

Superoxide in the neutrophil can also serve as a source of **singlet oxygen** as follows:

H+ + HO_2 + O_2^- → H_2O_2 + $^1O_2$

This example of spontaneous dismutation to produce $^1O_2$ has been proven by Khan (Khan, A.U. J Am Chem Soc. 1981; 103, 6516-6517).

H_2O_2 is also produced by gamma-glutamyl transpeptidase (GGT) and serves to protect U937 cells from apoptosis and stimulates proliferation.

10.5.1 Bleaches

Color and Bleach

Colored substances contain molecules with **chromophores, areas of the molecule that have double bonds between carbon atoms or oxygen atoms**. A good example is **beta carotene.**

Bleaches attack these chromophores in one of two ways.

Oxidizing bleaches, like **sodium hypochlorite (NaOCl), break the molecules at the double bond.** This results in either a shorter molecule that does not absorb visible light, or a molecule whose chromophores is either shorter or non-existent. A shorter chromophores will absorb light of a shorter wavelength than visible light (such as ultraviolet light), and so does not appear colored.

Reducing bleaches, such as lemon juice (in combination with sunlight) or sulfur dioxide, **convert the double bonds in the chromophores into single bonds,** eliminating its ability to absorb visible light. Sometimes the reaction is reversible, where oxygen in the air reacts with the molecule to repair the chromophores, and the strain returns.

Laundry bleaches fall into two categories. The first is what are called **"chlorine" bleaches.** The second are **"oxygen" bleaches.**

While pure chlorine gas will bleach colors, in laundry bleaches, **sodium hypochlorite or calcium hypochlorite are actually used, and they work by releasing oxygen**, not chlorine. The chlorine remains in solution, either as sodium chloride (table salt), or calcium chloride. These bleaches are made by bubbling chlorine gas through a solution of sodium hydroxide (lye) or calcium hydroxide (quicklime).

Chorine gas can be released if the bleach is mixed with an acid. To prevent this from happening, commercial bleaches leave extra alkalies in the solution to keep the pH very high (pH 12). This small amount of extra lye in the solution, along with the caustic nature of the hypochlorite itself, is what eats away the cloth if undiluted bleach is spilled on the clothing.

Another chlorine bleach often used is sodium dichloroisocyanurate.

Oxygen bleaches also work by releasing oxygen. Hydrogen peroxide is the active ingredient, either as itself, or as a product of reacting another ingredient with water to release hydrogen peroxide.

Oxygen bleaches, such as sodium carbonate peroxide (also called sodium per carbonate), sodium peroxide, or sodium perborate are made by reacting molecules with hydrogen peroxide. When the result is added to water, **the hydrogen peroxide is released.**

Borax also works by releasing **hydrogen peroxide** into the water.

Most oxygen bleaches work best in hot water. Additive such as tetra acetyl ethylene diamine allow the hydrogen peroxide to work in warm water (50° C).

Ultraviolet light from the sun is the most common hair-bleaching agent. Lemon juice is sometimes added to speed up the process of reducing the double bonds in hair pigments to single bonds.

However, **the most famous hair bleach is hydrogen peroxide** of peroxide blonde fame. Unlike sunlight and lemon juice, **peroxide is an oxidizing bleach**, and its effects are less easily undone.

The calcium hypochlorite or sodium dichloroisocyanurate used to disinfect swimming pools also bleaches hair, although (contrary to popular belief) it does not turn the hair green. It bleaches the hair, allowing **the green copper sulfate in the water to show in the hair.** The copper sulfate comes from the reaction of the copper pipes in the plumbing to the sulfuric acid used to neutralize the alkalies in the chlorination chemicals.

Dental bleaches are found in whitening toothpastes and in whitening gels or strips applied to the teeth. In toothpastes, **sodium carbonate peroxide** is generally used. In gels and strips, **carbamide peroxide** is used, often with tetra acetyl ethylene diamine as a bleach activator. **All of these products owe their bleaching action to the hydrogen peroxide** that is liberated when they are applied.

Skin lighteners, freckle and age spot removers, and other remedies for hyper pigmentation are not actually bleaches like the others listed so far. The active ingredient is **hydroquinones**, which **inhibits melanin formation** when applied to the skin. Since the effect is easily reversed by exposure to sunlight or ultraviolet light, a sunscreen is usually included in the formula.

Wheat flour normally becomes white by normal oxidation in air when stored for a few weeks. To speed up the process, **benzoyl peroxide** is used a bleaching agent.

Sulfur dioxide is a reducing bleaching agent that is used to preserve dried fruits.

Disinfecting

Oxidizing bleaches kill microbes by reacting with cell membranes and cell proteins. The most widely used is **sodium hypochlorite for household and hospital uses**, and **calcium hypochlorite for drinking water and swimming pool disinfecting.**

10.6 ULTRAVIOLET LIGHT AND HYDROXYL RADICALS

Ultraviolet (UV) light is not energetic enough to form .OH from H_2O, but it can cause the homolytic scission of H_2O_2 molecule. **Hence UV irradiation of H_2O_2 - containing systems can cause severe damage by making .OH**.

10.6.1 Miscellaneous Ultraviolet Light Factoids

- Ultraviolet blood irradiation is also called: photoluminescence, photopheresis, photo-oxidation, hemo-irradiation or even photodynamic therapy. It reportedly stimulates immunity and kills bacteria.

- ROS have been shown to be involved in all 3 stages of carcinogenesis and are produced by UV-A (315-400 nm) and UV-B (280-315 nm). UV-B is more efficient and UV-A is the main component of terrestrial sunlight and accounts for > 90% of the spectral energy in sunlight.

-UV-C and UV-B are absent from indoor light. Blue light has a visible spectrum of 500-381 nm and is half (50%) emitted from black light. Blue light waves inhibit cytochrome oxidase, which transports O_2 to photoreceptors and retinal cells, without it, cells die.

-UV DNA damage is repaired by "photolyase."

-O_2 itself does not absorb UV light. Skin photosensitizers absorb UV and pass the energy to O_2 to form $^1O_2$.

-UV light suppresses the natural defense system and causes immunosuppression.

-UV enhances NOS to produce NO· which causes vessel dilation and NO· blocks apoptosis of UV-A.

-Sunlight (UV light) is absorbed by surface waters and transient oxidants are formed such as ·OH, O_2^- and $^1O_2$. These species can degrade (oxidize) organic substances, i.e., phenols, polyaromatic hydrocarbons (PAHs) and pesticides.

-NO· protects membranes from UVA induced cell damage. **RMH Note: We may need to block NO· during cancer and plaque treatment.**

-UV irradiation of blood is FDA approved to treat cutaneous T cell lymphoma.

-All organic material is photodegradable at certain UV wavelengths and UV 100-280 nm destroys nearly all organics with ROS and $^1O_2$ and yields volatized CO_2 and H_2O.

-Excess sunlight to the skin leads to 1) DNA mutations 2) cell suicide or apoptosis and 3) immune suppression.

-UV radiation bands UV-C (<280 nm), UV-B (280-320 nm) and UV-A (320-400 nm). UV-B is 1000 times more damaging UV-A.

-Both UV-A and UV-B induce 8-hydroxydeoxyguanosine from guanosine by the action of $^1O_2$.

-UV light energy is insufficient to split water, but it can cleave H_2O_2 to yield .OH (Biochemistry of Oxidative Stress).

-UV-A (320-400 nm) is poorly absorbed by biomolecules, but can produce ROS via chromophores (i.e., porphyrins or flavins).

-UV radiation promotes lipid auto-oxidation.

-Under suitable conditions, UV and visible light can cause ionization of molecules, but usually it is from x-ray and gamma rays.

-Definition of terms:

> Phototherapy - light, UV, etc., is shown on to the skin, such as treating hyperbilirubinemia in babies.
> Photochemotherapy - uses a photosensitizer like, psoralin
> Photodynamic therapy - uses a photosensitizer given to the patient to produce $^1O_2$.
> Photo-oxidative therapy - also referred to as photo irradiative therapy, uses UV light shown on blood which is returned to the body.
> Bio-oxidative therapy - aerobic exercise.
> Autohemotherapy - ozone.
> Photodynamic effect - a photon is absorbed by a photosensitizer and raises it to its lowest triplet excited state, it diffused until it collides with O2 and raises it to its lowest singlet state.

-It is said that after UV light blood treatment, hemoglobin may give off light for months.

RMH Note: I do not have a scientific reference for verification of this.

-Our total skin surface is about 1.8 m^2, one of our largest organs.

-Light passing thru a transparent object, does not change the object.

Radiation damage:

-Direct Action - radiation produces DNA damage

-Indirect Action - radiation hits O_2 producing ROS producing DNA damage

-80% of a cell is H_2O

-H_2O and radiation produces .OH with nine electrons, one of which is unpaired and is a "free radical."

-2/3 of DNA radiation damage is from .OH in mammal cells.

10.6.2 Miscellaneous Iron Factoids

-Normal male ferritin 30-300 mg/l of blood; mean 127.

-Normal female ferritin 20-120 mg/l of blood; mean 46.

-For every mg of ferritin in blood, there is about 8 mg of ferritin stored in cells (Passwater interview).

-Hemosiderin - an iron storage compound.

-Iron is carried in blood by transferrin; normal adult has 200-400 mg transferrin/deciliter of blood.

-70% iron in hemoglobin

-10% iron in myoglobin

-20% iron stored in ferritin - ASA increases ferritin synthesis five times, if free iron is present.

-Hemochromatosis occurs between 3-6/1000 or 0.3 - 0.6% therefore, USA has between 600,000 to 1.6 million cases.

-Each heme group with iron atom binds 1 oxygen molecule, thus, hemoglobin can bind 4 oxygen molecules.

-Transferrin transport iron.

-Ferritin, stores intracellularly, Fe^{++} form, and can hold 4500 iron atoms.

-Formation of oxidized proteins depends upon the presence of iron or copper and requires H_2O_2 and the most sensitive residues are histidine, proline, lysine and arginine

-Some bacteria are attracted to magnetic field lines (magnetotaxis)

-Magnetite ($FeO \cdot Fe_2O_3$) is located in pigeon brains.

-Increased concentration of CO_2 + H^+ promote the release of O_2 from hemoglobin - "The Bohr Effect."

Some other noteworthy oxygen modification molecules to be aware of are:

10.7 OXIDES OF NITROGEN

Nitric oxide (.NO) and nitrogen dioxide (.NO_2) contain unpaired electrons and are therefore free radicals, whereas the 'laughing gas' nitrous oxide (N_2O) is not. **Nitrogen dioxide is a dense brown poisonous gas and a powerful oxidizing agent.** It is found in polluted air, smoke from burning organic materials, and at high levels in cigarette smoke. **Nitric oxide, on the other hand, is a colorless gas and a weak reducing agent**.

Singlet oxygen reacts with unsaturated lipids to form lipid hydroperoxides (LOOHs). Garry Beuttner's group found that beta carotene and vitamin E have only a minor antioxidant effect on $^1O_2$ induced membrane damage; whereas, **nitric oxide seems to be a powerful antioxidant** in lipid peroxidation.

Recently, biological interest in nitric oxide has centered around the observation that **nitric oxide is produced by:**

- **the cells lining our blood vessels (vascular endothelial cells),**
- **certain white blood cells that defend us against foreign organisms,**
- **and some cells in the brain, starting from the amino acid L-arginine.**

In blood vessels, **.NO relaxes muscles in the vessel wall, dilating the vessel and lowering blood pressure. It is sometimes called the 'endothelial-derived relaxing factor', or EDRF.** Organic nitrites such as nitroglycerin and amyl nitrite (a common constituent of the recreational drug 'poppers'), act by a similar mechanism. Although **.NO is biologically essential**, production of excess .NO in patients with severe infections can do harm (e.g., by lowering blood pressure too much and contributing to septic shock).

At body temperature, .NO can combine with oxygen to make .NO_2.

$$2.NO + O_2 \rightarrow 2 .NO_2$$

Among other reactions, **.NO_2 can pull off hydrogen atoms from membrane lipids and initiate lipid peroxidation.**

$$.NO_2 + lipid\ -H \qquad \rightarrow \qquad lipid + HNO_2$$

Hence, oxides of nitrogen are toxic in excess. Indeed, macrophages, cells which help defend us against foreign organisms by using **oxides of nitrogen as one of the mechanisms by which they can kill parasites. In small amounts, oxides of nitrogen (at least .NO) are useful. The same is true of many other free radicals, including $O_2^{.-}$**

As is true with many other demonized oxidizing agents, nitric oxide is a two edged sword in that it can be a prooxidant or antioxidant. It is thought that the antioxidant effect is due to its radical scavenging abilities (Buettner, G., Schafer, F., Kelley, E., Cueno, K., Venkataraman, S. and Wang, H. Nitric oxide as a cellular antioxidant. 2001, POL: ASP 29th Annual Meeting.). This dual type of reactivity only adds to the confusion of the overall consideration of antioxidants and the condition that the oxy-morons refer to as "oxidative stress." Many antioxidants can serve as pro-oxidants.

These inconsistent reactivities of antioxidants and oxidizing agents, make it difficult to say exactly what effect or effects they may produce, unless exacting specificities of the surrounding conditions are known.

10.8 OZONE

The pale blue gas ozone (O_3) provides an important protective shield in the stratosphere against solar UV radiation. At ground level, however, ozone is an unwanted toxic substance, generated in polluted urban air by the action of light on some of the chemicals present. Ozone can also be produced by some scientific equipment and sometimes by photocopying machines. Ozone is irritating to the eyes, nose, and lungs. Indeed, it can oxidize and damage proteins, DNA and lipids directly. **These are direct oxidations, O_3 is not a free radical and does not itself start free radical chain reactions.**

-Autohemotherapy is O_3 (ozone) blood treatment.

-Homozon is nascent ozone in magnesium oxide powder.

Also, please remember the recent work of Barbior, that shows that antibodies react with $^1O_2$ to yield O_3.

**"Singlet oxygen is spawned from the erotic mating ritual
between stately hydrogen peroxide and perky hypochlorite.
From this molecular true romance, is born the excited singlet love-child,
which, within micro-seconds,
rises to be a great leader
of electrons."**

R. M. Howes, M.D., Ph.D.

5/26/04

10.9 SINGLET OXYGEN (EXCYTOMERS)

Singlet molecular oxygen ($^1O_2$) is electronically excited oxygen which is formed in biological systems via enzymatic reactions, radical and non-radical reactions and photosensitization reactions. The photosensitization pathway is thought to be important in light-exposed tissue. The **half-life of singlet oxygen has been estimated to be 10^{-6} to 10^{-5} of a second or as 3-4 micro-sec.** $^1O_2$ can interact with target molecules either by transferring its excitation energy or chemical combination. **Preferential targets for chemical reactions are double bonds; e.g., in PUFAs or guanine bases in DNA.**

Although oxygen (O_2) has two unpaired electrons these electrons are arranged in such a way that O_2 **oxidizes most things very slowly at room temperature.** Indeed, one **theory of aging (the free radial theory)**, essentially states that aging is caused by the slow cumulative oxidation of body tissues over a lifetime. However, I disagree adamantly with this junk science theory.

By simple rearrangement of its electrons, it is possible to make O_2 much more reactive, converting it into singlet oxygen molecules, which are powerful oxidizing agents. For example, O_2 oxidizes lipids at an immeasurably slow rate, but singlet oxygen oxidizes them very fast into lipid peroxides. The rearrangement of electrons that produces singlet oxygen needs energy: the best established source of this energy involves **photosensitization reactions.** When solutions of several colored compounds (dyes and/or pigments) are illuminated, they absorb energy from the light. Some of this absorbed energy can be transferred to O_2, making singlet oxygen ($^1O_2$). This can be a particular problem in green plants: they must be illuminated to drive photosynthesis and convert carbon dioxide (CO_2) from the air into sugars, but the green photosynthetic pigment **chlorophyll can make $^1O_2$.** Compounds present inside the body that are capable of sensitizing $^1O_2$ production include **riboflavin (vitamin B2) and heme. It is generally believed that inside the body they are protected from light.** Others, such as myself, believe that there is considerable evidence to support the findings demonstrating the existence of biophotons and presently, their internal reactivity is unknown and usually not even considered. **I refer to these intracellular light emissions from the many excited state species (especially, singlet oxygen and excited carbonyls) as "nano-lightning."**

However, bright sunlight can damage milk because milk contains riboflavin. The complex reactions of **ozone with several biological molecules also make some singlet oxygen, and some $^1O_2$ is produced during lipid peroxidation.**

Several drugs (including **some tranquilizers, antibiotics and anti-inflammatory drugs), are photosensitizers and can cause skin damage if the patient sunbathes.** Something similar occurs in the porphyrias, a series of disorders in which photosensitizing pigments accumulate in the skin. One striking example is **congenital erythropoietic porphyria**, fortunately a rare disease. The condition presents at, or shortly after, birth with severe **sensitivity to light.** Extensive skin blistering with secondary infection leads to mutilation of exposed areas. The teeth (and bones) may be stained red due by the accumulated pigments and can glow in ultraviolet light. **Excess body hair growth may occur.** An interesting, if fanciful, theory is that these unfortunate individuals with hairy faces and shiny teeth who only ventured forth at night (to avoid the sun) gave rise to at least some of the werewolf legends. King George III of England may have suffered from porphyria, a disease that can be traced back through his ancestors James I and Mary Queen of Scots. The physicians of his day thought that he was suffering from **'evil humors,'** and treated him by blood-letting, using bloodsucking leeches.

Not all photosensitizing reactions are bad for us, however. A mixture of porphyrin derivatives known as **HPD ('hematoporphyrin derivative')** is used in cancer treatment. After injection of HPD, some tumors take it up and then become sensitive to damage and of being killed if they are illuminated. This method is being used to treat some forms of lung cancer, in which the tumor can be illuminated with light from a tube placed down the throat. Fiber optics are also being used.

Evidence has been presented for the **formation of singlet oxygen during the oxidation of NADPH by liver microsomes.** The evidence is based primarily on the enzyme-dependent formation of **dibenzoylethylene from diphenylfuran, a reaction which is specific for singlet oxygen.** The apparent formation of singlet oxygen is coupled to the occurrence of peroxidation of microsomal lipid, a phenomenon known to be associated with NADPH oxidation by the particles. Both the peroxidation of lipid and the apparent formation of singlet oxygen are related to the amount of Fe^{3+} present in the system and the results are consistent with the possibility that **the singlet oxygen formed by this system is derived from the breakdown of lipid peroxide** (King, M.M., Lai, E.K. and McCay, P.B. Singlet oxygen production associated with enzyme-catalyzed lipid peroxidation in liver microsomes. JBC 1975; 250(16): 6496-6502).

Ultraweak chemiluminescence (CL) is associated with the lipid peroxidation chain reaction. Oxidizing systems of fatty acids have been found to emit low levels of light. The excited species responsible for **this CL have been suggested as singlet molecular oxygen and triplet carbonyls.** Mechanisms for the generation of these excited species have been proposed whereby $^1O_2$ and excited carbonyls are formed in the termination step of lipid peroxidation by a "Russell type" mechanism. $^1O_2$ may then react with unsaturated fatty acids to produce excited carbonyls, while **quenching of triplet carbonyls by O_2 may produce $^1O_2$.**

The claim that the combination reaction of superoxide with hydrogen peroxide produces singlet oxygen has been in dispute and conflicting data has been reported (Kellogg, E.W. and Fridovich, I. Superoxide, hydrogen peroxide and singlet oxygen in lipid peroxidation by a xanthine oxidase system. JBC 1975; 250(22): 8812-8817).

Investigators studying the formation of active oxygen species and lipid peroxidation induced by hypochlorite found that tert-butyl hydroperoxide and methyl linoleate hydroperoxide reacted with hypochlorite to give peroxyl and/or alkoxyl radicals with little formation of $^1O_2$. In contrast, **the reaction of H_2O_2 with hypochlorite, gave $^1O_2$ exclusively** (Noguchi, N., Nakada, A., Itoh, Y., Watanabe, A., Niki, E. Arch Biochem Biophys 2002; 397(2): 440-447).

In 1965, Foote, et al. demonstrated that the product selectivities observed in oxygenation using the hypochlorite-hydrogen peroxide system were the same as those obtained in dye-sensitized photo-oxidation (Foote, C.S., Wexler, S. and Ando, W. Tetrahedron Lett 1965; 4111-4118). Results of additional studies of this type were also reported in 1968 by C. S. Foote.

It is stated in Singlet Oxygen $^1O_2$, edited by H. H. Wasserman and R. W. Murray, Volume 40, Academic Press, 1979, page 77 that the **hydrogen peroxide-hypochlorite method** of generating singlet oxygen has been of enormous importance in studies establishing the role of singlet oxygen in photosensitized oxidation. The spectroscopic evidence indicated that **both $^1\Delta_g$ and $^1\Sigma_g^+$ states of singlet oxygen are produced in this reaction.** Using methanol as solvent the efficiency of $^1\Delta_g$ singlet oxygen production can reach 80%

The method has limitations. It clearly cannot be used with substrates which react with hydrogen peroxide. It requires high alkalinity which can be a problem. The reagent has a limited solubility to organic solvents. Its optimum use requires alcohol solvents which are not useful for all substrates.

Adomas Ubanavicius in a paper entitled, "Free Radical Damage in Proteins," described the following pathways for formation of singlet oxygen:

Non-photochemical formation of $^1O_2$
1) Dismutation of $O_2^{\cdot-}$
$$HO_2^{\cdot} + O_2^{\cdot-} + H^+ \rightarrow {}^1O_2 + H_2O_2$$

2) Fenton type reaction
$$O_2^{\cdot-} + H_2O_{2\,(metal)} \rightarrow {}^1O_2 + OH^{\cdot} + OH^{-}$$

3) Reaction with hypochlorite

$$OCl^- + H_2O_2 \rightarrow {}^1O_2 + Cl^- + H_2O$$

4) Reaction with hydroxyl radicals

$$O_2^- + OH^- \rightarrow {}^1O_2 + OH^-$$

5) Reaction with diacyl peroxides

$$2O_2^- + R\text{-}C(=O)\text{-}O\text{-}O(=O)\text{-}C\text{-}R \rightarrow {}^1O_2 + RCO_2^-$$

Photochemical formation of ${}^1O_2$ requires a photon + a sensitizer:

Type I yields free radicals or radical ions

Type II yields ${}^1O_2$, which can further yield O_2^- and H_2O_2 by dismutation

10.9.1 Sources of ${}^1O_2$

In Wasserman and Murray's, 1979's book on Singlet Oxygen, page 598, they list the following sources of singlet oxygen and biological systems:

ENZYMES →	${}^1O_2$
$O_2 + {}^3$ SENSITIZER →	${}^1O_2$
$H_2O_2 + OCl^-$ →	${}^1O_2$
$H_2O_2 + O_2^-$ →	${}^1O_2$
OH. + O_2^- →	${}^1O_2$
O_2^- - e- →	${}^1O_2$
$O_2^- + Y^+$ →	${}^1O_2$
$O_2^- + O_2^-$ →	${}^1O_2$
$H_2O_2 + HO_2^-$ →	${}^1O_2$
OZONIDES →	${}^1O_2$
ENDOPEROXIDES →	${}^1O_2$
RCOO. + RCOO. →	${}^1O_2$

Adapted from Krinsky, N.I. Trends Biochem Sci 1977; 2: 35-38.

A metal source of singlet oxygen has been described as follows:

$$Fe^{2+} + O_2 \rightarrow Fe^{3+} + O_2^- \rightarrow {}^1O_2$$

RMH Note: With my singlet oxygen delivery system, for the treatment of arteriosclerotic plaque, cancer and AIDS, all that remains is oxidized particulate residues, O_2, NaCl and H_2O.

II OXYGEN EXCERPTS

Some of the following excerpts have been taken from **Methods in Enzymology, Vol. 319, Singlet Oxygen, UVA, and Ozone,** Eds. Lester Packer and Helmut Sies, Academic Press, 2000. **(Selective Book Review)**

Page 21- When **singlet oxygen** is generated by photosensitization in cells, it reacts rapidly with nearby biomolecules and is probably entirely consumed during this process rather than returning to the ground state.

Page 25 - ....very few of the **singlet oxygen** molecules generated actually reach the cells, **as singlet oxygen molecules exist ~4 μsec in aqueous solution; during this time they diffuse only about 100 nm.** The singlet oxygen-induced alterations are limited mainly to plasma membrane-associated molecules, as most of the singlet oxygen molecules reaching the cells encounter the membrane first and react with membrane components.

Page 29 - **The photochemical generation of hydrogen peroxide and singlet oxygen by irradiation of TiO_2 and ZnO has also been reported.** The cytotoxicity of irradiated TiO_2 to prokaryotic and eukaryotic cells has been ascribed to the production of these active oxygen species, especially to that of highly reactive hydroxyl radicals. **Despite their known photo reactivity, TiO_2 and ZnO has been widely used in sun screening and cosmetic products without complication. RMH Note: These facts bolster my position that hydrogen peroxide and singlet oxygen can be present in biological systems without producing harmful effects.**

Page 36 - ....removal of superoxide with a spin-trapping reagent was found to enhance the rate of formation of singlet oxygen, as **superoxide effectively quenches singlet oxygen.** Finally, it is noteworthy that **singlet oxygen is very toxic to prokaryotic cells but is almost nontoxic to eukaryotic cells. RMH Note: I believe that this is a most important observation.**

Page 38 - Photoexcitation of chromophores in the presence of oxygen often leads to the production of singlet delta oxygen by a bimolecular energy-transfer process involving the excited chromophores and ground-state triple oxygen, or $^3O_2$.

The quantum yield for singlet delta oxygen production is defined as the number of $^1O_2$ molecules formed per absorbed photon.

Page 49 - **Biological media in vivo is a micro-heterogeneous system as opposed to the homogeneous systems used to calculate $^1O_2$ yields in vitro. RMH Note: Keep in mind that biological media is also heterogeneous as it relates to O_2 concentrations.**

Page 59 - **Both heme-containing peroxidases and nonheme vanadium bromoperoxidases can produce singlet oxygen.** Peroxidases can also oxidize iodide anion. However, with hypoiodous acid, the reaction is endothermic and singlet oxygen is not produced. Singlet delta oxygen gives off light at 1270 nm, but its radiative rate is low due to quantum spin restrictions. Most deactivating collisions between H_2O and $^1O_2$ generate heat as a nonradiative transition. **Delta singlet oxygen is an electronically excited oxygen molecule with 23 kcal per mole more energy than ground state oxygen.** This energy can be released as a 1270 nm photon. **Singlet oxygen lifetime in water is only 3.1 μs but it is in a low steady state level in peroxidase systems.**

Page 64 - Under appropriate conditions,

chloroperoxidase,
eosinophil peroxidase,
horseradish peroxidase,
lactoperoxidase,
myeloperoxidase

and vanadium bromoperoxidases have been shown to produce 1270 nm chemiluminescence (mono-mol emission) characteristic of singlet oxygen. The singlet oxygen dimer has a 634 nm dimol emission.

Page 71 - The formation of $^1O_2$ in biosystems has been, in part, attributed to:

Phagocytosis
Photosensitization reactions
Recombination of peroxyl radicals (from lipid peroxidation)
Peroxidase-catalyzed reactions
Chemiluminescence:

$$^1O_2 \rightarrow {}^3O_2 + h\nu_{1268\,nm} \text{ (unique for } ^1O_2 \text{ in biosystems, monomer)}$$
$$^1O_2 + {}^1O_2 \rightarrow 2^3O_2 + h\nu_{634\,nm} \text{ (dimer)}$$

Page 86 - Photodynamic generation of $^1O_2$ occurs when an appropriate sensitizing agent is photoexcited in the presence of $^3O_2$. $^1O_2$ produced by endogenous sensitizers and 320-400 nm UVA radiation, which passes through the stratospheric ozone layer, is of particular biomedical interest because of its association with skin aging and cancer. However, when generated under carefully controlled conditions using exogenous sensitizers and light in the visible range (400 -700 nm), **$^1O_2$ can be exploited for therapeutic purposes, as for example, in antineoplastic photodynamic therapy (PDT).**

The lifetime of $^1O_2$ in pure water is 4-5 μsec, which corresponds to a mean diffusion distance of 90-100 nm. D_2O **enhances** $^1O_2$ **lifetime ~15-fold relative to** H_2O (Rodgers, M.A.J. and Snowden, P.T. J Am Chem Soc 1982; 104: 5541). However, **in a cell with quenchers abounding, $^1O_2$ lifetime is <50 nsec with a diffusion distance <10 nm from its point of origin, which is less than 0.1% of the radius of an average eukaryotic cell.**

RMH Note: **The lifetime of $^1O_2$, in water, varies depending upon the reference cited.**

Page 110 - The primary photosensitizers in cells are:

Flavines
Porphyrines
Chlorophylls
Quinines
Bilirubin
Retinal
Furocoumarins

Visible light and UVA (320-380 nm) of sunlight can produce $^1O_2$ in biological systems.

In cells, $^1O_2$ can be quenched by:

Carotenoids
Tocopherols
Plasminogens

Page 113- $^1O_2$ **has a much longer lifetime in the gaseous phase (about 10 times) than in a liquid phase and can diffuse "some millimeters" in air.**

Deuterated water by itself causes dramatic effects on the cytoskeleton of cells and arrests cells during interphase (Schroeter, D., Lamprecht, J., Eckhardt, R., Futterman, G. and Paweletz, N. Eur J Cell Biol 1992; 58: 365).

Page 118 - **All catalases are modified by $^1O_2$** but remain active and more acidic and fully active conformers arise.

Page 121 - **Deuterium substitution has been shown on several occasions to increase cell lethality triggered by photosensitization**, but is has rarely been used to demonstrate the involvement of singlet oxygen in transcription factor activation, excerpt for AP-2 activation after UV-A treatment of keratinocytes.

Page 130 - Singlet oxygen ($^1O_2$) is a mediator of UVA-induced expression of these proteins. AP-1, AP-2, and NF-kB are transcription factors found to be activated by UVA. NF-kB is also activated by $^1O_2$, and AP-2 is an integral part of signaling cascade leading from UVA via $^1O_2$ to an enhanced expression of ICAM-1.

More importantly, $^1O_2$ activates JNKs and p38-MAPK only when generated intracellularly. RMH Note: This is a very important point when one considers the therapeutic use of $^1O_2$, such as with my singlet oxygen delivery system.

Page 133 - a solvent effect exploitable in biological systems is the prolonged lifetime of $^1O_2$ in deuterium oxide (**D_2O, approximately 52 μsec) compared to H_2O (approximately 4 μsec)** (Foote, C.S. and Clennan, E.L. in "Active Oxygen in Chemistry " (C.S. Foote, J.S. Valentine, A. Greenberg and J.F. Liebman, eds., p 105 Blackie Academic, London, 1995). **The lifetime of $^1O_2$ depends on the polarity of the solvent.** It is highest (up to >1 μsec) in solvents lacking O-H and C-H moieties, such as $CDCl_3$ or CCl_4.

Page 154 - UVA (320-400 nm) represents more than 90% of the terrestrial UV solar energy. **$^1O_2$ can be produced in cells in "dark reactions" during lipid peroxidation and involve cellular oxidases (peroxidases, cytochromes).**

Page 155 - **$^1O_2$ and DNA interactions are based on quenchers or enhancers but there is no direct evidence of interaction between singlet oxygen and DNA in a cellular system. RMH Note: Please read this line again.**

Page 198 - Researchers have sought methods to generate pure $^1O_2$ in biological media. Up until now, only two anionic naphthalene derivatives, the endoperoxide of sodium 4-mthyl-1-naphthalenepropanoate MNPO$_2$ and of disodium 1,4-naphthalenedipropanoate NDPO$_2$1a, have been used to assess the antimicrobial activity of pure $^1O_2$. The first one kills the wild strain of the bacterium Escherichia coli, but is less effective against lycopene-producing strains, suggesting that lycopene protects E. coli against $^1O_2$ toxicity by scavenging $^1O_2$. The second one is able to inactivate efficiently extracellular enveloped viruses, but has no effect on intracellular viruses. **PDT produces ROS such as .OH, $O_2^{\cdot-}$, peroxy radical ROO. and $^1O_2$, not pure $^1O_2$. RMH Note: The preponderance of the data supports the generation of singlet oxygen with PDT.**

Page 204 - **The virucidal activity of both endoperoxides is actually due to $^1O_2$,** as preheated oxidized form H-NDPO$_2$ and H-DHPNO$_2$ were almost inefficient. Heating (thermolysis) of naphthalene endoperoxides was used to produced $^1O_2$

Page 209 - For PDT viral inactivation in general, lipid-enveloped viruses are more susceptible to PDT than non-enveloped viruses.

Page 216 - In recent years, considerable interest has been focused on the reaction of singlet oxygen with organic compounds and its toxicity toward living cells. Known $^1O_2$ generating systems, such as NaOCl-H$_2$O$_2$, (Kajiwara, T. and Kearms, D.K. J Am Chem Soc 1976; 15: 5886), **myeloperoxidase-hydrogen peroxide (H_2O_2)-halide ions**, and light-photosensitizer-$^1O_2$ systems **contain reactive oxygen species other than $^1O_2$** and often generate free radicals and therefore such systems cannot serve as pure $^1O_2$ generating reactions.

Page 226 - **The quenching of singlet oxygen can occur by synthetic compounds such as the following classes of pi or n-electron containing substrates:**

    olefins,

aromatic and heteroaromatic compounds,
amines,
sulfur compounds,
phenols,
metal chelates,
nonaromatic heterocycles,
and indigoids.

Singlet oxygen is quenched by or reacts with many organic and bioorganic molecules, which possess, in most cases, reactive pi electrons or lone pairs of sufficiently low ionization energy. The quenching process can be physical (the quencher enters a vibrational or an electronic excited state) or chemical (the quencher combines with oxygen or is oxidized by oxygen) in nature. Physical quenching may occur via triplet energy transfer or by simple catalysis of the singlet oxygen ($^1O_2$) $\rightarrow$ ground state oxygen ($^3O_2$) transition via spin-orbit coupling. Charge transfer interactions are important during the quenching process. **In many reactions, intermediates are involved, e.g., exciplexes, diradicals or zwitterions.**

11.1 AUTO-OXIDATION

Autoxidation (auto-oxidation) is a consequence of the aerobic internal milieu of the cell.

Some of the molecules that undergo autoxidation are the following:

**catecholamines,
hemoglobin,
myoglobin,
reduced cytochrome C
Thiol
Cu+
Fe++
Epinephrine
glutathione**

Autoxidation of any of these molecules results in ROS, **primarily superoxide**. Cooper or ferrous ion (Fe II) can also autoxidize to produce **superoxide** and ferric (Fe III).

Autoxidation of epinephrine and glutathione generate $O_2^{\cdot-}$ and H_2O_2.

11.1.1 Enzymatic Oxidation

The following enzymes are capable of producing large amounts of **oxygen free radicals**:

Xanthine oxidase
Prostaglandin synthase
Lipoxygenase
Aldehyde oxidase
Amino acid oxidase
Myeloperoxidase (uses H_2O_2 to oxidize chloride ions to form HOCl)

Strenuous exercise has been proposed to activate xanthine oxidase-catalyzed reactions and generate RONS in skeletal muscle and myocardium.

11.1.2 Oxidative Phosphorylation

Respiratory chain electron carriers can be blocked at three sites. They are inhibited by:

Site 1) Rotenone, piericydin, amytal, steroids, detergents, volatile anesthetics (halothane).
Site 2) Antimycin, hydroxyquinoline, BAL
Site 3) Cyanide, carbon monoxide, azide

Oxidative phosphorylation inhibitors include: rutamycin, oligomycin, and diciclohexicarbodiimide, inactivates both respiration and phosphorylation but does not interfere with electron transport in uncoupled mitochondria. Unlike direct inhibitors of the electron (cyanide, antimycin) they stimulate respiration.

Oxidative phosphorylation uncouplers include:

Substituted phenols (pentachlorophenol and dinitrophenol, **2-DNP**), thyroid hormones, carbonyl cyanide, phenylihydrazone, dicumarol, long chain fatty acids and antibiotics (valinomycin, gramicydin). **RMH Note: Many of these agents can be lethal because of the metabolic site of their action.**

11.2 SUBCELLULAR ORGANELLES

Prokaryocytes are cells that do not have a nucleus or internal membrane structures.

Eukaryocytes have a defined nucleus and intracellular organelles surrounded by membranes, such as yeast, fungi , plants and animals.

Superoxide has been shown to be produced by the following:

    Mitochondria
    Microsomes (endoplasmic reticulum)
    Peroxisomes
    Nuclei
    Chloroplasts (in plants)

The mitochondria are the main site of **superoxide production and can be enhanced by increasing the O_2 concentration or when the respiratory chain becomes fully reduced as happens in ischemia.**

Microsomes are responsible for 80% of the H_2O_2 produced in vivo at 100% hyperoxia sites. Peroxisomes produce H_2O_2 but not O_2^- , under physiological conditions. Peroxisomes are primarily in the liver but other organs contain them. **Peroxisomal oxidation of fatty acids has been recognized as an important source of H_2O_2 with prolonged starvation. This may be involved in increased longevity with caloric restriction.**

11.3 RESPIRATORY BURST

Phagocytic cells attack and destroy invading organisms and cancer cells by consuming large amounts of oxygen in a process called the "respiratory burst." Of the oxygen consumed, 70-90% is converted into the superoxide anion, which readily forms H_2O_2.

This respiratory burst is initiated by the activation of NADPH-oxidase by exposure to:

> **immunoglobulin-coated bacteria,**
> **immune complexes,**
> **complement 5a,**
> **or leukotrienes.**

The biosynthesis of leukotrienes is usually via 5-LO (5-lipoxygenase), which is a non-heme-containing dioxygenase that oxidizes polyunsaturated fatty acids to yield hydroperoxyl fatty acids with conjugated double bonds.

The heme-containing protein complex, NADPH oxidase, con produce large amounts of O_2^{-} and its derivative upon activation. In an inflammatory environment, H_2O_2 is produced by activated macrophages at an estimated rate of $2\text{-}6 \times 10^{-14}$ mol/h^{-1}/cell^{-1} and can reach as high as 10-100 mM in the vicinity of these cells (Nathan, C.F. and Root, R.K. Hydrogen peroxide release from mouse peritoneal macrophages: dependence on sequential activation and triggering. J Exp Med 146: 1648-1662).

11.4 LIPID PEROXIDATION

Lipids are a heterogeneous group of water-insoluable (hydrophobic), organic molecules that can be extracted from tissues by nonpolar solvents. Because of their insolubility in aqueous solutions, body lipids are generally found either compartmentalized, as in the case of membrane-associated lipids and droplets of triacylglycerol in adipocytes, or transported by plasma in association with protein as lipoprotein particles. Lipids are not only a major source of energy for the body, but also provide the hydrophobic barrier that permits partitioning of the aqueous contents of cells and subcellular structures. **Lipids with unsaturated double bonds can act as a trap for singlet oxygen and can also produce ROS, including $^1O_2$.** In addition, lipids provide many functions in the body, for example, some fat-soluable vitamins have regulatory or coenzyme functions, and the prostaglandins and steroid hormones play major roles in the control of the body's homeostasis. Theoretically, deficiencies or imbalances of lipid metabolism may lead to some of the major clinical problems encountered by physicians, for example, atherosclerosis and obesity.

Singlet oxygen ($^1O_2$) is known to be a product of a variety of reactions. Pioneering work by Dr. Steele and I, on microsomal lipid peroxidation (Howes, R.M. and Steele, R.H., Microsomal chemiluminescence induced by NADPH and its relation to lipid peroxidation, Res Commun Chem Path Pharmacol. July-Sept 1971, 2; 4 & 5:619-626) and aryl-hydroxylations (Howes, R.M. and Steele, R.H., Microsomal chemiluminescence induced by NADPH and its relation to aryl-hydroxylations. Res Commun Chem Path Pharmacol 1972; 3(2): 349-357), demonstrated evidence for the generation and participation of electronic excitation states, namely singlet oxygen. This was **the first demonstration of a functional generation of an electronic excitation state, exclusive of vision, in mammalian systems.** Our proposal, that **singlet oxygen is the identity of the long sought out "active oxygen" acting on the cytochrome P450 microsomal mixed function oxidases**, has recently been supported by the work of Yasui et al (Yasui, H., Deo, K., Ogura, Y., Yoshida, H., Shiraga, T., Kagayama, A. and Sakurai, H., Evidence for singlet oxygen involvement in rat and human cytochrome P450-dependent substrate oxidations, Drug Metab Pharmacokin 2002; 17(5): 416-426).

11.4.1 Howes' Observations

While studying widely divergent biological electronic excitation generating systems, such as the microsomal mixed function oxidases, the neutrophil respiratory burst (Howes, R.M., Allen, R.C., Su, C.T. and Hoopes, J.E. Altered polymorphonuclear leukocyte bioenergetics in patients with thermal injury. Surgical Forum, 1976; 27: 558-560), and proline hydroxylation for collagen biosynthesis, **I believed that these oxidative systems shared a point of convergence, expressed in the Howes Excytomer Pathway, involving superoxide anion and electronically excited singlet oxygen** (Howes, R.M., Steele, R.H. and Hoopes, J.E. The role of electronic excitation states in collagen biosynthesis. Persp In Biol and Med 1977; 20(4): 539-544). Furthermore, **I saw an additional commonality with generation of singlet oxygen produced by the steady-state physiological oxidative reagents containing an organic peroxide and the salt of hypohalous acid** (Howes, R.M., Steele, R.H. and Hoopes, J.E., Peroxide induced chemiluminescence in an in vitro proline hydroxylation system, 1976; 8(1): 77-84). Subsequently, I reasoned that the peroxide/hypochlorite oxidative system may represent an ideal method of singlet oxygen delivery for effectively treating premalignant and malignant lesions, while simultaneously eliminating many of the drawbacks associated, not only with PDT, but with all other conventional methods of cancer therapy. This work is presently in progress.

11.4.2 Singlet Oxygen's Role

Singlet oxygen can react with unsaturated lipids to form lipid hydroperoxides (LOOHs). These LOOHs can undergo free radical chain reactions leading to membrane leakage and cell death. There are various steps in these destructive pathways where antioxidants can intercept ($^1O_2$). Beta-carotene (b-Car), a singlet oxygen quencher, could prevent lipid damage at the initiation step. $^1O_2$ + b-Car $\rightarrow$ O_2 + b-Car* $\rightarrow$ O_2 + b-Car + heat. Vitamin E, a membrane antioxidant, can serve as a chain terminating antioxidant, reacting with the OLOOs radical formed during lipid peroxidation: OLOOs + Vit E $\rightarrow$ OLOOH + Vit Es radical. Nitric oxide (NO), a lipid soluble molecule that could also serve as chain terminating antioxidant during lipid peroxidation. **Nitric oxide seems to be a powerful antioxidant in lipid peroxidation. Glutathione peroxidase (PhGPx) is an outstanding membrane antioxidant protecting against this lipid peroxidation via removal of LOOH.** (Schafer, F.Q., Wang, H.P., Kelley, E.E., Cueno, K.L., Martin, S.M. and Buettner, G.R. Comparing [beta]-Carotene, Vitamin E and Nitric Oxide as membrane antioxidants. Biol Chem 2002; 383: 3).

Linoleic acid is the predominant polyunsaturated fatty acid (PUFA) in the human diet. The hydroxyoctadecadienoic acid (HODE) derivatives of linoleic acid, 9(S)-HODE, 9(R)-HODE and 13(S)-HODE, are the most widely distributed of the known linoleic acid metabolites. **HODEs can be generated enzymatically by cyclooxygenase, lipoxygenase and some cytochrome P450s.** However, the bulk of linoleic acid peroxidation, especially generation of 9-HODEs, occurs by non-enzymatic processes so that HODEs are excellent indicators of free radical mediated lipid peroxidation. **Some believe that in mammalian cells, free radicals are derived primarily from peroxide and singlet oxygen**, which are referred to as reactive oxygen species (ROS). ROS-derived free radicals include the superoxide anion and the hydroxyl radical. **Most ROS diffuse only a nanometer or so before reacting. Among the most important targets of free radical reactions in vivo are lipids, and the resultant oxidized lipids**, which can travel throughout the circulatory system, and are thought to be involved in arteriosclerosis.

I feel that the polyunsaturated fatty acids represent a biochemical "sink" or trap for singlet oxygen and this can result in a "deficiency state of excited singlet oxygen" which is manifested most markedly in obese patients. Consequently, obese patients are prone to infections and cancer, which would normally be held in abeyance and kept in check by singlet oxygen.

Researchers have long known that being overweight increases the likelihood that a woman will develop breast cancer. But a new study puts the risk into very real terms: pounds on the scale. Recent data indicates that **women who have gained more than 20 pounds since age 18 have a higher risk of developing breast cancer** after menopause than women who have kept their youthful figures (Fielgelson, H.S. et al. 21 pounds enough to raise breast cancer risk. Cancer Epidemiology Biomarkers and Prevention, 2004; 13(2): 220-224).

ACS researchers questioned more than 62,000 postmenopausal women about their height, current weight, weight at age 18 and use of hormone replacement therapy (HRT). After accounting for other breast cancer risk factors, like family history of the heart disease, exercise and alcohol use, they found that women who gained 21-30 pounds since age 18 had a 40% higher risk of breast cancer than women who'd stayed within 5 pounds of their teenage weight. **Those who had gained more than 70 pounds had double the risk.** (Lesser weight gain, between 6 -20 pounds, had little effect on risk, less than 10%).

The findings applied only to women who had never used hormone replacement therapy (HRT) or who were no longer using it. Among women who were using HRT at the time of the study, weight gain did not appear to influence risk, probably because **HRT "trumps" weight as a factor in breast cancer development.** Both HRT and excess fat raise estrogen levels, which increases the risk of breast cancer. But the researchers said HRT raises estrogen so much that even a lot of extra weight has only a minimal effect by comparison.

11.5 ESTROGEN

Millions of women have quit taking the estrogen-progestin combination since 2002, when federal scientists warned that those pills raised the risk of breast cancer (26% increase), strokes and heart attacks. It wasn't clear if taking estrogen alone was safe. Now (3/2/2004), **the NIH is telling 11,000 women that it is shutting down its study of estrogen-only use, because of increased risk of stroke and dementia**. I feel that these studies support my **Unified Theory** in that **estrogen-progestin or estrogen alone acts deleteriously through a single mechanism which decreases oxygen free radicals** and thereby makes these patients susceptible to many diseases. Studies have shown that estrogen acts as an antioxidant and therefore decreases the levels of reactive oxygen species and excitation states (Persky, A.M., Green, P.S., Stubley, L., Howell, C.O., Zaulyanov, L., Brazeau, G.A. and Simpkins, J.W. Protective effect of estrogens against oxidative damage to heart and skeletal muscle in vivo and in vitro. Proc Soc Exp Biol and Med 2002; 223(1): 59).

12 FREE RADICAL PATHOLOGY

12.1 FREE RADICALS AND ANTIOXIDANTS IN AGING AND DISEASE

If is difficult these days to open a popular science magazine or medical journal without seeing an article about the role of free radicals in human disease. Women's magazines contain articles about the use of 'antioxidant creams' to prevent aging of the skin, and health food stores are full of pamphlets and books describing how antioxidant or dietary supplements can prolong life, protect youth or prevent disease. Is there any truth in all of this?

Halliwell and Gutteridge **defined "antioxidants" as any substances that are able, at relatively low concentrations, to compete with other oxidizable substrates, thus, to significantly delay or inhibit the oxidation of these substrates** (Halliwell, B. and Gutteridge, J.M.C. *Free Radicals in biology and Medicine* (2nd ed.). Oxford, UK: Clarendon, 1989). This includes a vast array of compounds, such as amino acids and proteins, which serve as RONS scavengers. **Intracellular concentrations of free amino acids is on the order of 10^{-1} M and thus, they are important RONS scavengers**. Especially sensitive to attack are tryptophan, tyrosine, histidine and cysteine.

Three points are worth stating:

1. **There is no evidence that consuming more antioxidants will prolong the natural human life span**.

2. There is reasonable evidence that eating diets rich in fruits and vegetables decreases the incidence of cancer and heart disease. However, such diets contain thousands upon thousands of compounds and to try to attribute their benefits to a handful of chemicals is nonsense. Antioxidants present in such diets (including ascorbic acid, vitamin E and carotenoids), may cause this effect, or contribute to it.

Other factors may be equally or more important, however. For example, whole-grain cereals contain natural chelating agents (such as phytic acid), that might diminish iron uptake by the human gut. Some authors have suggested that high body iron stores may predispose to cancer and heart disease.

3. **Free radicals are formed in greater amounts during all human diseases (i.e., some degree of oxidative stress probably occurs in all diseases). This does not mean that free radicals cause disease, or that they contribute to its course. They may be there in a healing capacity.** Similarly, a number of toxins cause oxidative stress (Table 1), but it does not mean that this is the major mechanism by which they cause damage.

Significant research over the past decade has shown that ROS are not all bad for plants and animals and they assist survival by performing delicate balancing acts within the cell triggering reproduction and death (apoptosis). They also tell plants to prepare to adapt to stress-inducing conditions.

12.1.1 Oxidative Stress as a Cause of
Human Tissue Injury

What is the exact role played by oxygen-derived species in human disease? Some human diseases may be caused by oxidative stress. Thus, gamma-rays generate .OH by splitting water molecules:

$$H_2O \rightarrow .OH + H.$$

Many of the biological consequences of excess radiation exposure may be due to free radical damage to proteins, DNA and lipids, since .OH attacks all these molecules. The signs produced by chronic dietary deficiencies of selenium (e.g., Keshan's disease) or of tocopherols (neurological disorders seen in patients with defects in intestinal fat absorption) might also be mediated by oxidative stress. In the premature infant, exposure of the undeveloped retina to elevated concentrations of oxygen can lead to **retinopathy of prematurity**, which in most severe forms can result in blindness. Several clinical trials have documented the efficiency of a-tocopherol in minimizing the severity of the retinopathy, consistent with (**but by no means proving**) a role for lipid peroxidation. Another suggestion is that the risk of bleeding within the brains of premature infants may be minimized by giving a-tocopherol. Free radicals are also probably involved in the consequences of exposures to elevated O_2 concentrations, to certain toxins (Table 1), and in diseases that result in deficiencies of antioxidant defense enzyme or increases in the amounts of iron and copper in the body (Table 2).

12.1.2 Toxins that Cause Oxidative Stress

Table 1. Some Toxins that Impose Oxidative Stress in Human Tissues

Toxin	Consequences
Cigarette smoke	Rich source of free radicals. May contribute to destruction of lung elastic fibers (causing emphysema) and to lung cancer. However, cigarette smoke also contains hundreds of compounds.
Asbestos	Asbestos fibers contain iron and catalyze Conversion of H_2O_2 to .OH. It is speculated that this contributes to lung injury and lung cancer induced by this toxin.
Alcohol	Excess alcohol intake may deplete vitamin E and GSH in cells and increase iron uptake from the gut.
Adriamycin	A quinine drug, used to treat leukemias. Its major side-effect, heart damage, may involve free radicals.
Carbon tetrachloride	CCl_4 causes severe liver damage: lipid peroxidation is involved.
GSH-depleting agents	Anything that depletes GSH can make cells more prone to oxidative damage. Examples of drugs that can do this are **acetaminophen and cocaine**.
Metal ions	Poisoning by excess intake of **iron, copper, manganese, nickel, cadmium, chromium and lead may involve GSH depletion** and free radical generation.
Air pollutants	Ozone (O_3) and nitrogen dioxide ($.NO_2$) are powerful oxidizing agents. $.NO_2$ may induce peroxidation of lipids in the lung by abstracting hydrogen from polyunsaturated fatty acid side chains $$NO_2. + lipid\text{-}H \rightarrow HNO_2 + lipid.$$ O_3 can oxidize lipids and proteins directly. Sulphur dioxide (SO_2) toxicity has been suggested to involve free radicals.

12.1.3 Some Disorders to which Oxidative Damage may Contribute Significantly

(Table 2)

Ionizing-radiation-induced tissue injury
Consequences of chronic selenium deprivation
Consequence of inborn defects in antioxidant defense enzymes
Neurological disorders caused by chronic vitamin E deprivation (in diseases affecting intestinal fat absorption)
Retinopathy of prematurity (retrolental fibroplasia)
Tissue injury in copper-overload disease (Wilson's disease)
Tissue injury in iron-overload diseases (idiopathic hemochromatosis, thalassaemia)
Cataract induced by ionizing or ultraviolet radiation
Consequences of exposure to elevated O_2 levels
Ultraviolet-light-induced skin injury

12.2 TISSUE INJURY AS A CAUSE OF OXIDATIVE STRESS

Although oxidative stress may play an important role in some human disease, it is probably safe to say that most (and perhaps all) forms of tissue injury themselves lead to oxidative activity.

When body tissues are damaged, neutrophils and other phagocytes enter the damaged area. These cells become activated, releasing O_2^- and HOCl, that can help to remove foreign organisms at the injury site. However, this also imposes a stress on the surrounding tissues. For example, **HOCl can oxidize thiol (~SH) groups on proteins.** When tissues are crushed or torn, iron can be released from cells, both a free iron and in the form of heme-containing proteins (such as myoglobin), and as the storage protein ferritin. **Free iron can convert O_2^- and H_2O_2 into highly damaging .OH. O_2^- can cause a limited release of iron from ferritin, and H_2O_2 can release iron from heme proteins.** Heme proteins can accelerate lipid peroxidation. Since **the iron content of human tissues increases with age**, perhaps iron is mobilized in greater amounts as a result of injury and free radical damage becomes more severe in injured older tissues but **also keep in mind that oxygen consumption and hemoglobin levels decrease with age.**

Table 3. **Some Examples of Ischemic Injury in Human Disease**

Stroke
Myocardial infarction, angina pectoris
Reattachment of severed limbs
Frostbite
Shock due to excessive blood loss (O_2 supply to many body tissues is impaired)
Shock due to other causes (shock results in low blood pressure, which cuts O_2 supply to many tissues) Severe crash injury

12.2.1 Ischemia-Reoxygenation

All ischemic conditions reinforce the prime importance of maintaining normal oxygen levels in order to maintain a condition of health.

An apparently **"paradoxical" cause of oxidative stress** in human disease is ischemia-reoxygenation (Table 3). If body tissues are deprived of O_2, they are injured and will eventually die. This is because O_2 is needed for mitochondria to make the cell's energy currency (ATP) and mitochondria are the major source of ATP in most human cells. One example of this ischemia injury is the tissue damage resulting from application of a tourniquet to an injured limb for too long, cutting off the arterial blood supply. Stroke and myocardial infarction are other examples. In stroke, a blood clot forms in an artery in the brain, shutting off the blood supply to part of this organ. In a myocardial infarction (heart attack), a clot forms in one of the coronary arteries that supply the heart itself with blood.

Deprivation of blood flow, and the resulting deprivation of O_2 cause many metabolic changes. **Ischemic tissues become more acidic (their pH falls), ATP levels drop, and iron ions are released from storage sites.** Mitochondria may be disrupted. One change that has attracted much attention in the medical literature is that ischemic tissues increase their levels of xanthine oxidase, an enzyme that uses O_2 to oxidize xanthine and hypoxanthine into uric acid. The O_2 is converted into both O_2^- and H_2O_2 during this process. Hypoxanthine also accumulates in ischemic tissues because it is made as ATP levels drop.

When a tissue is ischemic, the O_2 supply must be restored as fast as possible before the cells die. For example, clot-dissolving agents such as streptokinase may be injected into patients who have suffered a heart attack **However, the restoration of O_2 (although essential), produces oxidative stress upon the tissue: this is the "paradox" of reoxygenation injury.** Damaged mitochondria may be 'leakier' than normal, so that, when they start working again, more electrons escape from the correct path in the electron transport chain and form $O_2^{.-}$. Once O_2 is available, xanthine oxidase can oxidize the accumulated hypoxanthine, **making $O_2^{.-}$ and H_2O_2.** If iron has been released within the tissue, .OH may form and worsen the damage. **The paradox is that, although restoring the O_2 is essential, the restoration adds an additional insult to the tissue in the form of so called oxidative stress.** Reoxygenation injury makes little difference if the tissue has already been killed by the ischemia but may be a significant additional source of injury after brief periods of O_2 deprivation. Another problem is that reoxygenation of badly damaged ischemic tissue can wash metal ions, xanthine oxidase, and other potential toxins into the bloodstream and injure other body tissues (Table 3).

If tissue injury leads to oxidative stress, does this then make a major additional contribution to the injury, or is it insignificant? The answer probably differs in different diseases (Table 4). Several diseases in which an important role for oxidative stress is envisaged by some, will now be briefly discussed.

Table 4. Some Disease in which Oxidative Stress is a Consequence of the Disease but Might Make Some Contribution to Tissue Injury

Atherosclerosis
Stroke (if reperfusion occurs before irreversible injury to tissue)
Myocardial infarction (if reperfusion occurs before irreversible tissue injury)
Rheumatoid arthritis
Inflammatory bowel diseases (Crohn's disease, ulcerative colitis)
Shock
Traumatic injury to brain and spinal cord

Rheumatoid arthritis and other chronic inflammations

Rheumatoid arthritis is a chronic inflammation of the joints, producing painful swelling and loss of mobility. It may result in disabling destruction of the joint. **The rheumatoid joint is a site of intense oxidative stress, for reasons unknown, large numbers of macrophages and neutrophils are present, releasing $O_2^{.-}$, H_2O_2, HOCl, .NO and other potentially damaging products.** Bleeding within the joint can raise its iron content, allowing .OH formation. **A comparable situation exists in the inflammatory bowel diseases, in which there is excessive accumulation and activation of phagocytes in the gut, causing severe damage.** Ulcerative colitis is one example.

A likely possibility that I envision is that the macrophages and neutrophils are present in large numbers in attempts to kill or oxidize stealth pathogens.

12.2.2 Brain and Spinal Cord Injury

In the test tube, damaged brain tissue undergoes lipid peroxidation very fast, one reason being that iron is very easily released from disrupted brain cells. In addition, **brain tissue is very rich in polyunsaturated fatty acid side chains, the levels of antioxidant defense enzymes in the brain are only moderate,** and the fluid surrounding the brain (cerebrospinal fluid), has little transferrin and so cannot bind released iron. **RMH Note: I find it very important that a critical organ, such as the brain, which has such a high oxygen consumption rate, has low levels of antioxidants. This alone argues against the free radical/oxidation theory.** Free radical reactions probably occur in damaged brain tissue after injury (e.g., that caused by a blow to the head). It has been **suggested that these reactions worsen** the consequences of initial injury to the brain or spinal cord, by spreading the damage into surrounding areas. Similar free radical reactions may occur after stroke, spreading the damage beyond the ischemia area.

12.3 ADULT RESPIRATORY DISTRESS SYNDROME (ARDS)

ARDS, acute respiratory failure due to clogging of the lungs with fluid (edema), can arise in patients with several different serious problems, including major infections, serious injury, severe shock, extensive burns and inhaling the contents of the stomach into the lungs. **The hallmark of ARDS is an accumulation of large numbers of neutrophils in the lung, where they are thought to become activated and produce $O_2^{\cdot-}$, H_2O_2 and HOCl.** It is widely believed that this oxidative stress contributes to the lung injury and edema in ARDS. Although the occurrence of oxidative stress has been demonstrated in ARDS patients, **there is as yet no direct evidence that it is a major contributor to the lung injury.**

12.4 EYE INJURY

The development of opacity of the lens of the eye (cataract) in old people involves oxidation and cross-linking of lens proteins. Its development can be accelerated, presumably by free radical mechanisms, as a result of exposure to ionizing radiation or to ultraviolet light. Bleeding within the eye or the accidental introduction of an iron object into the eye can cause severe damage, in which iron-dependent free radical damage has been implicated. For example, **the retina is rich in polyunsaturated fatty-acid side- chains and appears prone to undergo lipid peroxidation**.

12.5 RETINOPATHY OF PREMATURITY (ROP)

Retinopathy of prematurity (ROP) is a potentially blinding disease affecting the retinas in premature infants. The retinas are the light-sensitive membranes at the back of the eyes. In infants who are born prematurely, the blood vessels that supply the retinas are incompletely developed. Although blood vessel growth continues following birth, the vessels may sometimes develop in an abnormal, disorganized pattern, known as ROP. **In many affected infants, the changes associated with ROP spontaneously subside. This is another example of spontaneous regression and the body's ability for self-cure and follows my Unified Theory.** However, in others, ROP may lead to retinal detachment and visual loss. In addition, even in cases in which ROP changes spontaneously cease or regress, affected children may have an increased risk of certain eye (ocular) abnormalities, including nearsightedness, misalignment of the eyes (strabismus), and/or future retina detachment. Major risk factors of ROP include a low birth weight, premature delivery and exposure to high levels of supplemental oxygen following birth. However, **many babies on high supplemental oxygen do not develop ROP or any other ocular diseases. Keep in mind that a cause is always followed by its effect, if it is a true cause/effect relationship.**

12.6 HOW CAN OXIDATIVE STRESS BE TREATED?

Oxidative activity is probably an inevitable accompaniment of disease. This is as it should be and is consistent with my **Unified Theory.**   In some diseases, it may make a significant contribution to the disease pathology, whereas in others (perhaps most) it does not. **I firmly believe that the increase in oxidative metabolites is the body's attempt to control or cure respective disease processes.** How can disease-related oxidative stress be dealt with?

Eating a diet rich in fruits and vegetables will ensure adequate levels of antioxidant nutrients in the tissues and help the body to resist disease-related oxidative stress. I feel that the fact that **fresh fruits and vegetables contain significant quantities of hydrogen peroxide and that they contain large quantities of pigments such as chlorophyll**, tannins, flavonoids and carotenoids, that they also likely contain high levels of the products of excited state chemistry, all of which can be beneficial. Some believe, for example, if levels of vitamin E in the brain are subnormal, the consequences of a stroke, or of traumatic injury, that the damaging effects may well be more severe because uncontrolled lipid peroxidation could spread the injury to surrounding areas.

In general, trials of antioxidants in the treatment of human disease have given unimpressive results to date, except in disease in which oxidative stress may be causative (e.g., retinopathy of prematurity, hemolytic syndrome in premature babies, neurological degeneration caused by tocopherol deficiency in patients unable to transport fats through the gut, and Keshan's disease). Several speculative reasons can account for this:

1. **Oxidative stress may occur, but be unimportant in the pathology of that particular disease**.
2. Insufficient antioxidant has been used to reach the site of which it is needed or to remove enough radicals.
3. The wrong antioxidant has been used. Oxidative stress affects many different processes. If, in a particular situation, direct free radical damage to proteins or to DNA was the important injury mechanism, then an inhibitor of lipid peroxidation is unlikely to be protective.
4. Antioxidant has not been administered long enough.

12.7 THE AGING PROCESS: ARE FREE RADICALS INVOLVED?

We are all aging and will eventually die. The maximum human life span is probably around 110-120 years, but few people in the third world achieve it because of early death due to malnutrition, accidents or infection. In the USA and Europe, such deaths are rare. The few people who die under age 35 usually do so as a result of accidents, although deaths from AIDS are becoming significant. Older people in Europe and the USA more often die of myocardial infarction or cancer. **The incidence of cancer varies strikingly with age**. A few cancers occur in young people, such as cancer of the testis and some types of leukemia. For most cancers, however, the rate of incidence rises very sharply with age, i.e., an age-related disease. **It takes many years to accumulate all the different changes in DNA that are needed for most cancers to develop.**

The reasons for aging have been the subject of considerable speculation, but there is little or no hard information. Many years ago, it was realized that the basal rate of metabolism of animals (i.e., how fast the cells are working when the body is at rest) is approximately inversely related to their life span; in general, larger animals consume less O_2 per unit of body mass than do smaller ones, and they live longer. This data suggests that aging is somehow related to O_2 metabolism, and there have been many speculations that free radicals are involved. Thus, the faster O_2 is consumed by an organism, the more free radicals it might make.

The Free Radical Theory of Aging, as proposed by Denham Harman in 1956, postulates that accrual of macromolecular damage induced by reactive oxygen species is the central causal factor promoting the aging process. A large body of correlative evidence is possibly consistent with the predictions of this hypothesis; however, **there is no convincing evidence that free radicals cause the aging process. Antioxidant defenses do not appear to fail with age, nor is there any great accumulation of oxidatively damaged molecules. Feeding antioxidants to mammals in the laboratory has never been convincingly shown to make them live longer.** As one ages, tissues deteriorate, and this could lead to secondary free radical damage, as might all forms of tissue injury. Thus, claims that antioxidants, royal jelly, or any other potion will make you live longer awaits scientific support. Nevertheless, enhancing the antioxidant status of the body may possibly help prevent the development of age-related disease that appear to involve free radical-mediated processes.

12.8 LIPOFUSCIN

Postmitotic cells, such as neurons, cardiac myocytes, skeletal muscle fibers and retinal pigment epithelial cells **progressively accumulate** a brown-yellow, auto-fluorescent electron-dense material called **lipofuscin**, which is often called age pigment and considered a hallmark of aging. This is not only because the amount of lipofuscin **increases with age, showing an almost linear dependence, but also, and more importantly, because the rate of lipofuscin accumulation correlates with a shorter lifetime.** However, this same linear relationship or association can be shown for many other measurable parameters which have no known causal relationship to aging such as wrinkles, hair loss, blinking, etc. and makes this observation speculative.

Lipofuscin is a chemically and **morphologically polymorphous waste material**, originating from a variety of intracellular structures, and which accumulates at the primary site of waste disposal ~ **the lysosome**. What makes a small fraction of autophagocytosed material not degradable, resulting in its accumulation within lysosomes? It has been repeatedly shown that oxidative stress promotes lipofuscin formation, whereas antioxidant defense prevents it. In this regard, oxygen free radical mediated oxidation may make cellular components indigestible by lysosome enzymes.

Although senescent cells display a variety of functional disorders, it is still not clear to what extent such disturbances may be consequent to lipofuscin accumulation. However, the increased amounts of iron within lipofuscin granules may promote generation of ROS, sensitizing cells to oxidative injury through lysosome destabilization. As is true for all cellular functions, the capacity to produce lysosome enzymes for **autophagy** is not unlimited, and the attempts to digest large amounts of lipofuscin, accumulated within numerous secondary lysosomes, should eventually result in failure of essential lysosomal functions, such as autophagocytosis. In this regard, insufficient renewal of mitochondria might have the most serious consequences because (i) these organelles are vulnerable to their own production of superoxide, (ii) lack of normal mitochondria may result in reduced ATP generation, and (iii) the accumulation of damaged mitochondria may be a cause of additional oxidative damage, since they generate even more RONS.

"Obfuscation of scientific truth.
by the deceptive smoke of meaningless associations
and the arcane mirrors of manipulated data,
must be eschewed.
We must demand scientific exactitude."

R. M. Howes, M.D., Ph.D.

PART III - A CRITICAL REVIEW OF SELECTIVE ANTIOXIDANTS, VITAMINS...

13 THE FREE RADICAL PHANTASM: A PANOPLY OF PARADOXES

The scientific data concerning antioxidants, vitamins and dietary supplements is rife with contradictory claims, misstatements of fact and out and out lies. Profit or other forms of gain appear to be the primary motive for this area of deception.

Although initial studies with antioxidants held great promise, in keeping the heart and blood vessels healthy, rigorous recent studies have shown that antioxidant pills, such as vitamins A, C and E, are useless and possibly harmful.

13.0 PLACEBO

Unquestionably, the mind has great control over many physiological events, as was seen with "Beaumont's window." Physical disease triggered primarily by mental factors is called psychosomatic, from the Greek words *psyche*, meaning mind, and *soma*, meaning body. Studies have shown that the interactions between the mind and the body are complex, as is evidenced by **"the placebo effect."** When a new drug is tested on volunteers, some of them are given the drug and some of them get a chemically inert substance (a placebo) made to look the same as the drug. The term placebo was originally used as a derisive epithet to refer to treatment provided by non-physicians and not knowingly or deliberately prescribed by a physician.

In the 16th century, Montaigne observed that, physicians, in general, are a danger to their patients. Shakespeare's view was disclosed in Henry IV and Warwick, "a body… distempered… to his former strength may be restored with good advice and little medicine."

Many studies have shown that where a drug recipient knows what its effect is supposed to be, he or she may show that effect, even when they have received the placebo. **More than one third of patients suffering from pain of one sort or another, get relief from placebo analgesics** and doctors commonly prescribe harmless substances, knowing that patients, believing that the drug will cure them, will in fact be cured. Placebos have been used to successfully treat many conditions, including headaches, seasickness, insomnia and epilepsy and some cures have been effectuated even when the patient has known that the drug is a placebo. Please keep in mind that **some placebo's effectiveness may be related to the cost and/or unpleasantness of the treatment** and injected placebos seem to be more effective than oral ones. Visits to holy places and shrines, such as Lourdes, seem more effective among people who have to travel a long distance, than among those who live nearby.

Religiosity is a nearly universal human characteristic and played an important part in the history of medicine. In the Middle Ages, the Church focused on the healing powers of

Christ to weaken beliefs in Asclepios and in pagan rituals. Christ was referred to as the **Apothecary of the Soul** and medical treatment was scorned as interference in God's plan. This ultimately led to the medico-religious movement and to Phineas P. Quimby, a well known 19th century healer, whose famous patient was Mary Baker Eddy, the founder of **Christian Science**. Quimby stated, "But through a great many mistakes, and the prescription of a great many useless drugs, I was led to re-examine the question, and came in the end to the position I now hold: **the cure does not depend upon any drug, but simply upon the patient's belief in the doctor or the medicine.**"

Ironically, faith healers and psychic healers may have been historically more effective than traditional medical treatments because they allowed nature to take its course with self-cure; whereas, traditional medications not only were ineffective but also often harmed patients and even hastened their demise. This may well be the case in many forms of current medical practices.

Characteristics shared by placebo and quackery are: the changing theories of how the product works, what illness it is effective against, repackaging of the old treatment to fit the fad of the day and reliance on testimonials. This sounds like an apt description of current weight loss fads, beauty aids, vitamins, dietary supplements, hormone replacements, etc.

To illustrate the power of placebo, I present a quote of Alyce Green, Beyond Biofeedback, which is as follows:

"Occasionally, I had heard half-joking remarks about researchers in biofeedback sounding like snake-oil salesmen. It didn't bother me until one of our own doctors cautioned against the concept of biofeedback as a panacea. Then, I gave it serious thought. Why did biofeedback prove helpful in the treatment of so many and varied disorders? Suddenly, I realized that it isn't biofeedback that is the "panacea"-- **it is the power within the human being to self-regulate, self-heal, rebalance. Biofeedback does nothing to the person; it is a tool for releasing that potential.**"

Some of the following excerpts were taken or modified from: H. Brody, The Placebo Response. Harper Collins, 2000.

Ancient times utilized treatments, such as powdered mummy or crocodile dung in just as serious and logical manner as any of our modern pharmaceuticals. As was said by Arthur K. Shapiro, in 1969, "Since almost all medications until recently were placebos **(RMH Note: ...and most probably still are placebos),** the history of medical treatment can be characterized largely as the history of the placebo effect."

Shapiro states that the word **"placebo" is Latin for "I shall please"** and was first used in the Middle Ages referring to vespers sung for the dead. Benjamin Franklin was assigned to investigate, in France, the validity of Franz Anton Mesmer's theory of animal magnetism and likely introduced the concept of the "blind" control. Franklin and his fellow commissioners ruled that it was the imagination of the subjects, and not influences of any fluid, that accounted for mesmerism. The bad connotation of the placebo effect has carried over till today, although it is unquestionably an important factor for healing.

What I refer to as our body's system of **"self-cure," has previously been referred to as "spontaneous healing."** Plato believed in the healing power of words and that the spoken word's influence on an ill patient's mind might lead to a cure, even if the words were lies. We are all familiar with the power of suggestion. The writings of **Hippocrates**, which were likely a collection of writers, somewhat rejected the notion of persuasion and **believed that close adherence to the proper treatment acts as the healing agent. Reportedly, Hippocrates emphasized diet but discouraged fruits and vegetables. The Hippocratic triad consisted of bleeding, purging and starvation. Galen's humoral theory** of medicine shared beliefs with Chinese and Hindu ayurvedic medicine and allowed that mental influences were just as capable as physical influences in establishing a balance of the humors (sanguine, melancholy and phlegmatic). Paracelsus relied on the principle of *similia similibus curantur* ("like cures like"). In the 15th century, he also vigorously opposed the senseless poly-pharmacy of his day, observing that **medicine killed and nature healed.**

Today, as in the past, many physicians believe that cures secondary to the patient's imagination or to the power of suggestion is the work of quacks and charlatans; whereas, their own cures are due solely to skill, pharmaceuticals and in-depth medical knowledge. Placebo surgery has been described to relieve abdominal pain with a sham appendectomy or hysterectomy and thoracotomy has been used to relieve the pain of angina pectoris, all with reported good results. **Dr. Henry Beecher**, a Harvard anesthesiologist, hailed "the powerful placebo effect" and published his results using double-blind randomized trials in 1955. Medicine of the 20th century proceeded by primarily ignoring the effects of the mind on healing. I recall lectures by Dr. Galant, during my medical and graduate school studies, and his insistence that most of the effects (up to 90%) that we attributed to medications, were, in fact, due to the placebo effect. Being a student of both biochemistry and medicine and one who had amassed huge amounts of recallable cognitive data, I wondered, "How could a professor of psychiatry be so stupid? Didn't he know anything?" Subsequent years of experience, time, study and observation has taught me to **"open my mind"** to all such possibilities.

**"In order for the body to maintain homeostatic normalcy,
it's self-contained, chemical-cornucopia
must be stocked piled
with the component curatives which constitute**

a personal 'pharmacopoeia.'
We know this from observation,
yet, we tend to disavow its presence and
to ignore its impact.
And the wheel goes *round in circles.*"

R.M. Howes, M.D., Ph.D.

8/23/04

Interesting examples of the placebo effect are as follows:

- Dr. Robert Ader, University of Rochester, found that rats respond to the anti cancer-drug, cyclophosphamide, with a drop in the immune cell count; whereas, saccharin had no such effect. After co-administration of the two compounds, using a variety of schedules resulted in **many of the rats having a drop in immune cell counts to saccharin alone.** This effect could be strengthened (reinforced) or unlinked (extinction).

- Dr. Marianella Castes, a Venezuelan physician, conditioned 42 children to receive 2 daily doses of an active asthma medication, from an inhaler containing a vanilla aroma. After 15 days, **the conditioned group showed measurable improvement in lung function, when given the vanilla aroma, without the active medication.** Further, she showed that there could be a conditioned response to the metered-dose device (inhaler), if it was filled with water instead of any active medication.

- Studies have shown that if patients with pain were switched from an effective analgesic drug to placebo, the patients remained pain-free long past the "die-away" period of the active drug.

- Placebos were more effective when they followed active and effective drug therapy.

- Hypertensive patients taking beta-blockers maintained a normal pressure much longer when the beta-blocker was discontinued if the received a placebo, than if they got no medication at all. Similarly, the blood pressure response was far beyond the "wash out" period of the beta-blocker.

- Dr. Lawrence Egbert, Harvard anesthesiologist, studied 97 patients scheduled for major abdominal surgery in a double blind test. One group was extensively briefed on the post surgery pain expectations; whereas, the other group had a very limited pre-surgery visit. Neither the surgeons nor the nurses knew which patients were in which group. The **patients given the lengthy pre-surgery pain expectations used one-half as much pain medicine as the control group** and this group was discharged an average of 2 days earlier than the controls. Egbert argued that this was a **"placebo effect without the placebo."**

- Without a functioning cortex, there can be no placebo effect, e.g., therapeutic doses of atropine given to a decorticate subject, produces predictable effects on the gastrointestinal mucosal; whereas, the same dose , in a subject with an intact cortex, will have variable effects that are related to the subject's psychological state. This effect likely extends to drugs such as barbiturates, digitalis, thyroid hormone, and vitamins....surgery... and as an inevitable concomitant of all therapy.

- Physicians attribute the use of placebos to other physicians three times as often as they attribute it to themselves.

We must not forget **the nocebo effect (Latin for "I shall harm").**

Placebos can lower blood pressure, decrease pain, lower sugar in diabetes, relieve asthmatic attacks and perhaps shrink some malignant tumors.

The biochemical **"stress pathways"** have been implicated in the following disease processes: hypertension, hardening of the arteries, heart attacks, osteoporosis, memory loss, accelerated aging, stomach ulcers, fibromyalgia, chronic fatigue syndrome, eczema and vulnerability to infections. The stress may affect the hypothalamus, which lies outside the blood-brain barrier, to secrete corticotropin-releasing hormone (CRH), which causes release of cortisol. **Cortisol** can in turn raise blood sugar levels, cause salt and fluid retention and **reduce the body's inflammatory and immune responses.**

Dr. Robert Ader introduced the term **"psychoneuroimmunological"** response relative to mind-body interactions. It is believed that the conscious mind is powerless over the immune system, according the Dr. Brody and psychoneuroimmunology has taught us that **the immune system is responsive to nervous stimulation. Nervous stimulation seems to release IL-1, which causes the hypothalamus (which appears sensitive to incoming signals from the immune system) to release CRH, which triggers release of cortisol.** This seems to explain why people who have undergone stressful life changes, like death of a loved one, severe depression, or divorce, seem to be more prone to disease. Thus, the immune system seems to be affected by both the mind and the nervous system.

Drs. Gunver Kiele and Helmut Kiene, research institute in Freiburg, Germany, assert that there is no incontrovertible evidence for the placebo effect. **(RMH Note: How do they explain the mystery of the sugar pill?)**

During the 19th century, two outstanding scholars expressed their poignant views concerning pharmaceuticals and medicine as follows:

1) Sir Oliver Wendell Holmes said, "If the whole materia medica ... could be sunk to the bottom of the sea, it would be all the better for mankind and all the worse for the fishes."

2) Sir William Osler stated it this way, "The battle **against poly-pharmacy**, or the use of a large number of drugs (of the action of which we know little, yet we put them into bodies of the action of which we know less), has not been fought to a finish... the characteristics of the New School is firm in a few good well-tried drugs, little or none in the great mass of medicines still in general use... It is more concerned that a physician shall know how to apply the few great medicines which all have to use, such as quinine, iron, mercury, iodide of potassium, opium and digitalis, than that he should employ a multiplicity of remedies the action of which is extremely doubtful." However, the brilliant Dr. Osler used cupping, leeching, questionable drugs and venesection.

13.0.1 Antioxidants: A Panoply of Paradoxes

Studies of antioxidant biochemistry is particularly confusing because "nothing is cut and dried." **There exists a "panoply of paradoxes" created by intertwined multifactorial variables.** It is rarely pointed out that **many antioxidants become free radicals (pro-oxidants)** when they take electrons from the free radicals which they inactivate. Also, research shows that antioxidants taken individually do not provide a complete defense against free radicals, even theoretically because, even under the best of circumstances, no one antioxidant destroys or scavenges different free radical species. The chemical properties of each oxygen free radical is different and reacts differently with each proposed antioxidant. The properties of each antioxidant enzyme is quite different and some of them actually generate oxidants. Confusing terms and concepts are everywhere. With such confusion rampant, it makes the concept of "oxidative stress" a hodgepodge of conflicting data and terms and, in my opinion, renders it useless. In fact, **I believe that the "free radical phantasm" is counter productive to the advancement and understanding of oxygen metabolism.** The many silly metaphors used to describe free radicals defies common sense, in that they are so simplistic and so far removed from the complexities of the living/breathing cell.

The major antioxidants used to preserve food products are monohydroxy or polyhydroxy **phenol compounds** with various ring substitutions. These compounds have low activation energy to donate hydrogen. **The resulting antioxidant free radical does not initiate another free radical due to the stabilization of delocalization of radical electron. The resulting free radical is not subject to rapid oxidation due to its stability.** The antioxidant free radicals can also react with lipid free radicals to form stable complex compounds. Other antioxidants used on food preservation fall into two categories as follows: 1) natural antioxidant, such as tocopherols (delta, gamma, beta, alpha), nordihydroguaretic acid (NDGA), sesamol and gossypol and 2) synthetic antioxidants, such as butylated hydroxy anisole (BHA), butylated hydroxy toluene (BHT), propyl gallate (PG) and tertiary butyl hydroquinones (TBHQ).

Metal chelators deactivate trace that are free or salts of fatty acids by the formation of complex ions or coordination compounds and are compounds such as phosphoric acid, **citric acid**, ascorbic acid and ethylene-diamine-tetra-acetate (EDTA).

The efficiency of antioxidants are affected by: 1) activation energy, 2) oxidation-reduction potential, 3) stability to pH and 4) solubility. To have maximal efficiency, primary antioxidants are often used in combination with other phenolic antioxidants or with various metal chelating agents. Synergism of multiple antioxidants can occur.

Most studies show the benefits of eating fresh fruits and vegetables but they fail to point out that these fruits and vegetables are made up of thousands and thousands of complex compounds. Yet, studies are presented in a manner, which suggests that a mere handful of extracted vitamins and synthetic antioxidants are the verified agents responsible for the beneficial effects of fresh fruits and vegetables. **This is nonsense** and only recently have investigators attempted to determine the actual active chemical form of the respective vitamins and synthetic antioxidants.

Large epidemiological studies have attempted to compare groups of patients who are taking various antioxidants and to draw conclusions of disease causality from the data. We know that this step biases the data from the very beginning. Additionally, it is almost impossible, except at a few well-controlled academic dietary centers, to know all of the chemical constituents ingested in a wide array of diets. In a like manner, many drugs and pharmaceuticals affect antioxidant levels and their reactivity. These drugs must also be taken into account in evaluating data. For example, **pharmaceutical drugs that can cause antioxidant deficiencies** include acetohexamide, amitriptyline, amoxapine, **aspirin**, atorvastatin, benzthiazide, beta-blockers, bumetanide, cerivastatin, chlorothiazide, chlorpromazine, chlorpropamaide, chloestyramine resin, choline magnesium trisalicylate, choline salicylate, clomipramine, clonidine, colchicine, colestipol, corticosteroids, desipramine, doxepin, ethacrynic acid, fluphenazine, fluvastatin, furosemide, glimepiride, glimepiride, glipizide, haloperidol, hydralazine, hydrochlorothiazide, hydroflumethiazide, imipramine, indapamide, isoniazide, lovastatin, mesoridazine, methyclothiazide, methyldopa, metolazone, mineral oil, neomycin, nortiptyline, oral contraceptives, perphenazine, polythiazide, pravastatin, prochlorperazine, promazine, promethazine, protriptyline, quinethazone, simvastatin, thiethylperazine, thiroidazine, tolazamide, tolbutamide, torsemide, trichlormethiazide, trifluoperazine and trimipramine.

I am astounded at the level of the rhetoric of the uninformed, that is against oxygen free radicals, in their attempts to sell their even less informed customers their 21ˢᵗ century snake oil. Statements such as the following are a perfect examples:

" On a global scale, oxidative stress has claimed more lives than all of the wars and plagues throughout human history. It causes all of the degenerative diseases that go hand and hand with aging. Nothing causes more human misery or ends more lives prematurely". They go on to say, "To give you an idea of how much damage free radicals can do, consider that these renegade molecules strike and fracture every single one of your DNA molecules 10,000 times a day. About 9,900 of these breaks in the DNA strands are restored to normal by DNA repair enzymes. About 100, or 1%, escape the enzyme's notice. This unrepaired damage accumulates over time, setting the stage for atherosclerosis, cancer and other degenerative diseases. You can see why slowing the damage--by increasing antioxidant protection--translates into longer life span (www.bodyandfitness.com/Information/Health/antioxidant.html)."

This kind of intentional misuse of medico-scientific data is a classic example of the kinds of tripe that perpetuates the free radical/oxidation hoax. This illustrates the **"free radical phantasm."** It brings to mind a quote of the late Adlai Stevenson, (1900-1965), United Nations Ambassador, who said, **"There is nothing more horrifying than stupidity in action."**

More importantly, **the free radical/oxidation theory repeatedly does not hold up to scientific scrutiny and yet its proponents continue to push it for their own selfish reasons**.

In an article which appeared in the March 10, 2004 issue of JAMA, investigators analyzed the actual causes of death in the USA in 2000. Although most diseases and injuries have multiple causes and several factors and conditions that may contribute to a single death, **free radicals and/or oxidative stress is not mentioned a**

single time in the entire article. The authors state that, "Biological characteristics and genetic factors also greatly affect risk of death. In most studies we reviewed, low educational levels and income were associated with increased risk of cardiovascular disease, cancer, diabetes and injury." **(RMH Note: Thus, am I to deduce that people with lower educational and income levels have higher levels of O_2 consumption and consequently higher levels of RONS/excytomers, which the Free Radi-Crap theory states leads to cancer? Of course not, but that would be the conclusion of the oxy-morons.)** These authors conclude that smoking remains the leading cause of mortality. However, poor diet and physical inactivity may soon overtake tobacco as the leading cause of death. These findings, along with escalating healthcare costs and aging population, argue persuasively that the need to establish a more preventive orientation in the US healthcare and public health systems has become more urgent. (Mokdad, A.H., Marks, J.S., Stroup, D.F. and Gerberding, J.L. Actual causes in the United States, 2000, JAMA 2004; 291(10): 1238-1245).

13.0.2 Chemoprevention

Chemoprevention is a pharmaceutical approach to arresting or reversing the process of carcinogenesis during cancer's typically prolonged latent period (often 20 years or more) before invasion or metastasis occurs. Surging scientific and public interest in applying chemoprevention strategies to people in the general population that have been identified to carry even slight increases in the risk of developing cancer (e.g., genetic risk), is fueling the identification of exciting new chemopreventive agents. **Once we gain insight into cancer causation, then we can concentrate on prevention.** Some now argue that future development of chemopreventive agents offers greater potential for the long-term control of cancer than the much more widely studied and aggressively pursued chemotherapy agents. Attempts to use antioxidants as chemopreventative agents have failed.

13.1 SETTING THE RECORD STRAIGHT

13.1.1 Cardiovascular Disease

Because oxidative stress is believed to play an important role in the development of atherosclerosis, antioxidants such as beta-carotene and vitamin E have been touted and lauded for prevention of atherosclerosis progression and of adverse cardiovascular events and mortality. Countless books and lay publications constantly make claims that these agents can prevent cardiovascular disease and cancer. **Findings from randomized trials have failed to support this hypothesis, and some trial results have even suggested harmful effects of antioxidants.**

In a meta-analysis of large, randomized, controlled trials (7 on vitamin E, totaling 81,788 patients; 8 on beta-carotene, **totaling 138,113 patients),** Cleveland Clinic investigators assessed the effect of these antioxidants on all-cause and cardiovascular mortality. **In these trials, vitamin E did not reduce all-cause mortality compared with control treatment, nor did it decrease risk for cerebrovascular accident or cardiovascular death. Compared with control treatment, beta-carotene slightly -- but significantly -- increased risks for all-cause mortality and cardiovascular mortality.**

This huge quality study debunked the myths of the near miraculous healing powers of vitamin E. Instead, it clearly **showed no benefit** in the control or reversal of cardiovascular disease of in the prevention or control of strokes. More importantly, **the studies showed that beta carotene actually increases the risk of death and heart disease**. Incredibly, this work can not be found in the lay literature or on popular news programs.

These meta-analysis data show that beta-carotene and vitamin E fail to limit adverse cardiovascular events and that beta-carotene may actually increase risk for cardiovascular death. In view of these findings and recent U.S. Prevention Services Task Force recommendations (Journal Watch Cardiology, Aug 22, 2003), beta-carotene should not be used to prevent adverse cardiovascular events. **Current data are insufficient to indicate any cardiovascular benefit from vitamin E supplementation, so it should not be recommended routinely as preventive therapy.** (U.S. Preventive Services Task Force, Routine vitamin supplementation to prevent cancer and cardiovascular disease: recommendations and rationale. Annals 2003; 139: 51-55).

The U.S. Preventive Services Task Force (USPSTF) is a group of health experts that reviews published research and makes recommendations about preventive health care.

Cardiovascular disease (CVD) and cancer are two of the most common problems for Americans. Shortages of antioxidant vitamins (vitamins A, C. and E, beta-carotene and folic acid) are associated with the blood vessel changes that occur in CVD. Therefore, people have thought that taking these vitamins might reduce the chances of developing CVD. Similarly, information suggests that these vitamins might lower a person's chances of developing cancer. Many studies have examined associations between particular vitamins and CVD and cancer. The studies vary in quality and their **results often conflict**.

The USPSTF reviewed published studies to evaluate whether taking vitamins A, C and E, beta-carotene or folic acid (alone, in combination, or as part of a multivitamin tablet) lowers people's chances of developing CVD. The USPSTF rated the quality of each study to decide how heavily to weigh it in the recommendations. The review examining CVD appears in the 1 July, 2003 issue of Annals of Internal Medicine. In addition, the USPSTF performed another review to see whether taking the same vitamins lowers a person's risk for cancer. This review is available from the Agency for Healthcare Research and Quality (http://www.preventiveservices.ahrq.gov).

The authors of the review on CVD found that **the highest-quality studies did not show that vitamins consistently or meaningfully decreased CVD**. The highest-quality studies assigned people at random to take either vitamin supplements or a placebo pill. Placebo pills looked like the vitamin but contained no active ingredients. In these types of studies, the groups of people are similar in all regards except for taking vitamins. A fair number of studies with weaker designs suggested an association between taking vitamins and less CVD. However, in the weaker studies, the people who took vitamins may have had healthier behavior in general, such as better eating and exercise habits. The authors of **the article on vitamins and cancer found no convincing evidence that vitamins prevented cancer. In two high-quality studies, smokers taking beta-carotene supplements developed cancer more often than those who did not take beta-carotene.**

Supplementation with these nutrients has not been successful as a means of reducing cardiovascular morbidity and mortality. Studies have been done to assess the effectiveness of vitamin supplementation, specifically vitamins A, C and E; beta-carotene; folic acid; antioxidant combinations; and multivitamin supplements in preventing cardiovascular disease.

Some good-quality cohort studies have reported an association between the use of vitamin supplements and lower risk for cardiovascular disease. **Randomized, controlled trials of specific supplements, however, have failed to demonstrate a consistent or significant effect of any single vitamin or combination of vitamins on incidence of or death from cardiovascular disease**. (Morris, C.D. and Carson, S. Routine vitamin supplementation to prevent cardiovascular disease: A summary of the evidence for the U.S. Preventive Services Task Force. Ann Intern Med 2003; 139(1): 56-70).

To answer the question of vitamin supplementation for the prevention of cardiovascular disease, the USPFTF arrived at the following conclusions:

1. **Evidence is insufficient** to determine if vitamins A, C or E multivitamins with folic acid, or antioxidant combination reduce CVD risk.

2. **Beta-carotene should not be used for preventing CVD**; it does not decrease the risk for CVD, and **it may increase risk for lung cancer** and all-cause mortality in smokers, especially heavy smokers.

3. Vitamin supplements may nevertheless be beneficial for overall health in patients with dietary insufficiencies. Smokers should not take beta-carotene supplements, however, because of the potential risk.

These USPSTF guidelines conclude that **there is a lack of compelling data to show that routine vitamin supplementation is effective for primary or secondary prevention of cardiovascular disease**. The guidelines are consistent with a recent meta-analysis of studies on vitamin E and beta-carotene, which suggested that these 2 antioxidants do not reduce CVD risk and that beta-carotene may increase risk for all-cause and cardiovascular mortality. (Journal Watch Cardiology, Aug 22, 2003). (USPSTF. Routine vitamin supplementation to prevent cancer and cardiovascular disease: Recommendations and rationale. Ann Intern Med 2003; 139: 51-55).

13.1.2 Vitamin B

Data published in the New England Journal of Medicine on June 24, 2004, found a negative effect in a large study of stents with the use of vitamin B. **High doses of vitamin B, previously thought to help keep arteries clear after a coronary stent is inserted, actually do the opposite**, researchers found. Howard C. Hermann, University of Pennsylvania cardiologist, stated that **the latest results "raise the disturbing possibility that a therapy has previously been considered safe may actually be harmful."**

B vitamins are known to help reduce levels of homocysteine, an amino acid that has been linked to worsening coronary artery disease. In theory, getting rid of excess homocysteine in the body could help stents work better. Recent studies by German and Dutch researchers found the higher rate of "restenosis," in which arteries close up again, sent patients back for repeat surgery. Of those taking vitamins, 15.8% had to have repeat angioplasties, compared with only 10.6% of those taking the placebo.

Doctors will likely now be wary of high-dose, vitamin B therapy in heart patients, particularly those with stents.

13.1.3 Cancer

Since the hypothesis of Peto et al. (Peto, R., Doll, R., Buckley, J.D. and Sporn, M.B. Can dietary beta-carotene materially reduce human cancer rates? Nature 1981; 290: 201-209), in 1981 that beta-carotene might reduce the incidence of cancer, especially lung cancer, evidence that accumulated from observational studies that people eating more fruits and vegetables, which are rich in beta-carotene (a violet to yellow plant pigment that acts as an antioxidant and can be converted to vitamin A by enzymes in the intestinal wall and liver) and retinol (an alcohol chemical from of vitamin A), and people having higher serum beta-carotene concentrations had lower rates of lung cancer. Of the diverse components of fruits and vegetables, beta-carotene was considered the best candidate for a chemopreventive effect; its antioxidant activity provided a plausible mechanism. Epidemologic studies, strongly buttressed by chemoprevention bioassays using potent carcinogens in animals, made vitamin A and its analogues excellent candidates for chemoprevention in humans. In 1983, the National Cancer Institute approved a proposal to initiate pilot studies of the safety and feasibility of a chemoprevention trial of beta-carotene and retinol in smokers and in asbestos-exposed workers at high risk for lung cancer. After pilot studies showed successful recruitment, negligible toxicity and excellent adherence, a 10 times larger recruitment for testing efficacy was launched in 1988; stepwise recruitment was completed in September, 1994. Thus, **the beta-carotene and retinol efficacy trial (CARET)** tested the combination of 30 mg beta-carotene and 25,000 IU vitamin A against placebo in 18,314 men and women at high risk for lung cancer.

The CARET active intervention was stopped 21 months early because of clear evidence of no benefit and substantial evidence of possible harm; there were 28% more lung cancers and 17% more deaths in the active intervention group. (Omenn, G.S., Goodman, G.E., Thornquist, M.D., Balmes, J., Cullen, M.R. and Glass, A. et al. Effects of a combination of beta-carotene and vitamin A on lung cancer and cardiovascular disease [see comment citation in Medline]. N Engl J Med 1996; 334:1150-1155). Promptly after the January 18, 1996, announcement that the CARET active intervention had been stopped, preliminary findings from CARET regarding cancer, heart disease and total mortality were published.

The CARET findings of excess lung cancers and excess deaths in the intervention group receiving beta-carotene and vitamin A, including the 23% excess in lung cancers, in male smokers, confirm results reported in 1994: **The ATBC trial in 29,133 male smokers** in Finland found an **18% excess of lung cancer in participants receiving beta-carotene** (The effect of vitamin E and beta carotene on the incidence of lung cancer and other cancers in male smokers. The Alpha-Tocopherol, Beta Carotene Cancer Prevention Study Group [see comment citations in Medline]. N Engl J Med 1994; 330: 1029-1035), now updated to 16% excess. **Vitamin E had no effect and showed no interaction with beta-carotene in the ATBC study. The ATBC finding was largely dismissed and ignored** by those confident that the beta-carotene was responsible for the inverse association of fruit and vegetable intake with lung cancer risk (and heart disease risk, as well) in the epidemiologic literature. With these detailed results from CARET, the combined weight of the evidence is highly consistent and troubling. **These proven dangerous agents continue to be pushed upon the unknowing public.**

The long-awaited results from EUROSCAN (i.e., the European Study on Chemoprevention With Vitamin A and N-Acetylcysteine), the randomized two-by-two factorial **trial of vitamin A (retinyl palmitate) and N-acetylcysteine in patients with treated cancers of the lung or head and neck, show no benefit from either agent alone or from the combination.** Among 2592 participants who received maximal tolerable doses for 2 years with a mean follow-up of 49 months, 916 experienced recurrence, second primary tumor, or death. **The findings were analyzed exhaustively.** (van Zandwijk, N., Dalesio, O., Pastorin, U., de Vries, N. and van Trinteren, H. EUROSCAN, a randomized trail of vitamin A and N-acetylcysteine in patients with head and neck cancer or lung cancer. J Natl Cancer Inst 2000; 92: 977-986).

Hypothesis-driven chemoprevention of lung cancers, when put to the test of randomized large-scale clinical trails, **so far has been disappointing,** unlike important successes with selective estrogen receptor modulators for breast cancer and non-steroidal anti-inflammatory drugs and cyclooxygenase-2 inhibitors for familial colonic polyps. Once the carcinogenic processes have been initiated, prevention of cancers becomes much more problematic. **The most reliable methods of reducing the incidence of cancers depend on avoidance of known carcinogenic agents, including UV radiation, tobacco, alcohol, various infectious agents, medical exposures to certain pharmaceuticals and hormones, ionizing radiation, and environmental and occupational exposures to a moderately long list of chemicals.** (Goldman, L. and Bennett, J.C., editors. Cancer Prevention, Chap 190 in: Cecil textbook of medicine. 21st ed. Philadelphia, PA Saunders; 2000; pp. 1032-1035).

Retinoids are among the most promising classes of chemopreventative agents. Their many proliferation-suppressing, differentiation-enhancing cellular effects and actions on specific receptor targets in the nucleus have given them an extraordinary laboratory basis for clinical testing. Retinoids have reduced tumor incidence and tumor mass and have extended tumor latency when animals were treated before, during or -- most importantly -- after exposure to initiating and/or promoting agents. The International Agency for Research on Cancer has recently published a series of four handbooks of cancer prevention, covering non-steroidal anti-inflammatory drugs, carotenoids, vitamin A and then nine specific retinoids (including all-trans-retinoic acid, 13-cis-retinoic acid, 9-cis-retinoic acid, and 4-Hydroxyphenyl retinamide). Unfortunately, **none of these retinoids appears to have a therapeutic index or a pattern of biologic responses suggesting better results than the vitamin A ester retinyl palmitate produced in EUROSCAN.** Nevertheless, it is plausible that 13-cis-retinoic acid, 9-cis-retinoic acid and even retinyl palmitate may be effective in yet-to-be-defined subgroups of patients. Retinoid X receptor-selective agents do have the advantage of avoiding teratogenic side effects.

Lung cancer is a formidable foe. It is the leading cause of deaths due to cancers in both women and men. Treatment results are very disappointing in the majority of patients. The risk of lung cancer in former smokers does not fall upon cessation of smoking; it just stops increasing (thereby yielding slower relative risk, compared with continuing smokers). **Chemoprevention has yet to succeed, either in primary prevention in high-risk normal populations or in secondary prevention in patients with aerodigestive cancers.** Primary prevention trials with a-tocopherol with or without beta-carotene in the **Alpha-Tocopherol, Beta-Carotene (ATBC)** Trial in 29,133 smokers in Finland and with beta-carotene plus retinal palmitate in the **Beta-Carotene and Retinol Efficacy Trial (CARET)** in 18,254 smokers, former smokers and asbestos-exposed workers in the United States found striking increases in lung cancer incidence, pointing to beta-carotene as potent human carcinogen. After inconsistent results from four much smaller secondary prevention trials, EUROSCAN now shows no benefit from retinyl palmitate and/ or N-acetylcysteine in a large number of patients with previously treated lung or head and neck cancer, of whom 93% were current or former smokers.

The strategy of relying on low-cost vitamins and existing pharmaceuticals as potential cancer chemoprevention agents reflects both the desire to have **cost-effective approaches** for the general population and the fact that prevention has had a much lower priority to date than therapy for **investment by pharmaceutical companies** and even by national agencies. Successes are needed in chemoprevention to build confidence that we have the capability not only to design or discover effective agents but also to recruit study populations in which to demonstrate their efficacy. Basically, we need "positive controls" for the testing of larger numbers of new agents, based on mechanisms, validated intermediate end points, variation in subgroups of the population, and **cost-effectiveness in a cost-conscious health care environment.**

13.1.4 Miscellaneous Cancer Factoids

-Prostate cancer is the most common cancer in US men and second most lethal, killing 31,900 in 2000 (NCI, 1996).

-Most DNA (97%) does not code for anything.

-Leukemia is the most common childhood cancer.

-Cancer increased steadily between 1973 and 1996 overall, cancer incidence in US rose by 1.1%/yr or about 11,000 more cases per 1,000,000 people each year.

-Cancer is multi-stage 1) initiation (nitrosoamines) 2) promotion (PCBs) 3) progression.

-Meat and Cancer - suspected N-nitroso compounds

        Polycyclic aromatic hydrocarbons

        Heterocyclic amines (HCA)

-Humans inherit 3×10^9 base pairs of DNA from each parent.

-Therefore, each cell has 6×10^9 different base pairs, that can be a target for substitutions (mutations).

-Single base substitutions are more apt to occur when DNA is being copied; for eukaryotes that means during the S phase of the cell cycle (Mutations Website, J. Kimball).

-In humans and mammals, uncorrected errors (mutations) occur at the rate of about $1/50,000,000$ (5×10^7) nucleotides added to the chain. Therefore, with 6×10^9 base pairs in human cells, each new cell contains some 120 new mutations.

-Each new baby probably harbors at least one newly-arisen harmful mutation (maybe as high as 3).

-Anticancer quinones - anthrocyclines, such as doxorubicin or daunorubicin are affected by glutathione peroxidase activity (O_2 Paradox, page 470).

- Almost from inception, tumors shed cells in circulation. From animal models, it is estimated that a 1 cm tumor sheds > 1,000,000 cells/24 hrs into venous circulation. But the probability of a tumor becoming metastatic estimated at < 1: 1 million. (Merck Manual, Sec. 11, chap. 142).

- Theoretically, removal of a primary tumor can result in rapid growth of the metastatic lesions.

- Overall, cancer patients (cervix, head and neck cancer, bronchiogenic cancer, bladder and prostate cancer) with low hemoglobin levels have a lower local control and survival. Patients transfused to get Hgb levels above 13.5 g/dl showed significant improved local control rates (radiation).

-Chemicals causing cancer in lab animals reproductive organs such as the testes, breast, prostate, etc. (Toppari et al. 1996):

    DDT
    PCBs
    Dioxin
    Bispherol-A
    Phthalates

- Up to $750,000 worth of drugs can be sold to a single cancer patient.

- Gaston Naessen's 714-X satisfies cancers increased need for nitrogen and the attraction of camphor to cancer cells.

- Tumor cells have a H_2O_2 intolerance, due to insufficient peroxidase and catalase levels. Please remember that it is stated that tumor cells produce high levels of H_2O_2.

-Most anti-cancer treatments from radiation to chemo, produce oxidative events to kill cancer cells.

- In general, it has been said that if the body is too alkaline there will be bacteria problems and if it is too acid, there will be cancer problems.

- Diesel exhaust has 15 carcinogenic substances including: acetaldehyde; antimony compounds; arsenic; benzene; beryllium compounds; bis(2-ethylhexyl) phthalate; dioxins; and dibenzofurans; formaldehyde; inorganic lead; mercury compounds; nickel; POM (including PAHs); and styrene. (IARC) A cup of coffee has 9 carcinogens. A study published Aug.20. 2004 in the International Journal of Cancer stated, "Our study found that the risk of ovarian cancer increases with exposure to diesel exhaust." However, their studies did not support the previous findings suggesting an association between engine exhausts and risk of esophageal, testicular, kidney or bladder cancers. **RMH Note: This is just a glimpse of the confusion seen with epidemiologic associations. I am sure that they could also find associations, if they evaluated individuals wearing blue shirts, while driving Volvos or those wearing jeans and eating ice cream. Personally, I feel that much of this type of data clouds the real picture.**

- 20 HCAs (Heterocyclic amines)- food derived, have been identified as dietary carcinogens.

- **10^9 breast cancer cells are estimated to be the smallest body burden that, on average, can be detected by clinical and radiological means.**

- Micro-metastasis, a relative term, refers to a nodule containing 10^5-10^6 cells, will escape clinical and radiological detection, but will be a few hundred micrometers in diameter. (Tannock)

- Cancers with rare metastasis are brain, head and neck and cervix. **Most patients who die from cancer have subclinical metastatic disease at the time of diagnosis and most cancer deaths are due to metastasis.**

- Dietary fats affect cancer of breast, colon, prostate and pancreas. Tumor promotion is directly correlated to total amount of fat in the diet. **RMH Note: This is because fats (double bonds) trap RONS/excytomers and thus, increases cancer growth and aggressiveness.**

RMH Note: The free radical theory of aging states that the ROS leaked during oxidative metabolism cause DNA damage which accumulates to ultimately result in cancer in the elderly. If this is cancer's cause, then why are some newborns born with cancer or why does cancer develop in babies, especially leukemia? Also, why do many elderly patients die of heart disease, but are cancer free.

-Cancer incidence increases with approximately the fourth power of age.

-Studies link bladder cancer in women to diabetes and lack of physical activity. **RMH Note: I believe this is due to impaired PMN generation of RONS and $^1O_2$ and decreased oxygen uptake.**

- **Fraga calculated that 8.6×10^4 oxidized DNA residues are formed in one cell in a day and estimated that one oxidized DNA residue is formed for every 7.6×10^5 oxygen radicals (ROS) generated by aerobic cellular metabolism.**

The median age for diagnosis of cancer is 67 and the number of cancer cases will double by 2050.

-A low calorie diet increases life span and decreases cancer rate and it involves the SIR2 protein. It activates the pituitary adrenocorticotropic axis that leads to a decrease in the release of reproductive and mitogenic hormones (insulin, TSH, growth hormone, estrogen and prolactin).

-In the initiation phase of cancer, mutants either 1) activate cellular proto-oncogenes or 2) inactivate tumor-suppressor genes (Page 9).

-Four processes leading to cancer or DNA damage are: 1) oxidation, 2) methylation, 3) deamination and 4) depurination (Page 10).

-Total number of oxidative hits to DNA/cell/day is 10^4 in man and 10^5 in the rat (Page 11). **RMH Note: Lambin says, "on the oxygen paradox" that aging and cancer have a common cause. Then, how do you explain newborn or childhood cancer, if it is directly linked to aging. Or, how about the many elderly that at death, are cancer free. Thus, there is NO common cause.**

-1 in every 2000 O_2 molecules (0.44%) consumed is diverted to oxidize DNA and RNA.

-Brachytherapy - radioactive material put in the body.

-In Europe, 14% of all cancer patients are cured with radiotherapy as the sole treatment and 10% in combination with surgery or chemotherapy.

-About 50% of all cancer patients are treated with radiotherapy (Page 24).

-**Bleomycin requires free radicals for cell killing.**

14 DIABETES AND ANTIOXIDANTS

Free radicals are highly reactive molecular by-products produced in all cells as a result of normal metabolism, and are thought to participate in aging, and disease. (Harman, D. Free radical theory of aging. Mutat Res 1992; 275: 257-266), (Halliwell, B. and Gutteridge, J.M. Free radicals in biology and medicine. Oxford: Oxford University, 1989), (Shigenaga, M.K., Hagen, T.M. and Ames, B.N. Oxidative damage and mitochondrial decay in aging. Proc Natl Acad Sci USA 1994; 91:10771-10778). **This flawed theory is now being stringently applied by the oxymorons to diabetes mellitus (DM)**. Because of their essential role in cellular metabolism, mitochondria are the chief sources of free radical production. (Shigenaga, M.K. Hagen, T.M. and Ames, B.N. Oxidative damage and mitochondrial decay in aging. Proc Natl Acad Sci USA 1994; 91: 10771-10778), (Lenaz, G. Role of mitochondria in oxidative stress and aging. Biochem Biophys Acta 1998; 1366: 53-67).

14.1 BASIC BIOCHEMISTRY

Mitochondria are the sites of electron transport which is the process of passing electrons through the respiratory chain of proteins located in the inner mitochondrial membrane. This creates a transmembrane pH gradient that drives the production of ATP. This frequently (3-5%) results in an electron bonding to an oxygen molecule outside the respiratory chain. This single reduction, or transfer of a single electron, creates a molecule with unpaired electrons, referred to as a free radical. There is thought to be an inherent inefficiency in the process of transferring electrons through the chain, which increases with age and disease. Thus, many believe that aging and disease are associated with increased levels of free radicals, a condition known as **oxidative stress**. (Betteridge, D.J. What is oxidative stress? Metabolism 2000; 49: 3-8).

These free radicals are essentials of aerobic life and I strongly believe that they are products of intentional evolutionary design for the overall benefit of the organism.

Hyperglycemia is a hallmark of diabetes and elevated glucose levels are associated with increased production of RONS by several different mechanisms. Certain factors improve mitochondrial RONS production, such as activation of protein kinase C or NF-kB and the formation of advanced glycation end products and antioxidants appears to improve dysfunction of endothelial cells or increased platelet aggregation. However, all of the evidence linking free radicals to diabetogenesis is circumstantial.

14.2 MITOCHONDRIAL DAMAGE

Excessive production of free radicals or their inadequate neutralization by antioxidants, can lead to the in vitro damage of proteins, lipids, and DNA. Because of their proximity to the source of free radical production, mitochondrial constituents become primary targets of free radical damage. For example, it has been estimated that an individual produces approximately **1 kg of oxygen radicals per year, the consequence of which is approximately 100,000 oxidative "attacks" on mitochondrial DNA per cell each day** (Shigenaga, M.K., Hagen, T.M. and Ames, B.N. Oxidative damage and mitochondrial decay in aging. Proc Natl Acad Sci USA 1994; 91: 10771-10778). The cumulative and inevitable effect of these "attacks" on mitochondrial DNA is an increased frequency of mutations, (Michikawa, Y., Mazzucchelli, F., Bresolin, N., Scarlato, G. and Attardi, G. Aging-dependent large accumulation of point mutations in the human mtDNA control region for replication. Science 1999; 286: 774-779), which likely results in the production of proteins with impaired function. However, quick calculations of 5% RONS/day (out of the 250 gms of O_2 used each day) gives 4,563 gms or 4.5 kg/year. Seen another way, a 70 year old has produced 319.2 kgs of RONS in a life time or he has generated 4.45 times his body weight in free radicals in his life time, just from the electron transport chain alone. **Nonetheless, I am amazed that a human can survive in good health and free of major diseases for up to a century, while being assaulted or "attacked" by these oxidative mutagenic events, which I calculate to be ~7.5 times 10^{17} power over a 100 year lifetime. I believe that this fact alone, debunks the oxy-moronic free radical theory of aging. The overwhelming quantities of oxygen and its modifications can hardly be "detoxified" by milligram amounts of antioxidants.**

Because of the fundamental role that mitochondria play to fulfill physiological energy requirements, and the pathological repercussions that occur when this function is challenged, the pharmacological use of antioxidants is frequently recommended as a cure-all approach to supplement endogenous defenses.

Some believe that it is clear that increased oxidative stress is associated with a variety of pathological conditions including diabetes, atherosclerosis and cardiovascular disease, and neurodegenerative diseases. (Haffner, S.M. Clinical relevance of the oxidative stress concept. Metabolism 2000; 49: 30-34), (Baynes, J.W. and Thorpe, S.R. Role of oxidative stress in diabetic complications: A new perspective on an old paradigm. Diabetes 1999, 48: 1-9). Some even erroneously claim that it is a proven fact, however, **I believe that the data will show that they are wrong**. Oxidative stress is thought to play a causative role in the tissue and cellular damage in these diseases. In particular, diabetes mellitus is strongly associated with increased oxidative stress, (Paolisso, G., D'Amore, A., Volpe, C., Balbi, V., Saccomanno, F., Galzerano, D., Giugliano, D., Varricchio, M. and D'Onofrio, F. Evidence for a relationship between oxidative stress and insulin action in non-insulin-dependent (type II) diabetic patients. Metabolism 1994; 43: 1426-1429), (Giugliano, D., Ceriello, A. and Paolisso, G. Diabetes mellitus, hypertension and cardiovascular disease: Which role for oxidative stress? Metabolism 1995; 44: 363-368), (Nourooz-Zadeh, J., Rahimi, A., Tajaddini-Sarmadi, J., Tritschler, H., Rosen, P., Halliwell, B. and Betteridge, D.J. Relationships between plasma measures of oxidative stress and metabolic control in NIDDM. Diabetologia 1997; 40: 647-653), (Honing, M.L.H., Morrison, P.J., Banga, J.D., Stroes, E.S.G. and Rabelnk, T.J. Nitric oxide availability in diabetes mellitus. Diabetes Metab Rev 1998; 14: 241-249), (Packer, L. Oxidative stress, the antioxidant network and prevention of diabetes complications by a-lipoid acid. Environ Nutr Interact 1999; 3: 47-76), which could be a consequence of either increased production of free radicals or reduced antioxidant defenses. Nonetheless, **I will show that no causal relationship can be demonstrated between reactive oxygen species and diabetes.**

Persons with type II diabetes mellitus (DM), even without cardiovascular complications have a decreased maximal oxygen consumption (VO_2 max) and sub maximal oxygen consumption (VO_2) during graded exercise compared with healthy controls (Regensteiner, J.G., Bauer, T.A., Reusch, J.E., Brandedburg, S.L., Sippel, J.M., Vogelsong, A.M., Smith, S., Wolfel, E.E., Eckel, R.H. and Hiatt, W.R. Abnormal oxygen uptake kinetic responses in women with type II diabetes mellitus. J Appl Physiol 1998; 85(1): 310-317). **While developing my Unified Theory, I had predicted that such would be the case.**

Type II diabetes is associated with obesity and sedentary living; however, **maximal and submaximal O_2 consumption (VO_2) are lower in patients with type II diabetes than in non- diabetic individuals of similar age, gender, body composition, and self-reported physical activity. There is indirect evidence suggesting that exercise cardiac output may be impaired by Type 2 diabetes.** Up to 60% of individuals with Type 2 diabetes have impaired diastolic function, which is associated with reduced VO_{2max} in healthy subjects.

Peripheral O_2 delivery and extraction may also be affected by Type 2 diabetes. Type 2 diabetic patients have impaired nitric oxide-induced vascular function, which can result in impaired muscle blood flow during exercise. Moreover, Type 2 diabetic patients have reduced oxidative enzyme activity, increased percentage of type IIb fibers, and decreased percentage of type I fibers.

Maximal O_2 consumption (VO_{2max}) is lower in individuals with Type 2 diabetes than in sedentary nondiabetic individuals. This study aimed to determine whether the lower VO_{2max} in diabetic patients was due to a reduction in maximal cardiac out put (Q_{max}) and/or peripheral O_2 extraction. After II Type I diabetic patients and 12 no diabetic subjects, matched for able and body composition, who had not exercised for 2 years, performed a bicycle ergo meter exercise test to determine VO_{2max} sub maximal cardiac output, Q_{max}, and arterial-mixed venous O_2 (a-vO_2) difference were assessed. **Maximal workload, VO_{2max} and maximal a-vO_2 difference were lower in Type 2 diabetic patients** (P< 0.05). Q_{max} was low in both groups but not significantly different: 11.2 and 10.0l/min for controls and diabetic patients, respectively (P > 0.05) (Baldi, J.C., Aoina, J.L., Oxenham, H.C., Bagg, W. and Doughty, R.N. Reduced exercise arteriovenous O_2 difference in Type 2 diabetes. J Appl Physiol 2003; 94: 1033-1038). Again, **this illustrates the importance of basic oxygen metabolism and stresses the need to get normal levels of O_2 to the cells and consequently into the mitochondria, such that adequate levels of RONS/excytomers can be generated to maintain the homeostasis of the entire body, consistent with my Unified Theory.**

There is considerable **speculative evidence** to indicate that oxidative stress plays an important role in the etiology of diabetic complications. (Wolff, S.P., Juang, Z.Y. and Hunt, J.V. Protein glycation and oxidative stress in diabetes mellitus and aging. Free Rad Biol Med 1991; 10: 339-352), (Nourooz-Zadeh, J., Tajaddini-Sarmadi, J., McCarthy, S., Betteridge, D.J. and Wolff, S.P. Elevated levels of authentic plasma hydroperoxides in NIDDM. Diabetes 1995; 44: 1054-1058), (Jones, A.F., Winkles, J.W., Jennings, P.E., Florkowski, C.M., Lunec, J. and Barnett, A.H. Serum antioxidant activity in diabetes mellitus. Diabetes Res 1988; 7: 89-92), (Hartnett, M.E., Stratton, R.D., Browne, R.W., Rosner, B.A., Lanham, R.J. and Armstrong, D. Serum markers for oxidative stress and severity of diabetic retinopathy. Diabetes Care 2000; 23: 234-240), (Opara, E.C., Abdel-Rahman, E., Soliman, S., Kamel, W.A., Souka, S., Lowe, J.E. and Abdel-Aleem, S. Depletion of total antioxidant capacity in type 2 diabetes. Metabolism 1999; 48: 1414-1417). Many of the biochemical pathways (e.g., protein glycation, polyol pathway, glucose antioxidation) associated with hyperglycemia can result in increased free radical production. Some believe that oxidative stress is not only associated with complications of diabetes, but has been also linked to insulin resistance (**and everything else under the sun).** In vitro, oxidative stress seemingly causes insulin resistance at multiple levels (vide infra).

An additional potential target of oxidative stress is likely to be the B-cell. While **the process of glucose-stimulated insulin secretion is complex and is dependent upon many factors**, the critical importance of mitochondrial metabolism in linking stimulus to secretion is well established. Mitochondria are free radical generators and may be unwitting targets. Therefore, it is not surprising to learn that oxidative stress (e.g., H_2O_2) damages B-cell mitochondria and markedly blunts insulin secretion. (Maechler, P., Jomot, L. and Wollheim, C.B. Hydrogen peroxide alters mitochondrial activation and insulin secretion in pancreatic beta cells. J Biol Chem 1999; 274:

27905-27913). To make matters worse, **β-cells are particularly susceptible to oxidative attack because of their inherently low level of antioxidant defenses.** (Tiedge, M., Lortz, S., Drinkgern, J. and Lenzen, S.

Relation between antioxidant enzyme gene expression and antioxidative defense status of insulin-producing cells. Diabetes 1997; 46: 1733-1742). Consistent with this proposal, there is growing evidence to show that antioxidants including DHLA, vitamins C and E and N-acetyl-L-cysteine seem to exert a direct protective effect against free radical assault on insulin-secreting cells, along with providing a benefit against the damages of glucose-mediated toxicity in rodents with diabetes. (Tanaka, Y., Gleason, C.E., Tran, P.O., Harmon, J.S. and Robertson, R.P. Prevention of glucose toxicity in HIT-T15 cells and Zucker diabetic fatty rats by antioxidants. Proc Natl Acad Sci USA 1999; 96:10857-10862), (Kaneto, H., Kajimoto, Y., Miyagawa, J., Matsuoka, T., Fujitani, Y., Umayahara, Y., Hanafusa, T., Matsuzawa, Y., Yamasaki, Y. and Hori, M. Beneficial effects of antioxidants in diabetes: possible protection of pancreatic beta-cells against glucose toxicity. Diabetes 1999; 48: 2398-2406). In light of the negative physiological consequences commonly associated with increased oxidative stress, the idea of treating patients with type 2 diabetes pharmacologically with antioxidants to reduce oxidative stress is, perhaps unfortunately, gaining increasing experimental support and clinical acceptance. (Bursell, S.E. and King, G.L. Can protein kinase C inhibition and vitamin E prevent the development of diabetic vascular complications? Diabetes Res Clin Pract 1999; 45: 169-182). Yet, **the data is filled with contradictory studies and inconsistencies, just as in other areas of so called oxidative stress investigations.**

14.3 ARGUMENTS AGAINST ANTIOXIDANT DIABETOGENESIS

The theory regarding antioxidants and diabetes: Uncontrolled high blood sugar increases the oxidative load of diabetes, influencing complications, especially premature atherosclerosis.

So, in research, how do these antioxidants perform? In clinical research trials, **antioxidant supplement studies have failed to show significant benefits and in some cases report adverse outcomes**. Large randomized intervention trials failed to demonstrate any significant cardio protective effect of antioxidants. In two studies of beta-carotene an increased incidence of lung cancer was demonstrated. In those who smoked an **increased risk of heart disease** was seen. With regard to vitamin C, vitamin E, selenium and beta-carotene, large amounts hampered potential benefits of simvastatin (Zocor) and niacin on lipid profile. The anticipated increase in HDL (the "heart healthy" cholesterol) was blunted with the antioxidants. **One of the other problems is that when antioxidants are combined with statin/niacin combo therapy, they appear to nullify the rise in HDL cholesterol.** (Arter Throm Vas Biol 2001; 21:1320-1326). This article and the accompanying editorial **make a compelling case against recommending antioxidant supplements to prevent or treat coronary artery disease.**

We synthesize 3,000-4,000 mg of cholesterol/day and receive smaller amounts from the diet.

In summary, **there is no evidence of benefit from antioxidant supplementation in people with diabetes who do not have underlying deficiencies**. (Schwartz, N.L. Are supplemental antioxidants helpful in cardiovascular disease? Diabetes Education Center of the Midlands, Fall, 2003).

Classic CVD risk factors such as hyperglycemia, hypertension, dyslipidemia, and central obesity increase the risk of CVD in patients with type 1 diabetes, but do not fully explain the significantly higher incidence of CVD in type 1 diabetes. Thus, type 1 diabetes may lead to unique mechanisms for the onset and progression of CVD, as well as influencing mechanisms known for type 2 diabetes and the general population.

Recent data is vitro have implicated hyperglycemia-derived oxygen free radicals as mediators of diabetic complications. Overproduction of superoxide by the mitochondrial electron transport chain seems to activate pathways that have been suggested to be involved in the vascular complications caused by hyperglycemia. Despite the evidence of the role of oxidative stress in the development of cardiovascular complications in patients with diabetes clinical trials using **antioxidants have failed to demonstrate any beneficial effect**. Thus, research is needed to translate the basic science findings on oxidative stress into improved outcomes. (DHHS. NIH Guide: Progression of cardiovascular disease in type 1 diabetes. Dec. 4, 2003).

Oxidative stress is generally believed to play an important role in the initiation and progression of vascular disease. Dietary antioxidants, e.g., Vitamins A, C, E, have been recommended to reduce the impact of oxidative stress. However, **a recent large scale study failed to demonstrate a significant benefit for Vitamin E supplementation in patients with diabetes.** Additional studies may be necessary to clarify these unexpected findings. (Indiana State Department of Health, Cardiovascular Health & Diabetes Guidelines).

There is a discrepancy between the failure of clinical trials with antioxidants to improve diabetic vascular disease and the strong evidence in vitro and in preclinical models of the impact of oxidative stress in biochemical and cell biological changes in the diabetic tissue. It is necessary to try to understand the tissue-specific translation of oxidative stress into biological responses, and the inability of current antioxidants to exert potent effects.

While diabetes is increasing worldwide, so is our ability to combat many of its effects. Apart from major changes in lifestyle (weight control, exercise, not smoking), tight control of blood pressure is probably the most important measure to reduce deaths and heart disease. Better control of blood glucose, blood pressure, and lipid levels should ensure that one reduces the long-term effects of this disease.

There's no evidence that antioxidants or vitamin supplements are particularly valuable to diabetic patients. Adequate folic acid - usually achieved by eating plenty of green vegetables, or taking a supplement - will counter any high levels of blood homocysteine, which is sometimes seen in diabetic, as well as non-diabetic subjects.

Oxidative stress and oxidation of low-density lipoprotein (LDL) may be involved in the development of diabetic macroangiopathy and kidney disease. The urinary excretion of 8 hydroxydeoxyguanosine (8-OHdG), plasma concentrations of ascorbic acid, uric acid, a-tocopherol, and protein thiol, the plasma total peroxyl radical-trapping potential (TRAP), the level of autoantibodies against oxidized LDL (oxLDL-Ab), and the susceptibility of LDL to oxidation in a cohort of 87 NIDDM patients after nine years of disease duration was determined. Systemic oxidative stress, assessed by urinary 8 OHdG was increased in patients with NIDDM, but it was not reflected in the antioxidant activity of plasma. **High oxidative stress or LDL oxidation were not associated with the presence of CHD or diabetic kidney disease.** (Leinonen, J., et. al. Oxidative stress and LDL oxidation in patients with non-insulin-dependent diabetes mellitus (NIDDM). 1998, Poster. Website: www.oxyclubcalifornia. org).

14.4 OXIDATIVE STRESS, DIABETES AND EXERCISE

The following discussions are excerpted and based on materials from the following review article: (Atalay, M. and Laaksonen, D.E., Diabetes, oxidative stress and physical exercise. 2002; J Sports Sci Med 1: 1-14).

During moderate exercise oxygen consumption increased by 8-10 fold, and oxygen flux through the muscle may increase by 90-100 fold. Even **moderate exercise may increase free radical production and overwhelm antioxidant defenses**, presumably resulting in an oxidative insult (Sen, C.K. and Packer, L. Thiol homeostasis and supplements in physical exercise. Am J Clin Nutr. 2000; 72: 653S-669S).

It was first shown in 1978 by Dillard et al. (Dillard, C.J., Litov, R.E., Savin, W.M., Dumelin, E.E. and Tappel, A.L. Effects of exercise, vitamin E and ozone on pulmonary function and lipid peroxidation. J of App Physio 1978; 45: 927-932), that in humans, **even a moderate intensity of exercise increased the content of pentane, a lipid peroxidation byproduct, in expired air**. 1982 Davies et al. for the first time provided the direct evidence using electron paramagnetic resonance spectroscopy. In rats **exhaustive treadmill exercise increased the free radical concentration by 2- to 3-fold of skeletal muscle and liver**. (Davies, K.J., Quintanilha, A.T., Brooks, G.A. and Packer, L. Free radicals and tissue damage produced by exercise. Biochem Biophy Res Comm 1982; 107: 1198-1205). Further studies demonstrated that **strenuous exercise induces oxidative stress as measured by oxidative damage of lipids, proteins and even the genetic material**. (Ji, L.L. Antioxidants and oxidative stress in exercise. Proc Soc Exper Biol Med 1999; 222: 283-292), (Atalay, M. and Sen, C.K. Physical exercise and antioxidant defenses in the heart. Ann NY Acad Sci 1999; 874: 169-177). Thus, **regular physical exercise should induce many of the 100 diseases ascribed to oxidative stress but as we all know, exercise is good for us and is contrary to the beliefs of the free radical phobics..**

Diabetes mellitus (DM) is a syndrome characterized by abnormal insulin secretion, derangement in carbohydrate and lipid metabolism and is diagnosed by the presence of hyperglycemia. Diabetes is a major worldwide health problem predisposing to markedly increased cardiovascular mortality and serious morbidity and mortality related to development of nephropathy, neuropathy and retinopathy. The prevalence of type 2DM among adults varies from less than 5% to over 40% depending on the population in question. Due to increasing obesity, sedentariness and dietary habits in both Western and developing countries, **the prevalence of type 2 DM is growing at an exponential rate.** (Zimmet, P.Z., McCarty, D.J. and de Courten, M.P. The global epidemiology of non-insulin-dependent diabetes mellitus and the metabolic syndrome. J Diab Compl 1997; 11: 60-68). Type 1 DM is less common.

Increased oxidative stress as measured by indices of lipid peroxidation and protein oxidation has been shown to be increased in both insulin dependent diabetes (IDDM), and non-insulin dependent (NIDDM) (Cederberg, J., Basu, S. and Eriksson, U.J. Increased rate of lipid peroxidation and protein carbonylations in experimental diabetic pregnancy. Diabetologia 2001; 44: 766-774), even in patients without complications. Increased oxidized low density lipo-protein (LDL) or susceptibility to oxidation has also been shown in diabetes.

Despite strong experimental evidence indicating that oxidative stress may determine the onset and progression of late-diabetes complications, **controversy exists about whether the increased oxidative stress is merely associative rather than causal in DM**. This is partly because measurement of oxidative stress is usually based on indirect and nonspecific measurement of products of reactive oxygen species and partly because most clinical studies in DM patients have been cross-sectional. (Laaksonen, D.E. and Sen, C.K. Exercise and oxidative stress in diabetes mellitus. In: Handbook of Oxidants and Antioxidants in Exercise 2000; 1105-1136).

The mechanisms behind the apparent increased oxidative stress in diabetes are not entirely clear. Accumulating evidence points to a number of inter-related mechanisms, increasing production of free radicals such as superoxide or decreasing antioxidant status. These mechanisms include glycoxidation and formation of advanced glycation products, activation of the polyol pathway and altered cell26 and glutathione redox status and ascorbate metabolism antioxidant enzyme inactivation and perturbations in nitric oxide and prostaglandin metabolism.

Large prospective studies (Lakka, T.A., Venalainen, J.M., Rauramaa, R., Salonen, R., Tuomilehto, J. and Salonen, J.T. Relation of leisure-time physical activity and cardiorespiratory fitness to the risk of acute myocardial infarction. New Engl J Med 1994; 330: 1349-1554), suggest that regular exercise and physical fitness as measured by **maximal oxygen consumption have protective effects on cardiovascular disease and mortality. I believe that these protective are directly related to increased levels of reactive oxygen species and excitation states.** The relative benefits or risks of acute and chronic exercise in relation to oxidative stress in groups with increased susceptibility to oxidative stress such as diabetic patients are not known. Laaksonen et al., recently found **increased oxidative stress as measured by plasma thiobarbituric acid reactive substances (TBARS) at rest and after exercise in young men with type 1 DM.** Physical fitness as measured by maximal oxygen consumption (VO_2 max), however, was strongly inversely correlated with plasma TBARS in the diabetic men only, suggesting a protective effect of fitness against oxidative stress.

In vitro studies have suggested that **glycation itself may result in production of superoxide.** Oxidation has been hypothesized to result in generation of superoxide, H_2O_2 and through transition metal catalysis, hydroxyl radical. (Wolff, S.P., Jiang, Z.Y. and Hunt, J.V. Protein glycation and oxidative stress in diabetes mellitus and aging. Free Rad Biol Med 1991; 10: 339-352). Catalase and other antioxidants decrease cross linking and AGE formation.

Tissue glutathione is believed to play a central role in antioxidant defense. Glutathione is a tripeptide which has "free" sulfhydryl groups available to reduce H_2O_2 to water. The GSH is reduced by donating hydrogen to the hydrogen peroxide catalysed by glutathione peroxidase. The reduced glutathione (GSSG) is then oxidized by the reduction of NADPH catalysed by glutathione reductase. Reduced **glutathione detoxifies reactive oxygen species such as hydrogen peroxide and lipid peroxides directly or in a glutathione peroxidase (GPX) catalyzed mechanism.** Glutathione also regenerates the major aqueous and lipid phase antioxidants, ascorbate and a-tocopherol. Glutathione reductase (GRD) catalyzes the NADPH dependent reduction of oxidized glutathione, serving to maintain intracellular glutathione stores and a favorable redox status. Glutathione-S-transferase (GST) catalyzes the reaction between the -SH group and potential alkylating agents, rendering them more water soluble and suitable for transport out of the cell. GST can also use peroxides as a substrate.

Type 2 diabetic patients had decreased erythrocyte GSH and increased GSSG levels. (Jain, S.K. and McVie, R. Effect of glycemic control race (white versus black), and duration of diabetes on reduced glutathione content in erythrocytes of diabetic patients. Meta 1994; 43: 306-309).

It has to be clarified whether the levels are decreased in patients without complications and whether patients with complications have even lower levels. **The pathophysiological significance of decreased glutathione levels in DM remains to be shown.**

Changes in glutathione dependent enzymes in experimental diabetic models have been **contradictory.** Most studies show tissue and time dependent changes in enzyme activity. Even taking these factors into account, **no consensus can be found among studies about the impact of DM on glutathione dependent enzyme activity.** Changes in glutathione dependent enzymes in diabetic patients are **also inconsistent. Differences in results cannot be completely explained by study methodology. I believe that all of this confusion arises from the fact that investigators are trying to apply their data to the erroneous free radical oxidation theory of disease. Consequently, the data does not make sense, yet they are hell bound to make it fit the theory.**

Superoxide dismutase (SOD) and catalase are also major antioxidant enzymes. SOD exists in three different isoforms. Cu, Zn-SOD is mostly in the cytosol and dismutate superoxide to hydrogen peroxide. Extracellular (EC) SOD is found in the plasma and extracellular space. Mn-SOD is located in mitochondria. Catalase is a hydrogen peroxide decomposing enzyme mainly localized to peroxisomes or microperoxisomes. Superoxide may react with other reactive oxygen species such as nitric oxide to form highly toxic species such as peroxynitrite, in addition to direct toxic effects. Peroxynitrite reacts with the tyrosine residues in proteins resulting with the **nitrotyrosine production in plasma proteins, which is considered as an indirect evidence of peroxynitrite production and increase oxidative stress.** Although nitrotyrosine was not detectable in the plasma of healthy controls, nitro tyrosine was found in the plasma of all type 2 diabetic patients examined. Consistent with these results, plasma nitrotyrosine values were correlated with plasma glucose concentrations. Furthermore, exposure of endothelial cells high glucose leads to augmented production of superoxide anion, which may quench nitric oxide. Decreased nitric oxide levels result with impaired endothelial functions, vasodilation and delayed cell replication. (Giugliano, D., Ceriello, A. and Paolisso, G. Oxidative stress and diabetic vascular complications. Diab Care 1996; 19: 257-267).

Alternatively, superoxide can be dismutated to much more reactive hydrogen peroxide, which through the Fenton reaction can then lead to highly toxic hydroxyl radical formation. Decreased activity of cytoplasmic Cu,Zn-SOD and especially mitochondrial (Mn-) SOD in diabetic neutrophils was found. **There are reports disagreeing with these findings.** Red cell Cu,Zn-SOD activity was similar in type 1 and 2 DM patients compared to normal subjects irrespective of microvascular complications. Leukocyte SOD activity was similar between type 2 DM patients and healthy control subjects, despite increased lipid peroxidation and decreased ascorbate levels. Furthermore, increased red cell SOD activity and serum MDA levels were reported in patients of type 1 DM with normo- microalbuminuria and retinopathy compared to healthy subjects.

Red cell superoxide and catalase activities were decreased in 105 subjects with impaired glucose tolerance (IGT) and early hyperglycemia and also in type 2 DM patients. However, in another study red cell catalase and SOD activities were normal in 26 type 2 DM patients in poor glycemic control. EC-SOD activity was found to be similar in type 1 DM patients, despite somewhat higher plasma EC-SOD levels.

The wide variability among studies does not allow conclusions to be drawn as to whether SOD isoform in catalase enzyme activities are abnormal in diabetic patients. Again, differences in methodology or study design do not completely explain the conflicting findings among studies. Again, this is because the data is being forced to apply to the flawed free radical oxidative theory and it does not make sense.

Lipid peroxidation end-products are very commonly detected by the measurement of thiobarbituric acid reactive substances (TBARS). This assay has, however, been **criticized for the lack of specificity.** Lipid peroxidation as measured by lipid hydroperoxides have been shown to correlate closely with TBARS data in tissue samples. With proper caution, TBARS measurement may provide meaningful information. (Draper, H.H., Squires, E.J., Mahmoodi, H., Wu, J., Agarwal, S. and Hadley, M. A comparative evaluation of thiobarbituric acid methods for the determination of malondealdehyde in biological materials. Free Rad Biol Med 1993; 15: 353-363).

Use of TBARS as an index of lipid peroxidation was pioneered by Yagi et al., whose group also showed increased plasma TBARS levels in DM consistent with other's results. Similarly, increased plasma peroxide concentrations were reported in type 1 and type 2 DM patients. Diabetic red blood cells (RBC)s were shown to be more susceptible to lipid peroxidation as measured by TBARS in rats and humans. Oxidizabiltiy of plasma as measured by lipid hydroperoxides was greater in DM group, although baseline levels were similar in subjects with normal glucose tolerance, impaired glucose tolerance and type 2 DM. Furthermore, plasma TBARS level was significantly increased in type 2 DM with the duration of disease and development of complications.

The formation of conjugated dienes reflect early events of lipid peroxidation. Spectrophotometric assay of conjugated dienes, however, does not provide information on hydroperoxides in samples. Serum levels of a conjugated diene isomer of linoleic acid were higher in DM patients with microalbuminuria than control subjects. (Collier, A., Rumley, A., Rumley, A.G., Paterson, J.R., Leach, J.P., Lowe, G.D. and Small, M. Free radical activity and hemostatic factors in NIDDM patients with and without microalbuminuria. Diabetes 1992; 41: 909-913).

On the other hand, no difference in serum conjugated diene levels between otherwise healthy diabetic patients and healthy control subjects was noted. (Sinclair, A.J., Girling, A.J., Gray, L., Lunee, J. and Barnett, A.H. An investigation of the relationship between free radical activity and vitamin C metabolism in elderly diabetic subjects with retinopathy. Gerontology 1992; 38: 268-274).

Most published studies have found increased lipid peroxidation in both type I and type 2 DM patients. **Conflicting results have also been found, however, and they cannot be explained simply based on study design or methodology**. It is less clear whether lipid peroxidation is increased in DM even before development of micro- and macrovascular disease. **A causal role for lipid peroxidation in the development of diabetic macro- and microvascular complications is far from established**. Amen.

On the other hand, baseline lipid hydroperoxide levels were similar in 75 subjects with normal glucose tolerance, impaired glucose tolerance and type 2 DM. (Haffner, S.M., Agil, A., Mykkanen, L., Stern, M.P. and Jialal, I. Plasma oxidizability in subjects with normal glucose tolerance, impaired glucose tolerance and NIDDM. Diabetes Care 1995; 18: 646-653).

Incubation of LDL cholesterol with glucose at concentrations seen in the diabetic state increased susceptibility of LDL to oxidation as measured by TBARS and conjugated diene formation, Electrophoretic mobility and degradation by macrophages. (Kawamura, M., Heinecke, J.W. and Chait, A. Pathophysiological concentrations of glucose promote oxidative modification of low density lipoprotein by superoxide-dependent pathway. J Clin Invest 1994; 94: 771-778). Plasma TRAP (total peroxyl radical trapping potential) was lower and susceptibility of LDL to oxidation as measured by the lag phase of conjugated diene formation after initiation of LDL oxidation by the addition of **copper** was greater in poorly controlled subjects.

In contrast, there was no difference between type I diabetic patients and non-diabetic subjects in the susceptibility of LDL and VLDL cholesterol to oxidation in a number of studies. (Mol, M.J., de Rijke, Y.B., Demacker, P.N. and Stalenhoef, A.F. Plasma levels of lipid and cholesterol oxidation products and cytokines in diabetes mellitus and cigarette smoking: Effects of vitamin E treatment. Atherosclerosis 1997; 129: 169-176).

Most studies have found increased susceptibility of LDL cholesterol to oxidation in DM patients, although **some well-designed studies have had conflicting results**. Studies carried out to date **do not allow firm conclusions to be drawn** about whether LDL is more susceptible to oxidation in DM patients without complications than in healthy subjects, or about what effect complications and glycemic control have on the susceptibility of LDL to oxidation.

No clear consensus has been found concerning the presence of increased oxidized LDL antibodies for LDL cholesterol oxidizability or especially for indices of plasma or serum lipid peroxidation in DM patients. Although interesting results linking oxidized LDL antibodies to carotid atherosclerosis is the general population have been published, (Salonen, J.T., Yla Herttuala, S., Yamamoto, R., Butler, S., Korpela, H., Salonen, R., Nyyssonen, K., Palinski, W. and Wizlum, J.L. Autoantibody against oxidized LDL and progression of carotid atherosclerosis. Lancet 1992; 339: 883-887), similar conclusions cannot be drawn from studies in diabetic patients. Whether this is an argument against increased oxidative stress or its role in the pathogenesis of atherosclerosis in DM or against the use of oxidized LDL auto antibodies as a marker of lipid peroxidation of DM **remains unclear**.

Exercise is a major therapeutic modality in the treatment of DM (American Diabetes Association, 1998; Laaksonen et al., 2000).

Red cell GRD activity at rest was 15% higher in the diabetic group (p,0.05). However, erythrocyte Cu,Zn-SOD and catalase activities at rest were significantly lower in the diabetic group. Acute exercise increased erythrocyte Se-GPX activity modestly in the control group, but not in the IDDM group. Post-exercise Se-GPX activity was significantly higher in the control group compared to the IDDM group. Although acute exercise did not significantly affect GRD activity because of the higher resting values, post-exercise GRD activity was also higher in the IDDM group compared to the control group. Erythrocyte GST, Cu,Zn-SOD and catalase activities were similar in control and DM group after exercise. (Atalay, M. and Sen, C.K. Physical exercise and antioxidant defenses in the heart. Annals NY Acad Sci 1999; 874: 169-177).

Increased plasma TBARS in the diabetic men both at rest and after exercise, showing for the first time increased exercise induced oxidative stress in DM was found. These results also support previous studies suggesting that type I DM patients have increased lipid peroxidation even in the absence of complications. Decreased Cu,Zn-SOD activity coupled with increased superoxide production could exacerbate oxidative stress, especially if not compensated with increased catalase or Se-GPX activity. Superoxide may react with other reactive oxygen species such as nitric oxide to form highly toxic species such as peroxynitrite, in addition to direct toxic effects. Alternatively, superoxide can be dismutate to the much more reactive hydrogen peroxide, which through the Fenton reaction can then lead to highly toxic hydroxyl radical formation. Thus decreased catalase activity could also contribute to the increased oxidative stress found in the type I DM subjects. Increased glucose and hydrogen peroxide levels have also been shown to inactivate catalase. As reviewed above, **decreased red cell SOD and catalase activity have often, but not always, been found in DM patients**.

The strongly negative association between plasma TBARS and VO2 max suggests that good physical fitness may have a protective role against oxidative stress.

In a recent study in streptozotosin-induced experimental diabetic rats, our group showed that endurance training decreased lipid peroxidation measured by TBARS level in vastus lateralis muscle and increased glutathione peroxidase in red gastronomies muscle. However, endurance training increased conjugated dienes and decreased glutathione peroxidase activity in heart. Consistent with these results, decreased levels of cardiac antioxidants have been previously observed in endurance trained healthy rats. (Kihlstrom, M., Ojala, J. and Salminen, A. Decreased level of cardiac antioxidants in endurance trained rats. Acta Physiologica Scandinavica 1989; 135: 549-554). Acute exhaustive exercise induced oxidative stress measured as increased TBARS level in liver and increased dienes in heart. Increased TBARS levels in liver of untrained diabetic rats after acute exhaustive exercise are in agreement with a previous study carried out in normal rats. These results suggest that despite the adverse effects in heart, endurance training appears to up-regulate glutathione dependent antioxidant defense in skeletal muscle in experimental DM.

Diabetes pathology and complications can not be explained by traditional risk factors and the free radical oxidative theory.

14.4.1 Additional Antioxidant Confusion

Many experts are cautioning against the widespread use of antioxidants either for primary or secondary prevention of any disease entities, other than deficiency states, until convincing data from randomized trials is made available.

The term, the "French Paradox," became famous in 1991 when CBS's 60 Minutes reported an inconsistency in the lifestyles and rates of heart disease among people in France. In spite of a diet of rich foods - including more butter, cheeses, eggs and sauces, an estimated 15% of their daily calories obtained from saturated fats and less exercise - the rate of heart disease for French people is only 40% of that of Americans.

Countless publications have extolled the benefits of wine consumption for protection against heart disease and this protection has frequently been attributed to antioxidants (polyphenols) contained in the wine. Recent **studies refute the suggestion that benefits against heart disease are due to antioxidants in wine**. Two studies in the January, American Journal of Clinical Nutrition, report **no sign of reduced oxidation** within the arteries of heart-disease-prone mice given alcohol-free red wine. Nevertheless, the mice drinking that wine had fewer plaques in their arteries than drinking plain water did. (Croft, K.D. The chemistry and biological effects of flavonoids and phenolic acids. Annals of NY Acad Sci 1998; 854: 435-442). The scientists have removed the wine's alcohol content because **alcohol oxidizes fat** and would therefore affect the arterial oxidation they were tracking. Their results indicated that **the protective action of red wine polyphenols is independent of any antioxidant action of these compounds**. In contrast, other studies have indicated that the free radical, nitric oxide, has inhibited atherosclerosis. Even more damaging to the free radical/oxidation theory, **wine drinkers displayed more of the oxidation marker,** even though they had 60% fewer arterial plaques than did the non-wine drinkers. Many consider this situation to be another **"paradox," (more specifically, the French Paradox),** but it is readily explainable when one realizes that antioxidants do not work and that atherosclerosis is not caused by LDL oxidation. To further confuse the theory attempting to link oxidation to arteriosclerosis biochemist, Roland Stocker, has found that **atherosclerosis is not linked to oxidation of bad cholesterol (LDL)**. Once again, investigators are confused and perplexed because the results of their studies are not predictable based on the flawed free radical/oxidation theory. There is no paradox or confusion when you think outside of the erroneous free radical/oxidation theory. **It seems an impossibility for many scientists to open their minds and discard this disproven, outmoded and out dated theory.**

It has been suggested that increased intake of various antioxidant vitamins reduces the incidence rates of vascular disease, cancer and other adverse outcomes. 20,536 UK adults (aged 40-80) with coronary disease, other occlusive arterial disease, or diabetes were randomly allocated to receive antioxidant vitamin supplementation (600 mg vitamin E, 250 mg vitamin C and 20 mg beta-carotene daily) or matching placebo. **Allocation of this vitamin regimen approximately doubled the plasma concentration of alpha-tocopherol, increased that of vitamin C by one-third and quadrupled that of beta-carotene.** There were **no significant differences** in all-cause mortality (1446 [14.1%] vitamin-allocated vs. 1389 [13.5%] placebo-allocated), or in deaths due to vascular (878 [8.6%] vs. 840 [8.2%]) or non-vascular (508 [5.5%] vs. 549 [5.3%]0 causes. **Nor were there any significant differences in the numbers of participants having non-fatal myocardial infarction or coronary death** (1063 [10.4%] vs. 1047 [10.2%]), **non-fatal or fatal stroke** (511 [5.0%] vs. 518 [5.0%]), **or coronary or non-coronary revascularization** (1058 [10.3%] vs. 1086 [10.6%]). For the first occurrence of any of these "major vascular events," there were no material differences either overall (2306 [22.5%] vs. 2312 [22.5%]; event rate ratio 1.00 [95% CI 0.94-1.06]) or in any of the various subcategories considered. There were **no significant effects on cancer incidence or on hospitalization for any other non-vascular cause.** They found that among the high-risk individuals that were studied, these antioxidant vitamins appeared to be safe. But, although this regimen increased blood vitamin concentrations substantially, **it did not produce any significant reductions in the 5-year mortality from, or incidence of, any type of vascular disease, cancer or other major outcome.** (Heart Protection Study collaborative Group. MRC/BHF heart protection study of antioxidant vitamin supplementation in 20,536 high-risk individuals: A randomized placebo-controlled trial. Lancet 2002; 360(9326): 23-33).

15 THE "ANTIOXIDANT PARADOX"
(OR ANOTHER ATTEMPT TO HOLD ON TO THE
FLAWED FREE RADICAL/OXIDATION THEORY)

Oxidative stress is a term used to describe an imbalance between the production and destruction of reactive oxygen species (ROS), such as superoxide anions (O_2.-) and hydrogen peroxide (H_2O_2), thereby likely leading to cellular and tissue injury. The basic properties of oxygen are thought to be responsible for the destructive power of free radicals, in particular, their high reactivity. **Humans consume ~250 g of oxygen every day, and of this ~3-5% is converted to O_2.·** and other reactive species. (Rice-Evans, C.A. and Burdon, R.H. Free radical damage and its control. Amsterdam: Elsevier, 1994; 25-27). Many observational and epidemiological studies, although unable to establish a cause-and-effect relationship, suggest that increased dietary intake of naturally occurring antioxidant vitamins is associated with lower risk of cardiovascular disease. I will show that this association is misleading and confusing.

Vascular ROS formation is, in large part, initiated by the one-electron reduction of molecular O_2 and O_2.-, the production of which is increased in atherosclerosis. Potential cellular sources of O_2.- in blood vessels include **infiltrating phagocytic cells**, which contain the high-capacity O_2.- generating flavoenzyme NADPH oxidase, as well as **vascular endothelial cells, smooth muscle cells** (SMC) and **fibroblasts**. An earlier report suggested that endothelial cells may be responsible for the increased production of O2.· in hypercholesterolemia blood vessels (Ohara, Y., Peterson, T.E. and Harrison, D.G. Hypercholesterolemia increases endothelial superoxide anion production. J Clin Invest 1993; 91: 2546-2551). Using confocal microscopy to examine the cellular localization of O2. in situ, Miller et al. (Miller, F.J. Jr., Gutterman, D.D., Rios, C.D., Heistad, D.D. and Davidson, B.L. Superoxide production in vascular smooth muscle contributes to oxidative stress and impaired relaxation in atherosclerosis. Cir Res 1998; 82: 1298-1305), demonstrated that **SMC are a major source of RONS in blood vessels** from atherosclerotic rabbits. Similar studies also suggest that much of the O_2.· in atherosclerotic human coronary arteries is contained in the media and adventitia where it is presumably generated by SMC and fibroblasts.

It was shown recently **that a nonphagocytic NAD(P)H oxidase is a major source of RONS in cultured vascular cells** (Griendling, K.K., Sorescu, D. and Ushio-Fukai, M. NAD(P)H oxidase: Role in cardiovascular biology and disease. Circ Res 2000; 86: 494-501), **although xanthine oxidase, nitric oxide synthase, cytochrome *P*-450 and the mitochondrial electron transport chain may be important sources of RONS** in specific situations. Oxidation of LDL by endothelial cells in vitro is believed to be attenuated by over expressing (up-regulation) superoxide dismutase (SOD) in the cells, suggesting a role for O_2.· and/or its reaction products in this process. On the other hand, although **vitamin E rapidly reacts with lipid peroxyl radicals, it does not efficiently scavenge O_2.·.** Moreover, the localization of ROS within the deep layers of the blood vessel wall suggests that even if antioxidant vitamins were efficient scavengers of O_2.·, delivery to sites where they are most needed may be problematic and partly to blame for conflicting results.

O_2.· that exits from, or is produced outside of, vascular cells can be converted by extracellular SOD (ECSOD) to H_2O_2. In addition, O_2.· produced within the cell is converted by Cu/Zn SOD and Mn SOD to H_2O_2, which can readily cross cellular membranes. H_2O_2 present in the extracellular space can be, in turn, converted to the highly reactive species HOCl by the enzyme myeloperoxidase. Recent studies suggest that myeloperoxidase is localized to phagocytic cells in human atherosclerotic lesions. (Fu, X., Kassim, S.Y., Parks, W.C. and

Heinecke, J.W. Hypochlorous acid oxygenates the cysteine switch domain of pro-materializing (MMP-7): A mechanism for matrix metalloproteinase activation and atherosclerotic plaque rupture by myeloperoxidase. J Biol Chem 2001; 276: 41279-41287), (Sugiyama, S., Okada, Y., Subhead, G.K., Virmani, R., Heinecke, J.W. and Libby, P. Macrophage myeloperoxidase regulation by granulocyte macrophage colony-stimulating factor in human atherosclerosis and implications in acute coronary syndromes. Am J Pathol 2001; 158: 879-891). **Actually, I believe that H_2O_2 combines with HOCL to form singlet oxygen, which can act to remove arteriosclerotic plaques as it does in PDT**. Moreover, analysis of amino acid oxidation products in LDL isolated from the human arterial wall **suggests** that HOCl is an important modifier of LDL in vivo. (Heinecke, J.W. Mass spectrometric quantification of amino acid oxidation products in proteins: Insights into pathways that promote LDL oxidation in the human arterial wall. FASEB J 1999; 13: 1113-1120). In vitro, HOCl reacts rapidly with apolipoproteins in LDL, yielding secondary reaction products, such as chloramines, that can induce lipid peroxidation (Hazell, L.J., Davies, M.J. and Stocker, R. Secondary radicals derived from chloramines of apolipoprotein B-100 contribute to HOCl-induced lipid peroxidation of low-density lipoproteins. Biochem J 1999; 339: 489-495). Additionally, myeloperoxidase converts L-tyrosine to tyrosyl radical, which can also induce lipid peroxidation in LDL particles. Curiously, in vitro, vitamin E failed to protect LDL against protein oxidation by myeloperoxidase and the HOCl-induced secondary lipid peroxidation proceeded less rapidly when the lipoproteins were depleted of a-tocopherol. These studies suggest that **vitamin E may not afford protection against myeloperoxidase-dependent oxidative modification of LDL**. This adds further damage to the free radical/oxidation theory.

Another ROS implicated in the oxidation of LDL in vivo is peroxynitrite (OONO-), the reaction product of O_2^- and nitric oxide. In vitro, **OONO--induced protein oxidation was found to be independent of the content of a-tocopherol in LDL particles. Moreover, the magnitude of OONO--induced lipid peroxidation was increased with increasing a-tocopherol content at oxidant-to-LDL ratios of <100:1.** (Thomas, S.R., Davies, M.J. and Stocker, R. Oxidation and antioxidation of human low-density lipoprotein and plasma exposed to 3-morpholinosydnonimine and reagent peroxynitrite. Chem Res Toxicol 1998; 11: 484-494). Thus, vitamin E also may not adequately protect against LDL oxidation by OONO-, an important oxidant species in the blood vessel wall, which further discounts the validity of the free radical/oxidation theory.

On the other hand, clinical studies of **vitamin E in humans have shown mixed results in regard to improvement in endothelial function in patients with atherosclerosis.** (Carr, A.C., Zhu, B.Z. and Frei, B. Potential antiatherogenic mechanisms of ascorbate (vitamin C) and a-tocopherol (vitamin E). Circ Res 2000; 87: 349-354). Thus, if improvement in endothelial function is important in preventing atherosclerosis and its complications, treatment with vitamin E alone may be of little value. I will show that **combinations of antioxidants are equally worthless in treating cardiovascular disease or cancer.**

Traditionally, high levels of RONS have been viewed principally as toxic mediators of cell and tissue injury. More importantly, however, **low levels of RONS have been identified as important regulators of cellular signaling pathways and gene expression in the vasculature.** For example, **RONS can induce the release of arachidonic acid and activate tyrosine kinases and mitogen-activated protein kinases, which are critical components of many intracellular signaling cascades, including those required for cell survival and growth.** In addition, **many cardiovascular genes are redox sensitive.** Redox regulation of gene expression occurs through multiple mechanisms, including activation of upstream signal transduction pathways and modulation of transcription factor binding activity. As RONS, nitric oxide and products formed via interactions among oxidant species (including H_2O_2) can mediate signal transduction, it is conceivable that very high doses of antioxidants could, "**paradoxically,**" produce harmful effects on cellular signaling processes. Here is this "paradox" nonsense again. In addition, the expression of antioxidant enzymes is up-regulated in disease states and by factors such as angiotensin II and tumor necrosis factor-a, indicative of an adaptive response to oxidative stress. By altering redox-mediated signaling, it is possible that antioxidant therapy could suppress this adaptive response, which may, "**paradoxically,**" increase the vulnerability of the blood vessel to oxidative injury. There is no "paradox" in that antioxidants do not offer cardiovascular protection and they can be quite harmful. Authors tend to gloss over increased mortality rates caused by antioxidants by spinning it to say that deaths were slightly augmented instead of telling it like it is, "**Antioxidant supplements killed a bunch of people and gave a lot of others cancer!**"

The oxidants may activate signaling cascades and gene expression that, once set in motion, no longer require the presence of RONS. This is likely what is seen in PDT and in my clinical work with my singlet oxygen generating system.

The lipophilic vitamin E is partitioned into cell membranes and may not adequately protect against oxidant stress in the aqueous cytosolic environment. Furthermore, vitamin E has eight diastereoisomers, which vary considerably in regards to bioavailability and antioxidant potency. Surprisingly, many clinical studies do not specify which isomer (or mixture of isomers) was administered to patients. Some of the stereoisomerisms possess important actions aside from their chain-breaking antioxidant effects, such as inhibition of protein kinase C, which could affect vascular function, and, perhaps, O_2^- production. (Freedman, J.E., Li, L., Sauter, R. and Keaney, JF. Jr. *a*-Tocopherol and protein kinase C inhibition enhance platelet-derived nitric oxide release. FASEB J 2000; 14: 2377-2379). Also, **it is almost unheard of for an author to point out the pro-oxidant activity of many of the so-called antioxidants**. So, I will do it for them.

The recognition that supplementation with antioxidant vitamins (in particular, **vitamin E) is of little or no benefit in preventing or treating atherosclerosis** in large-scale clinical studies in humans raises more questions that it answers. The cellular actions of ROS are quite complex, in that **low levels of RONS appear to be essential for cellular signaling.** Thus, antioxidant supplementation is likely to be harmful to those tissues that are not subjected to substantial oxidative stress. **This is even more threatening to individuals whose immunity is compromised, such as HIV patients, organ recipients who are immunosuppressed or the millions undergoing chemo therapy and irradiation for cancer.** Tragically, this is rarely, if ever, mentioned in the lay press.

15.1 ANTIOXIDANT HOAX

The subsequent materials have been excerpted from and based on the following paper: (Tran, T.L. Antioxidant supplements to prevent heart disease: Real hope or empty hype? Postgrad Med 2001; 109(1): 109-114).

Observational studies can show only an associative and not a causative relationship between antioxidant consumption, supplementation and reduced rates of disease, yet they are routinely presented as "proof."

15.1.0 Quackery

The word *quacksalver* was shortened to "quack" to describe one who boasts (quacks) about the virtues of salves and ointments dispensed by transparent imposters and swindlers. Arthur Summerfield remarked that, "More money was being made in medical quackery than in any other criminal activity." Oliver Wendell Holmes observed that, "Quackery and idolatry are all but immortal. Despite repeated exposures of quackery's fraudulence, extensive federal regulations, law enforcement and the belief that as people become more intelligent and medicine more scientific, quackery should disappear, **quackery is more extensive than ever before.**

The cancer therapy area is filled with fraudulent treatments as has been seen in purported cures for arthritis and the common cold. However, right at the top of the list of quack treatments are vitamins. As was said by Fishbein, in 1938, **"Public interest in vitamins has led to a more extraordinary exploitation than in any other field of medicine." I believe that that holds true today but at exponentionally greater numbers.**

15.2 EPIDEMIOLOGIC CONFUSION

A World Health Organization cross-cultural study (Gey, K.F., Puska, P. and Jordan, P, et al. Inverse correlation between plasma vitamin E and mortality from ischemic heart disease in cross-cultural epidemiology. Am J Clin Nutr 1991; 53(1): 326-345), which surveyed 12 different populations in Europe, showed a significantly lower rate of cardiac death in groups with high dietary intake of vitamin C or vitamin E. Independent studies from Finland and the United States (Luoma, P.V., Nayha, S. and Sikkila, K., et al. High serum alpha-tocopherol, albumin, selenium and cholesterol and low mortality from coronary heart disease in northern Finland. J Intern Med 1995; 237(1): 49-54), (Verlangieri, A.J., Kapeghian, J.C. and el-Dean, S., et al. Fruit and vegetable consumption and cardiovascular mortality. Med Hypotheses 1985; 16(1): 7-15), also demonstrated similar beneficial effects of a diet rich in antioxidants, including vitamin C and E, beta carotene and selenium. In fact, **the lay literature is filled with articles praising the countless benefits and blessings of vitamins, antioxidants and supplements.**

15.3 PROSPECTIVE COHORT STUDY EVIDENCE

15.3.1 The Nurses' Health Study

Outcomes of prospective cohort studies have been **inconsistent.** The Nurses' Health Study (Stampfer, M.J., Hennekens, C.H. and Manson, J.E., et al. Vitamin E consumption and the risk of coronary heart disease in women. N Engl J Med 1993: 328(20): 1444-1449), which surveyed more than **88,000 women over an 8-year period**, showed that women who consumed the highest amount of vitamin E for more than 2 years, in both diet and supplements, had a much lower risk of heart disease compared with those who took the lowest amount. However, use **of vitamin C and beta carotene supplements did not lead to any reduction in heart disease risk.** A similar study involving nearly 40,000 male health professionals (Rimm, E.B., Stampfer, M.J. and Ascherio, A., et al. Vitamin E consumption and the risk of coronary heart disease in men. N Engl J Med 1993; 328(20): 1450-1456), showed risk reductions of up to 40% in men with the highest vitamin E intakes. Use of beta carotene supplements led to smaller reductions in risk but only in smokers. **No benefit was shown for vitamin C supplements.** Most of these studies in the 80's and early 90's appeared to be supportive of the use of vitamins and supplements.

In contrast, the first National Health and Nutrition Examination Survey (Knekt, P., Reunanen, A. and Jarvinen, R., et al. Antioxidant vitamin intake and coronary mortality in a longitudinal population study. Am J Epidemiol 1994; 139(12): 1180-1189), reported a significantly lower risk of cardiovascular death in persons with high intakes of vitamin C. This study, however, did not take into consideration other antioxidants that the study participants might have consumed in addition to vitamin C. More **perplexing** is the Scottish Heart Health Study (Bolton-Smith, C., Woodward, M. and Tunstall-Pedoe, H. The Scottish Heart Health Study. Dietary intake by food frequency questionnaire and odds ratios for coronary heart disease risk. II. The antioxidant vitamins and fiber. Eur J Clin Nutr 1992; 46(2): 85-93), which reported significant benefits from vitamins C and E and beta carotene but **only in men; no benefit was observed in women. Even then, the data did not hold together and results were unpredictable. Yet, they clung to the flawed free radical/oxidative theory. They had to keep trying to make it work.**

Bias is inherent in the selection of participants and there are a myriad of ways to prejudice a study. People who consume large amounts of fruits and vegetables tend to have more healthful living habits. Diets rich in antioxidants are also lower in saturated fat and cholesterol and higher in fiber. The low incidence of heart disease in these subjects could be the result of their overall lifestyle rather than intake of antioxidants alone.

15.3.2 The Alpha-Tocopherol, Beta-Carotene Cancer Prevention (ATBC) Study

The Alpha-Tocopherol, Beta-Carotene Cancer Prevention (ATBC) Study (Viramo, J., Rapola, J.M. and Ripatti, S., et al. Effect of vitamin E and beta carotene on the incidence of primary nonfatal myocardial infarction and fatal coronary heart disease. Arch Intern Med 1998; 158(6): 668-675), examined the effects of **vitamin E and beta** carotene over a period of **5 to 8 years in more than 29,000 male smokers** in Finland. Overall, **no reduction in heart disease or death was found.** Moreover, **an increase in mortality from hemorrhagic stroke was found with use of vitamin E supplements. An increased incidence of cardiac death was also found in the group taking beta carotene supplements.** As a follow up, the August 2004 issue of the European Heart Journal, investigators (ATBC) report that **neither vitamin E nor beta carotene supplements protect male smokers against heart disease and the antioxidants may actually be harmful** and the data argues against the use of these antioxidants in male smokers. **Vitamin E had no effect during the post-trial period on first-ever major coronary events; whereas, beta carotene increased risk for major coronary events by 14%.**

Further, the August issue of journal *Stroke*, reported that vitamin E reduced the risk of stroke due to blockage of arteries supplying blood to the brain by 14%. On the other hand, **beta-carotene increased the risk of stroke rates due to bleeding in the brain by 62%. The odds of an artery-block stroke was increased by 13% in those who had taken vitamin E, and reduced by 3% for these given beta-carotene. The risk of bleeding stroke was increased by 1% in the vitamin E group, but by 38% for beta-carotene supplementation.** The researchers conclude that the apparent increased risks of bleeding **"are difficult to explain because of the absence of any plausible mechanism."**

Similarly, the Beta-Carotene and Retinol Efficacy Trial (Omenn, G.S., Goodman, G.E. and Thornquist, M.D., et al. Effects of a combination of beta carotene and vitamin A on lung cancer and cardiovascular disease. N Engl J Med 1996; 334(18): 1150-1155), which involved more than **18,000 men and women, showed that after an average of 4 years of supplementation, the combination of beta carotene and retinol (vitamin A) had no benefit and may have increased the risk of cardiac death. For God's sake, someone should have told the unknowing public, but instead, the advertising and marketing of these dangerous products proceeded full steam ahead. Ever since, it has basically been "grab the money and run."**

15.3.3 The Physicians' Health Study

The Physicians' Health Study (Hennieken, C.H., Buring, J.E. and Manson, J.E., et al. Lack of effect of long-term supplementation with beta carotene on the incidence of malignant neoplasms and cardiovascular disease. N Engl J Med 1996; 334(18): 1145-1149), which for **12 years followed more than 22,000 male physicians** in the United States, showed **no significant effect of beta carotene on heart disease.** Also, a randomized study of more than **29,000 residents in rural China** (Blot, W.J., Li, J.Y. and Taylor, P.R., et al. Nutrition intervention trials in Linxian, China: Supplementation with specific vitamin/mineral combinations, cancer incidence, and disease-specific mortality in the general population. J Natl Cancer Inst 1993; 85(18): 1483-1492), **over a 5-year period reported no significant benefit of vitamin C supplements in reducing cardiovascular mortality.**

Early results of studies on secondary prevention were encouraging. **The Cambridge heart Antioxidant Study** (Stephens, N.G., Parsons, A. and Schofield, P.M., et al. Randomized controlled trial of vitamin E in patients with coronary disease; Cambridge Heart Antioxidant Study. Lancet 1996; 347(9004): 781-786), showed that in patients with atherosclerotic heart disease confirmed by angiography, high doses of vitamin E could lower the risk of nonfatal heart attack and other cardiovascular events such as stroke, but **the overall mortality rate did not improve.** The ATBC study, mentioned earlier, also showed that persons with previous heart attack had a lower risk of recurrent heart disease when given vitamin E supplements. Again, **there was no improvement in the overall rate of mortality.** Vitamin E was also shown to slow down the progression of atherosclerotic plaque in patients with coronary artery disease in the **Cholesterol Lowering Atherosclerosis Study.** (Hodis, H.N., Mack, W.J. and LaBree, L., et al. Serial coronary angiographic evidence that antioxidant vitamin intake reduces progression of coronary artery atherosclerosis. JAMA 1995; 273(23): 1849-1854). Whether this reduction might lead to a lower risk of heart attack or death **remains to be proved. No benefit was observed with use of vitamin C supplements.**

15.3.4 The GISSI and HOPE Studies

With the release in 1999 of the **Gruppo Italiano per to Studio della Sopravvivenza nell'Infarto miocardico (GISSI)** (GISSI-Prevention Investigators. (Gruppo Italiano per lo Studio della Sopravvivenza nell'Infarto miocardico). Dietary supplementation with n-3 polyunsaturated fatty acids and vitamin E after myocardial infarction: Results of the GISSI-Prevenzione trial. Lancet 1999; 354(9177): 447-455), and the **Heart Outcomes Prevention Evaluation (HOPE)** (Yusuf, S., Dagenais, G. and Pogue, J., et al. Vitamin E supplementation and cardiovascular events in high-risk patients. The Heart Outcomes Prevention Evaluation Study Investigators. N Engl J Med 2000; 342(3): 154-160), the role **of antioxidants for secondary prevention is again in doubt**. The HOPE study reported **no reduction in heart attack, stroke, or death in patients with heart disease or diabetes after use of vitamin E supplements for more than 4 years**. Similarly, the GISSI trial, which followed **11,000 patients with recent heart attacks, showed no benefit from use of vitamin E supplements for up to 2 years**.

15.3.5 The Indian Experiment of Infarct Survival

When antioxidants were used in combination, the results were **also inconclusive**. **The Indian Experiment of Infarct Survival** (Singh, R.B., Niaz, M.A. and Rastogi, S.S., et al. Usefulness of antioxidant vitamins in suspected acute myocardial infarction (the Indian Experiment of Infarct Survival-3). Am J Cardiol 1996; 77(4): 232-236), suggested that a combination of vitamins A, C and E and beta carotene could be beneficial in preventing complications and cardiac events in patients with suspected heart attacks.

15.3.6 The Multivitamins and Probucol Study

The Multivitamins and Probucol Study (Tardif, J.C., Cote, G and Lesperance, J., et al. Probucol and multivitamins in the prevention of restenosis after coronary angioplasty. Multivitamins and Probucol Study Group. N Engl J Med 1997; 337(6): 365-372), however, showed that the **combination of vitamins C and E and beta carotene had no effect in reducing the rate of restenosis in patients after angioplasty**. Probucol has been pulled off the market due harmful effects and the likelihood of cardiac arrhythmias.

15.3.7 Dangers of Antioxidant and Vitamin Supplements

Randomized clinical trails have failed to show a consistent benefit from use of antioxidant supplements; some antioxidant supplements, **especially beta carotene, has caused increased deaths and cancer.**

The amount of antioxidants in supplements may be so high compared with that in the diet that it leads to toxic effects but there is little caution in the lay press regarding safe amounts.

It should be stressed that antioxidant supplements are not without severe or deadly adverse effects. High doses of **vitamin E may lead to hemorrhagic stroke**. Long-term use of **beta carotene supplements may increase the risk of heart disease and cancer**. Many medical and health organizations, including the **American Heart Association, have cautioned the public about the excessive use of antioxidant supplements, especially beta carotene, based on the overwhelming evidence that it might do more harm than good.** (Tribble, D.L. AHA Science Advisory. Antioxidant consumption and risk of coronary heart disease: Emphasis on vitamin C, vitamin E and beta-carotene. A statement for healthcare professionals from the American Heart Association. Circulation 1999; 99(4): 591-595).

Besides vitamins A, C and E and beta carotene, **other antioxidants are being promoted to prevent heart disease: flavonoids, coenzyme Q10 or ubiquinone (Ubiqgel), selenium (Sele-Pak, Selepen), and**

lycopene, to name a few. Compared with studies of the more common antioxidants, **studies of these substances are more scarce and even less conclusive. Because the antioxidant properties of these newer products are stronger than many of the older ones, they have an even greater potential for harm, disease and death. Yet, because they are patentable, they are vigorously promoted to an unknowing public.**

The notion that antioxidant supplements can prevent heart disease has not been proven or supported by current clinical evidence. To the contrary, it has been proven that they do not prevent heart disease.

Unfortunately, **epidemiological studies** are considered suboptimal for deciding whether a therapy works. In epidemiological studies, a population of patients is followed for a period of time, keeping track of which patients happen to be using the therapy in question and which do not. Outcomes are then compared between patients using and not using the therapy. Because there may be inherent (but unidentified) differences between those who use a therapy and those who do not, and because patients who choose to use a therapy might experience improvement due to a **"placebo effect,"** such studies are regarded as offering suggestive evidence, but not proof, of a treatment's effectiveness. With a placebo effect, a "treatment" that actually has no specific physiological benefit produces positive results because patients expect it to. **The placebo effect is now recognized as sometimes being quite powerful in alleviating symptoms, and has confounded the evaluation of countless therapies. Just as important is the fact that prejudicial intents by an investigator can give false results and result in a meaningless study.**

To "really" measure a treatment's effectiveness, randomized trials are usually considered necessary. In randomized trials, groups of "identical" patients (that is, as close to identical as possible) are randomly chosen to receive the treatment in question - those who are not randomized to receive the treatment are given placebo. Ideally, neither the patients nor their doctors are aware of whether they are actually receiving the treatment or placebo. Randomized trials, then, at least in theory, minimize any hidden, systematic differences between patients taking or not taking the treatment being studied, and eliminate any falsely positive outcomes that may result from a **"placebo effect"** (since patients taking either the actual treatment or the identical-appearing placebo ought to have the same degree of placebo effect).

During the last two years, a number of randomized trials using antioxidant vitamin supplements have finally been reported, and the **results have generally been disappointing. Because of the failure of randomized trials to demonstrate a benefit from taking antioxidants, both the American Heart Association and the Institute of medicine have release recent statements saying that, while a diet rich in antioxidant vitamins seem prudent, there is insufficient evidence to recommend using supplements of vitamin C, vitamin E, beta-carotene, selenium, or other antioxidants to prevent heart disease.**

Patients need to be made aware of the dangers of antioxidants, vitamins and supplements and they should be encouraged to prevent cardiovascular disease by cessation of smoking, eating a prudent diet containing fresh fruits and vegetables and to exercise daily.

A 2004 report in the journal *Arthritis & Rheumatism,* stated that **vitamin C may worsen arthritis.** Before scoffing at this report, please keep in mind the biphasic activity of ascorbic acid as both antioxidant and a pro-oxidant and how it is effected by dose levels. USDA recommends 90 mg of vitamin C to men and 75 mg to women. However, many health food stores may recommend 675 mg, considerably more than one needs.

Another 2004 report stated, **that antioxidant vitamins may be potentially harmful for the heart based on their ability to increase the secretion of very low-density lipoproteins in the liver cells** of experimental mice. However, Prof. Edward Fischer of New York Univ. School of Medicine was quoted in the *London Times* as not making recommendations on taking antioxidant vitamins at this time.

Some investigators have reviewed prospective epidemiological studies and randomized clinical trials (RCT) regarding the role of antioxidant vitamins (vitamins E and C and beta-carotene) in the prevention of cardiovascular diseases. Lonn and Yusuf reviewed prospective epidemiological studies and double-blind, randomized controlled trials (RCT)s with at least 100 participants were included in the review. Retrospective studies, geographical correlations and case series were excluded. **Eighteen studies with 295,311 participants were included in the review: 12 prospective observational studies and 6 RCTs of these studies, 7 (227,493 participants) assessed vitamin E, 12 (246,488 participants) assessed beta-carotene and 10 (186,985 participants) assessed vitamin C.**

In conclusion, RCTs remain **inconclusive with regard to the role of vitamin E in cardiovascular protection.** The large RCT of beta-carotene in primary prevention showed **no effect** associated with the use of beta-carotene and possibly a potential for harm. There were **inconclusive and insufficient epidemiological and clinical trial data with regard to the role of vitamin C in cardiovascular protection.** The authors recommend that widespread use of antioxidant vitamins in cardiovascular protection should not be instituted, and should await the results of further ongoing trials. (Lonn, E.M. and Yusuf, S. Is there a role for antioxidant vitamins in the prevention of cardiovascular disease: An update on epidemiological and clinical trials data. Can J Cardio 1997; 13(10): 957-965).

I believe that part of the reason that beta-carotene and vitamin E (tocopherols) had either no effect or an adverse effect on cancer and cardiovascular disease is that they are quenchers of singlet oxygen. Hence, they produce deficiencies or lowered steady state levels of RONS and singlet oxygen and allow for the progressive development of both cancer and CVD. Furthermore, antioxidant use should be contraindicated in immunologically compromised patients.

15.3.8 Miscellaneous Antioxidant Factoids

-Beta Carotene is a Vitamin A precursor.

-Synthetic Beta Carotene is all trans double bonds, it is not effective.

-Cytoplasmic SOD contains copper.

-Mitochondrial SOD contains manganese.

-Extracellular SOD has only 1/3000 activity of intracellular SOD (Lam).

-SOD blocks platelet secretion and thrombin-induced adhesion (O_2 Paradox, page 241).

-According to the oxidative theory of Harman, it doesn't make sense, that the prostate and breasts are two of the areas of highest incidence of cancer in men and women; yet, the most active antioxidants are concentrated there. Thus, they should, by the free radical theory, have the lowest incidence of cancer. Actually, they have the highest.

-Vitamin C is present in cells in micromolar quantities (1/1000 of glutathione).

-Vitamin E is present in cells in nanomolar quantities (1/1,000,000 glutathione).

-Mammalian cells have 4 main antioxidant mechanisms

  1. Chelating transition metal catalysts, transferrin
  2. Chain-breaking reactions, a-tocopherol
  3. Reducing concentration of reactive radicals, glutathione
  4. Scavenging initiating radicals, SOD (Lam).

-90% Vitamin E is contained in serum LDL & HDL.

-1 LDL contains 6 a-tocopherol molecules and 1000 PUFAs.

-1 molecule Vitamin E can protect 3000 PUFA from free radical injury.

-Glutathiol contains sulphur and selenium.

-1 Vitamin C molecule terminates 0.6 free radicals

-**Catalase, in most aerobic cells, in humans is highest in liver and kidney and lowest in brain, heart and skeletal muscle. Yet, heart, brain and skeletal muscle has a very high rate of utilization of oxygen and generates the highest levels of RONS/excytomers and still they have very low rates of cancer formation. This is directly contradictory to the free radical theory and in direct support of my Unified Theory.**

RMH Note: Others say that H_2O_2 is mutagenic and therefore, heart, brain and skeletal muscle should have higher levels of cancer incidence than liver and kidney. But this is not true. Also, if H_2O_2 is harmful, then these organs (i.e., heart, brain and skeletal muscle), should have high levels of catalase to control "mutagenic or toxic" levels of H_2O_2 from accumulating from high O_2 consumption and metabolism....but, it doesn't, heart, brain and skeletal muscle have low levels of catalase.

-Both of these factors argue against the theory of oxidative stress, cancer and aging.

-GSH itself can also undergo $O_2^{\cdot-}$ dependent chain oxidation and thus contribute to oxidative stress, but by a pathway involving sulfinyl radical that leads to the thiyl radical and regeneration of $O_2^{\cdot-}$, without H_2O_2 formation.

-Most cells rely on de novo synthesis of GSH (O_2 Paradox, page 225).

-There is a general trend towards richness in GPX a-SODs in epithelial linings (O_2 Paradox, page 253).

-Following fertilization, the zygote is not protected from ROS oxidative damage (in the rat) for 12 days till GPX, SODs develop. **RMH Note: Why doesn't the RONS from the maternal circulation cause irreparable harm to the fetus?** (O_2 Paradox, page 253).

-**Several tumor cell types have reduced SOD and CAT levels** (O_2 Paradox, page 434).

-Vitamin E deficiency can result in lipid oxidation and externalization of phosphatidyl serine (a cofactor in coagulation cascade) leading to hypercoagulability, hyper viscosity and microvascular occlusion like myocardial, cerebral, vascular and spleno-hepatic microcirculation (hemorrheological disorders). (O_2 Paradox 483).

-SOD is 4 orders of magnitude faster than disproportionation (O_2 Paradox, page 487).

-Glutathione peroxidase requires 4 molecules of selenium per molecule of enzyme protein.

-10-15% of cellular glutathione is in the mitochondrial organelle. This low molecular weight thiol (tripeptide) tries to keep a reducing media present.

- Catalase is found in peroxisomes and not in mitochondria. **RMH Note: I find it quite curious that this is the case, in that the greatest site of $O_2^{\cdot-}$ production (which is basically H_2O_2 production) is the mitochondrion and catalase is absent. I believe that this is another way that the body is telling us that it needs H_2O_2 or it would have catalase present.**

- After the discovery of SOD in 1969, the proposed damaging effects of O_2 radicals was known as the **"superoxide theory of O_2 toxicity."**

- Glutathione peroxidase (GPx) a Se-containing enzyme removes H_2O_2 by converting reduced glutathione (GSH) into oxidized glutathione (GSSG). Most of the glutathione is found intracellularly

$$H_2O_2 + 2GSH \text{ (reduced)} \rightarrow GSSG \text{ (oxidized)} + H_2O$$

- Short term deprivation of vitamin E and selenium cause no harmful effects. Long term deficiency of selenium causes Keshan's disease, which is a degenerative disease of the heart due to soil deficiency of selenium in Keshan District of Heilongjiang province of China. Excess selenium causes loss of finger and toe nails. (Lam)

- Clearly, antioxidants are important to human life but they are not elixirs of life. Should we all take dietary antioxidant and trace element supplements, make drug companies rich, live forever and be disease free? **In strict scientific terms, little or nothing is proved.** (Lam)

-Most tumor cells have lower levels of SOD.

-SODs pharmaceutical form is "orgotein."

-Primary auto-oxidants - i.e., phenolic antioxidants such as tocopherols (Vitamin E), propyl gallate (PG), butylated hydroxyanisole (BHA), butylated hydroxytoluene (BHT), and tertiary butyhydroquinone (TBHQ).

-Beta carotene scavenges only under partial pressures of O_2 significantly less than 150 torr (normal air) which is at physiological conditions. With higher tissue pressures, beta carotene becomes a pro-oxidant.

- **Flavonoids (**polyphenolics) categories (**over 4,000 identified**): flavonols, flavanones, catechins, chalones, flavons, isolators, anthocyanidins.

- Average daily intake of vitamin C is 70 mg, vitamin E is 7-10 mg, carotenoids is 2-3 mg and flavonoids is 50-800 mg.

- **The antioxidant activity of lager beer (flavonoids) is higher than grape juice, green tea, and red wine.**

16 ANTIOXIDANTS AND CANCER

A post intervention follow-up on incidence of cancer and mortality following a-Tocopherol and β-Carotene supplementation was presented in 2003. There conclusion was that **large-scale controlled trials have not produced consistent evidence for the efficacy of a-tocopherol or β-carotene in the prevention of cancer.** There is, however, consistent evidence **that β-carotene supplementation in smokers increases the risk of lung cancer and total mortality.** The cumulative experience of nearly 16 years and nearly 350,000 person-years of observation during the intervention and post intervention follow-up of participants in the ATBC Study suggests a symmetry in the effect of β-carotene on these events, with the disappearance of risk occurring within the time it became evident. Furthermore, the post trail follow-up did not reveal any late preventive effects on cancer.

Thus, the recommendations made at the time their initial trial results were reported remain appropriate: the possible preventive effect of a-tocopherol on prostate cancer **requires confirmation** from other trials before public health recommendations can be made for vitamin E. (The ATBC Study Group. Incidence of cancer and mortality following a-tocopherol and β-carotene supplementation. JAMA 2003; 290: 476-485).

In 2002, C. T. Ryan presented a brief summary on antioxidants and cancer prevention. She states that antioxidants which were once confined to the vocabulary of scientists and nutritionists, the word "antioxidant" is now plastered on everything from magazine headlines to grocery ads. Basically, antioxidant means "against oxygen." Even though diets rich in fruits and vegetables (and thus naturally high in antioxidants) are thought to protect against cancer, **there is no convincing evidence** that the same benefits can be achieved by taking antioxidants as supplements. Keep in mind that fresh fruits and vegetables are also high in hydrogen peroxide.

16.1 ANTIOXIDANT INTAKE AND CANCER RISK

With a biologically plausible mechanism and such strong evidence from laboratory and animal studies, **one would naturally expect human studies to show lower cancer risks among those who have higher antioxidant intakes. However, this has not been the case.** Observational studies and randomized controlled trials have both failed to convincingly demonstrate a link between antioxidant intake and cancer risk. In fact, I have to wonder how any RONS get through the gauntlet of cellular antioxidants and into the nucleus, such that, according to Ames, they produce 10,000 hits upon DNA daily upon every cell in the body. Below is a brief summary of several major antioxidants.

16.2 VITAMIN E

Alpha-tocopherol is believed to be the major lipid-soluble, chain-breaking biological antioxidant, which protects mammalian cellular membranes from oxidative damage. In 1922 Evans and Bishop discovered vitamin E and proposed that it was and essential micronutrient for reproduction in rats. Alpha-tocopherol is believed to be the form of vitamin E which has the greatest nutritional significance and is the form maintained in the human body and found in the blood and tissue.. Actually, **vitamin E defines a group of 8 antioxidants, four tocopherols (alpha, beta, gamma, and delta) and four tocotrienols (also, alpha, beta, gamma and delta).** Technically, the term **tocopherol** is a generic descriptor for all mono, di, and trimethyltocols and **is not synonymous with vitamin E**. Alpha-tocopherols and tocotrienols scavenge lipid peroxyl radicals in the phospholipid bilayer faster than they can react with adjacent side-chains or with membrane proteins.

Lipid peroxidation produces alpha-tocopherolquinone, which is found in trace levels in humans and is reduced to hydroquinones. Clinical work on vitamin E has been on going for decades and has also produced conflicting and confusing results. The Cambridge Heart Antioxidant Study (CHAOS), in 1966, reported that vitamin E supplementation (400-800 IU/day) in 2000 patients, for about 2 years, significantly reduced **the incidence of cardiovascular death and nonfatal myocardial infarction by a whopping 77%** (Stephens, N.G., Parsons, A., Schofield, P.M., Kelly,, F., Cheeseman, K., and Mitchinson, M.J. Randomized controlled trial of vitamin e in patients with coronary disease - Cambridge Heart Antioxidant Study (CHAOS). Lancet. 1996, 339: 781-786.). Additionally, vitamin E supplementation has been thought to enhance specific aspects of the immune response that appear to decline with age and was found to increase formation of antibodies in response to hepatitis B vaccine and tetanus vaccine in the elderly patients (Meydani, S.N. vitamin E supplementation and in vivo immune response in healthy elderly adults. A randomized controlled trial. JAMA. 1997. 277: 1380-1386.). Please keep in mind this data when I present data to the contrary subsequently.

Although vitamin E has been studied in relation to most of the major cancers, there is **no convincing evidence that taking vitamin E lowers risk.**

16.3 CAROTENOIDS

Beta Carotene is one of over 600 carotenoids found in plants.

16.3.1 β-carotene

Beta carotene is one of the orange dyes found in most green leaves, and in carrots. When leaves lose their chlorophyll in the fall, carotene is one of the colors left over in the leaf.

Beta carotene is used in foods to provide color (margarine would look as white as shortening without it). Another similar molecule, **annatto is used in cheeses**, and another famous carotenoid dye, **saffron is used to color rice and other foods.**

Beta carotene is sometimes added to products for **its antioxidant effects**, to keep fats from going rancid.

The body turns it into vitamin A, and beta carotene is sometimes added to foods or vitamin supplements as a nutrient.

The same long chains of **conjugated double bonds (alternating single and double bonds)** that give the carotenes their colors are also the reason them make good antioxidants. They can mop up oxygen free radicals and dissipate their energy.

16.3.2 Lycopene

Another colorful carotene is **lycopene**. This is the red molecule that gives **ripe tomatoes** their color. There are alternating double and single bonds between the carbon atoms. These are called **"conjugated" bonds, or "resonance" bonds**. The electrons in those bonds are not locked onto one atom, but spend their time bouncing from atom to atom. This gives the effect of something in between a double bond and single bond, more of a one and a half bond.

The **long chain of conjugated bonds acts like a wire**, allowing the electrical energy to move from one side of the molecule to the other. The energy can slosh around like water in a bathtub. Normally it takes quite a bit of energy to move an electron away from an atom. **X-rays, or high energy ultraviolet light can move an electron into a higher orbit in an atom,** but ordinary visible light does not usually have enough energy.

A molecule of **lycopene can absorb blue light** because the electrons are not orbiting a single atom, they are sloshing around orbiting many atoms, and **the energy needed to move them is a lot less than in a smaller molecule, or one without conjugated bonds.**

You can think of energy in a lycopene molecule as a wave sloshing in a bathtub, or the wave you can make with a jump rope. The lowest energy state (called the "ground" state) would correspond to the jump rope going around in the normal fashion.

Each end of the jump rope is a **"node,"** a place where the rope doesn't move. It is possible to get a jump rope to have three nodes, as you may have done as a child. It acts like there are two jump ropes, each one half the length of the other. The energy sloshing around in the lycopene molecule can do the same thing. Absorbing a photon of green light makes it act as if the molecule were two molecules, each half as long. The molecule has absorbed the green light. White light that is missing; its green light looks red. **Beta carotene absorbs blue light, so it looks orange.**

Another class of colored compounds are the anthocyanins. These molecules give color to flowers, blueberries, apples, and red cabbage. Anthocyanins are in the group of compounds known as **flavonoids**. **Over 4000 polyphenol flavonoids have been identified.**

Anthocyanins can change their color, depending on how acid or alkaline they are. In neutral conditions, the molecule has no charge. It absorbs yellow light, and appears purple. In an acid (pH less than 3), the acid donates a hydrogen nucleus, and the molecule becomes positive. The bond next to the oxygen becomes a double bond, and the molecule now absorbs green light, so it appears red. In an alkaline solution, the molecule donates a hydrogen nucleus, and a hydroxyl group becomes an oxygen atom with a negative charge. The molecule now absorbs orange light, and appears blue.

Like vitamin E, carotenoids have been studied extensively with no convincing evidence of a cancer-related benefit. Although serum studies suggest that high carotenoid levels may lower the risk of breast cancer, this is still under investigation. Similarly, there is some evidence that lycopene might reduce prostate cancer risk, but studies on this have focused on dietary intake, and the effects of supplementation **remain unclear**. Finally, while a number of observational studies support a link between high carotenoid intake and lower risk of lung cancer, **randomized trails have shown an increase in lung cancer risk among smokers taking beta-carotene supplements**.

- This is a most important revelation in the data because β-carotene is a very efficient scavenger of $^1O_2$. Thus, my **Unified Theory** would predict that a deficiency of the cancer-killing $^1O_2$ produced by excessive amounts of this antioxidant, will result in increased cancer rates. **My Unified Theory is supported by this important data and the Free Radi-Crap theory is further invalidated.**

16.4 VITAMIN C

William Porter stated that, "Of all the paradoxical compounds, vitamin C probably tops the list. It is truly a two-headed Janus, a Dr. Jekyll-Mr. Hyde, an oxymoron of antioxidants." Here we go with another **"paradox."** Controversy surrounded **Linus Pauling** and Ewan Cameron's work on mega-doses of vitamin C and cancer therapy and the battle continued until Dr. Pauling's death at 93 years of age in 1994. I had the pleasure of meeting him on a visit to Tulane School of Medicine, while I was in both Medical school and graduate school for biochemistry. Obviously, I was somewhat in awe of this biochemical genius but I do recall his bitterness toward the medical/pharmaceutical industry, which he referred to as **"the sickness industry."** I truly hated to see the conflict, which marred the life of this brilliant man. Also, since I was the first student in Tulane's history to complete an M.D. and a Ph.D. in biochemistry simultaneously, I remember his words ever so clearly that, **"Randy, it may take people like you to bridge the huge chasm, which presently exists, between the physician/clinician and the research scientist."** Reportedly, Dr. Pauling had worked himself (and his wife) up to ingesting 25,000 milligrams of vitamin C daily. Allegedly, both he and his wife died of cancer. Most are familiar with the story of Norman Cousins, who was reportedly terminal and checked himself out of the hospital and began a daily megadose regimen of **vitamin C and laughter**, thus, producing longevity and a cure.

Humans lack gulonolactone oxidase, which is necessary to synthesize vitamin C an**d H_2O_2 is produced as a by-product in the process.** Dr. Albert Szent-Gyorgii first isolated vitamin C and jokingly first named it "ignose," referring to its resemblance to sugar and to his ignorance as to its nature. We now know that it is an important co-factor, along with O_2, in collagen synthesis and in many vital metabolic steps. At least 8 iron or copper containing enzymes use vitamin C as a co-factor. Please keep in mind the fact that vitamin C is also a pro-oxidant, in that it aids oxidation of substrates. **Vitamin C can also kill malarial parasites and cancer cells in vitro.** It likely does so by increasing RONS/excytomer production like occurs with PDT.

There is some evidence for a protective effect of vitamin C on certain cancers. However, these studies have focused on dietary intake, and the perennial question remains: is the protective effect due to vitamin C itself or to the combination of vitamins and minerals found in fruits, vegetables and other vitamin C-rich foods?

Vitamin C inhibits cell division and growth through production of **hydrogen peroxide**, which damages the cells probably through an as yet unidentified free radical(s) generation/mechanism. Results also suggest that ascorbic acid is a potent anticancer agent for prostate cancer cells. (Maramag, C., Menon, M., Balaji, K.C., Reddy, P.G. and Laxmanan, S. Effect of vitamin C on prostate cancer cells in vitro: Effect on cell number, viability and DNA synthesis. Prostate 1997; 32(3): 188-195), (Menon, M., Maramag, C., Malhotra, R.K. and Seethalaskshmi, L. Effect of vitamin C on androgen independent prostate cancer cells (PC3 and Mat-Ly-Lu) in vitro: Involvement of reactive oxygen species-effect on cell number, viability and DNA synthesis. Cancer Biochem Biophys 1998; 16(1-2): 17-30).

16.5 SELENIUM

Though not an antioxidant itself, selenium is an essential cofactor for an antioxidant enzyme, glutathione peroxidase. As such, it has been studied extensively in relation to cancer risk, but again there has been **no convincing evidence of a cancer-related benefit**. In fact, evidence against a large and rapid impact of selenium comes from a fortification intervention that was implemented in Finland. Because of low selenium levels in the soil there (leading to low levels in foods), selenium was applied with fertilizer in the mid-1980's. Blood selenium levels rose rapidly after this, but there has been **no apparent decline in prostate and colon cancer incidence and mortality**. (Ryan, C.T. Taking antioxidants for cancer prevention: A leap of faith. Newsletter of the Harvard Center for Cancer Prevention 2002; 9(1)).

β-carotene and other carotenoids have been thought to have anti-cancer activity, either because of antioxidant activity or because of their ability to be converted to vitamin A. Nevertheless, two large scale intervention studies in humans using high doses of β-carotene found **that β-carotene supplementation resulted in more lung cancer** rather than less lung cancer among smoking and asbestos exposed populations. R.M. Russell states that, "It appears that the explanation of the apparent paradoxical effects of β-carotene on lung cancer is related to dose (if you are a ferret)." (Russell, R.M. The enigma of β-carotene in carcinogenesis: What can be learned from animal studies. Am Soc Nutri Sci 2004; 134: 262S-268S).

Both NAC and Lipoic Acid are Glutathione Precursors

Despite the well documented damaging effects of oxidative stress, treatment of human oxidant-induced diseases with antioxidants including n-acetylcysteine (NAC) has yielded **disappointing results** (Molnar, Z., Shearer, E. and Lowe D. N-Acetylcysteine treatment to prevent the progression of multi-system organ failure: A prospective, randomized, placebo-controlled study. Crit Care Med 1999; 27: 1100-1104). Although suboptimal dosing, inappropriate timing of administration and failure to reach the site of action are among cited reasons for lack of efficacy of antioxidants in clinical trials, emerging evidence indicates that oxidative stress also modulates immune responses. For example, patients with chronic granulomatous disease, an inherited disorder caused by defects in respiratory burst oxidase, develop severe noninfectious inflammatory granuloma in lung, skin and gastrointestinal tract. (Foster, C.B., Lehrnbecher, T., Mol, F., Steinberg, S.M., Venzon, D.J., Walsh, T.J., Noack, D., Rae, J., Winkelstein, J.A. and Curnutte, J.T. et al. Host defense molecule polymorphisms influence the risk of immune-mediated complications in chronic granulomatous disease. J Clin Invest 1998; 102: 2146-2155). In a model of allogeneic (from the same species) marrow transplantation, Yang and coworkers observed exuberant pulmonary and systemic inflammation in irradiated mice lacking phagocytic nicotinamide adenine dinucleotide phosphate-oxidase, a major source of reactive oxygen species, compared with the wild type mice. Importantly, exaggerated immune-responses in nicotinamide adenine dinucleotide phosphate-oxidase-deficient mice were associated with suppression of oxidation/nitrative stress, increased serum and lavage fluid levels of the proinflammatory chemokine, monocyte chemoattractant protein-1, and impaired clearance of exogenous recombinant macrophage inflammatory protein-1B from the circulation. **These results indicate that oxidative stress can function to suppress tissue-damaging inflammatory responses by inactivation of chemokines in vivo**.

A **word of caution** regarding the use of n-acetylcysteine during oxidant-mediated disease is **warranted**, because the hydrogen atom of the free sulfhydryl group of n-acetylcysteine may be extracted by radical intermediates to generate a thiyl radical that can further propagate free radical reactions. (Sagrista, M.L., Garcia, A.F., De Madariaga, M.A. and Mora, M. Antioxidant and prooxidant effect of the thiolic compounds N-acetyl-L-cysteine and glutathione against free radical-induced lipid peroxidations. Free Radic Res 2002; 36: 329-340).

Total inhibition of oxidant production may also be detrimental because of the important physiologic roles of reactive oxygen species in regulating the redox state, which is critical for cell growth/differentiation. (Pani, G., Colavitti, R., Bedogni, B., Anzevino, R., Borrello, S. and Galecotti, T. A redox signaling mechanism for density-dependent inhibition of cell growth. J Biol Chem 2000; 275: 38891-38899).

Taken together, these results are consistent with the notion that **extreme inhibition of reactive oxygen species is best avoided. Maintaining a threshold level of oxidative stress can be beneficial**, especially during chemokines-driven inflammatory disease. The challenge remains to accurately estimate the extent of oxidative stress required to inactivate inflammatory mediators without causing significant effector oxidant-mediated injury.

17 MEGAVITAMIN THERAPY (OR "ANTIOXIDANT STRESS," AS IT WOULD BE REFERRED TO BY OXY-MORONS)

Some of the following materials were excerpted from or based upon articles appearing in the following: www. bodytalkmagazine.com/vitamins.htm and www.wustl.edu/-compmed/CAM_MEG.htm and Cecil's Textbook of Medicine 22nd Edition.

Many chemical reactions occurring in the body inevitably produce free radicals. The body can, however, usually keep these free radicals under control and uses them in maintaining cellular homeostasis. Moreover, despite the long list of problems they cause, free radicals are not all bad. **They play an essential role in a healthy human body.** The body harnesses the power of the free radicals - the oxy radicals and ROS - for use in the immune system and in inflammatory reactions. Certain cells in these systems engulf bacteria or viruses, take up oxygen molecules from the bloodstream, remove an electron to create a flood of oxy radicals and ROS, and bombard the invader with the resulting toxic shower. **This aggressive use of toxic oxygen species is remarkably effective in protecting the body against infectious organisms**.

If a little bit of something is good for you, then a lot of it should be really good for you (more is better). This is this rationale behind megavitamin therapy. Since **RONS have been linked to all major diseases and degenerative conditions, including dandruff and hangovers**, antioxidant consumption has been successfully promoted with the general population. This has led many individuals to consume dangerously high doses of these antioxidants. Unfortunately, and not known to many people, is the fact that **when large amounts of antioxidant nutrients are taken, they can also act as pro-oxidants by inducing stress** (Podmore, I.D., Griffiths, H.R., Herbert, K.E., Mistry, N., Mistry, P. and Lunec, J. Vitamin C exhibits pro-oxidant properties [letter], Nature 1998; 392: 559), (Palozza, P. Pro-oxidant actions of carotenoids in biologic systems. Nutr Rev 1998; 56: 257-265). Reportedly, all major vitamins (e.g., A, C, and E) and flavonoids can serve as pro-oxidants. Also, according to Palozza, pro-oxidant activity can induce either beneficial or harmful effects in biosystems.

Megavitamin therapy is the use of vitamins in doses that exceed the Recommended Daily allowance (RDA). **Megadose therapy is the use of vitamins in doses that are ten times greater than the RDA dose (5 times with vitamin D).** Both therapies are often used preventatively based on the belief that intakes of certain vitamins and minerals in amounts greater than the RDA may reduce the risk of developing some diseases. In addition, megavitamin therapy has been used as a treatment for diseases such as cancer, heart disease, schizophrenia and the common cold. However, some megavitamin therapy regimens produce adverse effects and are unsafe, while others are not supported by conclusive evidence and may be ineffective.

Everyday some new "potion" is aggressively marketed with an exotic sounding name or with outlandish claims that encourage individuals to take almost toxic levels of vitamins, antioxidants and dietary supplements. The theory they project is that these agents are good for you, therefore, the more of them you ingest, the healthier you will be, but, this is wrong. Please remember the wisdom of Paracelsus, "only the dosage makes the poison," in regards to everything that you ingest.

The following is a selective list of some common antioxidants and vitamins and their known risks and adverse effects:

17.1 VITAMIN A
(RETINOID COMPOUNDS/RETINOL)

Unless you have celiac disease or cystic fibrosis, a deficiency of vitamin A is rare in Western countries, as your liver stores enough supplies to get you through the months. It needs fats in the gut to be absorbed. A balanced diet containing dairy foods, eggs and fish should provide adequate amounts of A. Fruits and yellow and green veggies contain beta-carotene, which is converted to vitamin A in the body (remember that, beta-carotene was thought to help prevent lung cancer but recent trials in the US were stopped after the **incidence of lung cancer actually increased**).

The RDA for vitamin A is 1000 retinol equivalents. (1 retinol equiv. = 1 microgram = 3.33 IU). Vitamin A is essential for embryogenesis growth and epithelial differentiation. However, consumption of 7500 -15000 microgram/day can result in liver toxicity. There is an **increased prevalence of defects associated with cranial-neural-crest tissue in babies** born to pregnant women who take more than 3000 microgram/day of preformed vitamin A. However, there is no evidence that doses lower than 3000 microgram/day produce adverse effects in adults, including pregnant women and the elderly.

Hypervitaminosis A, which most often affects adolescents taking excessive dosages for acne, causes increased intracranial pressure, which, if prolonged, **can result in visual loss**. A normal adult diet supplies around 5000 units of vitamin A per day (adult minimum is 2500 units, children 1000-2500 per day). **Taking unnecessary supplements can lead to chronic toxicity which causes vomiting, headache, scaly skin, hair loss, tender bones, enlarged liver, anemia, cracked lips. It's worse in kids - arrested growth and headaches. Pregnant women can have malformed children.**

17.2 VITAMIN B6 (PYRIDOXINE)

The RDA for pyridoxine is 2 mg/day. Both deficient and excess intake of pyridoxine can **cause neurologic disturbances**. Daily intake of over 500 mg/day has been shown to **cause sensory neuropathy**. Doses of up to 200 mg/day are not associated with adverse effects.

Alcoholics or people who don't have a balanced diet may need B6 supplements, but outside that, there's no valid reason for popping extra pills. The recommended amount per day is 2.5 mg (50 mg during pregnancy). Taking over 100 mg per day can lead to **nerve toxicity. Over 2000 mg per day will lead to toxic nerve damage**.

A **severe sensory polyneuropathy** affects persons taking pyridoxine in mega doses (2 to 6 g/day for 2 to 40 months). Doses in excess of 100 mg/day are never indicated and are unwise, because the lower limit of toxicity has not been defined. Improvement follows pyridoxine withdrawal but typically requires months to years.

17.3 VITAMIN C (ASCORBIC ACID)

Ascorbic acid (vitamin C) **does not cure colds or cancer**, and we only need around 25-40 mg per day (more if you're pregnant, smoke, have an unbalanced diet or medical deficiency).

The RDA for ascorbic acid is 60 mg/day. Doses of vitamin C greater than 1000 mg have been shown to inhibit the chemical synthesis of nitro amines (animal carcinogens) in the gastric contents, and both clinical and epidemiological studies suggest that high intakes of vitamin C may reduce the risk of risk factors for diseases such as heart disease and cancer, especially when combined with high intakes of vitamin E. Vitamin C is one of the most controversial vitamins **and studies can be found to support most any position one cares to take.** In my opinion, this aspect of the data only serves to weaken all of the data on vitamin C and it must be kept in mind **that it can serve also as a prooxidant.** Please refer to papers of Dr. Linus Pauling and the Pauling Institute for further discussions of high dose vitamin C therapy.

Unsubstantiated reports of adverse side effects of high intake of vitamin C have claimed kidney stone formation, uricosuria, mutagenicity, iron overload and conditioned scurvy. However, no controlled study of vitamin C toxicity in humans has been undertaken and the existing reports seem to have little factual basis. The most common side effect of high doses of vitamin C is transient gastrointestinal distress and doses greater than 1 g/day have not conclusively been shown to produce any adverse effects.

Taking high doses of vitamin C can actually **create a dependency**, or your body gets used to dealing with the extra load. If you suddenly stop taking vitamin C, the body still operated in "big load" mode and actually destroys C more quickly. Ironically, a condition called **'rebound scurvy'** occurs. You may also be **prone to kidney stones**.

A recent study showed that **mega-doses of vitamin C might actually speed up hardening of the arteries.** Researchers from the University of Southern California studied 573 outwardly healthy middle-aged men and women. About 30% of them regularly took various vitamins. The study found no clear-cut sign that getting lots of vitamin C from food or a daily multivitamin does any harm. But **those taking vitamin C pills had accelerated thickening of the walls of the big arteries in their necks. The more they took, the faster the buildup.**

The only consistent aspect of antioxidant activity, is its inconsistency, other than for the treatment of deficiency states.

The Institute of Medicine in the US reports there's a total lack of evidence to show large doses of antioxidants protect us from disease. In the case of vitamin C, doses of over 2000 milligrams can cause diarrhea, and **mega doses may even accelerate cancer growth and harden the arteries.** The University of Pennsylvania found large doses of vitamin C triggered the release of DNA-damaging chemicals in the body, which may lead to cancer. The Institute of Medicine has set recommended daily doses of vitamin C for women at 75 milligrams and 90 mg for men. Smokers should add another 35 mg.

To add further to the confusion, Barry Haliwell of the National University of Singapore wrote an article in Lancet, explaining why large doses of **antioxidant vitamins sometimes prevent cancer and sometimes causes it**. Every chemical reaction in the body releases chemicals called free radicals that damage tissue, which releases certain metals into the cell fluid. Antioxidants convert these free metals, which are harmless, to powerful oxidants that cause further cell damage. So sometimes antioxidants protect cells and other times, they damage them. For example, paraquat is a powerful cancer-causing chemical. If you give vitamin C to animals before giving them paraquat, the vitamin C prevents cells damage and helps protect them from cancer, but if you give these same animals vitamin C after they take paraquat, **the vitamin C spreads the cancer.** The paraquat causes cells to release large amounts of minerals and the vitamin C then causes these minerals to damage cells and spread the cancer. For this reason, and others, **the American Cancer society advises patients not to take large doses of vitamin A, E, C and selenium.**

I believe that one of the most important reasons not to take large doses of antioxidant vitamins is that free radicals of oxygen and singlet oxygen can kill cancer cells and have been shown to be able to dissolve arteriosclerotic plaques. Logically, although theoretical, taking high doses of antioxidants would be working against this natural protective activity.

17.4 VITAMIN D
(CALCIFEROL, CHOLECALCIFEROL)

Sunshine makes our bodies produce vitamin D. Fish and dairy products contain small amounts. The only reason you may need D supplements is if you're housebound, or have a medical problem.

There's no recommended daily dose as our bodies look after that department, however **too much (over 4000 units per day over a few months) can cause elevated blood calcium accompanied by a nasty batch of symptoms ranging from headaches to calcium deposits in ligaments and skin. Your bones will eventually weaken.**

In the past, vitamin D has been used to treat tuberculosis, rheumatoid arthritis and skin disorders. **Doses greater than 2.5 mg/day have been associated with adverse effects such as hypocalcaemia, hyperphosphatemia, bone demineralization, calcifying tendonitis and skeletal pain.** Hypercalcemia and hypercalciuria associated with high intake of vitamin D are **potential causes of kidney and heart damage.**

Hypervitaminosis D, from excessive vitamin D intake, malignant or granulomatous disease, hyperparathyroidism, or other endocrinopathies, **causes life-threatening hypocalcaemia with bone, kidney and neurologic disease.** Symptoms include **weakness, lassitude, impaired memory, dementia, depression, paranoia, hallucinations, delirium and coma.** Treatment includes saline administration, furosemide diuresis and sometimes corticosteroids.

17.5 VITAMIN E
(TOCOPHEROLS, TOCOTRIENOLS)

There is not evidence that vitamin E prevents heart attack, stroke, aging or improves sexual function but there is some evidence that we may need small supplements due to inadequate intake. Large daily doses can cause diarrhea.

Over 1000 mg of vitamin E per day **can increase the risk of hemorrhage** and the Institute of Medicine says 15 mg or 22 International Units per day is adequate.

Although the recommended daily allowance of vitamin E is 30 IU, most supplements contain 200 to 800 IU. Reports of **possible toxicity include hemorrhagic stroke in men who smoke and acceleration of disease in patients with retinitis pigmentosa.**

I believe that the reason that beta carotene and vitamin E have been shown to increase cancer and cardiovascular disease is because of their affinity to especially quench or inhibit $^1O_2$ but it may likely affect other RONS.

17.6 FOLIC ACID

The RDA for folic acid is 180 microgram/day. An intake of 400 mg/day has been shown to reduce the risk of neural tube defects. In addition, folic acid is thought to decrease the plasma concentration of homocysteine, thereby perhaps reducing the risk of heart disease. Folic acid in non-toxic and intakes up to 1000 microgram/day are without known adverse effects. However, intakes greater than 5000 microgram **may mask pernicious anemia**.

17.7 NIACIN

Niacin is used to treat hyperlipidemia, and **large doses can be associated with flushing, vomiting, diarrhea, hepatic dysfunction, lactic acidosis, delirium and retinal maculopathy.**

17.8 SELENIUM

The RDA for selenium is 70 microgram/day. **Adverse effects on the hair, nails, liver, nervous system and teeth have been associated with doses exceeding 910 microgram/day** and some side effects occur at intakes as low as 600 microgram/day. No adverse effects have been associated with doses of 200 microgram/day.

According to Time Magazine, March 29, 2004, even the omega-3 fatty acid supplement may be contaminated with mercury, dioxins, DDT and PCB's. Also, a new study has found rising levels of a flame retardant in samples of cod-liver oil.

Since the benefits of many antioxidants and dietary supplements are in question, as is their safety, **clinicians should exert restraint in over indulgence of prescribing of these types of therapy without scientific rationale.**

17.9 SUPPLEMENT DIRTY DOZEN

The Consumers Union warned Americans in the April 12, 2004 issue of Time magazine that they should avoid the following dietary supplements that may cause cancer, kidney or liver damage or even death: aristolochic acid (birthwort), comfrey, germander, androstenedione, chaparral, kava, bitter orange, organ or gland extracts, lobelia, pennyroyal oil, scullcap and yohimbe. They also warn that some may interfere with prescription medicine and one should stay away from all supplements for weight loss.

An alternative view that I have developed relative to the benefits of a vegan diet is that it produces the effects that I would expect to see if the body had adequate levels of ROS and excited states (O_2 excytomers), which would manifest itself as lower levels of diabetes, cancer, CVD and increased life span. Consumption of meat with its saturated fats reverses the effects of being a vegan. It appears that nuts and PUFAs are in part responsible for the effects seen:

PUFA + RONS $\rightarrow$ lipid peroxides, which can interact to form $^1O_2$

Also, I need to view biological systems with near total disregard of the actions of exogenous "antioxidants" since they likely have little in vivo effect, even though they can manifest dramatic effects in vitro.

17.10 VITAMINS LINKED TO ASTHMA

The July 2004 issue of the Journal of the Americal Academy of Pediatrics, published a report, from the Children's National Medical Center in Washington, on more than **8,000 infants and found a possible link between the use of multivitamin supplements and the risk of asthma and food allergies.** It found "an association between early infant multivitamin intake and asthma among black infants and an association between early infant multivitamin intake and food allergies in formula-fed infants."

The investigators said that **more than 50% of all toddlers in the United States are taking multivitamins,** which are also added to infant formula. They also reported that certain vitamins may cause cell changes that can increase the odds of an allergic response when certain antigens are encountered. Recommendations for vitamin supplementation and the actual multivitamin formulation may need to changed to reduce these risks.

UTOPIA CONNECTIONS

My studies of the biochemical intricacies connecting reactive oxygen radicals and excited states has led me to the following unifying concepts:

- RONS and excited states have levels or ranges, which I prefer to call zones, which determine certain biological outcomes, relative to the appearance of cancer and infection. Zones of RONS/excytomers appear to be multi-phasic (at least triphasic) and to exhibit non-linearity. In general, these zones refer to the whole organism but due to the cellular heterogeneity of tissue and/or organs necessitates that they be considered on an individual basis at times.

- Howes' **TRIPHASIC ZONES OF RONS/EXCYTOMERS**

- **Apoptosis Zone** - the **highest zone (hyper-zone)** of RONS and excited states. Based on the results of thousands and thousands of papers and patients **(humans),** it is well established that very high levels of RONS and excited states which can be produced by PDT, many chemotherapeutic drugs, radiation and the Howes Singlet Oxygen delivery system, RONS/excytomers **will kill cancer.** Also, a hyper-stimulated immune system (respiratory burst), such as is seen in spontaneous regression of cancer, **kills cancer.**

- **Abeyance Zone** - the **middle zone (mid-zone)** of RONS and excited states. Based on the fact that millions and millions of people **(humans)** go through life without the manifestation of cancer is evidence, par excellence, for the existence of this mid zone of RONS and excited states, which **holds cancer cell development in abeyance.** It is an accepted scientific fact that all aerobic cells undergo exponential numbers of potentially mutagenic oxidative damaging events on a continual basis yet, **millions do not manifest or develop continual infections or tumors in a life time.** This is the zone of RONS/excytomer **homeostasis.** We know that we can exist in this state for many years and for some, for a life time.

- **Allowance Zone** - the **lowest zone (hypo-zone)** of RONS and excited states. This zone is based on the millions of cases of patients **(humans)** with immunosuppression (acquired or innate) and on genetic diseases such as chronic granulomatous disease, the elderly, obesity and diabetes. We know that low levels of RONS and excited states **allow the development of cancer.**

"With regards to cancer and atherosclerosis, the inflammatory cell has been convicted of guilt by association and oxygen has been strung up by a rush-to-judgement scientific lynch mob."

R. M. Howes, M.D., Ph.D.

5/9/04

**"Give me the power to induce fever
And I will cure all diseases."
Parmenides (ca 540-480 B.C.)**

PART IV - OXYGEN METABOLISM

"With regards to cancer and atherosclerosis,
the inflammatory cell has been convicted of
guilt by association and oxygen has been
strung up by a rush-to-judgement
scientific lynch mob."

R. M. Howes, M.D., Ph.D.

5/9/04

18 INFLAMMATION AND OXYGEN MODIFICATIONS

18.1 ATHEROGENESIS, ATHEROSCLEROSIS

By the interpretations of many, there is compelling evidence for the importance of inflammation and atherosclerosis at both the basic and clinical level which has evolved in parallel. Accumulating data indicate that insights gained from the **link between inflammation and atherosclerosis** can yield predictive and prognostic information of considerable clinical utility (Libby, P., Ridker, P.M. and Maseri, A. Inflammation and atherosclerosis. Circulation 2002; 105: 1135-1143).

Good cardiopulmonary fitness is associated with slower progression of early atherosclerosis in middle aged men (Lakka, T.A., et al. Cardiorespiratory fitness and the progression of carotid atherosclerosis in middle aged men. Ann Intern Med — Abstracts 2001; 134(1): 12). **I interpret this data to mean that improving oxygen consumption increases the levels of RONS/excytomers that can stall or reverse the effects of plaque formation.**

18.2 ATHEROGENESIS AND INFLAMMATION: THE USUAL VIEW

In a variety of animal models of atherosclerosis, signs of inflammation occur simultaneously with incipient lipid accumulation in the artery wall. For example, blood leukocytes, mediators of host defenses and inflammation, localize in the earliest lesions of atherosclerosis, not only in experimental animals but in humans as well. The basic science of inflammation biochemistry applied to atherosclerosis has afforded considerable new insight into the mechanisms underlying this recruitment of leukocytes. The normal endothelium does not in general support binding of white blood cells. However, early after initiation of an atherogenic diet, patches of arterial endothelial cells begin to express on their surface selective adhesion molecules that bind to various classes of leukocytes. In particular, **vascular cell adhesion molecule-1 (VCAM-1)** binds precisely the types of leukocytes found in early human and experimental atheroma, the moncyte and T lymphocyte. Not only does VCAM-1 expression increase on endothelial cells overlying nascent atheroma, but mice genetically engineered to express defective VCAM-1 show interrupted lesion development (Cybulsky, M.I., Iiyama, K and Li, H., et al. A major role for VCAM-1 but not ICAM-1 in early atherosclerosis. J Clin Invest 2001; 107: 1255-1262).

Of note, the foci of increased adhesion molecule expression overlap with sites in the arterial tree are particularly prone to develop atheroma. Considerable evidence suggests **that impaired endogenous atheroprotective mechanisms occur at branch points in arteries,** where the endothelial cells experience disturbed flow. In addition to inhibiting natural protective mechanisms, disturbed flow can augment the production of certain leukocyte adhesion molecules (e.g., **intercellular adhesion molecule-1 [ICAM-1]).** Augmented wall stresses may also promote the production by arterial smooth muscle cells (SMC's) of proteoglycans that can bind and retain lipoprotein particles, facilitating their oxidative modification and thus promoting an inflammatory response at sites of lesion formation (Lee, R.T., Yamamoto, C. and Feng, Y., et al. Mechanical strain induces specific changes in the synthesis and organization of proteoglycans by vascular smooth muscle cells. J Biol Chem 2001; 276: 13847-13851).

Once adherent to the endothelium, the leukocytes penetrate into the intima. Once resident in the arterial wall, the blood-derived inflammatory cells participate in and perpetuate a local inflammatory response. The macrophages express scavenger receptors for modified lipoproteins, permitting them to ingest lipid and become foam cells. In addition to MCP-1, **macrophage colony-stimulating factor (MC-SF)** contributes to the differentiation of the blood monocytes into the macrophage foam cell. T-cells likewise encounter signals that cause them to elaborate inflammatory cytokines such as gamma-interferon and lymph toxin (tumor necrosis factor [TNF] B) that in turn can stimulate macrophages as well as vascular endothelial cells and SMCs. As this inflammatory process continues, the activated leukocytes and intrinsic arterial cells can release fibrogenic mediators, including a variety of peptide growth factors that can promote replication of SMCs and contribute to elaboration by these cells of a dense extracellular matrix characteristic of the more advanced atherosclerosis lesion.

It is felt that inflammation processes not only promote initiation and evolution of atheroma, but also contribute decisively to precipitating acute thrombotic complications of atheroma. Most coronary arterial thrombi that cause fatal acute myocardial infarction arise because of a physical disruption of the atherosclerotic plaque. The activated macrophage abundant in atheroma can produce proteolytic enzymes capable of degrading the collagen that lends strength to the plaque's protective fibrous cap, rendering that cap thin, weak, and susceptible to rupture. Gamma-interferon arising from the activated T-lymphocytes in the plaque can halt collagen synthesis by SMCs, limiting its capacity to review the collagen that reinforces the plaque. Macrophages also produce a tissue factor, which is the major procoagulant and trigger to thrombosis found in plaques. Inflammatory mediators regulate tissue factor expression by plaque macrophages, demonstrating an essential link between arterial inflammation and thrombosis (Libby, P and Simon D.I. Inflammation and thrombosis the clot thickens. Circulation 2001; 103: 1718-1720).

18.3 OXIDATION OF LIPOPROTEINS

For almost a century, many have **regarded lipids as the sine quine non of atherosclerosis**. Over the last few decades, a plausible model linking lipids and inflammation to parthenogenesis has emerged. **According to the oxidation hypothesis, low-density lipoprotein (LDL) retained in the intima, in part by binding to proteoglycan, undergoes oxidative modification.** Lipid hydroperoxides, lysophospholipids, carbonyl compounds, and other biologically active moieties localize in the lipid fraction of atheroma. These modified lipids can induce the expression of adhesion molecules, chemokines, proinflammatory cytokines, and other mediators of inflammation in macrophages and vascular wall cells. The apoprotein moieties of the lipoprotein particles can also undergo modification in the artery wall, rendering them antigenic and capable of inciting T-cell responses, thus activating the antigen-specific adaptive limb of the immune response. In some experimental situations, administration of antioxidants can retard the progression of atherosclerotic lesions that develop in the face of hyperlipidemia.

Although attractive, theoretically compelling, and supported by a considerable body of experimental evidence, the relevance of **the LDL oxidation hypothesis to human atherosclerosis remains unproven**. Chemical analysis of the types of modified lipids and **proteins extracted from human atheroma do not necessarily correspond to the compounds derived from lipoproteins oxidized in vitro that have furnished much of the evidence linking oxidized lipoproteins to inflammation.** Most cell culture studies of biological effects of oxidized LDL have used material generated by transition metal mediated oxidation, conditions that some find of **dubious in vivo relevance**. **Hypochlorous acid** mediated derivation of lipoprotein constituents may bear closer relationship to human atherosclerosis than oxidative modification catalyzed by transition metals (Hazen, S.L., Hsu, F.F. and Gaut J.P., et al. Modification of proteins and lipids by myeloperoxidase. Methods Enzymol 1999; 300: 88-105). The leukocyte enzyme myeloperoxidase produces hypochlorous acid within the atheroma. **Clinical trials have repeatedly failed to validate the concept that antioxidant vitamin therapy can improve clinical outcomes**. Thus, "the jury is still out" on the applicability of LDL oxidation hypothesis to patients.

18.4 DYSLIPIDEMIA

Other lipoprotein particles such as very low-density lipoprotein (VLDL) and intermediate-density lipoprotein also have considerable atherogenic potential (Diehtl, W., Nilsson, L. and Goncalves, I., et al. Very low-density lipoprotein activates nuclear factor kB in endothelial cells. Circ Res 1999; 84: 1085-1094). High-density lipoprotein (HDL) protects against atherosclerosis. Reverse cholesterol transport effected by HDL likely accounts for some of its atheroprotective function. However, **HDL particles also can transport antioxidant enzymes such as platelet-activating factor acetylhydrolase and peroxidase, which can break down oxidized lipids and neutralize their proinflammatory effects.**

18.5 HYPERTENSION

Hypertension follows closely behind lipids on a list of classical risk factors for atherosclerosis. Increasing evidence supports the view that, like atherosclerosis itself, inflammation may participate in hypertension providing a pathophysiological link between these two diseases. Angiotensin II (AII), in addition to its vasoconstrictor properties, can instigate intimal inflammation. For example, AII elicits the production of superoxide anion, a reactive oxygen species, from arterial endothelial cells and SMCs. AII can also increase the expression by arterial SMCs of proinflammatory cytokines such as Interleukins (IL)-6 and MCP-1 on endothelial cells (Kranzhofer, R., Schmidt, J. and Pfeiffer, et al. Angiotensin induces inflammatory activation of human vascular smooth muscle cells. Arterioscler Thromb Vasc Biol 1999; 9: 1623-1629).

18.6 DIABETES

Diabetes is yet another risk factor for atherosclerosis of growing importance. The hyperglycemia associated with diabetes can lead to modification of macromolecules, for example, by forming advance glycation end products (AGE) (Schmidt, A.M., Yan, S.D. and Wautier, J.L., et al. Activation of receptor for advance glycation end products: A mechanism for chronic vascular dysfunction in diabetic vasculopathy and atherosclerosis. Circ Res 1999; 84: 489-497). Beyond the **hyperglycemia, the diabetic state promotes oxidative stress mediated by reactive oxygen species and carbonyl groups** (Baynes, J.W. and Thorpe, S.R. Role of oxidative stress in diabetic complications: A new perspective on an old paradigm. Diabetes 1999; 48: 1-9). As in the case of hypertension, inflammation links diabetes to atherosclerosis.

18.7 OBESITY

Obesity not only predisposes to insulin resistance and diabetes, but also contributes to **atherogenic dyslipidemia. High levels of free fatty acids originating from visceral fat** reach the liver through the portal circulation and stimulate synthesis of the triglyceride-rich lipoprotein VLDL by hepatocytes. Adipose tissue can also synthesize cytokines such as TNF-a and IL-6 (Yudkin, J.S., Stehouwer, C.D. and Emeis, J.J., et al. C-reactive protein in healthy subjects associations with obesity, insulin resistance and endothelial dysfunction: A potential role for cytokines originating from adipose tissue. Arterioscler Thromb Vasc Biol 1999; 19: 972-978). In this way obesity itself promotes inflammation and potentiates atherogenesis independent of effects on insulin resistance or lipoproteins.

Obesity is associated with a wide variety of diseases ranging from arteriosclerotic vascular disease to cancer and diabetes. The reason for this is not known. On 2/22/04, I had another epiphany during my rest period. After returning to bed from a trip to the restroom secondary to nocturia, I realized that such a short trip had resulted in my having to mouth breathe to compensate for an oxygen debt secondary to the effort expended on the trip. Then it occurred to me that all obese people have an enormous oxygen requirement above that of people of normal weight. Likely, the need to provide energy to maintain all of these extra oxygen-requiring aerobic fat cells puts their bodies at constant risk of falling into an oxygen deficient state relative to people of normal weight. In other words, **they have proportionately less oxygen available to fight infections and cancer.** It is common knowledge that obese patients have higher rates of infection, heart problems and cancer. My explanation has the hallmarks of simplicity and clarity. In fact, these obese patients may normally have slightly reduced oxygen tensions, than that of normal weight patients, and this reduction in overall oxygen levels sets the stage for the allowance of the many disease states associated with obesity. This further implies that oxygen supplementation in obese patients could be used prophylactically to prevent disease development or progression.

Additionally, in my opinion, **the presence of excess lipids, which can act as a sink for free radicals and especially excited oxygen, could serve to reduce the levels of RONS and excytomers such that obese individuals are prone to a spectrum of diseases, just as is the case in smokers.**

A report on 8/23/04, by American Cancer Society epidemiologist, Eugenia Calle, indicates that **obesity raises the risk for nine types of cancer.** With two thirds of the nation overweight, this is an important bit of information. **Fat is known to increase the risk of developing cancers of the colon, breast, uterus, kidney, esophagus, pancreas, gallbladder, liver and top of the stomach.** Fat cells are metabolically active and **after menopause, fat becomes the leading source of estrogen.** Obese men are 50% to twice as likely as lean men to get colon cancer and for women, the risk is 20-50%. Apparently, hormones play a role in the obese patient, but **I feel that the unsaturated lipids in circulation and those in situ, can act as a trap for RONS/excytomers, decrease their availability and allow for development of infections and cancer.**

18.8 INFECTION

Infectious agents might also conceivably furnish inflammatory stimuli that accentuate atherogenesis (Libby, P., Egan, D. and Skarlatos, R. Roles of infectious agents in atherosclerosis and restenosis: An assessment of the evidence and need for future research. Circulation 1997; 96: 4095-4103). **Many human plaques show signs of infection by microbial agents such Chlamydia pneumoniae.** Chlamydiae, when present in the arterial plaque, may release lipopolysaccharide (endotoxin) and heat shock proteins that can stimulate the production of proinflammatory mediators by vascular endothelial cells and SMCs and infiltrating leukocytes alike (Kol, A, Bourcier, T. and Lichtman, A.H., et al. Chlamydial and human heat shock protein 60s activate human vascular endothelium, smooth muscle cells and macrophages. J Clin Invest 1999; 103: 571-577). **Epidemiological studies of infection, however, have yielded mixed results, with little prospective evidence that antibodies directed against chlamydeous pneumoniae, Helicobacter pylori, herpes simplex virus or cytomegalovirus in predicting vascular risk.**

In August of 2004, at the European Society of Cardiology, Dr, Christopher Cannon, of Brigham's Women's Hospital, said that negative results from two new major studies, with each study involving over 4,000 patients, had closed the door on studies which proposed that "antibiotics could prevent heart attacks." **Despite growing evidence that inflammation plays a key role in cardiovascular disease, scientists have failed to show that fighting these infections with antibiotics can prevent heart attacks.** The studies used Tequin (gatifloxacin) and Zithromax (azithromycin). They said that these results are leading investigators to refocus on things that they know work, such as anti-platelet therapy, beta blockers, ACE inhibitors and statins, although Zocor results were not statistically significant.

I interpret the data showing the presence of bacteria in plaques to indicate that levels of RONS and singlet oxygen are insufficient to kill the bacteria and to dissolve the plaques. I see this as being analogous to the situation in which chronic inflammation is being accused of being causal of cancer, in that I believe that sufficient levels of RONS and singlet oxygen would kill both the bugs and kill the cancer. The inflammatory cells are present in an attempt to dissolve the plaque, to kill pathogenic organisms or to kill pro-neoplastic or neoplastic cells.

18.9 ACUTE CORONARY SYNDROME (ACS)

The mechanisms of ACS encompass elements of thrombosis and vasoconstriction superimposed on atherosclerotic lesions. **Thrombosis may beget vasospasm**. Local thrombus formation generates serotonin, thromboxanes A and thrombin. Each of these thrombosis-associated mediators can cause vasoconstriction not only at the site of thrombosis, but also downstream. Even aggressive thrombolytic, anticoagulant, and/or antiplatelet agents or interventional therapy, in patients with ACS still have a 12% to 16% incidence of major cardiac events at 4 to 6 months after hospital discharge (Cannon, C.P., Weintraub, W.S. and Demopoulos, L.A., et al. Comparison of early invasive and conservative strategies in patients with unstable coronary syndromes treated with the lipoprotein IIb/IIIa inhibitor tirofiban. N Engl J Med 2001; 344: 1879-1887).

Oxygen has been dubbed the center of the chemical revolution but more importantly, it is the center of aerobiosis. The demonization of oxygen, which is the essential element of life, has been referred to as the essential element of death. I vehemently disagree.

18.10 CHRONIC INFLAMMATION
AND CANCER

The following material has been excerpted from: Shacter, E. and Weitzman, S.A. Chronic inflammation and cancer. Vol. 16, No. 2 (February 2002).

Much of our understanding of the association between chronic inflammation and cancer is illustrated through inflammatory bowel disease and colon carcinogenesis. Patients with either **chronic ulcerative colitis or Crohn's disease have a five to sevenfold increased risk of developing colorectal carcinoma** (Ekbom, A., Helmick, C. and Zack, M., et. al. Ulcerative colitis and colorectal cancer. A population-based study. N Engl J Med 1990; 323: 1228-1233). It is generally thought that **the colitis must persist for a least 8 years to significantly increase the risk of cancer** (Choi, P.M. and Zelig, M.P. Similarity of colorectal cancer in Crohn's disease and ulcerative colitis: Implications for carcinogenesis and prevention. Gut 1994; 35: 950-954). **Neoplasia generally appears after a median duration of approximately 15 years.** Shacter and Weitzman believe that increased cancer incidence is associated with increased duration of the inflammation.

Some animal models demonstrate experimentally that chronic inflammation predisposes to the development of various forms of cancer. For example, marmosets have a high incidence of spontaneous colitis and a high incidence of colon cancer as well. Skin cancer is induced by administration of carcinogens such as dimethylbenzanthracine (DMBA) followed by repeated administration of tumor promoters such as phorbol myristate acetate (PMA) or benzoyl peroxide, which induce inflammation and the production of various inflammatory mediators. Intraperitoneal introduction of mineral oils (e.g., pristane), or plastic discs into BALB/c mice promotes the formation of **chronic granulomatous tissue** and the development of plasmacytomas (Potter, M. Indomethacin inhibition of pristane plasmacytomagenesis in genetically susceptible inbred mice. Adv Exp Med Biol 1999; 469: 151-156).

18.11 INHIBITION OF APOPTOSIS

Except during development and tissue regeneration, normal tissues exhibit a precise balance between the rate of cell division and cell death. Disruption of this balance in favor of excess growth signals possible oncogenesis. **Because dead or dying cells are rarely detected in normal tissue, it is thought that normal (programmed) cell death occurs through a controlled process called apoptosis.**

Apoptotic cells have unique morphologic and biochemical characteristics that distinguish them from necrotic cells. The main physiologic difference between apoptosis and necrosis is in how the cells affect the surrounding tissues: **Cells dying by apoptosis are recognized and taken up by phagocytic cells before they have an opportunity to lyse and release their content into the tissue.** The phagocytes degrade the cells with minimal environmental disturbance and no induction of inflammation. In contrast, **cells dying by necrosis lyse before being taken up by phagocytes, thereby causing an inflammatory response that can cause incidental damage to the surrounding tissue.**

Treatment with **chemotherapeutic drugs or depletion of growth factors usually kills tumor cells by inducing apoptosis,** (Hickman, J.A. Apoptosis induced by anticancer drugs. Cancer Metastasis Rev 1992; 11: 121-139), **whereas high levels of oxidants, chemicals, or severe hypoxia usually induce necrotic death. Cells that have become resistant to apoptosis have a greatly increased risk of being or becoming neoplastic.** An appreciation for the strong association between reduced apoptosis and tumorogenesis was advanced by the discovery that the oncogene bcl-2, which mediates B-cell tumorogenesis, acts by inhibiting normal B-cell apoptosis.

We know that many different oncogenes act by inhibiting apoptosis, thereby conferring a survival advantage to preneoplastic and malignant cells. By the same token, normal tumor-suppressor genes such as p53 and Rb promote apoptosis in response to toxic stimuli, inducing appropriate death in a damaged cell. **Any agent that prevents cells from dying in response to toxic stimuli can have the effect of promoting tumorogenesis by allowing proliferation of an abnormal cell.**

18.12 REACTIVE OXYGEN AND NITROGEN INTERMEDIATES

When phagocytes (neutrophils, eosinophils, monocytes, macrophages) are exposed to an inflammatory stimulus (e.g., bacteria), they become activated and begin to generate large quantities of reactive oxygen and nitrogen intermediates. **Reactive oxygen intermediates, also generically referred to as oxidants, are derivatives of molecular oxygen such as superoxide, hydrogen peroxide, hypochlorous acid, singlet oxygen and hydroxyl radical.** Under normal circumstances, phagocyte-derived oxidants serve a protective function by killing invading bacteria and parasites. Many believe that they can also have detrimental effects, causing tissue damage and contributing to the development or progression of numerous disease including cancer (Babior, B.M. Phagocytes and oxidative stress. Am J Med 2000; 109: 33-44). The same is true for reactive nitrogen intermediates, which are generated by inflammatory phagocytes through the enzymatic synthesis of nitric oxide by an inducible nitric oxide synthase and the subsequent interaction with molecular oxygen or reactive oxygen intermediates (Grisham, M.B., Jourd'heuil, D. and Wink, D.A. Review article: Chronic inflammation and reactive oxygen and nitrogen metabolism - implications in DNA damage and mutagenesis. Aliment Pharmacol Ther 2000; 14(1): 3-9).

Reactive oxygen and nitrogen intermediates have varying degrees of reactivity and diffusability that influence their mutagenic potential (Aust, A.E. and Eveleigh, J.F. Mechanisms of DNA oxidation. Proc Soc Exp Biol Med 1999; 222: 246-252). Superoxide is the primary product of the phagocytic oxidative burst and is generated by a membrane-associated nicotinamide adenine dinucleotide phosphate (NADPH) oxidase. **Superoxide is not particularly reactive with biomolecules and cannot diffuse across cell membranes.** It rapidly dismutates - either spontaneously or catalytically through the action of superoxide dismutase - **to hydrogen peroxide, which also is not particularly reactive on its own.** However, **hydrogen peroxide can diffuse significant distances and cross cell membranes like water.**

The biological danger from superoxide and hydrogen peroxide comes when there is a redox-active transition metal present, such as iron (Fe) or copper (Cu). Interaction of Fe^{2+} or Cu^{1+} with hydrogen peroxide generates highly reactive radicals such as the hydroxyl or ferryl radicals. **Superoxide serves as a source of hydrogen peroxide and acts also to maintain the transition metals in the reduced state, thus supporting radical formation**. The hydroxyl radical is too reactive to diffuse any significant distance and will react with the first molecule with which it comes in contact. Hence, **the site where the hydroxyl radical is formed is also the site of its damage.**

DNA contains a significant amount of bound iron and copper. If and when phagocyte-derived hydrogen peroxide diffuses into the nucleus of the target cell, it theoretically interacts with the transition metal on the DNA, forming a radical and giving rise to strand breaks and base modifications.

18.13 HYPOCHLOROUS ACID

In addition to synthesizing superoxide and nitric oxide, **activated neutrophils, monocytes and eosinophils generate large quantities of hypochlorous acid**, the active ingredient in household bleach. The formation of hypochlorous acid from hydrogen peroxide and chloride is catalyzed by **myeloperoxidase, which comprises approximately 5% of the total protein of neutrophils,** or by the homologous eosinophil peroxidase. **Hypochlorous acid is a strong oxidant that also has the ability to diffuse across cell membranes, and although it is not thought to cause DNA strand breaks, it can theoretically cause DNA base modifications leading to mutations.**

18.14 LINES OF EVIDENCE

According to Shacter and Weitzman, support for the theory that phagocyte-derived oxidants contribute to mutagenesis and carcinogenesis comes from several lines of evidence.

- Inflammatory phagocytes have the capacity to induce oxidative and nitrosative DNA damage and mutagenesis in neighboring cells. Thus, co-incubation of cells with activated neutrophils or macrophages fosters the induction of strand breaks and oxidative base damage. The most common mutations induced by reactive oxygen and nitrogen intermediates are based modifications leading to point mutations. Prominent among these is **8-oxo-2-deoxyguanosine (8-oxodG),** which is misread by DNA polymerase to generate GC-to-TA transversions. In addition, oxidants cause the formation of gross chromosomal abnormalities such as sister chromatid exchanges, deletions and inversions (Weitberg, A.B., Weitzman, S.A. and Clark, E.P., et al. Effects of antioxidants on oxidant-induced sister chromatid exchange formation. J Clin Invest 1985; 75: 1835-1841).
- **Incubation with activated neutrophils or macrophages results in neoplastic transformation of fibroblasts and epithelial cells** (Weitzman, S.A., Weitberg, A.B. and Clark, E.P., et.al. Phagocytes as carcinogens: Malignant transformation produced by human neutrophils. Science 1985; 227: 1231-1233), (Tamatani, T., Turk, P. and Weitzman, S.A., et.al. Tumorigenic conversion of a rat urothelial cell line by human polymorphonuclear leukocytes activated by lipopolysaccharide. Jpn J Cancer Res 1999; 90: 829-836). **The induction of chromosomal damage and neoplastic transformation by activated phagocytes can be inhibited with antioxidant compounds,** indicating that oxidants are mediators of phagocyte-mediated cell transformation.
- **The types of mutations found in some tumor cells are reflective of oxidative damage.** For example, the GC-to-TA transversions that are induced by reactive oxygen and nitrogen intermediates are commonly found in Ras codons 12, 13, and 61, leading to activation of the oncogene, and in "hot spots" in the tumor-suppressor genes p53 and Rb.
- Tumor promoters such as PMA and benzoyl peroxide are known for their ability to activate the oxidative burst of neutrophils and macrophages and PMA causes oxidative base damage in the skin (Wei, H. and Frenkel, K. In vivo formation of oxidized DNA bases in tumor promoter-treated mouse skin. Cancer Res 1991; 4443-4449). This represents a possible common mechanism of tumor promotion by these agents. **Compounds that inhibit tumor promotion in the mouse skin cancer model also inhibit the respiratory burst of phagocytes.**
- **Chronic inflammation is accompanied by increased production of tissue reactive oxygen and nitrogen intermediates.** Evidence of this process is documented in studies of the markers of oxidative activity in vivo. Thus, oxidatively and nitrosatively modified DNA and proteins are present in chronically inflamed tissue or the body fluids of patients with chronic inflammatory conditions. The likely source of the oxidative activity is the polymorphonuclear neutrophils and macrophages recruited as part of the inflammatory response. **Markers of oxidative damage are also elevated in tumor tissues** (Ray, G. Batra, S. and Shukla, N.K., et. al. Lipid peroxidation, free radical production and antioxidant status in breast cancer. Breast Cancer Res Treat 2000; 59: 163-170), **but it is unclear whether these are caused by oxidants generated by inflammation-associated leukocytes or whether**

the damaging oxidants come from the tumor cells themselves (Szatrowski, T.P. and Nathan, C.F. Production of large amounts of hydrogen peroxide by human tumor cells. Cancer Res 1991; 51: 794-798). **Please re-read the above highlighted sentence.**

In addition, the inducible form of **nitric oxide synthase**, thought to be responsible for the generation of nitric oxide in inflamed tissues, is up-regulated in chronically inflamed tissues, including gastric tissue associated with H pylori infection. **While increased expression of inducible nitric oxide synthase is seen in inflammatory bowel disease, it is unclear whether it actually promotes or attenuates the inflammatory condition,** because knockout mice display an increased susceptibility for colitis (Mashimo, H. and Goyal, R.K. Lessons from genetically engineered animal models: IV. Nitric oxide synthase gene knockout mice. Am J Physiol 1999; 277: G745-G750).

Overall, although **there is some disagreement as to whether phagocyte-derived oxidants contribute to tumorogenesis** (Collins, A.R. Oxidative DNA damage, antioxidants and cancer. Bioessays 1999; 21: 238-246), there is a significant body of experimental data supporting the conclusion that they do.

18.15 MECHANISMS OF TUMORIGENESIS

Many different mechanisms have been proposed to explain how **prostaglandins** promote tumorogenesis. These mechanisms are briefly described below:

- Prostaglandins can stimulate cell proliferation.
- PGE_2 induces synthesis of cytokines such as IL-6 that serve as tumor growth factors.
- Synthesis of prostaglandins is coupled with formation of DNA-reactive by-products with mutagenic potential, e.g., formation of malondialdehyde from prostaglandin G_2.
- COX enzymes can catalyze the oxidative metabolism of xenobiotics, leading to the formation of genotoxic mutagens.
- Prostaglandins can induce angiogenesis, which is required for growth and metastasis of tumors. Some evidence of this comes from the demonstration that NSAIDs inhibit angiogenesis in vitro. It has been suggested that these drugs may not be acting entirely through the inhibition of PGE_2 synthesis because the addition of exogenous PGE_2 fails to overcome the inhibitory effect of the NSAIDs. However, the concentrations of NSAIDs required to inhibit prostaglandin-independent angiogenesis in vitro are quite high (e.g., 250 to 500 μM of indomethacin) and are unlikely to be achieved in vivo. In contrast, inhibition of prostaglandin synthesis by NSAIDs occurs at concentrations that are achieved in vivo (e.g., 1 μM or less for indomethacin).
- In addition to serving as proinflammatory mediators, prostaglandins are also immunosuppressive. By inhibiting the functions of T-cells and macrophages, they may decrease immune surveillance and thereby allow nascent tumor cells to escape detection by the immune system.
- Prostaglandins may inhibit apoptosis of tumor cells by increasing expression of the ant apoptotic oncogene bcl-2 or by removing arachidonic acid, which is thought to be proapoptotic.
- Prostaglandins can stimulate cell signaling through peroxisome-proliferator-activated receptor delta, a transcription factor that regulates proliferation-associated genes.

18.16 NSAIDS AND NOVEL AGENTS

Chronic intake of NSAIDs may reduce carcinogenesis by inhibiting production of prostaglandins, cytokines and angiogenic factors. **Note that NSAIDs do not eliminate inflammation, but rather act by reducing the production of selected inflammatory factors.** Hence, **unlike steroids, they do not suppress elements of the immune response that are necessary for tumor depletion such as T cells, NK cells and macrophages.** COX-2 selective inhibitors may provide a safer method of chemoprevention than older NSAIDs such as aspirin and indomethacin, which also inhibit COX-1 activity and cause gastric lesions. **Recent alerts in 2004, indicate that drugs such as Celobrex and Vioxx, COX-2 inhibitors, cause alarming rates of gastric bleeding.**

18.17 DIETARY ANTIOXIDANTS

Eating a diet rich in fruits and vegetables is thought to be the best and safest means of preventing cancer. Epidemiologic studies suggest that diets high in fruits and vegetables are strongly associated with a lower incidence of different forms of cancer. This approach to cancer prevention has been reviewed elsewhere (Blumberg, J.B. Considerations of the scientific substantiation for antioxidant vitamins and beta-carotene in disease prevention. Am J Clin Nutr 1995; 62: 1521S-1526S). **Please keep in mind that the thousands of compounds in fresh fruits and vegetables is a far cry from the usual synthetic dietary supplements available today.**

The Food and Nutrition Board of the Institute of Medicine recently examined the role of oxidants in disease in order to determine whether dietary antioxidants inhibit the development of chronic disease such as atherosclerosis and cancer (see http://books.nap.edu/books/0309061873/html/index.html). **The panel of experts concluded that, at present, there are insufficient human data to conclude that dietary antioxidants, such as vitamins C and E, carotenoids and selenium, can prevent cancer.**

If antioxidants are involved primarily in initiation through the induction of DNA damage, and this occurs years (or decades) before tumor outgrowth begins, then administration of antioxidants over a narrow window of time later in life would likely be ineffective. Studies of NSAID inhibition of colon cancer indicate that the drugs must be taken for many years in order to lower tumor incidence. The same may hold true for antioxidant supplements.

18.18 REVIEW OF SHACTER/WEITZMAN ARTICLE BY KRYSTYNA FRENKEL, PH.D. FOLLOWS:

Initially, oxidative stress triggers the adaptation by up-regulating antioxidant defenses. However, a prolonged exposure to reactive oxygen and nitrogen species, cytokines and other inflammatory factors overwhelms those protective defenses, while pathways that favor growth of mutated cells are activated. These include increased formation of prostaglandins, which enhances cell proliferation by up-regulating cytokine Interleukins (IL)-6 that serves as a growth factor, and down-regulating pathways that lead to apoptosis by activating transcription factor NF-kappaB and bcl-2 oncogene.

Anti-inflammatory agents, such as aspirin, non-steroidal anti-inflammatory drugs (NSAIDs), and cyclooxygenase (COX)-2 inhibitors, suppress the neoplastic process and, at the same time, decrease oxidative stress, oxidative DNA base damage and prostaglandin and cytokine formation. They also decrease angiogenesis and up-regulate pathways leading to apoptosis. This has been shown to occur in both animal models and in humans.

Overall, Drs. Shacter and Weitzman present a compelling rationale well grounded in experimental facts that strongly support their main thesis that chronic inflammation unleashes a plethora of agents, such as cytokines, prostaglandins, chemotactic factors, reactive oxygen and nitrogen species (which cause the mutations in neighboring cells), as well as changes in gene expression favoring the activation of oncogenes and down-regulation of tumor suppression genes.

18.19 SELECTIVE REVIEW OF SHACTER/WEITZMAN ARTICLE BY ALAN B. WEITBERG FOLLOWS:

The association between chronic inflammation and tumorogenesis continues to be well documented in the literature, even though the full spectrum of intra- and extracellular intermediates in this process remains to be elucidated. The ones that have been elucidated, however, likely participate in the initiation as well as promotion and progression of carcinogenesis. These pro-neoplastic inflammatory mediators include the reactive oxygen and nitrogen intermediates, prostaglandins and cytokines that act via several mechanisms to promote the transformed phenotype. **It is probable that multiple molecular and biochemical events must occur over time for cancer to develop (e.g., DNA damage, promotion of cell proliferation and angiogenesis, inhibition of repair enzymes, inhibition of apoptosis).**

Although the association between chronic inflammation and cancer is well described, cause and effect remain to be proven, perhaps because definitive causative inflammatory mediators have not been completely identified. One can imagine extracellularly generated radical species that interact with the cell membrane to produce a series of intracellular radicals, which careen through the cytoplasm, initiating serial oxidation-reduction events that terminate at the site of nuclear DNA. In the process, cell signals are distorted, repair mechanisms interrupted, and DNA damaged. Some cells die, some repair the damage faithfully, but others miscue, and the preneoplastic genotype eventuates. Obviously identifying the causative intermediate in this process is difficult and thus, **establishing the link between inflammation and cancer has been elusive.**

An especially interesting aspect of research in this area involves the role of stimulated human phagocytes whose normal salutary biological role is to thwart infection. The chronicity of that stimulation, however, may result in too much of a good thing, with DNA damage being induced in the target cells, as in ulcerative colitis. This is aptly discussed by authors, although **notably only a minority of patients with ulcerative colitis develop malignancies.**

Dr. Shacter and Weitzman appropriately review the known anticancer effects of antioxidants and oxygen radical scavengers in the reliable clinical trials published to date. **The results are inconclusive**, but we have yet to define the effective doses of the agents based on measurements of biological end points.

As demonstrated with vitamin C, its pro- and antioxidant effects are dose-dependent, and thus, more is not necessarily better. Mechanism-based chemoprevention trials should be refined (e.g., using animal models involving transgenic mice), so that the expected molecular or biochemical effect of the agent being studied can be measured and correlated with its anticancer effect or lack thereof.

**"Fatuous condemnation of the beneficence of dioxygen,
is tantamount to
the evasion of sunshine
for fear of a longing to go out-of-doors,**

to denouncing bodily nourishment
perchance for fear of choking and
to the damnation of love
for fear
of a broken heart."

R. M. Howes, M.D., Ph.D.

5/31/04

19 OXYGEN METABOLISM

Oxygen homeostasis is controlled in higher organisms by a tight regulation of the red blood cell mass and respiratory ventilation. Carotid bodies are sensory organs that detect changes in arterial blood oxygen levels and they are composed of glomus type I chemoreceptor cells that release neurotransmitters in response to hypoxia. Changes in the electrical activity in the efferent fibers relay the sensory information to the brain stem neurons that regulate breathing. Changes in O_2 concentration, RONS levels or K^+ are likely involved in control of respiration and ventilation.

The **red blood cell mass is regulated by the hormone erythropoietin**, which is mainly produced by kidney and liver cells following stimulation with hypoxia. Oxygen sensing mechanisms are still unclear.

19.0 CARDIORESPIRATORY FITNESS AND CANCER MORTALITY

Data on the relationship between cardiorespiratory fitness and cancer mortality was obtained on 9039men (19-59 yr) and showed a highly significant association of cardiorespiratory fitness and cancer mortality in Japanese men (Swada, S.S., Muto, T., Tanaka, H., Lee, I.M., Paffenbarger, R.S. Shindo, M. and Blair, S.N. Cardiorespiratory fitness and cancer mortality in Japanese men: A prospective study. Med. Sci Sports Excer 2003; 35(9): 1546-50). **I believe that this is another study that directly supports my Unified Theory, in that low O$_2$ levels lead to low RONS/excytomer levels and thus, lead to increased cancer rates.**

19.0.1 Cardiorespiratory Fitness and Stroke Risk

Just as cardiopulmonary fitness has been associated with decreasing rates of atherosclerosis, it has been shown that low cardiorespiratory fitness was acuminated with an increased risk for any stroke and ischemic stroke. The VO2 max was one of the strongest predictors of stroke (Kurl, S., et al. Cardiorespiratory fitness and risk for stroke in men. Arch Intern Med 2003; 163: 1682-1688). **This also supports my Unified Theory.**

Some of the following material has been excerpted from or is based on material in an article by Stephen Levin, Ph.D., entitled, **Oxygen and Life: Original Hypothesis concerning Oxygen Deficiency as a Cause of Disease States** at www.healingpeople.com .

19.1 OXYGEN DEFICIENCY STATES (OXYGEN STARVATION)

"We are presently at a climatic phase of evolution where daily human activity has turned the tide and caused **oxygen in the atmosphere to decrease** rather than increase. Modern technology with excessive burning of carbon-based fuels, such as that by automobiles and for the generation of electricity and heat, our most precious element in the universe for living organisms, to decrease. A consistent and devastating consequence or environmental insults **causes an oxygen deficit by a reduction of oxygen in both our atmosphere and in our bodies**. Physical insults to living organisms such as disease or any damaging force can cause an oxygen deficiency. Excessive inflammation and immunological system functions require the use of oxygen. Increased oxygen utilization is a signpost of stress. **Low oxygen in body tissue is a sure indicator of pathology.**"

"We can look at oxygen deficiency or oxygen starvation as the single greatest cause of all disease." **RMH Note: I agree with the importance of ground state oxygen but I believe that the free radical oxygen modifications and excitation states (RONS/excytomers) are of greater importance for fighting infections and cancer. Additionally, one could have adequate levels of ground state oxygen and yet not be able to generate adequate levels of reactive oxygen species or excitation states.**

Evidence of Oxygen Starvation

- We are starving in our cities as we combust oxygen in our automobiles and industries.
- We are starving in our office buildings as we improve insulation to save heating costs.
- We are starving due to reduced oxygen-generating plants and forests that are destroyed every day.
- We are starving due to pollutants that combine with and use up oxygen in our atmosphere.
- We are starving because the pollutants that we eat, drink and breathe must be detoxified by the addition of oxygen in our bodies.

19.2 OXYGEN DEFICIENCY: AN INTEGRAL ASPECT IN ALL DISEASE STATES

Any stress causes oxygen deficiency. Stress resulting from toxic environmental chemicals requires the use of oxygen to detoxify chemical pollutants. Emotional stress produces adrenaline and related adrenal hormones that require oxygen to detoxify. Physical trauma reduces circulation and subsequent oxygen supply to cells and tissues. Infection utilizes free radical forms of oxygen modifications to combat bacteria, fungi and viruses, functioning as a killer of these invading pathogens. Hence, **oxygen deficiency** will result from any excessive stress and forms the basis of a unifying principle in stress and illness. Dr. Levine believes that hypoxia is the condition of reduced oxygen in body tissues, which is the eventual result of all degenerative disease processes. He feels that toxicity of hypoxia is due to selective free radical formation that occurs during and after hypoxia.

- Oxygen deficiency is probably the biggest cause of cancer and cardiovascular diseases.
- Oxygen is the breath of life and everyday there is less of it for breathing.
- It is known that utilization of oxygen in our atmosphere has risen tremendously due to industry and other polluting aspects of modern society.
- Scientists have determined that **oxygen concentrations in our atmosphere are being reduced by about 0.8% every 15 years**.
- In all illnesses, oxygen will become less available for primary respiration as it is used up in inflammatory, immunologic and detoxification processes.
- In modern technological societies most people consume diets that are excessively acidic -emphasizing such foods as meats, coffee, soda pop and alcohol. This causes an acid constitution where there is an excess of positively charged hydrogen ions (H+). When excessive numbers of hydrogen ions are in the tissue environment, they will combine with (and thus utilize) oxygen, resulting in an oxygen deficiency state. **Diets high in fats, especially polyunsaturated fats, will also cause an increase in oxygen utilization.** Unsaturated fats contain available double bonds which attract oxygen to them causing the formation of fatty acid (peroxides). These peroxides can be damaging to the cells and use up oxygen, thus making it less available for its primary function of respiration. Thus, we can see that the typical modern day stressors all tend to use up oxygen. Oxygen is the great detoxifier for both our bodies and for our environment. **RMH Note: More technically, the active detoxifying form is not ground state oxygen but is an oxygen modification such as reactive oxygen species or excited states (RONS/excytomers).**

Oxygen is the single most important substance for life and should be used regularly as a medicine to treat the sick. **RMH Note: I believe that exercise serves to provide a "dose" of reactive oxygen species and excitation states. Hence, they (RONS) and exercise are good for you.** However, new methods of oxygen delivery must be developed and utilized in this country. Inhalation of pure oxygen is inadequate because the lung tissue may be damaged by high-tension oxygen delivered by mouth, if for prolonged periods or at high concentrations. **RMH Note: Data from NASA indicates that astronauts can inhale pure oxygen for prolonged periods without untoward effects. Consequently, a lot of the pure oxygen scare may not be justified. I have been told many antidotal stories by fellow physicians of the salutary effects of prolonged use of 100% O$_2$.**

Oxygen solutions have been used by Russian athletes and should also be utilized regularly to treat many of our chronic inflammatory degenerative disease. In large part, the reason these approaches have not been utilized is that such modalities would be **difficult to patent and large pharmaceutical (profit driven) companies would rather market new drugs that they develop and can own.** Such drugs may have marginal and limited benefits along with considerable side effects. Why not develop better ways to deliver oxygen to damaged tissues?

19.3 OXYGEN FREE RADICAL METABOLISM (RONS)

Free radicals are an integral part of metabolism and are formed continuously in the body. Many sources of stress, heat, irradiation, hyperoxia, inflammation and any increases in metabolism including exercise, injury and even repair processes lead to increased production of free radicals and associated reactive oxygen or nitrogen species (RONS/excytomers). Evidence is accumulating that **free radicals have important functions**, in part, in the signal network of cells including induction of growth and apoptosis and as **killing tools used by immunocompetent cells.** Allegedly, endogenous and nutritional antioxidant systems may have to be adjusted to ensure adequate removal of radicals during stress to prevent damage to membranes, proteins, or nucleic acids. Excessive stress may induce DNA damage in the form of oxidized nucleosides, strand breaks, or DNA-protein cross links. Possible consequences of DNA damage may be repair, apoptosis/necrosis, or defective repair leading to DNA sequence alterations and possibly to the development of cancer or, in case of mitochondrial DNA, to metabolic dysfunction. **Excessive exercise will also induce DNA damage in peripheral leukocytes.** The good message is that moderate stress in form of regular exercise/training may have protective effects against exercise-induced DNA damage. Up-regulation of endogenous antioxidant defense systems and complex regulation of repair systems such as heat shock proteins (HSP 70, HSP 27, HO 1) may be seen in response to training and exercise. Up-regulation of antioxidants and modulation of the repair response may be, or may not be, mechanisms by which exercise can beneficially influence our health. **I believe that the beneficial effects of exercise may be due to the increased levels of RONS/excytomers. Massive intervention into the natural redox state by pharmaceutical doses of exogenous antioxidants should be regarded with caution due to the ambiguous role of free radicals in regulation of growth, apoptosis and cytotoxicity by immunocompetent cells.** (Fehrenbach, E. and Northoff, H. Free radicals, exercise, apoptosis and heat shock proteins Exerc Immunol Rev 2001; 7: 55-89).

So called oxidative stress is allegedly induced by a wide range of environmental factors including UV stress, pathogen invasion (hypersensitive reaction), xenobiotic action (drugs, pesticides, herbicides) and oxygen shortage. Oxygen deprivation stress in plant cells is distinguished by three physiologically different states, transient hypoxia, anoxia and reoxygenation. Generation of reactive oxygen species (ROS) is characteristic for hypoxia and especially for reoxygenation. Of the ROS, hydrogen peroxide (H_2O_2) and superoxide O_2^- are both produced in a number of cellular reactions, including the iron-catalysed Fenton reaction, and by various enzymes such as lipoxygenase, peroxidases, NADPH oxidase and xanthine oxidase. The main cellular components susceptible to damage by free radicals are lipids (peroxidation of unsaturated fatty acids in membranes), proteins (denaturation), carbohydrates and nucleic acids. Consequences of hypoxia-induced oxidative stress depend on tissue and/or species (i.e., their tolerance to anoxia), on membrane properties, on endogenous antioxidant content and on the ability to induce the response in the antioxidant system. Effective utilization of energy resources (starch, sugars) and the switch to anaerobic metabolism and the preservation of the redox status of the cell are vital for survival. The formation of RONS/excytomers is prevented by an antioxidant system: low molecular mass antioxidants (ascorbic acid, glutathione, tocopherols), enzymes regenerating the reduced forms of antioxidants, and ROS-interacting enzymes such as SOD, peroxidases and catalases. In plant tissues, and following ingestion in many animal tissues, many phenolic compounds (in addition to tocopherols) are potential antioxidants: flavonoids, tannins and lignin precursors may work as RONS/excytomer-scavenging compounds. Antioxidants act as a cooperative network, employing a series of redox reactions. Interactions between ascorbic acid and glutathione, and ascorbic acid and phenolic compounds are well known. **The pro-oxidant activity of ascorbic acid is also well known.** Under oxygen deprivation stress, some contradictory results on the antioxidant status have been obtained. **Experiments on over expression of antioxidant production do not always result in the enhancement of the antioxidative defense and hence increased antioxidative capacity does not always correlate positively with the degree of protection.** Blokhima et al., present a consideration of factors which possibly affect the effectiveness of antioxidant protection under oxygen deprivation as well as under other environmental stresses. Such aspects as compartmentalization of RONS formation and antioxidant localization, synthesis and transport of antioxidants, the ability to induce the antioxidant defense and cooperation (and/or compensation) between different antioxidant systems are the determinants of the competence of the antioxidant system (Blokhima, O., Virolainen, E. and Fagerstedt, K.V. Antioxidants, oxidative damage and oxygen deprivation stress: A review. Ann Bot (Lond). 2003; 91: 179-194).

19.4 FREE RADICAL PECKING ORDER

Free radicals are species with one or more unpaired electrons. The unpaired electron results in a species that can be highly reactive. Free radicals have a wide range of reactions; **two broad classes of reaction are electron transfer and addition reactions resulting in covalent bond formation**. Free radicals can be classified as reducing (donating an electron to an acceptor) or oxidizing (accepting an electron from a donor). Because of the wide range of reactivities of radicals, **there is a thermodynamic hierarchy or pecking order for electron transfer reactions** (Buettner, G.R. The pecking order of free radicals and antioxidants: Lipid peroxidation, a-tocopherol and ascorbate. Arch Biochem Biophys 1993; 300: 535-543). Table 1 is arranged with the most oxidizing radicals at the top and most reducing at the bottom. **This pecking order predicts the flow of electrons.** This thermodynamic hierarchy helps predict which species might react with each other. **In general, the radical species higher in the pecking order steal electrons from the reduced species lower in the pecking order.**

The pecking order predicts that peroxyl radical will react with vitamin E (tocopherol):

ROO. + TOH → ROOH + TO.
Ascorbate + TO. → Ascorbate.- + TOH

eliminating the dangerous ROO. and generating the much less reactive tocopheroxyl radical. This radical must be removed because it can also do damage, albeit very slowly. TO. can be recycled by ascorbate, which is lower in the pecking order, producing the ascorbate radical that is even less reactive. Because vitamin E is located in lipid structures, this reaction also moves the radical from lipid regions into aqueous environments where enzymes can detoxify and recycle ascorbate radical back to ascorbate.

TABLE I. **One-electron reduction potential at pH 7.0 for selected radical couples.**

Redox couple	E /mV
HO., H+/H$_2$O	+2310
RO., H+/ROH (aliphatic alkoxyl radical)	+1600
ROO., H+/ROOH (alkyl peroxyl radical	+1000
GS./GS- (glutathione)	+920
PUFA., H+/PUFA-H (bis-allylic-H)	+600
HU.-, H+/UH2- (Urate)	+590
TO., H+/TOH (Tocopherol)	+480
H$_2$O$_2$, H+/H$_2$O$_2$, HO.	+320
Ascorbate.-, H+/Ascorbate monoanion	+282
Fe(III)EDTA/Fe(II)EDTA	+120
O$_2$/O$_2$.-	-330
Paraquat2+/Paraquat.+	-448
Fe(III)DFO/Fe(II)DFO (Desferal)	-450
RSSR/RSSR.- (GSH)	-1500
H$_2$O/e-az	-2870

(Buettner, G.R. and Schafer, F.Q. Free Radicals, Oxidants and Antioxidants. Teratology 2000; 62: 234).

This shows that vitamin E is a more potent oxidizer than hydrogen peroxide and that both vitamin E and C are more potent oxidizers than superoxide anion. Also, note the ranking of PUFA and glutathione, which are quite high in the list. I believe that this is extremely important data.

19.5 ANTIOXIDANT SYSTEMS

To control the level of RONS and to protect cells under stress conditions, tissues contain several enzymes scavenging RONS (SOD, CAT, peroxidases and glutathione peroxidase), detoxifying LP products (glutathione S-transferases, phospholipid-hydroperoxide glutathione peroxidase and ascorbate peroxidase), and a network of low molecular mass antioxidants (ascorbate, glutathione, phenolic compounds and tocopherols).

19.5.1 Enzyme Antioxidants

Superoxide dismutase
Catalase
Glutathione peroxidase
Glutathione S-transferases
Phospholipid-hydroperoxide glutathione peroxidase
Ascorbate peroxidase
Monodehydroascorbate reductase
Dehydroascorbate reductase
Glutathione reductase

Antioxidant Defense

19.5.2 RONS Scavenging Agents

RONS Scavenging Agents   **Sequestration of transition metal ions**

- Glutathione   Transferrin
- Uric acid   Ferritin
- Ascorbic acid   Metallothioneins
- Albumin   Ceruloplasmin
- Phenolic Compounds
- Tocopherols

A whole array of enzymes is needed for the regeneration of the active forms of the antioxidants such as, monodehydroascorbate reductase, dehydroascorbate reductase and glutathione reductase. It is also possible in different tissues, different mechanisms are involved in the protection against so called oxidative stress. **Please remember that knock out mice, for some of the antioxidant enzymes, develop normally and that diets given to mice, which are deficient in antioxidants, also have no problems in development. Again, this is data which should forever put to rest the flawed free radical/oxidation theory of aging and disease (aka,**

the Free Radi-Crap theory). However, investigators overlook it and continue to try to force the data to fit the erroneous theory.

Phospholipid hydroperoxide glutathione peroxidase (PHGPX) is allegedly a key enzyme in the protection of the membranes exposed to oxidative stress and it is inducible under various stress conditions. The enzyme catalyzes the regeneration of phospholipid hydroperoxides at the expense of GSH and is localized in the cytosol and the inner membrane of mitochondria of animal cells. PHGPX can also react with H_2O_2 but this is a very slow process. Until now, most of the investigations have been performed on animal tissues.

Functioning of GSH as antioxidant under oxidative stress has received much attention during the last decade. **A central nucleophilic cysteine residue is responsible for high reductive potential of GSH**. It scavenges cytotoxic H_2O_2 and reacts non-enzymatically with other ROS: **singlet oxygen**, superoxide radical and hydroxyl radical (Larson, R.A. The antioxidants of higher plants. Phytochem 1988; 27: 969-978). The central role of GSH in the antioxidative defense is due to its ability to regenerate another powerful water-soluable antioxidant ascorbic acid (AA), via the ascorbate-glutathione cycle (Noctor, G., Arisi, A.C.M., Jouanin, L., Kunert, K.J., Rennenberg, H. and Foyer, C.H. Glutathione: biosynthesis, metabolism and relationship to stress tolerance explored in transformed plants. J Exper Botany. 1998; 49: 623-647).

The ability to donate electrons in a wide range of enzymatic and non-enzymatic reactions make AA the main ROS-detoxifying compound in the aqueous phase. AA can directly scavenge superoxide, hydroxyl radicals and **singlet oxygen** and reduce H_2O_2 to water via ascorbate peroxidase reaction. In addition, AA carries out a number of non-antioxidant functions in the cell.

Please keep in mind the fact that nearly all of these antioxidants and the antioxidant enzymes, serve multiple functions within the cell and do not necessarily serve only as an antioxidant.

-Oxygen scavengers - react with O_2 and remove O_2 from the system, i.e., ascorbic acid, ascorbyl palmitate, sulfites, erythroid acid and sodium erythorbate.

-Chelating agents (sequestering agents) - citric acid, amino acids, ethylene diaminetetra-acetic acid (EDTA) and certain phosphoric acid derivatives can chelate metallic ions, which catalyze lipid oxidation and retard oxidative decomposition of lipids.

.OH scavengers are ethanol, mannitol, formate, benzoate, thiourea, DMSO and azide.

19.6 ANTIOXIDANT HAZARDS

Even with an impressive antioxidant system perpetually in place, **the body automatically maintains steady state levels of RONS and excited states.** In fact, **if one were to give enough antioxidants to stop or remove all RONS and excited states, then the organism would die. I can not emphasize this point strongly enough. Free radicals and excited states are not only characteristic of the life process but are an essential for its maintenance.** Data from hundreds of thousands of patients now **clearly demonstrate the potential hazards of antioxidant supplements.** Consequently, the ingestion of small quantities **of antioxidant supplements are working against the natural processes occurring in the living/breathing cell, if they are having any effect at all.** The lack of a beneficial effect of antioxidants on the body helps explain the wide spectrum of contradictory experimental results seen in the current scientific and medical literature. This approach emphasizes the point that ROS and excited states are needed in the performance of important and essential biological and chemical functions.

In reviewing the materials needed for the assimilation of this book, I have been struck by the fact that **the body has a multitude of pathways leading to the synthesis of hydrogen peroxide.** In fact, the data leads to the conclusion that **hydrogen peroxide synthesis is a programmed salutary necessity** and it is not a "leak," "mistake," or "intracellular disaster" as is so frequently promoted by marketers selling 21st century snake oil.

The fact that we are alive and breathing, means that the free radicals and the excited states are winning, even though we try to extinguish their healing energies with antioxidants.

As has been the case in the history of medicine, we frequently work against the body's innate healing capabilities. Medical history clearly points out we repeatedly try to block the body's ability for self-cure. Only after prolonged periods of faulty practice do we realize the folly of our ways.

Convincingly, RONS/excytomers play a crucial role in many lifesaving biological mechanisms. Phagocytic cells protect us from deadly microorganisms, killing them by producing **an antibacterial avalanche of RONS.** When neutrophils and other phagocytic cells engulf bacteria, they greatly increase consumption of oxygen ("respiratory burst"), which is rapidly transformed to **RONS/excytomers that kill the dangerous intruders. This fact alone would contraindicate the use of antioxidants.** NADPH supplies electrons, required for the reduction of oxygen and the formation of RONS. In turn, NADP+ receives electrons from the pentose cycle pathway by NADPH oxidase through cytochrome b245. Importantly, by a burst of RONS/excytomers, **phagocytes kill not only invading bacteria, but also cancer cells** (Halliwell, B. and Cutteridge, J.M.C. Free radicals in biology and medicine. Oxford: Oxford University Press, 1999), (Alexander, P. Can antioxidants facilitate cancer induction? Oxidation reactions involved in host-mediated destruction of cancer cells. In Nygaard OF, Simic MG (Eds) Radioprotectors and anticarcinogenes. New York: Academic Press, 1983; 575-584). **Excessive antioxidants scavenge these beneficial RONS/excytomers and can thereby interfere with the protective functions of phagocytes** (Cedro, K., Klosiewicz-Wasck, B. and Wasek, W. Inhibitory effect of vitamins C and E on the oxygen free radical production in human polymorphonuclear leucocytes. Eur J Clin Invest 1994; 24: 316-319). **We must stop trying to inhibit the very system which is protecting us from infections and cancer.**

Detoxification reactions, processed by the cytochrome P450 family, are dependent on the integrity of the microsomal ROS-generating system. **Dr. R. Steele and I (Dr. R. M. Howes) were the first to show that this system is capable of generating electronic excitation states of singlet oxygen, in mammals.** NADPH and

NADH supply reducing equivalents for the reduction of cytochrome b5 and cytochrome P450. The latter oxidizes hydrophobic toxic substances, steroids and drugs, transforming them into hydrophilic ones, which are removed from the body. In view of the pivotal role of ROS in the functioning of the cytochrome P450 complex, **it is reasonable to suggest that excessive antioxidants could interfere with the important cell function**. Data supports this suggestion (Ghosh, M.K., Mukhopadhyay, M. and Chatterjee, I.B. NADPII-initiated P450-dependent free-iron-dependent microsomal lipid peroxidation: Specific prevention by ascorbic acid. Mol Cell Biochem 1997; 166: 35-44).

Production of RONS/excytomers is essential for a number of biochemical reactions involved in the synthesis of prostaglandins, hydroxylation or proline and lysine, oxidation of xanthine and other oxidative processes. Increase of ROS concentration by depletion of antioxidants enhances apoptosis and thereby inhibits tumor growth. Excessive antioxidants decrease ROS levels, inhibit apoptosis and suppress the elimination of cancer cells induced by anticancer drugs. Yet, **investigators are hell-bent to incriminate this most important system, all in the name of conforming to the fallacious free radical theory, and marketers push their antioxidant supplements upon an unknowing public harder than ever.**

19.7 APOPTOSIS, FREE RADICALS AND CANCER

Apoptosis, sometimes called "a guardian angel" or "cell policeman," is a cell suicidal altruistic mechanism targeted to **selectively eliminate cancerous and other cells that threaten our health and life.** It appears to be the sacrifice of the "bad" cells to save the integrity and life of the whole organism. Apoptosis is carried out by a multistage chain of reactions in which **RONS/excytomers act as triggers and essential mediators** (Kerr, J.F.R., Winterfold, C.M. and Harmon, B.V. Apoptosis, its significance in cancer and cancer therapy. Cancer 1994; 73: 2013-2026), (Blackstone, N.W. and Green, D.R. The evolution of a mechanism of cell suicide. Bio Essays 1999; 21: 84-88). Recently, it became evident that **mitochondria play a crucial role in apoptosis** (Kroemer, G., Zamzami, N. and Susin, S.A. Mitochondrial control of apoptosis. Immunol Today 1997; 18: 44-51). Schematically, apoptosis signals, which arise in cancer cells, promote accumulation of the p53 protein that triggers the release of ROS, cytochrome C and a few other regulators from mitochondria. The latter activate a cascade of proteolytic enzymes, called caspases, that digest a number of pivotal cell proteins and promote a caspase-activated deoxyribonuclease. Cleavage of the critical proteins and DNA results in apoptotic cell death. Importantly, **most anticancer drugs and radiation kill cancer cells by inducing apoptosis** (Hickman, J.A. Apoptosis induced by anticancer drugs. Cancer Metast Rev 1992; 11: 121-139). Mutations in the p53 gene make cancer cells resistant to apoptosis and, accordingly, to anticancer drugs.

19.8 HARMFUL EFFECTS OF ANTIOXIDANTS

Because of the pivotal role of ROS in triggering apoptosis, **antioxidants can inhibit this protective mechanism by depleting RONS/excytomers** (Verhaegn, S., Adrain, J., McGovan, J., Brophy, A.R., Fernandes, R.S. and Gotler, T.G. Inhibition of apoptosis by antioxidants in the human IIL-60 leukemia cell line. Biochem Pharmacol 1995; 40: 1021-1029). Salganik states that this is why **antioxidants could interfere with the therapeutic activity of anticancer drugs that kill cancer cells by apoptosis.** His data demonstrate that, indeed, apoptosis induced in human breast cancer cells by **cisplatin, a widely applied anticancer drug, is accompanied by an increase in RONS generation.** We have further demonstrated that the powerful antioxidant **alpha-tocopherol inhibits RONS generation and apoptotic death of breast cancer cells induced by cisplatin.** It appears that antioxidants might inhibit the therapeutic activity of anticancer drugs in patients (Labriola, D. and Linvingston, R. Possible interaction between dietary antioxidants and chemotherapy. Onocolgy 1999; 13: 1003-1012). **It has been repeatedly demonstrated that antioxidants can be counter productive to maintaining good health.**

He reasoned that if depletion of RONS by antioxidants suppresses apoptosis, then **a rise in RONS concentration could enhance the apoptotic death of cancer cells.** The concentration of RONS can be increased by enhancing RONS generation or by depleting antioxidants. We tried to increase RONS accumulation by depleting antioxidants. Experiments to verify this reasoning were performed at the University of North Carolina at Chapel Hill (Salganik, R.I., Albright, C.D., Rodger, J., Kim, J., Zeisel, S.H., Sivashinskiy, M.S. and Van Dyke, T.A. Dietary antioxidant depletion: Enhancement of tumor apoptosis and inhibition of brain tumor growth in transgenic mice. Carcinogenesis 2000; 21: 909-914). Transgenic mice developing brain tumors were fed a diet depleted of antioxidants, while control mice were fed a standard diet. **The antioxidant-depleted diet significantly increased RONS/excytomers concentration in brain tumors that, in turn, led to a dramatic increase in apoptotic death of brain tumor cells.** Because of intensive apoptosis, a sharp decrease in tumor volume resulted. Importantly, **an enhancement of apoptosis was not observed in normal tissues of animals fed the antioxidant-depleted diet. Neither weight loss nor changes in behavior or pathology of normal tissue were found in mice fed the antioxidant-depleted diet for four months.** Similar results were obtained in transgenic mice developing mammary tumors. The data indicate that **antioxidants scavenging RONS can interfere with cancer cell killing apoptosis and vice versa; an increase of RONS concentration could enhance apoptosis,** thereby **selectively removing cancer cells.** Currently, clinical studies are in preparation to verify this presumption (Salganik, R.I. The benefits and hazards of antioxidants: Controlling apoptosis and other protective mechanisms in cancer patients and the human population. J Am Coll Nutr 2001; (5 Suppl): 464S-472S). I have been arguing this point for some time. The effects of RONS and excitation states appear to be selective against infections and cancer. All of this data fits nicely with my Unified Theory.

Since RONS have been implicated in the pathogenesis of many clinical disorders such as adult respiratory distress syndrome, ischemia-reperfusion injury, atherosclerosis, neurodegenerative diseases and cancer, **gene knockout mice deficient in copper-zinc superoxide dismutase (CuZnSOD) and GSHPx-1** have also been generated in the laboratory. **These mice developed normally and showed no marked pathologic changes under normal physiologic conditions.** In addition, **a deficiency in these genes had no effects on animal survival under hyperoxia.** (Ho, Y.S., Magnenat, J.L., Gargano, M. and Cao, J. The nature of antioxidant defense mechanisms: A lesson from transgenic studies. 1998; 106(5): 1219-1228). These transgenic studies clearly demonstrate that mice can develop quite normally and suffer no ill effects under hyperoxia conditions, which should produce considerable oxidative stress.

R.I. Salganik states that an excessive intake of antioxidants can be as harmful as a lack of these protective entities. Unfortunately, widely advertised and poorly controlled application of antioxidants can lead to unwanted consequences to our health. Some **trials have failed to demonstrate protective or anticancer properties of combinations of antioxidants, vitamins E, C, A and beta-carotene, commonly found in supplements** (Salganik, R.I. Biochemical aspects of ecology: Mechanisms of the damage and defense of genetic structures. In Ione KG (ed) Chemistry, Ecology, Health. New York: Nova Science Publishers, Inc. 1995; 31-52). **He states that for people with a low RONS level, high doses of antioxidants can be deleterious suppressing the already low rate of RONS generation and the RONS-dependent cancer preventive apoptosis. I concur whole heartedly.**

An excess of antioxidants, which interferes with apoptosis, also can be cancer-promoting in people who are constantly exposed to the effect of environmental carcinogenic factors (tobacco smoke, industrial pollutants), which result in a high accumulation of pre-cancerous and cancerous cells. **In cancer patients, an excess of antioxidants can interfere with the therapeutic activity of anticancer drugs, which kill cancer cells by RONS-dependent apoptosis.**

At last, **it appears that others are beginning to rethink the role of antioxidants**. It has been long over due.

The scavenging of O_2^- is achieved through an upstream enzyme, SOD, which catalyzes the dismutation of superoxide to H_2O_2. **This reaction has a 10,000-fold faster rate than spontaneous dismutation** (Bowler, et al., 1992). The enzyme is present in all aerobic organisms and in all subcellular compartments susceptible of oxidative stress.

ROS have recently been considered as possible signaling molecules in the detection of the surrounding oxygen concentration. (Semenza, G.L. Perspectives on oxygen sensing. Cell 1999; 98: 281-284).

Both O_2^- and the hydroperoxyl radical $HO_2.$ undergo spontaneous dismutation to produce H_2O_2. Although **H_2O_2 is less reactive than O_2^-**, in the presence of reduced transition metals such as $Fe2+$ in a chelated form (which is the case in biological systems), the formation of OH. can occur in the Fenton reaction. (Blokhina, O., et al. 2003).

Peroxidases, besides their main function in H_2O_2 elimination, **can also catalyze O_2^- and H_2O_2 formation** by a complex reaction in which NADH is oxidized using trace amounts of H_2O_2 first produced by the non-enzymatic breakdown of NADH. Next, the NAD radical formed reduces O_2 to O_2^-, some of which dismutates to H_2O_2 and O_2 (Lamb, C., and Dixon, R.A. The oxidative burst in plant disease resistance. Ann Rev Plant Phys and Plant Mole Biol 1997; 48: 251-275). **Thus, peroxidases and catalases play an important role in the fine regulation of RONS concentration in the cell through activation and deactivation of H_2O_2** (Elstner, E.F. Metabolism of activated oxygen species. In: Davies DD, ed. Biochemistry of plants. 1987 Vol. 11 London: Academic press, 253-315). Lipoxygenase (LOX, linoleate:oxygen oxidoreductase, EC.1.13.11.12) reaction is another possible source of ROS and other radicals. It catalyses the hydroperoxidation of polyunsaturated fatty acids (PUFA) (Rosahl, S. Lipoxygenases in plants - their role in development and stress response. Zeitschrift fur Naturforschung. 1996 51c: 123-138). The hydroperoxyderivatives of PUFA can undergo autocatalytic degradation, producing radicals and thus initiating the chain reaction of lipid peroxidation (LP). **In addition, LOX-mediated formation of singlet oxygen (Kanofsky, J.R., et al. 1986) or superoxide has been shown.** Lipoxygenases represent another potential enzymatic source **of singlet oxygen.**

Changes in O_2 electronic configuration can lead to the formation of highly reactive singlet oxygen. Under aerobic conditions, the **reaction of oxygen with linoleic acid radicals** (formed by the interaction of linoleic acid with lipoxygenase-3 in its oxidized state) **represents a second mechanism for the formation of peroxy radicals. The Russell mechanism predicts that one molecule of singlet oxygen will be produced for every two peroxy radicals.** (Russell, G.A. J Am Chem Soc 1957; 79: 3871-3877).

$$2RR'CHOO. \rightarrow RR'CHOH + RR'CO + {}^1O_2 \text{ (singlet delta oxygen)}$$

Under aerobic conditions, the maximum number of peroxy radicals that may be formed is equal to the sum of the initial concentrations of 13-hydroperoxylinoleic acid and linoleic acid. Viewed in this manner, the lipoxygenase-3 system produced 12+/- 0.4% of the theoretical yield. The decrease in singlet oxygen yield at low oxygen concentrations is consistent with the known decomposition of peroxy radicals into oxygen and alkyl radicals that occurs at low oxygen conditions.

Several apoplastic plant enzymes may also lead to ROS production under normal and stress conditions. **Other oxidases, responsible for the two-electron transfer to dioxygen (amino acid oxidases and glucose oxidase) can contribute to H_2O_2 accumulation**. Also an extracellular germin-like oxalate oxidase catalyses the formation of H_2O_2 and CO_2 from oxalate in the presence of oxygen. Amine oxidases catalyze the oxidation of biogenic amines to the corresponding aldehyde with a release of NH_3 and H_2O_2.

Lipid peroxidation is a natural metabolic process under normal aerobic conditions and it is one of the most investigated consequences of RONS action on membrane structure and function. PUFA, the main components of membrane lipids, are susceptible to peroxidation. The idea of LP as a solely destructive process has changed during the last decade. It has been shown that **lipid hydroperoxides** and oxygenated products of lipid degradation as well as LP initiators (i.e., RONS) **can participate in the signal transduction cascade** (Tarchevskii, I.A. Regulatory role of degradation of biopolymers and lipids. Fiziologiya Rastenii 1992; 39: 1215-1223).

19.9 RETHINKING ANTIOXIDANTS

Perhaps, the most extreme view that I have seen relative to the chemistry of antioxidants, was seen in the following paper by Andras Matkovics, An overview of free radical research in Acta Biologica Szegediensis, 2003, Volume 47(1-4): 93-97. Matkovics states the following:

"A great number of data shows than **any antioxidants can be transformed to a prooxidant**, especially if it is given in a high dose and without other antioxidants. When being not able to step in to the chain of electron transport the antioxidant will be saturated and become a free radical source. Probably this is the explanation of the failure of the "Natural" Cancer prevention Trial (Peterson, K. "Natural" Cancer Prevention Trial Halted. Science 1996; 271: 441-442). Later **it was experimentally proved that high doses of beta-carotene produce superoxide radicals**."

"It can, thus, be stated: "A single antioxidant is not an antioxidant!" (Tulok, I. and Matkovics, A. Antioxidants a megelozesben es a gyosyitasban. Hazio Tvk Szle 1997; 2: 446-450).

"A new term called "**antioxidative stress**" has also been introduced. This includes all adverse effects of antioxidants and the indirect disadvantages of them. For example, the beneficial action of exercise by the induction of aortic catalase activity and endothelial nitric oxide synthase expression was counteracted by the administration of vitamin E. (Meilhac, O., Ramachandran, S., Chiang, K., Santanam, N. and Parthasarathy, S. Role of arterial wall antioxidant defense in beneficial effects of exercise on atherosclerosis in mice. Arterioscler Thromb Vasc Biol 2001; 21: 1681). It means that an adaptive reaction may be hindered by the administration of an antioxidant. Certainly the physiological free radical reactions must not be blocked. The antioxidants have a Janus face! **RMH Note: Antioxidants are two faced**.

**"The verity of the nature of oxygen radicals
can only be realized by acknowledgement of the condition
resultant to their absence: death and rigor mortis.
The way of the radical
is the way of life."**

R. M. Howes, M.D., Ph.D.

6/11/04

20 HYPOXIA AND HYPOXEMIA

Because of the importance that I place on oxygen modifications and excited states, as they relate to cancer development, cancer control and cancer kill, I will now consider the data concerning hypoxia and hypoxemia relative to my **Unified Theory**.

Hypoxia is a pathological condition in which the body as a whole (generalized hypoxia) or region of the body (tissue hypoxia) is deprived of adequate oxygen supply. Hypoxia is often associated with high altitudes, where it is called altitude sickness. Symptoms of generalized hypoxia depend on its severity and speed of onset. They include headaches, fatigue, shortness of breath, nausea, unsteadiness and sometimes even seizures and coma.

Hypoxia has been noted to be present before initiation of treatment in cervix, head and neck, pancreas, brain, and breast tumors and sarcomas. (Coleman, C.N. and Mitchell, J.B. Radiation modifiers, in Chabner BA, Longo DI (eds): Cancer Chemotherapy and Biotherapy: Principles and Practice. Philadelphia, PA Lippincott Williams & Wilkins, 2001; 707-751), (Koong, A.C., Menta, V.K. and Le, Q.T., et al. Pancreatic tumors show high levels of hypoxia. Int J Radiat Oncol Biol Phys 2000; 48: 919-922).

- Hypoxemia is the relative deficiency of O_2 tension in arterial blood; this is more significant as the partial pressure of O_2 goes below 70 mm Hg

20.1 CAUSES OF HYPOXEMIA
(THESE ARE NOT MUTUALLY EXCLUSIVE)

Hypoventilation (decreased O_2 delivery from the environment to the lungs)

- Drugs (narcotics, barbiturates)
- Thoracic wall trauma
- Pleural space disease (pneumothorax, hemothorax, pleural effusion, diaphragmatic hernia)
- Central nervous system trauma
- Upper airway obstruction (foreign body, laryngeal paralysis, edema, neoplasia)
- Neuromuscular disease (polyradiculoneuritis, myasthenia gravis)

Diffusion impairment (thickened alveolar septa or decreased transit time of blood through pulmonary capillaries prevents equilibration of oxygen between alveolus and blood [pulmonary edema, pulmonary fibrosis])

Ventilation/perfusion mismatching (blood flow is inadequate at the alveolar level to allow gas exchange even though adequate fresh gas is being delivered or blood flow/gas exchange is adequate but fresh gas is not).

- Atelectasis
- Alveolar pneumonia
- Pulmonary edema
- Pulmonary thromboembolism
- Asthma

Arteriovenous shunting (extreme form of pulmonary ventilation/perfusion mismatching that happens when pulmonary blood bypasses ventilated lung tissue before returning to circulation).

- Atelectasis and lung lobe consolidation (O_2 may help correct)
- Arteriovenous fistula (O_2 may help correct)
- Right-to-left-intracranial shunt

Low fractional inspired oxygen concentration

- High altitude
- Administration of nitrous oxide

Toxins

- Carbon monoxide
- Methemoglobin
- Hypoxia is a relative deficiency of O_2 in the tissues, and can be caused by many factors (including hypoxemia).

Thus, according to my **Unified Theory**, any and/or all of these above factors may play a contributory role in inflammation or cancer causation or cure. This high number of variables makes analysis very difficult.

Emad El-Omar , professor of gastroenterology, University of Aberdeen, UK says, "I personally believe that chronic inflammation is the root of all evil." However, even the definition of inflammation is problematic. Randall S. Johnson, associate professor of biological sciences, UC-San Diego found that **eliminating the ability of WBCs**

to respond to low oxygen levels blocks inflammation from developing in mice. Specifically, they found that HIF-1 inactivation blocked the inflammatory response in mice.

Investigators have proposed a link between inflammation and cancer for a long time. Robert Strieter, David Geffen School of Medicine, UC Los Angeles, said, "Another example that we as pulmonologists think about in the periphery of the lung is a tumor that develops in conjunction with a nearby scar, suggesting that at one time there was an inflammatory process. However, **I interpret this to mean that the scar tissue is an area of lowered O$_2$ partial pressure and of lowered O$_2$ consumption and thus, it is predisposed to allow for the development of both decreased inflammation and increased cancer.** This **Unified Theory** approach could be extrapolated to observations with hypertrophic scars and keloids, in which they act as tumors by exhibiting progressive and uncontrolled growth and cell multiplication.

Severe anemia and acute hemorrhage, where the amount of hemoglobin is reduced and the relative contribution of dissolved O$_2$ to overall O$_2$ content in blood is greater, followed by therapy.

- Therapy for severe anemia requires replacement of hemoglobin (RBCs and/or O$_2$ carrying plasma-phase hemoglobin solution such as Oxyglobin ®)
- Supplemental oxygen may not be beneficial for the above cases, if the patient also has low cardiac output, hypotension, hyperthermia, or problems with cellular O$_2$ uptake. Correction of the underlying circulatory problem via Extravascular volume expansion, positive inostropes, or pressor agents is necessary.

20.2 TUMOR HYPOXIA

Tumor **hypoxia has been shown to affect the malignant progression** of transformed cells and their response to therapy. It has also experimentally been shown **to promote tumor progression through the selection of tumor cells with diminished apoptotic potential, stimulate proangiogenic gene expression, and increase metastatic potential**. (Brown, J.M. and Giaccia, A.J. The unique physiology of solid tumors: Opportunities (and problems) for cancer therapy. Cancer Res 1998; 58: 1408-1416). Past studies have demonstrated a strong correlation between pretreatment tumor pO_2 and tumor control and survival in patients with head and neck squamous cell carcinomas (HNSCC). (Brizel, D.M., Dodge, R.K., Clough, R.W. and Dewhirst, M.W. Oxygenation of head and neck cancer: Changes during radiotherapy and impact on treatment outcome. Radiother Oncol 1999; 53: 113-117). Studies have also indicated that **hypoxia increases tumor invasiveness and dissemination in human solid tumors** (Fyles, A.W., Milsevic, M., Wong, R., Kavanagh, M.C., Pintilie, M., Sun, A., Chapman, W., Levin, W., Manchul, L., Keane, T.J. and Hill, R.P. Oxygenation predicts radiation response and survival in patients with cervix cancer. Radiother Oncol 1998; 48: 149-156).

20.3 HEAD AND NECK SQUAMOUS CELL CARCINOMA

Head and neck squamous cell carcinomas (HNSCC) is the fifth most common malignancy worldwide. These tumors arise from diverse anatomical locations, including oral cavity, or pharynx, larynx and hypo pharynx, but have common epithelial origin and etiological association with tobacco and alcohol exposure. Despite modern intervention, the five year survival rate for this disease has improved only marginally over the past decade (Greenlee, R.T., Hill-Harmon, M.B., Murray, T. and Thun, M. Cancer statistics, 2001. CA - Cancer J Clin 2001; 51: 15-36), and recurrent disease is observed in ~50% of the patients.

In a recent study on HNSCC **the median tumor pO$_2$ was consistently lower than that of normal s.c. tissues from the same patient, for all patients**. (Le, Q.T., Sutphin, P.D., Raychaudhuri, S., Ching, S., Yu, T., Terris, D.J., Lin, H.S., Lum, B., Pinto, H.A., Koong, A.C. and Giaccia, A.J. Identification of osteopontin as a prognostic plasma marker for head and neck squamous cell carcinomas. Clinc Cancer Res 2003; 9: 59-67).

The impact of hypoxia in increasing radiation resistance to a variety of biologic end points has been known for almost 70 years. It was demonstrated 35 years ago that **hypoxia limited the radio-curability of murine tumors. That hypoxia exists in human tumors was demonstrated 45 years ago by Thomlinson**, (Hall, E.J. Radiobiology for the Radiologist. Philadelphia, PA Lippincott Williams & Wilkins, 2000), who observed that necrosis occurred in tumor cells greater that 150 umol/L from blood vessels, which is the approximate diffusion distance of oxygen. This diffusion-limited hypoxia was felt to be an important reason for the inability of radiation therapy to achieve local tumor control, and consequently, an extensive laboratory and clinical effort was undertaken to overcome this effect starting with the use of hyperbaric oxygen in the mid-1960s.

It must kept in mind that molecules other than oxygen are also abnormally distributed within tumor cells, when compared to normal cells. In general, there are two types of hypoxia: 1) chronic or diffusion-limited hypoxia, where tumor cells are too far from a functional vessel and 2) acute/intermittent or perfusion-limited hypoxia, where there is abnormal periodic flow within a tumor vessel. Overall, hypoxia relates to molecular biology, biochemistry, physiology, angiogenesis and imaging. **Hypoxic cells are radio- resistant, requiring two or three times the radiation dose to kill them compared to the same cells in a eu-oxic state.** Hypoxia can be of two types: 1) chronic hypoxia, which is diffusion limited and 2) acute hypoxia, which is perfusion limited.

Tumor oxygen status is a reliable prognostic marker that impacts malignant progression and outcome of tumor therapy. However, tumor oxygenation is heterogeneous and cannot be sufficiently described by a single parameter. It is influenced by several factors including microvessel density (MVD), blood flow (BF), blood volume (BV), blood oxygen saturation, tissue pO$_2$, oxygen consumption rate, and hypoxic faction. Hypoxia-inducible factor-1 (HIF-1) is a transcription factor that plays a critical role in tumor growth by increasing resistance to apoptosis and the production of angiogenic factors such as vascular endothelial growth factor (VEGF). (Welsh, S.J., Williams, R.R., Birmingham, A., Newman, D.J., Kirkpatrick, D.L. and Powis, G. The thioredoxin redox inhibitors 1-methylpropyl 2-imidazolyl disulfide and pleurisy inhibit hypoxia-induced factor 1a and vascular endothelial growth factor formation. Molecular Cancer Therapeutics 2003; 2: 235-243).

Hypoxia is a feature inherent in solid tumors as is increased energy demand and diminished vascular supply. Tissue hypoxia is a characteristic property of cervical cancers that **makes tumors resistant to chemo- and radiation therapy.** Erythropoietin (Epo) is a hypoxia-inducible stimulator of erythropoiesis. Acting via its receptor (EpoR), Epo up regulates bcl-2 and inhibits apoptosis of erythroid cells and rescues neurons from hypoxic damage. In addition to human papillomavirus infection, increased bcl-2 expression and decreased apoptosis are thought to play a role in the progression of cervical neoplasia. (Acs, G., Zhang, P.J., McGrath, C.M., Acs, P., McBroom, J., Mohyeldin, A., Liu, S., Lu, H. and Verma, A. Hypoxia-inducible erythropoietin signaling in squamous dysplasia and squamous cell carcinoma of the uterine cervix and its potential role in cervical carcinogenesis and tumor progression. Am J Path 2003; 162: 1789-1806).

The present understanding of the changes in cellular function during hypoxia are rather complex. **The hypoxia-inducible factors (HIF-1a and HIF-2a)** (Semenza, G.L. HIF-1: Using two hands to flip the angiogenic switch. Cancer Metastasis Rev 2000; 19: 59-65), dimerize with the constitutively expressed HIF-1B subunit to bind to a hypoxia-responsive element to **activate a wide array of genes, including those involved in anaerobic metabolism, cell cycle arrest, differentiation, stress adaptation, angiogenesis and others**. These can result in profound alterations on tumor and cellular phenotype, including an obvious role in angiogenesis by upregulation of angiogenic factors such as vascular endothelial growth factor.

Hypoxia, with or without reoxygenation, is a mediator of malignant progression, with mechanisms that include selection pressure, genomic instability, genomic heterogeneity, decreasing apoptotic potential, increasing angiogenesis, and a chaotic microcirculation. Radioresistance of hypoxic cells is well established. Clinically, **hypoxic tumors tend to do worse in terms of both local recurrence and distant metastases.** (Fyles, A., Milosevic, M. and Hedley, D., et al. Tumor hypoxia has independent predictor impact only in patients with node-negative cervix cancer. J Clin Oncol 2002; 20: 680-687). This has been reported after surgical resection as well as after radiation therapy. (Nordsmark, M. and Overgaard, J. A confirmatory prognostic study on oxygenation status and loco-regional control in advanced head and neck squamous cell carcinoma treated by radiation therapy. Radiother Oncol 2000; 57: 39-43). Hypoxia may also adversely effect chemotherapy response. (Telcher, B.A. Hypoxia and drug resistance. Cancer Metastasis Rev 2001; 155: 837-846).

20.4 BIOCHEMICAL AND CLINICAL ASPECTS

Materials in the following section have been excerpted from and based upon the following paper, Hockel, M. and Vaupel, P. Tumor hypoxia: Definitions and current clinical, biologic and molecular aspects. J Natl Cancer Instit 2001; 93(4): 266-276.

Hypoxia in tumors is primarily a pathophysiologic consequence of structurally and functionally disturbed micro-circulation and the deterioration of diffusion conditions. **Tumor hypoxia appears to be strongly associated with tumor propagation, malignant progression and resistance to therapy**, and it has thus become a central issue in tumor physiology and cancer treatment. Biochemists define it as O_2-limited electron transport and physiologists and clinicians define it as a state of reduced O_2 availability of decreased O_2 partial pressure that restricts or even abolishes functions of organs, tissues or cells. For the purposes of applications to my **Unified Theory**, I am ultimately concerned with the levels of RONS and excited states (excytomers) that are generated intracellularly, thus, I must consider all factors that can affect these levels.

Traditionally, **tumor hypoxia has been considered a potential therapeutic problem because it renders solid tumors more resistant to sparsely ionizing radiation**. (Hall, E.J. editor. Radiobiology for the radiologist 4th ed. Philadelphia, PA Lippincott; 1994). More recent experimental and clinical studies (Vaupel, P. and Kelleher, D.K. editors. Tumor hypoxia: Pathophysiology, clinical significance and therapeutic perspectives. Stuttgart (Germany): Wissenschaftliche Verlagsgesellschaft; 1999), suggest that **intratumoral oxygen levels may influence a series of biologic parameters that also affect the malignant potential of a neoplasm.**

Sustained hypoxia in a growing tumor may cause cellular changes that can result in a more clinically aggressive phenotype. (Hockel, M., Schlenger, K., Aral, B., Mitze, M., Schaffer, U. and Vaupel, P. Association between tumor hypoxia and malignant progression in advanced cancer of the uterine cervix. Cancer Res 1996; 56: 4509-4515). **During the process of hypoxia-driven malignant progression, tumors may develop an increased potential for local invasive growth, perifocal tumor cell spreading** (Hockel, M., Schlenger, K., Hockel, S. and Vaupel, P. Hypoxic cervical cancers with low apoptotic index are highly aggressive. Cancer Res 1999; 59: 4525-4528), **and regional and distant tumor cell spreading**. Likewise, hypoxia may cause intrinsic resistance to radiation and other cancer treatments may be affected. (Sethi, T., Rintoul, R.C., Moore, S.M., MacKinnon, A.C., Salter, D. and Choo, C., et al. Extracellular matrix proteins protect small cell lung cancer cells against apoptosis: A mechanism for small cell lung cancer growth and drug resistance in vivo. Nat Med 1999; 5: 662-668).

Hypoxia-induced or hypoxia-mediated changes of 1) the **proteome (i.e., the complete set of proteins within a cell at a given time)** of the neoplastic and stroma cells and 2) the genome of the genetically unstable neoplastic cells may explain the fact that tumor oxygenation is associated with disease progression, a link that has been demonstrated for a variety of human malignant tumor types.

With hypoxia and because of finely tuned regulatory processes, increases in tissue O_2 consumption are generally matched by an increase in blood flow and, therefore, do not usually lead to hypoxia unless the system regulating blood flow fails to meet the increased O_2 demand of the tissue in question. **In solid tumors, oxygen delivery to the respiring neoplastic and stroma cells is frequently reduced or even abolished by a deteriorating diffusion geometry, severe structural abnormalities of tumor microvessel, and disturbed microcirculation.** (Vaupel, P., Kallinowski, F. and Okunieff, P. Blood flow, oxygen consumption and tissue oxygenation of human breast cancer engrafts in nude rats. Cancer Res 1987; 47: 3496-3503).

20.5 SOLID TUMOR HYPOXIA

When an unrestricted supply of oxygen is available, for most tumors, the rate of O_2 consumption (respiration rate) and adenosine triphosphate (ATP) production is comparable to that found in the corresponding normal tissue, despite the deregulated organization of cells in malignant tumors. To maintain a sufficient energy supply for membrane transport systems and synthesis of chemical compounds, an adequate supply of O_2 is required.

In hypoxia, **the mitochondrial O_2 consumption rate and ATP production are reduced,** which hinders inter alia active transport in tumor cells. Specifically, major effects of the reduced production of ATP are 1) collapse of Na+ and K+ gradients, 2) depolarizaiton of membranes, 3) cellular uptake of Cl-, 4) cell swelling, 5) increased cytosolic Ca2+ concentration, and finally, 6) decreased cytosolic pH, resulting in intracellular acidosis in tumor cells.

20.6 HYPOXIA (OXYGEN) THRESHOLD LEVELS

On the basis of experimental results from isolated engrafted human breast cancer tissue, **tumor tissue hypoxia with reduced O_2 consumption rates is expected when the O_2 partial pressure in the blood at the venous end of the capillaries (end-capillary blood) falls below 45-50 mmHg** (Table1). This critical threshold, however, has been validated only under the following boundary conditions: a tumor blood flow rate of 1 mL/g per minute, a hemoglobin concentration of 140 g/L, and an arterial O_2 partial pressure of 90-100 mmHg. Reducing the perfusion rate to 0.3 mL/g per minute yields an hypoxic tissue fraction of approximately 20%. When the hemoglobin concentration falls below 100 g/L or the normal O_2 content of arterial blood decreases (hypoxemia), the relative proportion of hypoxic tissue substantially increases in the experimental tumor system described.

Conditions for normoxemia are Hb content = 140 g/L, MRO_2 = 30 uL/g per min, TBF = 1 mL/g per min

Table 1. Critical O_2 partial pressures below which adequate metabolic functions in solid tumors (metabolic hypoxia) cannot be maintained

Critical pO_2, mmHg	Entity measured	Parameter of interest
45-50	End capillary blood	O_2 consumption rate
8-10	Tissue (global)	ATP levels
~5	CHO cells	ATP per cell
0.5-1	CHO cells	O_2 consumption rate
0.5.-2	Ehrlich ascites cells	O_2 consumption rate
8-10	Neuroblastoma cells	O_2 consumption rate
~0.5	Isolated mitochondria	O_2 consumption rate
0.02-0.07	Cytochromes	Oxidation status

Median O_2 partial pressures of less than 10 mmHg result in intracellular acidosis, ATP depletion, a drop in the energy supply and increasing levels of inorganic phosphate.

Oxidative phosphorylation for ATP formation will continue to a cellular O_2 partial pressure of 0.5-10 mmHg [Table 1]. Certainly, the threshold O_2 partial pressure below which oxidative phosphorylation ceases is dependent on the cell line investigated and its respiratory capacity, the type of medium and substrate chosen, the temperature and pH of the suspending medium, and even the type and accuracy of the setup used to measure O_2 consumption rates.

Mitochondrial oxidative phosphorylation is limited at O_2 partial pressures of less than approximately 0.5 mmHg [Table 1]. Above this threshold, mitochondria should function physiologically.

Cytochromes aa_3 and c in ascites cells require O_2 partial pressures of greater than 0.02-0.07 mmHg [Table 1] to maintain respiration. At O_2 partial pressures above this range, cytochrome are fully oxidized.

From this rather rudimentary summary of critical O_2 partial pressures for metabolic hypoxia, **there does not appear to be a single hypoxic threshold that is generally applicable**. Hypoxic thresholds range from 45-50 mmHg in end-capillary blood to 0.02 mmHg in cytochrome, as was seen with xenografted human breast cancer tissue. Furthermore, such data on hypoxic thresholds in a given tissue do not take into consideration the existence of severe heterogeneities even on a microscopic level related to variable O_2 demands and O_2 supply.

In general, a number of key findings have been described as follows: 1) **Most tumors have lower median O_2 partial pressures than their tissue of origin;** 2) many solid tumors contain areas of low O_2 partial pressure than cannot be predicted by clinical size, stage, grade, histology and site; 3) tumor-to-tumor variability in oxygenation is usually greater than intratumoral variability in oxygenation; and 4) **recurring tumors have a poorer oxygenation status than the corresponding primary tumors.**

Anoxia/hypoxia-induced proteome changes in neoplastic and stroma cells may lead to the arrest or impairment of neoplastic growth through molecular mechanisms, resulting in cellular quiescence, differentiation, apoptosis and necrosis. **Cells exposed to hypoxia are generally arrested at the G1/S-phase boundary.** (Giaccia, A.J. Hypoxic stress proteins: Survival of the fittest. Semin Radiat Oncol 1996; 6: 45-58). **Under anoxia, most cells are arrested immediately, regardless of their position in the cell cycle.**

Hypoxia can induce programmed (apoptotic) cell death in normal and neoplastic cells. The level of p53 in cells increases under hypoxic conditions, and **the increased level of p53 induces apoptosis by a pathway involving Apaf-1 and caspase-9 as downstream effectors.** (Soengas, M.S., Alarcon, R.M., Yoshida, H., Giaccia, A.J., Hakem, R. and Mak, T.W., et al. Apaf-1 and caspace-9 in p53-dependent apoptosis and tumor inhibition. Science 1999; 284: 156-159). However, hypoxia also initiates p53-dependent apoptosis pathways involving hypoxia-inducible factor-1 (HIF-1), genes of the BCL-2 family, and other unidentified genes. (Shimizu, S., Eguchi, Y., Kosaka, H., Kamiike, W., Matsuda, H. and Tsujimoto, Y. Prevention of hypoxia-induced cell death by Bel-2 and Bel-xL. Nature 1995; 374: 811-813). **Below a critical energy state, hypoxia/anoxia may result in necrotic cell death, a phenomenon seen in many human tumors** and experimental systems.

Hypoxia stimulates the transcription of glycolytic enzymes, glucose transporters (GLUT1 and GLUT3), angiogenic molecules, survival and growth factors (e.g. vascular endothelial growth factor [VEGF], angiogenin, platelet-derived growth factor-B, transforming growth factor-B, and insulin-like growth factor-II), enzymes, proteins involved in tumor invasiveness (e.g., urokinases-type plasminogen activator), chaperones, and other resistance-related proteins. At the same time, hypoxia-induced inhibition of gene expression has been demonstrated for cell-surface integrins facilitating tumor cell detachment. Again, **I take issue with the term "stimulates" in that the best term here should be "allows". If something isn't there (oxygen), then it can not induce something else since it is not there but its absence can "allow" for subsequent events.**

Nuclear factor kB (NFkB) is another transcriptional factor that can be activated by hypoxia. The threshold for activation of NFkB in AG1522 cells occurs after 3 hours at an O_2 partial pressure of about 15 mmHg. Thus, **the critical O_2 levels necessary for hypoxia-induced gene expression are probably in the range of 1-15 mmHg.** Below these levels, mRNA levels often rise almost exponentially to a maximum value.

Critical O_2 tension below which typical cellular function in solid tumors progressively <u>cease or anticancer treatments are impaired as a result of an inadequate O_2 availability</u>

Critical O_2 tension mmHg	Function or parameter observed
30-35	Effectiveness of certain (passive) immunotherapy
15-35	Cell death with photodynamic therapy
25-30	Cell death on exposure to x- and y-radiation
10-20	Binding of hypoxia markers
1-15	Proteome changes
0.2-1	Genome changes

20.7 METASTASIS

Tumor spread can occur **locally** (through direct invasion of neighboring tissue and organs), **perifocal spread** (through migration of single neoplastic cells and microfoci into the interstitial space, lymphatic space involvement and perineural invasion), **regional spread** (through metastasis to the lymph nodes), and **distant spread** (through hematogenous metastasis or dissemination into body cavities, such as the peritoneum and pleura). Hypoxia can drive progression of a malignant tumor which is a consequence of 1) an increasing neoplastic cell load, 2) micro-environment-induced (epigenetic) phenotypic changes in neoplastic and stroma cells and 3) genotypic changes and clonal selection of neoplastic cells (Cheng, K.C. and Loeb, L.A. Genomic instability and tumor progression: Mechanistic considerations. Adv Cancer Res 1993; 60: 121-156).

Hypoxia-mediated clonal expansion of tumor cells with diminished apoptotic potential has been shown both experimentally and clinically, such as occurs in hypoxic surgical scars as a major pathogenetic event for local recurrences, despite cell free margins on complete surgical excisions. In general, hypoxia-induced changes are detectable at an O_2 partial pressure of less than 1 mmHg, which is one order of magnitude below the O_2 partial pressures associated with proteome changes. **RMH Note: It is stated that hypoxia "induces" an increased mutation rate; however, I feel that induction requires the presence of an inducing factor (not its absence) and hence, I feel that hypoxia "allows" for genomic changes instead of inducing them.** Hypoxic oxygen levels limits the cells ability to produce adequate amounts of reactive oxygen species and electronic excitation states (RONS/excytomers) to keep newly developed cancer cells in abeyance. My **Unified Theory** approach assumes that the intracellular metabolic machinery of the electron transport system is functioning properly.

Reynolds et al. (Reynolds, T.Y., Rockwell, S. and Glazer, P.M. Genetic instability induced by the tumor microenvironment. Cancer Res 1996; 56: 5754-5757), used a mouse tumor cell line carrying a chromosomally based l phage shuttle vector for reporting mutations. After exposing these cells to an O_2 partial pressure of less than 1 mmHg for 4 hours, they detected a mutation rate that was 3.4-fold higher than the rate in similar cells cultured under standard atmospheric conditions. Here, again, **lower levels (deficiency states) of O_2 resulted in increased mutation rates, consistent with my Unified Theory.**

A study reported in the June 25 issue of *Cell* said that a protein called Twist orchestrates gene activity and facilitates the spread of some breast cancers. Twist binds to DNA, switching on some genes and turning off others and it induces cells to disengage from their surroundings and float freely and allow for metastasis.

20.8 HYPOXIC TUMOR RESISTANCE

Hypoxic O_2 partial pressures in a tumor present a severe problem for X and Gamma radiation because the presence of ground state O_2 increases DNA damage with "an oxygen enhancement effect." **It requires 3 times more radiation to kill cancer cells in the absence of O_2 than it does in the presence of normal levels of O_2.** Hypoxia-associated resistance to photon radiotherapy is multifactorial. The presence of molecular oxygen increased DNA damage through the formation of oxygen free radicals, which occurs primarily after the interaction of radiation with intracellular water.

Oxygen dependence has also been established for a number of chemotherapeutic agents such as cyclophosphamide, carboplatin, doxorubicin, etc. and levels are different for each agent. Hypoxia can impart resistance to many chemotherapeutic agents (Teicher, B.A, Holden, S.A., Al-Achi, A. and Herman, T.S. Classification of antineoplastic treatments by their differential toxicity toward putative oxygenated and hypoxic tumor subpopulations in vivo in the FSaII murine fibrosarcoma. Cancer Res 1990; 50: 3339-3344). Tissue **acidosis is frequently found in hypoxic tumors with a high glycolytic rate** (Wike-Hooley, J.L., Haveman, J. and Reinhold, H.S. The relevance of tumor pH to the treatment of malignant disease. Radiol Oncol 1984; 47: 687-696).

Photodynamic Therapy-mediated tumor cell death also requires the presence of oxygen and **cells are not killed under anoxic conditions.** The critical threshold below which progressively reduced cell death was observed varied from 15 to 35 mmHg, probably **because of the reduced production of singlet oxygen ($^1O_2$)** species and different sensitivities to the treatment in different cell lines (Table 3 and Table 4). (Henderson, B.W. and Fingar, V.H. Relationship of tumor hypoxia and response to photodynamic treatment in an experimental mouse tumor. Cancer Res 1987; 47: 3110-3114), (Chapman, J.D., Stobbe, C.C., Arnfield, M.R., Santus, R., Lee, L. and McPhee, M.S. Oxygen dependency of tumor cell killing in vitro by light-activated Photofrin II. Radiat Res 1991; 126: 73-79). This means that because of the utilization of oxygen by PDT, it is a self-limiting process. In contrast, the **Howes Singlet Oxygen Delivery System** brings its own oxygen supply with it and is, therefore, not self-limiting.

PDT prodrugs, such as ALA, may be further limited because conversion of the prodrug to the active photosensitizer appears to be less effective under hypoxic conditions.

Additionally, **tumor hypoxia can dramatically effect cytokines (interferon gamma and tumor necrosis factor-a) and alter Interleukins 2-induced activation of lymphokine-activated killer cells**.

20.9 PATIENT PROGNOSIS
AND HYPOXIA

Studies have demonstrated that tumor hypoxia is independent of patient and tumor characteristics such as, patient age, menopausal status, and parity, International Federation of Gynecology and Obstetrics (FIGO) stage, clinical tumor size, histopathological and grade of malignancy. In advanced cancer of the uterine cervix, hypoxic tumors had larger extensions, more frequent (occult) parametrial spread and more lymph-vascular space involvement than no hypoxic tumors of the same clinical stage and size. **Tumor oxygenation is the strongest independent prognostic factor**, followed by FIGO stage and the disadvantage in outcome for patients with hypoxic tumors was independent of the mode of primary treatment (radiation therapy or radical surgery).

Critical oxygen or O_2 levels that characterize the upper limit of the hypoxic range (below which activities or specific functions of tumor cells progressively change) are as follows:

Immunotherapies, PDT, X and gamma radiation requires 25-30 mmHg O_2.

Binding of hypoxic markers, cellular ATP synthesis and cellular O2 consumption rate is about 10-15 mmHg O_2.

Mechanisms at the subcellular and molecular levels such as, gene amplification, genomic instability and loss of apoptotic potential occurs at less than 20 mmHg O_2.

Mitochondrial O_2 consumption requires about 1 mmHg O_2 and oxidation of the cytochromes requires about 0.05 mmHg O_2.

20.9.1 Hypoxia Miscellaneous Factoids

-Hypoxia has been seen in cervical cancer, squamous cell cancer of the head and neck, melanoma, breast, sarcoma and recently in prostate cancer (Page 13).

-Hypoxia promotes angiogenesis, metastasis and selection of cells with a more malignant phenotype (Page 14). **RMH Note: According to my Unified Theory, lower levels of oxygen lead to deficiency levels of RONS/excytomers, which "allows" the development or progression of cancer.**

-Another O_2 **Paradox:** O_2 contributes significantly to initial mutations through oxidative damage, but lack of O_2 promotes metastasis, angiogenesis and selection of cells with a more malignant phenotype (Page 20).

-Hb concentration is directly related to outcome of radiotherapy of cancer. **RMH Note: This would be predicted. O_2 (RONS/excytomers) are needed to kill cancer.**

-Carbogen (95% O_2 and 5% CO_2) and nicotinamide reduce hypoxia and increases radiotherapy (Page 28).

-Hypoxia sensitizers to improve radiotherapy (i.e., nimorazole, a widespread antimicrobial) and is used in Denmark to treat head and neck cancer.

-Another O_2 paradox: cancer is mainly initiated by mutations due to oxidative damage but radiotherapy can cure cancer by producing DNA damage with oxidative free radical damage. **RMH Note: There is no paradox, ROS and $^1O_2$ do not cause cancer. Their absence "allows" cancer to develop.**

-Erythropoietin (EPO), is a glycoprotein hormone produced by the kidney in response to hypoxia to stimulate RBC production in bone marrow.

-Bioreductive drugs (take advantage of hypoxia, i.e, TPZ tirapazamine) forms a radical to produce DNA damage and kills regardless of p53 status. When O_2 is restored, the TPZ radical is oxidized back to less toxic form (Page 30).

-Another **O_2 paradox:** hypoxia increases malignancy of tumors and increases treatment resistance, but induction of severe, acute hypoxia (anoxia) also has a therapeutic effect (Page 36). **RMH Note: Since these cells still require some O_2 or they die, hypoxia is better than no "oxia" at all.**

U.T.O.P.I.A.

-In hypoxia, the O_2 sensor, is a prolyl hydroxylase.

-HIF-1, induces expression of more than 30 known genes, including EPO, VEGF, NOS2, Flt-1, GIUT-1 & 3, PK-M and IGF-2 (Page 37).

-Tumor hypoxia stimulates expressing of vascular endothelial growth factor (VEGF) and hypoxia-inducible factor-1a (HIF-1a).

-Interleukin-8 (IL-8) is a member of the CαC chemokines and originally it was called, "neutrophil-activating peptide," but is also activates lymphocytes and monocytes and angiogenesis factor. It is inducible in tumors by hypoxia. **RMH Note: I believe that hypoxia induces the release of H_2O_2 to compensate for low O_2 levels, for an effect similar to that seen by dripping H_2O_2 to maintain viability of heart cells by the Baylor Research Group.**

-HIF-1α is regulated by a proline hydroxylase.

20.10 HYPERTHERMIA

Hyperthermia can also effect tumor cell survival and cell lines vary considerably in their intrinsic heat sensitivity. In addition, cell cycle position, intracellular pH, nutrient deprivation, and ATP depletion can affect cell survival after a heat treatment. (Vaupel, P.W. and Kellecher, D.K. Metabolic status and reaction to heat of normal and tumor tissue. In: Seegenschmiedt, M.H., Fessenden, P. and Vernon, C.C. editors. Medical radiology - diagnostic imaging and radiation oncology, thermo radiotherapy and thermo chemotherapy. Berlin and Heidelberg (Germany) and New York (NY): Springer; 1995: 157-176). At 43°C hyperthermia, hypoxia per se may not cause cell death as long as concomitant changes in the nutritional and/or bioenergetic status of the cells do not occur. (Gerweck, L.E., Richards, B. and Jennings, M. The influence of variable oxygen concentration on the response of cells to heat or X irradiation. Radiat Res 1981; 85: 314-320).

Recent studies show clear evidence that **hypoxia (defined as the fraction of measured O_2 partial pressures of <5 mmHg) is a statistically significant adverse prognostic factor of disease-free survival.** Similarly, poor outcomes have been shown to be associated with low oxygen tensions in advanced squamous cell carcinomas of the uterine cervix. Also, **tumor hypoxia appears to adversely effect the prognosis of patients with primary and metastatic squamous cell carcinomas of the head and neck** (HNSCC).

In summary, there is a wide range of hypoxia in malignant tumors, but they all appear to have hypoxic thresholds, below which, activities and functions become progressively restricted. These O_2 levels can encompass O_2 partial pressures from 35 mmHg (start of reduced cell death in conventional photodynamic therapy or restricted efficacy of some immunotherapy) to 0.02 mmHg (below this level, cytochromes aa3 and c are no longer fully oxidized) with all other critical O_2 levels for specific cellular functions or activities distributed in between.

Considerable data indicates that low O_2 in tumor cells is an adverse prognostic sign and this would be in direct contradiction to the Free Radi-Crap theory of aging and oxidative stress. Low tumor O_2 is associated with:

increased aggressiveness of primary cancerous lesions
their ability to metastasize
and an increased resistance to treatments with:
irradiation,
chemotherapeutics,
surgery

The lowered O_2 levels generate lowered levels of RONS/excytomers, which "allows" the cancer to grow and metastasize; whereas, high levels of RONS/excytomers from PDT, irradiation, chemotherapeutics or the Howes Singlet Oxygen Delivery System, kill the

cancerous cells. Get it?....high levels of RONS/excytomers kills cancer and low levels "allows" cancer to grow. This directly supports my Unified Theory. Also, remember the above work of Reynolds, who showed that low levels of O_2 resulted in a 3.4 fold **increase of mutations,** which again supports my Unified Theory and is contradictory to the Free Radi-Crap theory.

21 CANCER, HEREDITY AND ENVIRONMENT

21.0 CANCER UNDEFEATED

Samuel S. Epstein, M.D., Professor of Environmental Medicine, University of Illinois School of Public Health released the following statement: At a highly publicized March 12, Washington, DC press briefing, the National Cancer Institute (NIC) and American Cancer Society, (the cancer establishment), together with the Centers of Disease Control and Prevention, released a "Report Card" announcing the recent reversal of "an almost 20-year trend of increasing cancer causes and death," as detailed in a current issue of the journal Cancer. "These numbers are the first proof that we are on the right track," enthused NCI director, Dr. Richard Klausner. This news received extensive and uncritical nationwide media coverage. These claims were based on a comparison between NCI's published statistics for 1973-1990 and 1973-1995. However, the more recent information remains unpublished and, according to senior NCI statistician Dr. Lyn Ries, is still being analyzed. More importantly, a critical review of the Cancer publication is hardly reassuring. **The claimed reversal in overall mortality rates is not only minimal but exaggerated**. It is largely due to a reduction in lung cancer deaths from smoking in men, reflecting personal lifestyle choices, and to improved access to healthcare rather than to any improvements in treatment and survival rates. Additionally, **any true decline would be considerably less if the mortality rates were appropriately based on the current age distribution of the US population**, rather than that of 1970, with its relatively higher representation of younger age groups, as misleadingly calculated by NCI.

These criticisms are in general consistent with those detailed in a May, 1997 New England Journal of Medicine article, **"Cancer Undefeated,"** by former NCI epidemiologist, Dr. John Bailar. **The claimed reversal in the incidence of cancers of "all sites" is minimal and statistically insignificant, as are similar claims for leukemia and prostate cancer.** Even this minimal reduction of prostate cancer is highly questionable as admitted by the Report Card authors: "The decreased incidence rates (of prostate cancer) may be the result of decreased utilization of PSA screening tests -- during the early 1990's." While there were significant reductions in the incidence of lung, colon/rectum and bladder cancers, **there were significant and sharp increases in uterine cancer, melanoma and non-Hodgkin's lymphoma.** Moreover, there was no decline in breast cancer, rates which remain unchanged at their current high level. Curiously, **no reference at all was made to testicular cancer in young adults nor to childhood cancer, whose rates have dramatically increased in recent decades.** The Report Card apart, there are disturbing questions on the reliability of NCI's incidence statistics. This is well illustrated by wild reported variations since 1973 for the percent changes in the incidence of childhood cancer: 1973-1980, +21%; 1973-1989, +10%; 1973-1990, +1%; 1973-1991, -8%; 1973-1994, +31%. The Report Card's optimistic and misleading assurances, the latest in a series of smoke and mirror break through since 1971 when **President Nixon launched the "War Against Cancer,"** are designed to divert attention from the escalating incidence of cancer which ahs reached epidemic proportions. Cancer now strikes 1 in 2 men and 1 in 3 women, up from an incidence of 1 in 4 a few decades ago. Meanwhile, **our ability to treat and cure most cancer, apart from relatively infrequent cancers particularly those of childhood, remains virtually unchanged.**

The Report Card is also designed to neutralize criticism of NCI's intransigent fixation on diagnosis, treatment and basic genetic research, coupled with indifference to prevention which receives minimal priorities and resources -- less than 5% of NCI's budget. Further illustrative is the fact that NCI has never testified before congress or regulatory agencies on the substantial published evidence on the wide range of carcinogenic industrial contaminants of air, water, the workplace and consumer products -- food, household products and cosmetics -- and on the need to prevent such avoidable and involuntary exposures. Nor has NCI recognized the public's right-to-know of such critical information, which plays a major role in escalating cancer rates, and to develop community outreach prevention programs. Finally, the Report Card is designed to further buttress aggressive lobbying by the cancer establishment and cancer drug industry for a major increase in NCI's budget from the current $2.6 billion, up from $223 million in 1971, to the requested $3.2 billion in 1999. In my opinion, this data clearly indicates that a unique new approach needs to be implemented in the pursuit for a cancer cure. Our present outdated system has not and is not working. The pandemic of cancer rages on.

21.0.1 Nature vs. Nurture (DNA)

For many years it was believed that genes were the major factor involved in a person's risk of developing cancer. However, new evidence suggests that **environmental factors - such as tobacco, diet, infection, alcohol, drugs, chemicals and radiation - may play a larger role**. Sometimes it seems that genetics is the reason, especially when certain types of cancers run in families, but it's really not clear whether shared genes or a shared environment are to blame.

Data reported in the June, 2004 issue of *Nature Neuroscience* demonstrated, for the first time, that nurture can alter nature. **Different mothering styles in rats can change the activity of specific genes that in turn govern the way the brain responds to stress**, according to researchers at McGill University in Montreal. These effects, which occur as early as the second week of life in the rat, are still present in adulthood.

The researchers wanted to understand how genes respond to nurturing environments and whether that alters the way an animal responds to stress later in life. They looked at changes in the molecular processes in adult rats whose mothers had licked and groomed them, and compared them to adults whose mothers had shown little interest in their pup's grooming. The brains of the adults showed signs of change based on the attention the pups received from the mother, in that the animals that received more attention were more explorative and less anxious. Thus, **nurture does alter nature**.

21.1 TWINS AND GENETIC RESEARCH

Studying identical and non-identical twins is the ideal way, at this stage, to separate genetic factors from environmental factors in the development of disease. **Identical twins share the exact same genes, while non-identical (fraternal) twins share around half.** If, for example, a disease is caused by genetic factors alone, then **it could be assumed that identical twins will develop the disease in the same part of their body at around the same time and with the same frequency.** Therefore, if genes play a significant role in cancer, then cancer rates should be higher among identical twins.

Indeed, the nature-versus-nurture debate has waged for decades. A study published in the July 13, 2000 issue of the New England Journal of Medicine, provides some answers to the underlying question: Is biology destiny?

Researchers studied **44,788 pairs of twins** from Sweden, Denmark and Finland to tease out the roles of genes and environmental influences in the cause of 11 common types of cancer.

21.2 SWEDISH TWIN STUDY

They compared rates of stomach, colorectal, pancreas, lung, breast, cervix, uterus, ovary, prostate and bladder cancers, as well as leukemia.

The study found more than 10,000 cancers among their group of over 90,000 people. By calculating the incidence of the same cancer in both twins, the researchers were able to roughly estimate the role of genetic factors. **Generally, if one of the pair developed cancer, the odds of the other twin developing the same cancer were less than 15 percent.** This means that, based on the results of this study, **environment has the greatest influence on the development of cancer.**

Overall, the data show that 58 to 82 percent of risk in the 11 types of cancer was attributable to environmental influences not shared by both twins. **The researchers concluded that genes actually play a relatively minor role in most cancers; environmental factors (and I believe the redox status of the cell and its DNA) are the principal determinants of who gets cancer.**

21.3 CANCERS WITH STRONG GENETIC COMPONENT

According to the research, cancers that seem to be influenced the most by genes (estimated percentage of genetic contribution also shown) include:

- Prostate cancer - 42 percent
- Colorectal cancers - 35 percent
- Stomach cancer - 28 percent
- Breast cancer - 27 percent
- Lung cancer - 26 percent

These are also the most common human cancers, other than cancer of the skin.

In the New England Journal of Medicine study, genes did play a significant role in breast, colorectal and prostate cancers, contributing 27, 35 and 42 percent of risk, respectively. But, according to the researchers, genes alone cannot be fully responsible for these relatively high risks, suggesting that **there are still major holes in our current understanding of the genetics of cancer.**

The research, however, did not explore specific types and degrees of exposure to environmental factors, such as cigarette smoking or diet. This means that the interaction between genes and environment in the development of cancer was not fully explored.

21.3.1 Genetics and Breast Cancer

Scientists believe that breast cancer has a genetic component, since many women with breast cancer have family members with a positive history for breast cancer. Breast cancer is the most common cancer diagnosed in women after skin cancer and is the second leading cause of cancer deaths in women after lung cancer.

Mutations (inherited genetic variations) of 2 genes (segments of DNA that are biologic units of heredity) appear to account for about %5 of breast cancers diagnosed annually in the America. JAMA, 2004; 292(4): 522, presented advise for patients with genetic positive results as follows:

BRCA1 and BRCA2

- BRCA1 and BRCA2 (BReast CAncer 1 and 2) are genes that have been discovered to play a role in some breast cancers.
- Most women have 2 normal copies of the BRCA1 and BRCA2 genes.
- An estimated 250,000 women in the United States have a mutation in one of these genes.
- Women in general have about a 12% chance (1 in 8 women) of developing breast cancer. Women with a BRCA1 or a BRCA2 mutation have up to an 87% lifetime risk of breast cancer. However, this means that at least 13% of women with these mutations will not develop breast cancer.
- Women with BRCA1 or BRCA2 mutations also have an increased lifetime risk of cancer of the ovaries - up to 54% for BRCA1 and up to 27% for BRCA2.

- Women who test positive for BRCA1 or BRCA2 mutations should undergo further screening and take additional precautions, including frequent and early breast self-examinations, clinical breast examinations (performed by a doctor), and regular mammograms. They may consider other risk reduction options including the use of chemopreventive agents, such as tamoxifen, surgical removal of the ovaries, or surgical removal of the breasts.
- Men with a BRCA2 mutation also have an increased risk of breast cancer - a 6% lifetime risk compared with the average lifetime risk of 0.1% in US men.

Genetic Testing

Genetic testing can determine whether a person has a specific genetic mutation that can increase the risk of certain disease or disorders. Genetic test can detect mutations in the BRCA1 and BRCA2 genes. Because most breast cancers are not caused by genetic mutations, genetic testing may only be of value if you believe you are at a high risk of having a BRCA1 or BRCA2 mutation. You are morel likely to have these mutations if:

- there are 3 or more women with breast cancer in a single generation of your family
- women develop breast cancer at a young age in your family (younger than 50 years)
- breast cancers in the family are often found in both breasts
- there are cases of breast and ovarian cancer in the same family

It is interesting to consider the variability of cancer characteristics, as it relates to their cells of origin. For instance, primary bone cancer is very rare, occurring in approximately 2,500 new cases diagnosed in the United States yearly. More often, bones are the sites of tumors that have spread from another organ, such as the breasts, lungs and prostate. However, these cancers occur more frequently in children and young adults, especially in those who have had radiation or chemotherapy treatments for other conditions. Children with hereditary retinoblastoma of the eye are at higher risk of developing osteosarcoma as are adults with Paget's disease, a non-cancerous disease characterized by abnormal development of new bone cells. Interestingly, benign tumors do not spread and are rarely life-threatening. It has also been said that many malignant cancers are lethal because of their ability to metastasize. **I feel that the redox status of a potential metastatic site must be favorable (low levels of RONS/ex-cytomers) for a metastatic cell to "take and grow."**

21.4 LUNG CANCER AND THE ENVIRONMENT

A study published in the International Journal of Cancer (August 2002), showed that **diet can reduce the risk of developing lung cancer in women who have never smoked.** A study of German women showed that exposure to tobacco smoke is estimated to cause up to 85 percent of all lung cancer. Women exposed to the highest amount of environmental tobacco smoke increased their risk by 2.6 times, and certain occupational exposures doubled the risk. However, high consumption of fresh vegetables and cheese decreased risk by 50 and 70 percent respectively. Other studies have also reported lower lung cancer rates in people consuming vegetables daily, even in smokers.

These results are similar to the conclusions of previous research, according to an editorial that accompanied the study. For example, **breast cancer rates** among women who have recently immigrated to the United States from rural Asia are similar to those among women in their homelands. These rates are approximately 80 percent lower than those among third-generation Asian-American women, who have rates similar to those among Caucasian women in the United States. This **suggests a strong impact of the environment on cancer risk.**

Many recent observations seem to contradict that idea that mutations to a few specific genes lie at the root of all cancers (W. Gibbs, Scientific American, The science of staying young: Untangling the roots of cancer. Vol. 14, No. 3, 2004, p. 64). This is especially important when considering RONS/excytomers as mutagenic agents. The mere fact that they can alter DNA under certain conditions does not necessarily mean that they cause cancer.

In addition, data comparing cancer incidence among identical twins (twins with identical genetic make-up) show that the rate of concordance (agreement) is usually less than 15 percent. In other words, the likelihood is low that a cancer in one twin will also develop in the other.

21.5 ANEUPLOIDY AND CANCER

The word "aneuploidy" once referred to an abnormal number of chromosomes but now it is used in a broader sense that encompasses chromosomes with truncations, extensions or swapped segments. Also, **it appears that the oncogene/tumor suppressor gene hypothesis has failed**, despite two decades of studies to identify a particular set of gene mutations that occurs in every instance of any of the most common and deadly kinds of human cancer. **The list of cancer-related mutations has grown to more than 100 oncogenes and 15 tumor suppressor genes.** This may mean that each tumor is unique, since many new molecular markers are being identified (W. Gibbs, Untangling the roots of cancer. Sci Amer 2004; 14(3): 65). In fact, in some cancers, tumor suppressors are not mutated at all. Their output is simply reduced and this condition is called **"haploinsufficiency."**

At a recent meeting of over 70 scientists, there exists considerable controversy as to whether one can blame tumorogenesis on chromosomal gains and losses. When it comes to chromosomal alterations as being a direct causal link to cancer formation, **the jury is still out** (Appraising aneuploidy as a cancer cause. Sci. News 2004; 18(5)).

Biologists have estimated that it takes the cooperation of over 10 million billion cells to keep a human being healthy over the course of an 80-year life span.

21.6 CONCLUSIONS

While genetics may mean that some people are more vulnerable to cancer than others, environmental factors determine which of these people will develop the disease. The major study of cancer rates in twins supports the current belief that most cancers are caused by environmental factors, such as diet and smoking. However, the high rates of genetic influence in some cancers, such as prostate cancer, indicate that more research is needed.

This may help to explain why the discovery of over 25 so-called cancer genes (for example, the BRCA1 and BRCA2 breast cancer susceptibility genes) has been met with ambivalence. I also interpret this to mean that merely because RONS are implicated in producing DNA mutations, this does not necessarily translate to an direct causal relationship to cancer development. Many factors other than DNA determine the cell's fate. This is beautifully illustrated by cases involving identical twins.

It may just be that the nature-versus-nurture debate is now obsolete. Ultimately, genetic and environmental factors interact with one another to determine cancer risk, and we now know that biology is not destiny. The future lies in researching new ways to manipulate both genes and environment to help us control cancer.

Things to remember

- Comparing cancer rates between twins helps to distinguish between genetic and environmental factors.
- The cancers with the highest genetic contribution include prostate, colorectal, stomach, breast and lung cancers (which are the most common cancers, excluding skin cancer).
- Latest research supports current thinking that most cancers are caused mainly by environmental rather than genetic factors, but we realize that it is a combination of factors and variables that ultimately causes cancer.

The annual 2004 conference of the World Cancer Research Fund International and the American Institute for Cancer Research stated that **women who exercise, don't smoke and eat a vegetable-rich diet may be able to cut their cancer risk by 30%. I believe that this is good common sense advise.**

22 NADPH OXIDASE, SUPEROXIDE ANION AND H$_2$O$_2$

Some of the following material was excerpted or modified from the following paper: (Babior, B.M. **NADPH oxidase: An update.** Blood 1999; 93(5): 1464-1476).

The O$_2^-$ generated by this enzyme (NADPH) serves as the starting material for the production of a vast assortment of reactive oxidants, including oxidized halogens, free radicals, H$_2$O$_2$ and singlet oxygen. These oxidants are used by phagocytes to kill invading microorganisms. **I feel that the production of O$_2^-$ may well be the main source of H$_2$O$_2$ and ultimately ^{1}O$_2$ for the cell's well being, even though O2.- is produced by many other enzymatic reactions.**

When phagocytosis takes place, the plasma membrane is internalized as the wall of the phagocytic vesicle, with what was once the outer membrane surface now facing the interior of the vesicle. From this location, the enzyme pours O$_2^-$ into the vesicle, and the rapid conversion of this O$_2^-$ into its successor products bathes the internalized target in a lethal mixture of corrosive oxidants.

Kinetic competence is the gold standard for determining metabolic sequences, and there is no escape from the fact that the rate of reduction of the heme is far too slow for it to participate in any meaningful way as an electron carrier for the oxidase.

In resting cells, the membrane associated oxidase components are located exclusively in intracellular organelles and the active oxidase in the plasma membrane is delivered there by membrane fusion events. It is further implied that vesicles whose membranes contain the active oxidase, cycle between the interior of the cell and the plasma membrane.

Barbior states that the oxidase enzyme system may act as a "battery" because of the "electric current" it theoretically creates.

There is a very large body of evidence showing that this O$_2^-$ is the precursor of the powerful oxidants the phagocytes use as microbicidal agents.

Phosphorylation is an essential element in the activation of the NADPH oxidase.

Chronic granulomatous disease (CGD) is an inherited immune deficiency in which phagocytes from affected patients are unable to manufacture O$_2^-$ All cases so far have been found to result from a deficiency of one of 4 oxidase-specific proteins: p47^{PHOX}, p67^{PHOX}, p22^{PHOX}X, or gp91^{PHOX}.

Recent findings have confirmed the speculation that NADPH oxidase of much lower activity has widespread tissue distribution than that of the WBC, showing clearly that a low-activity NADPH oxidase is present in a variety of nonphagocytic cells, most of which are derived from the embryonic mesoderm, and that this oxidase is a source of second messengers. **This is a most important observation because it increases the role of O$_2^-$ H$_2$O$_2$ and ^{1}O$_2$ beyond the bounds of phagocytes and distributes their role through out tissues and organs of the body.**

An **NADPH oxidase** similar to the one found in phagocytes has been reported to occur in **all three layers of the aorta** (endothelial cells, aortic smooth-muscle cells and fibroblasts from aortic adventitia), all of which produce O_2^-. It was postulated that the O_2^- generated by the aorta was functioning as a blood pressure regulator by consuming nitric oxide, a well known hypotensive agent with which it reacts at a diffusion-limited rate.

In joint tissues, O_2^- production has been detected in **synoviocytes** (both type A and type B) and in **chondrocytes**.

There is evidence that NADPH oxidase serve as components of oxygen sensors in various tissues. Erythropoietin production in some hepatoma lines appears to be regulated by O_2^- and $p22^{PHOX}$, the *a*-subunit of cytochrome b_{558} has been detected immunologically in **renal peritubular fibroblasts and in cells of the liver**, both of which may be sources of erythropoietin. In **the lung**, pulmonary neuroepithelial bodies have been proposed as airway oxygen sensors.

Inhibition of O_2^- and H_2O_2 production by diphenylamine iodonium is generally regarded as presumptive evidence for an NADPH oxidase. Furthermore, the K+ current in these cells increased when the cells were exposed to H_2O_2. **These results suggest that the cells contain an NADPH oxidase whose output is a function of the ambient oxygen tension and whose dismutated product (i.e., H_2O_2) regulates the flow of current through the K+ channel, the latter representing the signal by which the oxygen tension is communicated to the rest of the organism.**

22.1 CHOLESTEROL AND CONSEQUENCES OF STATINS AND COVER UP

It is estimated that **20 million patients are currently taking statin drugs to lower their cholesterol levels.** Pharmaceutical companies want to increase this number to 40 million patients and double the dosages up to 80 mg./day. However, the statin drugs are not without harmful side effects. A few years back, it was recommended that I take Lipitor, due to a cholesterol level in excess of 300. Within 4 days of taking this drug, my thigh muscles became too sore to permit walking. Obviously, I immediately stopped taking the statin drug, whereupon, the symptoms abated but the strength of my muscles have yet to return to 100%, some three years later. Additionally, my 82 year old mother started taking statins, subsequent to aortic valve replacement and she developed thigh muscle pain but she was kept on the drug for sometime thereafter by her physician. Curiously, she also began to develop early signs of Alzheimer's disease and even though the statins were stopped a year or so later, she has gone on to develop full stage three Alzheimer's disease. I truly believe that there is a high probability that these two occurrences were directly related.

22.2 STATIN SIDE EFFECTS

According to Kilmer McCully, M.D., former Harvard physician, there are many side effects of statin drugs, which he describes in his book, "The Heart Revolution." Statins can decrease ubiquinone (coenzyme Q 10) and weaken heart muscle and result in heart failure. **Ubiquinone** serves as a vital and necessary electron carrier to our ultimate respiratory enzyme, cytochrome oxidase. Other effects include liver toxicity, jaundice, bloating, diarrhea, and memory loss. Most important is the fact that **all statin drugs have been proven to cause cancer in laboratory animals** and may pose the same threat for patients. Thus, experts have recommended that the statin drugs be used only in people with a short life expectancy of 5-10 years. Unbelievably, drug companies are now trying to get children on statin drugs and to double the daily dosage in adults. Baycol was pulled off of the market, due to the harmful side effect of severe rhabdomyolysis, only to be replaced by a bevy of even more powerful statins.

22.3 STATINS AND MEMORY LOSS

In 2004, former astronaut, aerospace medical research scientist, flight surgeon and family doctor, Dr. Duane Graveline, published "Lipitor, Thief of Memory: Statin Drugs and the Misguided War On Cholesterol, Infinity Publishing. In his book, Dr. Graveline tells of his personal experience of total global amnesia secondary to ingestion of statin drugs. He makes a persuasive case for **the bogus demonization of cholesterol by pharmaceutical companies and of attempts to cover up their harmful side effects**. This scenario is **strikingly parallel to the situation with antioxidants**, which I have described in detail. In fact, I believe that it is possible that patients may exacerbate the harmful effects of statins with the concomitant usage of high doses of antioxidants.

The mechanism of action of statin drugs is the inhibition of HMG-CoA reductase and its subsequent reduction of cholesterol synthesis. Please keep in mind that cholesterol plays an essential role in brain metabolism and synaptic formation (Pfrieger, F. Brain Researcher discovers bright side of Ill-famed Molecule. Science, 9 November, 2001). **Cholesterol is the most abundant organic molecule in the brain**. Cholesterol is a synaptogenic factor, which is produced by the glial cells, which are the biochemical sources of cholesterol for the brain. A strong statin drug can wipe out 40% of this cholesterol synthesis and a similar percentage of the vital ubiquinone and dolichols as collateral damage.

Unquestionably, statins reduce cholesterol levels but there is a growing concern among researchers that cholesterol reduction is not leading to significant reductions in cardiovascular disease mortality and an increasing awareness of their harmful effects. Dr. Uffe Ravnskov published his book, The Cholesterol Myth: Exposing the fallacy that cholesterol and saturated fat cause heart disease, New Trends Publishing, Inc. 2000, in which he reported on the PROSPER trial in Lancet. He found that **statistical tricks were used to color the results and to cover up the fact that there was an increase in cancer deaths which offset the slight decrease in deaths from cardiovascular disease**. Ravnskov summarizes that statin drug therapy is reported to be almost as effective for women as for men, despite the fact that most studies have shown that cholesterol is not a risk factor for women. Also, the elderly are protected just as much as younger individuals, although all studies have shown that high cholesterol is only a weak factor for men over 50 years. More and more, **clinical investigators are expressing the notion that an elevated homocysteine level is a strong independent risk factor for the development of arteriosclerotic disease** (Boushey, C.J. et al., A quantitative assessment of plasma homocysteine as a risk factor for vascular disease. JAMA, 1995; 274: 1049-57).

Jay Cohen stated that, "Each time an individual takes a new drug, it is the beginning of an experiment." (Cohen, J.S., The Case Against Drug Companies. Tarcher/Putnam, 2001). One should also read the 2004 book by Harvard Medical School lecturer and editor in chief at the New England Journal of Medicine, Dr. Marcia Angell, "The Truth About the Drug Companies : How They Deceive Us and What to do About It." Dr. Angell points out that drug companies spend 2-3 times as much on marketing as they do on research. Further, she points out that drug companies now sponsor most drug studies and they have the sole authority to decide whether or not to publish negative results or side effects. **Now, the FDA acts as a spokesperson for the drug companies**, instead of a watch dog for the consumer. Obviously, this is a dangerous situation but it is not likely to change in the near future. The pharmaceutical companies have a strong influence over physicians and legislative bodies. Hence, my caveat is to read the PDR carefully, keeping in mind that it may not have full disclosure of harmful effects and to remember that none of these so called "medicines" have a singular activity in the body and in the living/breathing cell.

Dr. Mary Enig, an expert in lipid biochemistry has stated, "The idea that saturated fats cause heart disease is completely wrong, but the statement has been "published" so many times over the last three or more decades that it is very difficult to convince people otherwise unless they are willing to take the time to read and learn what all the economic and political factors were that produced the anti-saturated-fat agenda." Also, Dr. George Mann, prior professor of medicine and biochemistry at Vanderbilt University, stated in a 1977 article in the Journal *Nutrition Today* stated, "The diet-heart idea is the greatest scientific deception of our times…never in the history of science have so many costly experiments failed so consistently." With increasing frequency, we are currently seeing more and more medical transgressions, which have been spawned by the pharmaceutical industry.

23 HYDROGEN PEROXIDE PHYSIOLOGY, BIOCHEMISTRY AND FACTS

23.1 H$_2$O$_2$ FACTS

H$_2$O$_2$ is a naturally occurring substance. Surface water concentrations of H$_2$O$_2$ have been found to vary between 51-231 mg/L, increasing both with exposure to sunlight and the presence of dissolved organic matter (IARC. 1985. International Agency for Research on Cancer. Hydrogen Peroxide. In: IARC Monographs on the Evaluation of Carcinogenic Risk if Chemicals to Humans: Allyl compounds, Aldehydes, Epoxides and Peroxides, Vol. 36. IARC, Lyon, pp. 285-314).

Endogenous hydrogen peroxide has been found in plant tissues at the following levels (mg/kg frozen weight):

> potato tubers, 7.6
> Green tomatoes, 3.5
> Red tomatoes, 3.5
> Castor beans in water, 4.7 (IARC, 1985)

Reportedly, the best way to get H$_2$O$_2$ from your fruits is to use a juicer and drink the juice within 10 minutes before the H$_2$O$_2$ auto-oxidizes such as with carrots. Cranberry juice is said to be loaded with H$_2$O$_2$ as is the tops of beets and watermelon. Uncooked vegetables and fruits contain natural H$_2$O$_2$ and cooking breaks it down. This is likely one of the major factors which responsible for the frequent articles recommending a high intake of fresh fruits and vegetables. **The colostrum of mother's milk is high in H$_2$O$_2$, which is thought to activate the newborn's immune system and protect the undeveloped immune protective system of the baby.** Perhaps this is a corollary to the formation of bactericidal amounts of H$_2$O$_2$ when glucose is oxidized in the presence of penicillium notatum (General Biochemistry, Fruton & Simmonds 577.1 F944 p. 339).

Gaseous H$_2$O$_2$ is recognized to be a key component and product of the earth's lower atmospheric photochemical reactions, in both clean and polluted atmospheres. Under severe smog conditions, daytime levels of H$_2$O$_2$ as high as 0.18 ppm have been reported, but atmospheric night-time levels of 2-5 ppb did not correlate to smog intensity (IARC, 1985). Atmospheric H$_2$O$_2$ is also believed to be generated by gas-phase photochemical reactions in the remote troposphere (IARC, 1985).

23.2 PHARMACOKINETICS

H_2O_2 is a normal product of metabolism. It is readily decomposed by catalase in normal cells. H_2O_2 is normally present in the aqueous humor of the eye and is thought to be a major oxidant in the formation of cataracts. However, the lens exists in an unusual environment. It is an avascular tissue and nutrients are supplied by the aqueous humor which bathes the lens. The aqueous humor contains high concentrations of ascorbic acid (up to 20Xs that of plasma) and relatively high concentrations of H_2O_2. In addition, the lens contains extremely high levels of the intracellular reducing agent, glutathione.

In experimental animals exposed to H_2O_2, target organs affected include the lungs, intestine, thymus, liver and kidney, suggesting its distribution to those sites. In toxicity studies, **using massive doses of H_2O_2**, in rabbits and cats following I.V. doses of H_2O_2, the lungs were pale and emphysematous. Following intraperitoneal injection of H_2O_2 in mice, pyknotic nuclei were induced in the intestine and thymus. Degeneration of hepatic and renal tubular epithelial tissue was observed following oral administration of H_2O_2 to mice (IARC, 1985). **H_2O_2 has been detected in the human breath at levels ranging from 1.0 ug/L to 0.34 ug/L (IARC, 1985), and even in the breath of babies.** H_2O_2 is decomposed in the bowel before absorption (IARC, 1985). **When applied to tissue, solutions of H_2O_2 have poor penetrability** (HSDB. 1995. Hazardous Substances Data Bank. Medlars Online Information Retrieval System, National Library of Medicine).

H_2O_2 is produced metabolically in intact cells and tissues. It is formed by the reduction of O_2 either directly in a two-electron transfer reaction, often catalyzed by lipoproteins, or by an initial one-electron step to O_2 followed by dismutation to H_2O_2 (IARC, 1985). **H_2O_2 has been detected in serum and in intact liver** (IARC, 1985).

H_2O_2 as a human food additive is generally regarded as safe and may be used as a component of articles for use in packaging, handling, transporting or holding food in n accordance with prescribed conditions [FDA 21 CFR 175.105 (4/1/93)].

H_2O_2 has been used on fresh fruits and vegetables for decades. It has been used in dentistry and oral hygiene for decade upon decade. It has been used on wounds for three quarters of a century on millions and millions of wounds. **All of these umpteen examples of H_2O_2 application and ingestion have been essentially without adverse effects.**

23.3 ACUTE TOXICITY

In 5 persons who accidentally drank 50 mL of a 33% H$_2$O$_2$ solution, symptoms included stomach and chest pain, retention of breath, foaming at the mouth and loss of consciousness. Later, motor and sensory disorders, fever, micro hemorrhages and moderate leukocytosis were noted. **All recovered completely within 2-3 weeks** (IARC, 1985). In my opinion, this represents the low toxicity of H$_2$O$_2$ and demonstrates the body's ability to handle excess amounts of H$_2$O$_2$. **Alternative medicine clinics around the world have given thousands upon thousands of I.V. doses of H$_2$O$_2$ without untoward effects** and many have extolled the benefits of H$_2$O$_2$. Dr. Kurt Donsbach and the late Dr. Charles Farr praised the use of H$_2$O$_2$ I.V., even though both received pressure from organized medicine, legal authorities and the pharmaceutical industry not to do so.

A characteristic whitening of the skin occurs after topical application of H$_2$O$_2$ (1-30%), which is believed the result of avascularity of the skin produced by H$_2$O$_2$ acting microembolically in the capillaries (IARC, 1985). H$_2$O$_2$ as a topical gel or a liquid is used to cleanse minor wounds or minor gum inflammation (HSDB, 1995).

Hydrogen peroxide is potentially one of the most beneficial, yet most maligned, substances in medical and scientific history. Again, the literature in this area of science is marked by inconsistency of data, misinterpretation, lies and confusion. However, **I firmly believe that there are extremely important facts discovered by Baylor scientists which have been essentially over-looked (whether purposely or unintentionally) for nearly a half of a century.** This is disturbingly reminiscent of the important work of Dr. William Coley (Coley's toxin), which fell into obscurity for nearly a century.

Basically, hydrogen peroxide (peroxide or H$_2$O$_2$) is a non-radical of rather low reactivity and has a proven record of safety for over a century, especially when compared to modern pharmaceuticals which are responsible for significant numbers of adverse reactions (reportedly, hundreds of thousands annually) and deaths. I realize that **any substance, medicine, substrate, co-factor, nutrient, supplement, mineral chemical or reagent can be harmful,** if administered to a cell, tissue, organ or an organism and if it is in the wrong concentration, location, etc. (too much or too little or in the wrong place at the wrong time). **A damaging case or scenario can be built against any man-made or naturally-occurring substance, if one is allowed to control its amounts, location and timing relative to the cell, tissue or organism being evaluated or considered. I believe that this is one of the main problems with in vitro experimentation.**

23.4 PEROXIDE DISTORTIONS

The following information was excerpted from the **Memorial Sloan-Kettering website** www.mskcc.org and fortunately it contained a disclaimer which stated "Memorial Sloan-Kettering Cancer Center make no warranties nor express or implied representations whatsoever regarding the **accuracy,** completeness, timeliness, comparative or controversial nature, or usefulness of any information contained or referenced on this website. Memorial Sloan-Kettering does not assume any risk whatsoever for your use of this website or the information contained herein. Health-related information changes frequently and therefore information contained on **this website may be outdated, incomplete or incorrect (and I agree with their assessment).**

23.5 CLINICAL SUMMARY

Unproven alternative therapies and products offered over the internet and at clinics in Mexico, the U.S. and Europe. The term "oxygen therapy" refers to any product or treatment based on the false theory that cancer, infections, HIV and degenerative diseases are caused by oxygen deficiency. Such therapies purport to deliver high levels of oxygen to tissues and thereby kill cancer cells, estimate pathogens, stimulate metabolism and produce "oxidative detoxification." They include: **hydrogen peroxide** therapy, involving intravenous infusion, ingestion, colonic administration, or soaking in hydrogen peroxide solution; ozone colonics and ozone autohemotherapy, in which blood is bubbled with ozone and reinjected; hyperbaric oxygen chambers; and "oxygenated" water, pills and solutions. **No scientific evidence supports their marketing claims**; studies show that oxygen neither prevents nor inhibits cancer growth and tumors grow rapidly in tissues that are well supplied with oxygen. Even if "oxygenated" products contain the oxygen levels they claim, oxygen is not likely to be absorbed through the gastrointestinal tract. Ingestion or use of hydrogen peroxide enemas can cause lethal gas embolism and colitis-induced sepsis and gangrene, while its **intravenous injection has led to acute hemolytic crisis and death.** Transmission of blood-borne viruses such as hepatitis C and HIV is reported after treatment with contaminated autohemotherapy devices. Oxygen radicals released by ozone and hydrogen peroxide may be mutagenic. The American Cancer Society urges cancer patients not to seek treatment with hydrogen peroxide, ozone therapy, or other "hyperoxygenation" therapies. Oxygen therapies should not be recommended.

Information from the Hazardous Substances Data Bank (HSDB), a database of the National Library of Medicine's TOXNET system (http://toxnet.nlm.nih.gov) **indicates in general, ingestion, ocular or dermal exposure to small amounts of dilute hydrogen peroxide will cause no serious problems.**

However, in treatment of corneal ulcerations, particularly in herpetic dendritic keratitis, 20% solution has been applied, after local anesthetic, every two hours as a localized cautery to the ulcer, and **has been reported to have had good effect in numerous patients**. In one instance a 10% solution was dropped on one eye of a patient after application of cocaine, and this eye was normal by the next day. (Grant, W.M. Toxicology of the Eye. 3rd ed. Springfield, IL Charles C. Thomas Publisher, 1986: 493). Ocular exposure to household strength (3%) solutions usually requires little more than thorough irrigation, **since serious complications are rare.**

23.6 MUTAGENCITY

Pregnant rats were fed a diet containing up to 10% hydrogen peroxide. Maternal and fetal weights were reduced but no significant malformations were reported. (Shepard, T.H. Catalog of Teratogenic Agents. 5th ed. Baltimore, MD The Johns Hopkins University Press, 1986: 296). **Hydrogen peroxide was mutagenic to Salmonella** typhimurium TA92 and TA102 and was positive in a forward mutation test in Salmonella typhimurium SV50. (IARC. Monographs on the Evaluation of the Carcinogenic Risk of Chemicals to Man. Geneva: World Health Organization, International Agency for Research on Cancer, 1972 - Present. (multicolumn work); p V36 301 (1985)).

The International Agency for Research on Cancer (IARC) has determined that hydrogen **peroxide is not classifiable as to its carcinogencity to humans. Even though accusations against H_2O_2 have been wide spread, there is no verified data, in man, that H_2O_2 in any way causes or promotes cancer in vivo. The WHO-IARC said, "There is inadequate evidence in humans for the carcinogenicity of hydrogen peroxide."**

Again, according to the Memorial Sloan-Kettering website, oxygen therapies are based on the false concept that cancer and other degenerative diseases are caused by oxygen deficiency resulting from air pollution, processed foods, toxin buildup, emotional distress and water fluoridation. Proponents cite Otto Warburg's finding of lower metabolism rates in cancer cells to conclude that cancer cells operate on an anaerobic level and therefore will be selectively destroyed by the oxygen liberated by hydrogen peroxide, ozone, and "oxygenated" products. Laboratory studies show that oxygen neither prevents nor inhibits cancer growth, that tumors grow rapidly in tissues that are well supplied with oxygenated blood, and that the absence of oxygen does not stimulate tumor growth in vitro or in vivo.

This supports my Unified Theory, in that, ground state oxygen is of little reactivity and it requires alterations of its electron structure to be of tumoricidal benefit.

According to Sloan-Kettering, exogenous hydrogen peroxide undergoes an exothermic decomposition reaction upon contact with catalase in human blood, liberating oxygen and water. It shows no antitumor effects at non-lethal concentrations in animal models **RMH Note: This is not true.** Intravenous administration of hydrogen peroxide results in no decrease in Escherichia coli bacteremia in rabbits or free human blood. **RMH Note: This is not true.** Typical intra-arterial administration produces only 2.9 ml of oxygen per 100 ml of blood per minute, an insignificant addition considering that normal adult metabolism requires between 200 and 250 ml of oxygen each. However, **they fail to point out that 2 ml of 3% H_2O_2 can release 20 ml of oxygen micro-bubbles. Hydrogen peroxide has a half-life of 0.75 to 2.0 seconds in human blood. Refer to section 24.0.**

Ozone exhibits broad antiviral activity via peroxidation of phospholipid and lipoproteins in the viral envelope. Although ozone effectively kills HIV in vitro, it does not reduce viral load in human studies. Ozone incubation of free human blood has been recorded to result in immonomodulatory effects, but it is unknown whether these effects occur in vivo. Ozone gas has a half-life of about 40 minutes in dry air at 22° C.

24.0 BAYLOR UNIVERSITY MEDICAL CENTER H_2O_2 RESEARCH

24.0.1 Hydrogen Peroxide Clinical History
(Human and Animal)

RMH Note: I feel that this work is of such significance that I have gone to great lengths to obtain and summarize this most important work. In fact, I have contacted both Dr. Urschel and Dr. Mallams in regard to these experiments.

In the early sixties, Baylor University Medical Center investigators studied five dogs, rats with Walker 256 rat sarcoma and four human patients and found that:

- none of the patients showed adverse clinical effects secondary to intra-arterial hydrogen peroxide
- no adverse local or systemic toxic effects were encountered in animals or humans
- there was no significant imbalance in acid-base or cation-anion equilibrium
- early evidence in these studies would suggest an increased therapeutic ratio in malignant tumors to ionizing irradiation.

(Mallams, J.T., Finney, J.W. and Balla, G.A. The use of hydrogen peroxide as a source of oxygen in a regional intra-arterial infusion system. Southern Med J 1962; 55: 230-232).

Studies by Nathan and Cohn have shown that **hydrogen peroxide contributes to the lysis of tumor cells by macrophages and granulocytes in a variety of experimental conditions.** (Nathan, C.F. and Cohn, Z.A. Antitumor effects of hydrogen peroxide in vivo. J Exp Med 1981; 154: 1539-1553).

Further, they found that glucose oxidase covalently coupled to polystyrene microspheres (GOL), produced H_2O_2 at an average rate of 3.6 nmol/min per 10^9 beads under standard assay conditions. Injection of 1.3×10^{10} to 1.1×10^{11} GOL i.p. prolonged the survival of mice by 27% after injection of 10^6 P388 lymphoma cells in the same site, consistent with **destruction of 97.6% of the tumor cells.** Placing mice for several hours in 100% O_2, the probable rate-limiting substrate for GOL, afforded a 42% prolongation of survival from P388 when the inoculum was 10^5, 10^4, or 10^3 cells, GOL led to long term survival **(presumed cure) of 23%, 77% and 92% of the mice,** respectively, consistent with reduction of the injected tumor dose to <10 cells. Subcutaneous growth of 10^5 P388 cells (~300 lethal dose to 50% of mice) was suppressed in 83% of mice by admixture of GOL with the tumor cell inoculum. GOL alone had no effect against a more peroxide-resistant tumor, P815 . However, P825 cell glutathione reductase could be inhibited in vivo by well-tolerated doses of the antitumor agent. 1,3-bis(2-chloranthy)-1-nitrosourea (BCNU). BCNU alone cured few mice with P815. Together, BCNU and GOL apparently cured 86% of mice injected with 10^6 P815 cells i.p. The protective effect of GOL was abolished by boiling it to inactivate the enzyme, by co-injection of catalase coupled to latex beads, or by delaying the injection of tumor cells for 3 h, by which time the beads had formed aggregates. Soluble glucose oxidase, in doses threefold higher than that bound to GOL, had no detectable antitumor effect. **A single injection of preformed H_2O_2 readily killed 388 cells in the peritoneal cavity,** but only at doses nearly lethal to the mice. In contrast, GOL had very little toxicity, as judged by the normal appearance of the mice for over 400 d, gross and microscopic findings at autopsy, and various blood test. GOL injected i.p. remained in the peritoneal cavity, where it was gradually organized into granulomata by macrophages, without generalized inflammation. **Thus, an H_2O_2-generating system confined to the tumor bed exerted clear-cut antitumor effects with little toxicity to the host.**

24.0.2 Interferon Inducing Activity of H_2O_2

The activated macrophages have a major role in the immune response as regulatory cells which can enhance or suppress immune reactions. (Rosenthal, A.S. Regulation of the immune response - role of the macrophage. N Engl J Med 1980; 303: 1153). With natural killer (NK) cells, the activated macrophages induced by various stimulants, including adjuvants such as bacillus Calmette-Guerin (BCG), Corynebacterium parvum, or polyanions, show dual effects of suppression and augmentation on the activity of NK cells. Also, **these activated macrophages produce oxidative metabolites such as hydrogen peroxide, which is responsible for sterilizing action against microorganisms and cytotoxic activity against tumor cells** (Murray, H.W., Juangbhanich, C.W., Nathan, C.F. and Cohn, Z.A. Macrophage oxygen-dependent anti-microbial activity: The role of oxygen intermediates. J Exp Med 1979; 150: 950), (Nathan, C.F., Silverstein, S.C., Brukner, L.H. and Cohn, Z.A. Extracellular cytolysis by activated macrophages and granulocytes: Hydrogen peroxide as a mediator of cytotoxicity. J Exp Med 1979; 149: 100). Little investigation, however, has been done on the action of hydrogen peroxide against the immune response. Metzger, et al. (Metzger, Z., Hoffeld, J.T. and Oppenheim, J.J. Macrophage-mediated suppression: Evidence for participation of both hydrogen peroxide and prostaglandins in suppression of murine lymphocyte proliferation. J Immunol 1980; 124: 983), demonstrated that macrophage-suppression effects on murine lymphocyte proliferation were mediated by release of hydrogen peroxide. Fisher and Bostick-Bruton (Fisher, R.I. and Bostick-Bruton, F. Depressed T cell proliferative responses in Hodgkin's disease: Role of moncyte-mediated suppression via prostaglandins and hydrogen peroxide. J Immunol 1982; 129: 1770), demonstrated that hydrogen peroxide and prostaglandin produced by activated macrophages, suppressed human T cell proliferation stimulated by phytohemagglutinin (PHA); furthermore, Zoschke and Messner (Zoschke, D.C. and Messner, R. Phagocytic cell-derived hydrogen peroxide and T cell regulation. Clin Res 1982; 30: 544A), reported that exogenous hydrogen peroxide suppressed T cell response stimulated by concanavalin A. **These reports suggest that hydrogen peroxide regulates immune responses.**

24.0.3 Tumoricidal Activity of H_2O_2

Investigators have shown that hydrogen peroxide-generated by TNF-activated PMNs was also cytotoxic and tumoricidal. (Shau, H. Cytostatic and tumoricidal activities of tumor necrosis factor-treated neutrophils. Immunol Lett 1988 17(1): 47-51).

Studies support the internalization and degradation of receptor bound C-reactive protein by U-937 cells (human monocytic cell line**): induction of H_2O_2 production and tumoricidal activity.** (Tebo, J.M. and Mortensen, R.F. Internalization and degradation of receptor bound C-reactive protein by U-937 cells: Induction of H_2O_2 production and tumoricidal activity. Biochem Biophys Acta 1991; 1095(3): 210-216).

Hydrogen peroxide (HP) is routinely used during microsurgical procedures to augment hemostasis after intracranial tissue resection. Elsewhere in the body, HP is used to kill the resection margin of tumor cells; in vitro studies support these clinical uses. Although HP appears to have tumoricidal effects in vitro, it should be used with caution in humans because of risks of collateral injury with **3% H_2O_2** to surrounding normal brain. HP may prove most beneficial for discrete lesions, such as pituitary tumors and metastases. (Mesiwala, A.H., Farrell, L., Santiago, P., Ghatan, S. and Silbergeld, D.L. The effects of hydrogen peroxide on brain and brain tumors. Surg Neurol 2003; 59(5): 398-407).

Mast cells, when supplemented with H_2O_2 and iodide, are cytotoxic to mammalian tumor cells as determined by 51Cr release, and transmission and scanning electron microscopy. H_2O_2 at the concentration employed (10(-4)M) initiates mast cell degranulation, and mast cell granules (MCG), which contain a small amount of endogenous peroxidase activity, are toxic to tumor cells when combined with H_2O_2 and iodide. This toxicity is greatly increased by binding eosinophil peroxidase (EPO) to MCG surface. These reactions may play a role in the host defense against neoplasms. (Henderson, W.R., Chi, E.Y., Jong, E.C. and Klebanoff, S.J. Mast cell-mediated tumor-cell cytotoxicity. Role of the peroxidase system. J Exp Med 1981; 153(3): 520-533).

Several anti-cancer drugs are known to bring about their tumoricidal actions by a free radical dependent mechanism. A majority of the studies reported that adriamycin, mitocmycin C, etc., augment free radical generation and lipid peroxidation process in vitro. Our results reported here suggest that following chemotherapy both stimulated and unstimulated human polymorphonuclear leukocytes generate increased amounts of **superoxide anion and hydrogen peroxide.** This was accompanied by increased formation of lipid peroxidation products as measured by thiobarbituric acid assay. **These results confirm that many anti-cancer drugs augment free radical generation and lipid peroxidation even in an vivo situation.** (Sangeetha, P., Das, U.N., Koratkar, R. and Suryaprabha, P. Increase in free radical generation and lipid peroxidation following chemotherapy in patients with cancer. Free Radic Biol Med 1990; 8(1): 15-19).

Ascorbic acid, when given at sufficiently high dosages, has demonstrated preferential cytotoxicity to tumor cells in vitro and in vivo. Levels required to be cytotoxic in vivo to tumor cells are not attainable via oral administration. Cytotoxic effect requires intravenous administration of 50 Gms or more and is likely due to its pro-oxidant activity at these levels.

It is hypothesized **that ascorbic acid exhibits cytotoxic activity via a prooxidant effect. There is a 10 to 100 fold greater content of catalase in normal cells than in tumor cells.** Due to this, **cancer cells reach high levels of intracellular hydrogen peroxide leading to their destruction, while normal cells are protected.** (Matsuda, T., Kuroyanagi, M., Sugiyama, S., Umehara, K., Ueno, A. and Nishi, K. Role of hydrogen peroxide for cell death induction by sodium 5,6-Benzylidene-L-ascorbate. Chem Pharm Bull 1994; 6: 1216-1225), (Mizuno, M., Minato, K., Ito, H., Kawade, M., Terai, H. and Tsuchida, H. Anti-tumor polysaccharide from the mycelium of liquid-cultured Agaricus Blazel Mill. Biochem Mol Biol Int 1999; 47: 707-714).

Studies support the point that antioxidants (including flavonoids and other phenolics) can induce oxidative stress in cancer cells and that some or many of their effects seen in vitro may be due to induction of such stress. Beta carotene at levels just above those seen in human plasma **was shown to induce apoptosis in human adenocarcinoma cells in vitro via a free radical-mediated mechanism.** Vitamin C was cytotoxic to several cell lines in vitro, **again due to free radical generation.** These papers highlight the need to consider redox effects when discussing the in vitro actions of antioxidant compounds. (Halliwell, B., Clement, M.V., Ramalingam, J. and Long, L.H. Hydrogen peroxide: ubiquitous in cell culture and in vivo? IUBMB Life 2000; 50(4-5): 251-257), (Palozza, P. Calviello, G., Serini, S., et al. Beta carotene at high concentrations induces apoptosis by enhancing oxy radical production in human adenocarcinoma cells. Free Radic Biol Med 2001; 1,30(9): 1000-1007), (Clement, M.V., Ramalingam, J., Long, L.H. and Halliwell, B. **The in vitro cytotoxicity of ascorbate depends on the culture medium used to perform the assay and involves hydrogen peroxide.** Antioxid Redox Signal 2001; 3(1): 157-163).

Of particular interest was the finding that **liposome-encapsulated glucose oxidase, a H_2O_2-generating compound, eradicated 46% of IL-5-transected tumors.** (Samoszuk, M.K., Wimley, W.C. and Nguyen, V. Eradication of Interleukins-5 transfected J558L plasmacytomas in mice by hydrogen peroxide-generating stealth liposomes. Cancer Res 1996; 56: 87-90). **This suggest that EPO from eosinophils and locally produced H_2O_2 might cooperate to damage tumors under some conditions.** Because eosinophil-stimulated macrophages can be a source of H_2O_2 and eosinophils and macrophages are both abundant during localized production of IL-4 by tumor cells, it is interesting to speculate that macrophage-eosinophil interplay induces tumor cell cytotoxicity through the production of these molecules.

Various investigators have studied the value of H_2O_2 and shrinking the size of tumors (Aronoff, B.L., et al. Cancer 1965; 18: 1250), and have studied treatment advantages and **increased tumor cytotoxicity by the use of regional H_2O_2 infusion.** (Mallams, J.T., Balla, G.A. and Finney, J.W. Regional oxygenation and irradiation in the treatment of malignant tumors. Prog in Clin Cancer 1965; 1: 137).

Polymorphonuclear leukocytes (PMN) of mice can destroy tumor cells effectively in vitro in the presence of antitumor polysaccharide, linear beta-1, 3-D-glucan from Alcaligenes faecalis var, myxogenes IFO 13140 (TAK), and some other immonomodulators. **Hydrogen peroxide is important for these cytotoxicities** whereas, unlike the results with TAK, **the H$_2$O$_2$: halide:myeloperoxidase system may partly participate in the cytotoxicity with some immunomodulators**. (Morikawa, K., Kamegaya, S., Yamazaki, M. and Mizuno, D. Hydrogen peroxide as a tumoricidal mediator of murine polymorphonuclear leukocytes induced by a linear beta-1,3-D-glucan and some other immonomodulators. Cancer Res 1985; 45(8): 3482-3486).

It was found that the (Nitric Oxide) NO-mediated loss of cell viability was dependent on both NO and hydrogen peroxide (H$_2$O$_2$). Somewhat surprisingly, superoxide (O$_2$.-) and its reaction product with NO, peroxynitrite (-OONO), did not appear to be directly involved in the observed NO-mediated cytotoxicity against this cancer cell line. A recent report utilizing NO donor compounds indicated that **NO was particularly tumoricidal in the presence of hydrogen peroxide (H$_2$O$_2$) and not O$_2$.-.** There is evidence confirming the original observations of Ioannidis and de Groot (Ioannidis, I. And de Grott, H. Cytotoxicity of nitric oxide in Fu5 rat hepatoma cells: evidence for cooperative action with hydrogen peroxide. Biochem J 1993; 296(Pt2): 341-345), indicating **that the combination of NO and H$_2$O$_2$ was particularly cytotoxic to a human ovarian cancer cell line.** (Farias-Eisner, R., Chaudhuri, G., Aeberhard, E. and Fukuto, J.M. The chemistry and tumoricidal activity of nitric oxide/hydrogen peroxide and the implications to cell resistance/susceptibility. J Biol Chem 1996; 271(11): 6144-6151).

Studies demonstrate that **a combination of sub-lytic concentrations of chemically generated NO and H$_2$O$_2$ leads to death of murine lymphoma cells, in part, via induction of apoptosi**s. (Filep, J.G., Lapierre, C., Lachance, S. and Chan, J.S.D. Nitric oxide cooperates with hydrogen peroxide in inducing DNA fragmentation and cell lysis in murine lymphoma cells. Biochem J 1997; 321: 887-901). In vitro studies have suggested that a reaction of **NO gas and H$_2$O$_2$ produces singlet oxygen or hydroxyl radicals**. (Kanner, J., Harel, S. and Granit, R. Arch Biochem Biophys 1991; 289: 130-136), (Noronha-Dutra, A.A., Epperlein, M.M. and Woolf, N. FEBS Lett 1993; 321: 59-62). Nevertheless, this has not yet been demonstrated in cell cultures.

24.1 HYDROGEN PEROXIDE AND ARTERIOSCLEROSIS

I ascribe such importance to the Baylor group that I have included their references, at times, in a replicative manner because I do not want any reader of this tome to miss them.

24.2 INTRA-ARTERIAL H$_2$O$_2$ REGIONAL OXYGENATION

The intra-arterial infusion of hydrogen peroxide has been employed by Baylor University investigators as a method of regional oxygenation in the management of a variety of diseases (Urschel, H.C., Jr., Finney, J.W., Balla, G.A. and Mallams, J.T. Regional oxygenation of the ischemic myocardium with hydrogen peroxide. Surgical Forum, Amer Coll of Surg Cling Congress XV 1964; 273), (Urschel, H.C., Jr., Finney, J.W., Morales, A.R., Balla, G.A., Race, G.J. and Mallams, J.T. Cardiac resuscitation with hydrogen peroxide. Ann of Thorac Surg 1966; 2: 665), (Urschel, H.C., Jr., Finney, J.W., Balla, G.A., Race, G.J. and Mallams, J.T. Effects of hydrogen peroxide on the cardiovascular system. Proc Third Intl Conf on Hyperbaric Med 1966; 307), (Finney, J.W., Balla, G.A., Jay, B.E., Race, G.J., Urschel, H.C., Jr., Greenlee, R.G. and Mallams, J.T. Removal of cholesterol and other lipids from human athermanous arteries by dilute hydrogen peroxide. Angiology 1966; 17: 233), (Finney, J.W., Urschel, H.C., Jr., Balla, G.A., Race, G.J. and Mallams, J.T,. Protection of the ischemic heart with DMSO alone or in combination with hydrogen peroxide oxide. Ann of the NY Acad Sci 1967; 151: 231-241), (Balla, G.A., Finney, J.W., Aronoff, B.L., Byrd, D.L., Race, G.J., Mallams, J.T. and Davis, G. Use of intra-arterial hydrogen peroxide to promote wound healing. I. Regional intra-arterial therapy - technical surgical aspects. II. Wound healing - clinical aspects. Amer J surg 1964; 108: 621), (Finney, J.W., Collier, R.E., Balla, G.A., Tomme, J.W., Wakely, J., Race, G.J., Urschel, H.C., D'Errico, A.D. and Mallams, J.T. The preferential localization of radioisotopes in malignant tissue by regional oxygenation. Nature 1964; 202: 1172). In some **patients so treated with hydrogen peroxide, a decrease in the severity of their atherosclerosis was observed**. This phenomenon was studied and confirmed by both in vitro and in vivo experimentation. (Finney, J.W., Jay, B.E., Race, G.J., Urschel, H.C., Mallams, J.T. and Balla, G.A. Removal of cholesterol and other lipids from experimental animal and human athermanous arteries by dilute hydrogen peroxide. Angiology 1966; 17: 223).

Several patients who have been infused intra-arterially with hydrogen peroxide as an adjunct to irradiation therapy in the management of their malignant disease have undergone postmortem examination. In all cases studied to date, the patients received hydrogen peroxide infusion through a retrograde catheter in the abdominal aorta as an adjunct to irradiation therapy over periods of time ranging from 4 - 16 weeks. During this time, **the individuals were given daily infusions of 250 ml of hydrogen peroxide in "Ionosol-T" with a peroxide concentration ranging from 0.24% to 0.48%.**

Upon gross examination, **the segment of the aorta being infused with hydrogen peroxide was found to be different from the area not being infused. This difference was marked by a decrease in the number and severity of atheromatous plaques and an increase in flexibility and elasticity of the vessel.** Ordinarily one expects to find an increase in number and severity of the athermatous lesions from the thoracic to the abdominal aorta. In these patients, **where the H$_2$O$_2$ infusion catheter was in the abdominal aorta below the renal arteries, there was lack of raised lesions from the point of the catheter to the bifurcation, and the iliacs were relatively free of gross disease except from some intimal and subintimal fibrosis.** In my opinion, this observation is of most importance since it is both dramatic and in humans.

Histologic evaluation of Oil Red O stained sections showed a decrease in total subliminal lipid deposits in the aorta below as compared to that above the H$_2$O$_2$ infusion catheter tip. When weighed samples of the vessels were extracted and total lipids determined, it was found that approximately a 50% reduction in total lipids (10 - 40% decrease in cholesterol and 20 - 50% decrease in cholesterol esters) had

occurred in the area being infused with hydrogen peroxide. This data further emphasizes the importance of this research data. Obviously, H_2O_2 has unique clinical importance in the treatment of arteriosclerosis that has thus far been over-looked or ignored.

In vitro studies confirmed the elution of lipid from human atheromatous aortas when incubated with either hydrogen peroxide or saline under high oxygen tension.

Serum lipid studies were conducted in various patients being infused intra-arterially with hydrogen peroxide. Venous blood samples were collected from the cubital vein immediately before and after the infusions with a total time lapse between the two sample of 20 - 30 minutes. **It was noted that the total increase in circulating lipids following the intra-arterial infusion of H_2O_2 seemed to be directly proportional to both the severity of disease and concentration of hydrogen peroxide infused.**

Routine blood work was done on alternate days; this included complete blood count (CBC) and platelet and reticulocyte counts. They demonstrated elevation in all the formed elements as noted previously when the carotid arteries have been infused by hydrogen peroxide.

Although the early clinical improvement was slight and the changes subtle, it can be stated that the patient was in no way clinically worse and it not demonstrate progression of the patient's symptoms which were marked prior to H_2O_2 infusion. **Apparent diminution of the vertebral artery stenosis and less delay in filling time of the vertebral compared to the carotid artery were observed.** This occurred with the severest limitations for infusion which probably will be encountered. These included minimal blood flow past a severe stenosis in a small vessel system which has a higher susceptibility to spasm and with the catheter a moderate distance from the lesion.

24.2.1 Human Studies

Human Studies: (Finney, J.W., George, M.S., Balla, A, Race, G.J. and Mallams, J.T. Peripheral blood changes in humans and experimental animals following the infusion of hydrogen peroxide into the carotid artery. Angiology 1965; 16: 62). In the human series studied (137 patients), the catheter varied in size and location, depending upon the tumor site. To March 1, 1964, 33 patients have been treated for malignant tumors of the head and neck, 13 of whom had the catheter placed in either the **common or internal carotid artery.** In the other 20, the catheter was placed into **the external carotid** via either the superficial temporal or superior thyroid artery. For the most part, the remaining 104 patients have been **treated for malignancies involving the liver, bladder, ovary, pancreas, endometrium, colon or cervix, with the catheters passed retrograde through the femoral artery to the appropriate level in the aorta.** This clinical approach should be used with the Howes Singlet Oxygen Delivery System, albeit with appropriate caution.

24.2.2 Animal Studies

Animal Studies. The animals infused with 10.0 ml of 0.12% hydrogen peroxide in "Ionosol-T" into the right common carotid artery showed an increase in circulating platelets within the first 24 hour period. The time of maximum response was between 24 to 72 hours; maximum counts varied from 600,000 to 900,000 platelets with an average preinfusion count between 200,000 to 300,000. The counts generally returned to approximately the preinfusion levels between the fifth and eighth day.

An increase in circulating platelets and reticulocytes has been observed in rabbits following the infusion of hydrogen peroxide in "Ionosol-T" into the common carotid artery.

An increase in one or more of the formed elements in the peripheral circulation (Platelets, reticulocytes, or white blood cells) has been noted in 11 of 13 patients being infused with a solution **of hydrogen peroxide into either the internal or common carotid artery.** In one of 20 patients being infused into the external carotid, and two of the 104 patients being infused into the aorta, **a significant increase in platelet levels was measured.** As of March 1964, **the Baylor group had studied 137 patients under the H_2O_2 infusion protocol and 33**

had been treated for head and neck malignancies, 13 of whom had H$_2$O$_2$ infused into the common internal carotid artery. In 11 of the 13 cases, a marked change in the peripheral blood picture was observed and 2 of the other 104 patients demonstrated a significant change in peripheral blood, both of which were being treated for carcinoma of the bladder.

24.3 H₂O₂ CARDIAC RESUSCITATION

The following information was excerpted from a paper by Urschel et al., (Urschel, H.C., Jr., Morales, A.R., Finney, J.W., Balla, G.A., Race, G.J. and Mallams, J.T. **Cardiac Resuscitation with Hydrogen Peroxide**. 1966; 2(5): 665-682).

Many clinical cardiac arrhythmias or situations of cardiac arrest are associated either primarily or secondarily with local or systemic hypoxia and anoxia. In addition to standard methods of cardiac resuscitation, hyperbaric oxygenation (OHP) has been employed both experimentally and clinically to improve myocardial oxygenation in these situation. Due to the technical and physiological problems inherent with OHP, studies were undertaken in Baylor University Medical Center laboratory to determine the feasibility of administering intravascular oxygen in a regional or systemic system. This approach employees dilute concentrations of hydrogen peroxide given by a variety of routes to provide oxygen. Hydrogen peroxide under the influence of catalase and peroxidases is degraded to oxygen and water. Human blood and tissues contain excess quantities of both enzyme systems. **Hydrogen peroxide provides from 3 to 8 atmosphere equivalents of oxygen which is administered in solution**, thus avoiding the necessity of lung transport. Therapy can be provided regionally, avoiding the pulmonary and CNS toxicity problems of hyperbaric chambers. It can be given continuously over long periods of time by a single physician without expensive equipment and large teams, and also avoids the compression-decompression hazards of OHP.

Many clinical and experimental applications of hydrogen peroxide have been demonstrated. In over 300 patients regional intra-arterial hydrogen peroxide has potentiated the effect of radiation therapy in situations of malignancy involving the head, neck, pelvis and retro-peritoneum (Mallams, J.T., Balla, G.A. and Finney, J.W. Regional oxygenation and irradiation in the treatment of malignant tumors. Prog Clin Cancer 1965; 1: 137). **Increased localization of radioactive isotopes in malignant tumors has been achieved by regional and intra-arterial infusion of hydrogen peroxide** (Finney, J.W., Collier, R.E., Balla, G.A., Tomme, J.W., Wakley, J., Race, G.J., Urschel, H.C., D'Errico, A.D. and Mallams, J.T. The preferential localization of radioisotopes in malignant tissue by regional oxygenation. Nature 1961; 202: 1172) (Finney, J.W., Balla, G.A., Collier, R.E., Wakely, J., Urschel, H.C. and Mallams, J.T. Differential localization of isotopes in tumors through the use of intra-arterial hydrogen peroxide: Part I: Basic science. Amer J Roentgen 1965; 94: 783). **Peripheral bone marrow stimulation has been obtained by carotid artery infusion of hydrogen peroxide experimentally and clinically.** (Finney, J.W., Balla, G.A., Mallams, J.T. and Race, G.J. Peripheral blood changes in humans and experimental animals following the infusion of hydrogen peroxide into the internal carotid artery. Angiology 1965; 16: 62). **Wound healing has been markedly accelerated by the intra-arterial administration of hydrogen peroxide** (Balla, G.A., Finney, J.W., Aronoff, B.L., Byrd, D.L., Race, G.J., Mallams, J.T. and Davis, G. Use of intra-arterial hydrogen peroxide to promote wound healing: Part I: Regional intra-arterial therapy - technical surgical aspects. Part II: wound healing - clinical aspects. Amer J Surg 1964; 108: 621). **Significant reduction in the morbidity and mortality of experimental and clinical Clostridium welchii infections has been achieved by intra-arterial hydrogen peroxide** (Bradley, B.E., Jr., Vedros, N.A., Defalco, A.J., Lawson, D.W., Vineyard, G.C. and Urschel, H.C. The effect of intra-arterial hydrogen peroxide in rabbits infected with clostridum perfringens. J Trauma 1965; 6: 799). **Arteriosclerotic plaques have been markedly reduced and have even disappeared following the intra-arterial infusion of hydrogen peroxide** (Finney, J.W., Balla, G.A., Jay, B.E., Race, G.J., Urschel, H.C., Greenlee, R.G. and Mallams, J.T. Removal of cholesterol and other lipids from human atheromatous arteries by dilute hydrogen peroxide. Angiology 1966; 17: 223). **The reversal of many**

types of shock has been achieved by infusion of hydrogen peroxide into the thoracic aorta (Urschel, H.C., Jr., Finney, J.W., Morales, A.R., Balla, G.A., Mallams, J.T. and Race, G.J. Myocardial protection during aortic cross clamping with hydrogen peroxide [Abstract], Circulation 1964; 30: 172), (Urschel, H.C., Jr., Finney, J.W., Balla, G.A., Race, G.J. and Mallams, J.T. Effects of hydrogen peroxide on the cardiovascular system. In Proceedings of the Third International Conference of Hyperbaric Medicine; 1965).

The time required to remove all hydrogen peroxide from the blood system when one-sixth of the total volume is 0.5% hydrogen peroxide is less than 0.1 second in human blood and 0.2 second in rabbit blood. This total peroxide volume would not be encountered under in vivo conditions; therefore, the life of the peroxide molecule in the vascular system would be considerably shorter than this.

It has also been shown that **the time of maximum oxygen concentration in a dilute blood system was at a point immediately following the complete disappearance of hydrogen peroxide from the solution.**

Elevated oxygen tensions have been observed during the intra-arterial infusion of hydrogen peroxide under a variety of experimental conditions in both animals and humans. In animals being infused into the thoracic aorta, samples collected from the femoral artery revealed a total oxygen content equivalent to 4 to 6 atmospheres of pressure. In humans who were being infused into the thoracic aorta, blood samples were collected from the femoral artery and showed an oxygen content equivalent from 2 to 4 atmospheres of pure oxygen.

It has been repeatedly observed that high concentrations of oxygen are present on both the arterial and venous side of a regional system being infused with dilute hydrogen peroxide solutions. The rate of the diffusion and final concentration in a given tissue will ultimately govern the degree to which the peroxide will exert its beneficial effect.

Studies indicate that exogenously generated superoxide anion by xanthine/xanthine oxidase reaction is spontaneously converted to H_2O_2, **which dilates human coronary arteries through vascular smooth muscle hyperpolarization.** Superoxide is converted to H_2O_2 likely by superoxide dismutase within vascular cells and dilates human coronary arterioles through a different pathway involving the activation of guanylate cyclase. These findings suggest that exogenously and endogenously produced H_2O_2 may elicit vasodilation by different mechanisms (Sato, A., Sakuma, I. and Gutterman, D.D. mechanism of dilation of reactive oxygen species in human coronary arterioles. Am J Physiol, 2003, 285: H2345-H2354).

24.4 DIRECT MYOCARDIAL PO$_2$ MEASUREMENTS

The myocardial tissue oxygen tension was measured during (1) the intra-arterial infusion of hydrogen peroxide into the coronary arteries, and (2) the direct application of hydrogen peroxide to the epicardium. Using 5-pound giant New Zealand rabbits, a catheter was passed retrograde from the right carotid artery to the coronary ostia.

24.5 OXYGENATION OF THE ISCHEMIC OR ANOXIC MYOCARDIUM OF SMALL ANIMALS

24.6 TRACHEAL OCCLUSION

Employing 5- to 7-pound giant New Zealand rabbits, the myocardium was rendered anoxic by tracheal cross-clamp. These animals were divided into three groups of 10 each: (1) hydrogen peroxide infused into the coronary arteries, (2) hydrogen peroxide perfused intrapericardially, and (3) the carrier solutions administered in each of the 2 routes without hydrogen peroxide, this group serving as controls. In all animals, the arterial blood pressure, pH, and electrocardiogram were monitored, and solutions were normothermic.

In the first group, tracheotomies were performed and the animals were intubated and placed on the Byrd respirator breathing 100% oxygen for 15 minutes. A small No. 90 polyethylene catheter was inserted into the right common carotid artery and passed retrograde to the coronary ostia. **The trachea was cross-clamped, and hydrogen peroxide from 0.06% to 0.48% in Ionosol-T solution was infused through the carotid catheter into the coronary ostia. Blood pressure reached 0 in an average of 15 minutes and the pH dropped to 7 in an average of 9.5 minutes. In these animals, neither nodal block nor cardiac arrest was observed during the 120-minute period of monitoring.** Occasionally, reversible evidences of ischemia appeared in the electrocardiogram.

In the second group, tracheotomies were performed and the animals were intubated and placed on the Byrd respirator breathing 100% oxygen. The left chest was opened and two No. 5 French catheters were inserted and sutured into the pericardium. The pericardium and chest were closed and the animals were taken off the respirator for 30 minutes prior to the tracheal occlusion. Following cross-clamping of the trachea, **the pericardium was perfused in a closed system with 0.06% to 0.48% hydrogen peroxide in Ionosol-T solution. Blood pressure fell to 0 in an average of 12.5 minutes and pH reached 7.0 only after a prolonged period of time. In these animals neither nodal block nor cardiac arrest was observed during the 120 minutes of monitoring.**

The third group of control rabbits were equally divided, each half being treated as one of the previously treated groups except that only **the carrier solution without hydrogen peroxide was administered.** In both groups of control rabbit's the blood pressure dropped to 0 in an average of 8 minutes and the pH to 7.0 in an average of 6 minutes. **In all control animals, ischemic changes in the electrocardiograms, as noted by nodal block or arrhythmias, appeared in an average of cardiac arrest was 13 minutes, the range being from 10 to 16 minutes. All animals developed cardiac arrest and following failure to standard resuscitative methods, most of them could be resuscitated by simply adding hydrogen peroxide to the heart by whichever route of carrier solution administration was being employed.**

In 10 rabbits, a catheter was inserted retrograde through the right carotid artery into the base of the aorta. The left chest was opened, the pericardium opened and a variety of coronary arteries were ligated, including the circumflex, the anterior descending, the right coronary, or a combination of these. **Dilute hydrogen peroxide in concentrations ranging from 0.06% to 0.72% was infused retrograde into the coronary arteries by a slow drip at the time of ligation.** Ionosol-T was used as the carrier solution. **Specific cardiographic abnormalities, associated myocardial ischemia such as S-T segment elevation, elevation or depression of the T-wave, nodal block and ventricular tachycardia or fibrillation could readily be reversed and often repeatedly so in a given animal by application of the peroxide. A drop in blood pressure associated with cardiac arrhythmias could also be reversed with similar therapy,** but less consistently.

In another group of 10 animals, the left chest was opened, the pericardium was incised and a similar group of coronary arteries and branches were ligated. Ventricular fibrillation usually followed in several minutes. **After cardiac massage, which was carried on for 15 minutes with no reversal of fibrillation, hydrogen peroxide in concentrations from 0.06% - 0.72% in Ionosol-T carrier solution at normal temperature was added directly to the epicardium. Reversal of arythmia to regular sinus rhythm in 7 to 10 animals was accomplished. Blood pressure was frequently reversed simultaneously.**

Ligation of the right coronary artery with 50% of the anterior descending vessel produced the most consistent ischemic lesion.

Two groups of 10 pigs each were studied, one group to evaluate the effect of hydrogen peroxide during coronary artery ligation and the other to serve as the control. The animals were anesthetized with intravenous Pentothal and curare. Tracheotomies were performed and the pigs were placed on a Byrd respirator with 100% oxygen. In the first group a sternal-splitting incision and pericardiotomy were carried out. Arterial cannulas were placed in the left femoral artery and vein for monitoring venous and arterial blood pressure. The electrocardiogram was constantly monitored, as was the tissue oxygen tension of the myocardium, by a IL-125 electrode inserted into the left ventricular myocardium. **Two plastic No. 190 polyethylene catheters were sutured into the pericardium,** the inflow over the apex and the outflow near the atria interiorly. The apical catheter was attached to a Harvard constant infusion pump and a steady flow of Hank's solution with **0.06% hydrogen peroxide at 37°C was constantly infused at the rate of approximately 400 cc per hour.** Following the placement of the cannulas, the right coronary artery was ligated 1 cm from the ostia and the anterior descending coronary artery was ligated at a point 50% of its length on the anterior part of the heart. The homozygous vein was ligated. The pericardium was closed tightly and the infusion began following the ligation of the vessels. The apical catheter served as an outflow.

The second group of 10 pigs were treated identically, with the exception that only Hank's solution **without hydrogen peroxide was employed for the pericardial perfusion.**

In 10 control animals ventricular fibrillation occurred between 2 and 32 minutes in all but 1 animal, with **an average time of 12 minutes.** In 7 animals resuscitation was successful employing cardiac massage and defibrillation. Two animals could not be resuscitated. Following the return of regular sinus rhythm, mean blood pressure remained less than the control value of 100 mm Hg in all but 3 animals, the average being from 30 to 70 mm Hg mean arterial blood pressure. These animals developed ventricular fibrillation many times and could be resuscitated until their death; however, they never maintained a normal arterial blood pressure, in 2 animals, which developed ventricular fibrillation and in 1 animal which did not, mean arterial blood pressure returned to 100 mm Hg. One of these animals survived for two hours before fibrillating and expiring. The other 2 animals continued for three hours and were sacrificed. The length of survival was from 2 minutes to two hours, with the average being 20 minutes, excluding 2 animals that remained alive and were sacrificed.

Comparison of Control and H_2O_2 Treated Pigs after Coronary Artery Ligation

	Control*	H_2O_2 Treated
Incidence of ventricular fibrillation	9 of 10	5 of 10
Average onset time of ventricular fibrillation	12 min	20 min
Reversibility of ventricular fibrillation	7 of 9	10
Average number of shocks to reverse ventricular fibrillation	5	1 to 2
Normal mean arterial blood pressure	4 of 10	9 of 10
Myocardial tissue oxygen Tension	Less than control	Normal or greater than control

*Received carrier solution only.

In animals treated with 0.06% hydrogen peroxide in Hank's solution, ventricular fibrillation occurred in only one-half of the animals between 5 and 30 minutes, with an **average time of 20 minutes. Five animals never developed ventricular fibrillation. All of those which did were easily resuscitable with cardiac massage and electrical defibrillation. All except 1 maintained normal blood pressures with a mean of 100 mm Hg. Nine H$_2$O$_2$-treated animals lived 3 hours and were sacrificed.** One animal with an average blood pressure of 75 mm Hg died 2 hours after coronary artery ligation.

In all the animals used as controls, following a terminal episode when no blood pressure or cardiac activity could be obtained with the standard methods of resuscitation, dilute solutions of hydrogen peroxide were added to the myocardium. In 4 animals resuscitation could be obtained in spite of massive infarctions and systemic acidosis. No toxicity was demonstrated during the period of therapy.

24.7 HUMAN OBSERVATIONS

Because of the apparent advantages in myocardial support during situations of anoxia, hydrogen peroxide was employed in a 60-year old white female. She developed vascular collapse of unknown etiology and was unresponsive to the conventional methods of resuscitation. A cardiac catheter was passed through the right brachial artery to the root of the aorta. Electrocardiogram and blood pressure were monitored. **Within 1 minute after the infusion of 0.12% hydrogen peroxide, the electrocardiogram reverted from a nodal rhythm to a regular sinus rhythm, and the mean arterial pressure increased 35 to 70 mm Hg within 3 minutes.** In 10 minutes after cessation of the infusion, the electrocardiogram again reverted to nodal rhythm and the blood pressure dropped. This sequence of events was carried out six times during the course of one evening. Each time the reversal of the electrocardiographic abnormalities and hypotension was achieved with hydrogen peroxide.

24.8 POTENTIATION OF THE H$_2$O$_2$ EFFECT ON THE ISCHEMIC MYOCARDIUM BY DMSO

Because of the limitation of diffusion in the thick ventricle and because of the effect of vasoconstriction when oxygen is given intra-arterially, the possible advantage of combining peroxide with an agent such as **dimethyl sulfoxide, which both increases diffusion and in dilute solution acts as a vasodilator.**

The pilot experiments simply showed 0.06% hydrogen peroxide was adequate in maintaining the rabbit myocardium, but a smaller percent could be used in combination with dimethyl sulfoxide to achieve almost the same myocardial protection,. **Dimethyl sulfoxides alone was not adequate to maintain the ischemic myocardium.**

As was the case with peritoneal perfusion, the oxygen content of the portal vein blood approximated that of 100% saturated arterial blood. No attempt has been made to date to adjust carbon dioxide content by this procedure.

24.9 VENTILATION OF RABBITS WITH A H$_2$O$_2$ AEROSOL

In these studies, rabbits were anesthetized with pentobarbital sodium, intubated and placed on 100% oxygen on a Byrd respirator. The chest was opened between the fourth and fifth intercostals space. The pericardium was slit and a flanged PE-90 catheter was secured into the left atrium by a purse-string suture. The chest was closed and the animal was allowed to breath 100% oxygen for 30 minutes prior to the aerosol. **Concentrations of hydrogen peroxide from 1% to 6% in normal saline were nebulized as an aerosol. Following nebulization therapy, the left atrial blood of these animals was found to be "supersaturated" with oxygen, containing quantities equivalent to that expected with oxygen at 3 atmospheres absolute pressure.** If this value were exceeded, small bubbles began to appear in the samples collected. **The 1% aerosol, which was least irritating, provided as good arterial oxygen concentration as did the higher concentrations.**

Although this report is involved predominantly with pilot data, certain observations warrant comment. Dilute solutions of hydrogen peroxide provide a supersaturation of oxygen in plasma and tissue fluids equivalent to from 2 to 12 atmospheres.

In the concentrations and rates of application employed in these experiments, no evidence of intravascular emboli or capillary obstruction have been noted, nor has oxidation of tissue been a problem. It is necessary to employ vasodilators with the intra-arterial use of hydrogen peroxide, since arterial spasm is produced by this method.

Both peritoneal and rectal perfusion of hydrogen peroxide provide high concentrations of oxygen in the portal vein and inferior vena cava. If the lungs are intact, this oxygen is promptly lost in one passage through the pulmonary circulation.

Long-term toxicity studies employing hydrogen peroxide intravascular or by direct application to organs on twenty four hours of constant therapy do not demonstrate significant changes in rabbits followed for two months.

24.10 DIMETHYL SULFOXIDE APPEARS TO ENHANCE THE DIFFUSION OF OXYGEN THROUGH TISSUE

Dr. Hugh E. Stephenson, Jr., (Columbia, MO): There is little question but that hydrogen peroxide can oxygenate the myocardium and the blood in the coronary arteries when applied directly to these structures. **I think Dr. Urschel and his group are especially to be congratulated for pursuing this subject in view of earlier pessimism expressed by previous reports on hydrogen peroxide.** For example, there is the German pharmacologist, Richter's report, in 1941 on an irreversible myocardial effect produced by hydrogen peroxide. There is the 35-year old patient reported by Sellers and Lillehei four years ago who developed a cardiac arrest following the direct application of hydrogen peroxide. These authors worried about the cell membrane integrity and the adverse enzymatic activity and denaturation of protein by hydrogen peroxide.

Other complications such as hemiplegia following irrigation of the chest with hydrogen peroxide and gas embolism following hydrogen peroxide enemas sometimes caused the heart to stop in systole. In spite of these reports, **Dr. Urschel and his group have shown that hydrogen peroxide can be a definite adjunct in our armamentarium for cardiac resuscitation, if used properly.** I think it is important to emphasize the decimal point when using hydrogen peroxide, because accuracy of concentration is of great importance.

The pro-oxidant effect of H_2O_2 can be dramatically effected by its concentration.

Again, **Dr. Urschel and his group are to be commended for showing us how to effectively use hydrogen peroxide in resuscitation.**

24.11 H₂O₂ ELUTION OF CHOLESTEROL AND LIPIDS FROM HUMAN ATHEROMA

The following material was excerpted or modified from: Finney, J.W., Jay, B.E., Race, G.J., Urschel, H.C., Mallams, J.T. and Balla, G.A. **Removal of cholesterol and other lipids from experimental animal and human atheromatous arteries by dilute hydrogen peroxide**. Angiology 1966; 17: 223-228.

Hydrogen peroxide is broken down very rapidly when introduced into the blood stream in both rabbits and humans; **in dilute solutions, intravascular hydrogen peroxide has no unacceptable deleterious effect on formed blood elements** (with the exception of dogs, where, due to an apparent deficient in RBC and plasma catalase, methemoglobin is produced); (Mallams, J.T., Balla, G.A. and Finney, J.W. Regional oxygenation and irradiation in the treatment of malignant tumors. Progress in Clinc Cancer 1965; 1: 137), and **the breakdown of hydrogen peroxide by biological fluids results in the supersaturation of these fluids with oxygen** (Jay, B.E., Finney, J.W., Balla, G.A. and Mallams, J.T. The supersaturation of biologic fluids with oxygen by decomposition of hydrogen peroxide. Texas Rep Biol & Med 1964; 22: 106). **The magnitude of the supersaturation is equivalent to several atmospheres of oxygen.**

Kann, Mengel, and others have shown that the formation of lipid peroxides is one sequela to exposure to oxygen at high pressure. The authors have noted a reduction in the subintimal lipid deposits and atheromatous plaques in the arteries of individuals being infused intra-arterially with hydrogen peroxide.

This paper reports the results of 3 different approaches.

1. Chemical and histologic evaluation of aortas taken at postmortem from patients who had been treated with intra-arterial hydrogen peroxide as an adjunct to external irradiation in the management of their malignant disease.

2. In vitro studies of human aortas incubated with hydrogen peroxide.

3. In vivo studies of the total serum lipids in animals and humans before and immediately following the intra-arterial infusion of hydrogen peroxide.

Several patients who have been infused intra-arterially with hydrogen peroxide as an adjunct to irradiation therapy in the management of their malignant disease have undergone postmortem examination. During the autopsy, the catheter was left in place, the aorta was split longitudinally, and the tip of the catheter marked. Sections were prepared from the aorta immediately above and below tip for comparative histologic evaluation by oil red-O and H and E stains.

All patients were being **infused into the abdominal aorta with 0.48 percent hydrogen peroxide in Ionosol T**. Venous samples were taken before and during the last minute of infusion and the results of the two samples compared. During the entire infusion period (20 minutes), the patient was reclined and relaxed.

The evaluation of aortas taken at postmortem from patients who had been treated with intra-arterial hydrogen peroxide showed the following changes:

In all cases studied to date, the patients have received hydrogen peroxide infusion alone as an adjunct to other modes of therapy for a variety of conditions over extended periods of time ranging from 4 to 16 weeks. During this time, the individuals received daily infusions of 250 ml of hydrogen peroxide in Ionosol T with **a peroxide concentration ranging from 0.36 to 0.48 percent.**

Upon gross examination, the segment of the aorta being infused was found to be different from the area not being infused. **This difference was marked by a decrease in the number and severity of atheromatous plaques, and an increase in flexibility and elasticity of the vessel.** Histologic evaluation by oil red-O stained sections **showed a decrease in total subliminal lipid deposits.** When weighed samples of the vessels were extracted and total lipids determined, **it was found that approximately a 50 percent reduction in total lipids had occurred in the area being infused with hydrogen peroxide.** In my opinion, this work is some of the most exciting work in the last 50 years!

In vitro studies on human aortas incubated with hydrogen peroxide, the results indicate a bi- or multiphase reaction which starts immediately with the elution of relatively large quantities of cholesterol, cholesterol esters, phospholipid, triglyceride and free fatty acids: the total concentration of these components in the supernatant fluid decreases over a period of the next few hours. This decrease if followed by a subsequent increase in total concentration at 12 to 24 hours. **The same general results have been obtained with human aorta in saline exposed to oxygen at five atmospheres absolute pressure.**

The elution of lipids from the arterial wall by dilute hydrogen peroxide has been accomplished by in vitro and in vivo procedures. In view of the extremely short life of hydrogen peroxide in the vascular system in vivo, and the preliminary data indicating a similar effect by oxygen at five atmospheres absolute pressure in vitro, it is postulated that the effects noted in both in vivo and in vitro studies are due primarily, if not solely, to a very high oxygen environment. **I believe that this data indicates the signaling capability of H_2O_2 because ,even though it is present for a very short time, it can activate processes which occur sometime later. This effect is being reported with increasing frequency for many of the RONS/excytomers.**

One additional observation should be made with respect to gross and microscopic examinations of aortas taken at autopsy from patients who had been treated for extended periods of time with intra-arterial hydrogen peroxide. **Some patients expired within a few weeks and some expired between 6 months and 1 year after the last infusion. The vessels of both groups showed the same gross and microscopic differential between the infused and noninfused areas. Therefore, it seems probable that the noted effect is not transitory in nature.**

These results are so important that I will repeat them as follows:

Gross and microscopic examination of aortas taken at autopsy from patients who had been treated with intra-arterial hydrogen peroxide for extended periods of time showed an increase in elasticity, a decrease in subluminal lipid deposits and a reduction in number and severity of atheromatous lesions in the infused areas when compared to the noninfused area.

In vitro studies conducted with human aorta incubated with dilute hydrogen peroxide for various periods of time demonstrated the elution of cholesterol, cholesterol esters, phospholipid, triglyceride and free fatty acids from the arterial wall.

In vivo studies have been carried out in experimental animals and humans in which total serum lipids were determined before and immediately after the intra-arterial infusion of hydrogen peroxide. The results show a rise in total lipids, with the most marked increase noted in patients with clinical atherosclerotic disease.

24.12   ISCHEMIC HEART PROTECTION WITH DMSO AND H$_2$O$_2$

The following information was excerpted from the following paper: (Finney, J.W., Urschel, H.C., Balla, G.A., Race, G.J., Jay, B.E., Pingree, H.P., Dorman, H.L. and Mallams, J.T. **Protection of the ischemic heart with DMSO alone or DMSO with hydrogen peroxide**. Ann NY Acad Sci 1967; 151: 231-241).

While oxygen delivered at high pressure is a promising investigative area, there are a number of problems inherent in such procedures. Some of these problems are: 1) limited duration of patient exposure due to CNS and pulmonary toxicity; 2) compression and decompression hazards; and 3) the expense and space requirements of hyperbaric systems. Due to the technical and physiological problems inherent in the hyperbaric procedures, studies were undertaken in the laboratory to **determine feasibility of employing a regional system for cardiac resuscitation following coronary artery occlusion**. Since hydrogen peroxide under the influence of catalase and peroxidases is degraded to oxygen and water, and since blood and tissues contain relatively large quantities of both enzyme systems, **hydrogen peroxide was evaluated as a source of oxygen**. From previous studies reported from the laboratory, one report remains pertinent to this discussion, i.e., **it has been shown that catalase-containing fluids (blood or other body fluids) become supersaturated with oxygen following their breakdown of exogenous hydrogen peroxide.**

It was obvious at the conclusion of the study that hydrogen peroxide alone (0.06%) could supply an adequate amount of oxygen to the ischemic heart of small animals. It was found, however, that when the procedure was applied to larger animals (swine), although improvement in the monitoring parameters could be noted, it became evident that due to the thickness of the myocardium, a sufficient amount of oxygen was not penetrating deeply enough into the left ventricle or septum to afford adequate protection.

It is of interest to note that in the animals treated with DMSO alone, the right ventricle shows a more extensive infarction than the control and also part of the septum shows a more diffusely infracted area when compared to the acute infarction in the control series. In the "peroxide only" series, the stain indicated the maintenance of reasonable activity in both the right and left ventricles; however, the septum showed evidence of infarction. In the last group, **where DMSO and H$_2$O$_2$ were combined, it seems as though the oxygen from the H$_2$O$_2$ breakdown is allowed to diffuse into the septum as well as into both the left and right ventricles**.

At this point, it is not possible to draw any definite conclusion from this data; however, it seems a trend has been established, and from the staining procedures, it would appear that the combination of DMSO and H$_2$O$_2$ will afford more protection than either reagent alone.

24.12.1 Summary

In summary, the following points should be made:

1. **Dilute solutions of hydrogen peroxide can be used as an oxygen source to maintain or resuscitate the anoxic heart of small animals. This can be accomplished by either pericardial perfusion or coronary infusion via the retrograde catheterization of the right carotid artery and passing the catheter to the coronary ostia.**

2. **Pericardial perfusions of dilute solutions of hydrogen peroxide alone serve to maintain a functional heart in large animals.** By the Nitro BT staining technique, it was found that even during the pericardial perfusion of dilute solutions of hydrogen peroxide in large animals, the septum remained essential anoxic.

3. **By adding DMSO to the dilute hydrogen peroxide being perfused to the pericardium in large animals following coronary artery ligation, results indicate the maintenance of a functioning heart.** By the Nitro BT staining technique, it has been shown that DMSO may aid in the diffusion of oxygen into the thick myocardium, thus affording a higher degree of protection from anoxia.

24.13 INTRA-ARTERIAL H$_2$O$_2$ PROMOTES WOUND HEALING

The following was excerpted from: (Balla, G.A., Finney, J.W., Aronoff, B.L., Byrd, D.L., Race, G.J., Mallams, J.T. and Davis, G. **Use of intra-arterial hydrogen peroxide to promote wound healing.** Am J Surg 1964; 108: 621-629).

The ever increasing use of the intra-arterial route of administration of drugs has necessitated the development of surgical techniques to insert and position plastic catheters into regional arteries accurately with minimal damage to the vessel. **During the past two and half years, intra-arterial infusions have been employed in approximately 150 cases** and the current techniques, as they have evolved with increasing experience, are reported. The open surgical approach for introducing the catheters used for long range therapy has proved to be the most successful in this study. The catheter selected is made from polyvinyl, No. 5 French, with a moderately thick wall, and is 36 inches in length. The tissue reactivity to this material has been minimal. These catheters have been left in human arteries for as long as seven months with no gross or microscopic damage to the vessel. Occasionally, there is a small deposit of fibrin within the vessel along the course of the catheter; however, these deposits have been without sequelae.

The peroxide solution is prepared daily as follows: to 250 cc of "Ionosol T" in 5% dextrose is added 25 to 50 mg of **Priscoline**. Then 5 to 40 cc of 3% pharmaceutical grade hydrogen peroxide is added. **This results in approximate concentrations of 0.06 to 0.48 percent peroxide solution**. This solution is then transferred to the Peroset infusion bag.

During the early studies in the treatment of patients with intra-arterial hydrogen peroxide and irradiation therapy, two observations were made. In some of the patients, **not only did the tumor respond more rapidly to irradiation, but also it was found that the wounds would heal at a much faster rate and with less scar formation**. As a result of this, wounds that were refractory to conventional modes of therapy were treated with intra-arterial hydrogen peroxide either alone or in combination with intra-arterial antibiotics. The major reasons given for delays in wound healing are: 1) inadequate nutrition, 2) necrotic tissue, 3) foreign bodies, 4) bacterial infections, 5) interference with blood supply, 6) lymphatic blockage and 7) diabetes mellitus. Many of these factors that interfere with wound healing can be combined under the broad, general term of "tissue anoxia." It was believed that if tissue anoxia could be altered by regional super oxygenation, an increased healing rate could be achieved. The patients used in this study were those who have exhibited delayed wound healing that has been refractory to conventional modes of therapy. The techniques used were daily or twice daily infusions of intra-arterial antibiotics (Mallams, J.T., Finney, J.W. and Balla, G.A. The use of hydrogen peroxide as a source of oxygen in regional intra-arterial infusion system. South Med J 1962; 55: 230), (Balla, G.A., Hutton, S.B., Mallams, J.T., Aronoff, B.L., Byrd, D.L., Finney, J.W. and Race, G.J. Retrograde catheterization of the external carotid artery via the superficial temporal artery for the treatment of head and neck malignancies by continuous intra-arterial infusion. Am Surgeon 1963; 29: 265), (Balla, G.A., Finney, J.W. and Mallams, J.T. A method for selective tissue oxygenation utilizing regional intra-arterial infusion techniques. Am Surgeon 1963; 29: 496), (Finney, J.W., Mallams, J.T. and Balla, G.A. Increased available oxygen through regional intra-arterial infusion. Proc Am Assoc Cancer Res 1962; 3: 318), (Mallams, J.T., Balla, G.A., Finney, J.W. and Aronoff, B.L. Regional oxygenation and irradiation. Head and Neck. Arch Otol 1964; 79: 155),

(Balla, G.A., Mallams, J.T., Hutton, S.B., Aronoff, B.L. and Byrd, D.L. The treatment of head and neck malignancies by continuous intra-arterial infusion of methotrexate. Am J Surg 1962; 104: 699).

It is apparent with the results shown in these cases that the introduction of three factors, either singly or in combination, has definitely altered the character of the rate of healing of these wounds. **First**, intra-arterial antibiotics are a more effective way of combating regional infections than systemic antibiotic therapy. A much larger concentration of the antibiotic can be administered by this method into the regional area. This has been accomplished with minimal side effects from the regionally-given large doses of the antibiotics employed. Second, **regional super oxygenation using intra-arterial hydrogen peroxide has apparently increased regional oxygen and beneficially influenced the tissue utilization of oxygen in these patients**. This would demonstrate the ability of wounds to heal when states of tissue anoxia are corrected. **Third,** intra-arterial Priscoline promotes regional vasodilation which may be beneficial. Many of these patients were treated with conventional bed rest, elevation, systemic antibiotics and saline compresses without materially affecting the course of their wounds prior to the treatment of intra-arterial hydrogen peroxide. Several patients were admitted to have their leg amputated as a last resort, only to find that with this relatively conservative approach, not only could their wounds be healed but also normal function could be obtained. A detailed study to try to ascertain tensile strength of wounds, amount of scar formation and actual rapidity of wound healing in calibrated wounds in animals has not been made at this date. Suffice it to say, that **the best objective evidence of tissue utilization of oxygen, which is really the heart of any study involving super oxygenation, has been that wounds, which would previously not heal, would heal with super oxygenation**. This would certainly indicate that the oxygen being supplied to the area has exercised a beneficial effect in these patients.

24.14 ADDITIONAL PAPER - H$_2$O$_2$ CARDIAC RESUSCITATION

Ventricular fibrillation or cardiac arrest resulting from myocardial ischemia or anoxia in hearts which could not be resuscitated by conventional techniques **could be reversed to regular sinus rhythm by the regional application of dilute hydrogen peroxide**. Hydrogen peroxide is converted to high atmospheric equivalents of oxygen, and with regional application systemic oxygen toxicity is avoided.

Ventricular fibrillation or cardiac arrest was produced in 40 rabbits by tracheal occlusion or circumflex coronary artery ligation. **Regional application of 0.12 to .24% hydrogen peroxide via coronary artery infusion or epicardial application returned the heart to regular sinus rhythm and elevated blood pressure to normal, in contrast to ten control animals who could not be resuscitated with standard methods.** The procedure was repeated in ten goats undergoing anterior descending coronary artery ligation. The electrocardiogram, arterial and venous pressure, pH and myocardial tissue oxygen tension were monitored. Myocardial tissue oxygen tension values increased from two to six times control values following hydrogen peroxide application. Low molecular weight dextran and papaverine improved effective coronary artery infusion of hydrogen peroxide. Dimethyl sulfoxide (DMSO) may improve diffusion in the thick myocardium.

Following the failure of conventional resuscitation methods, hydrogen peroxide was employed in one human case with temporary reversal of ventricular fibrillation to regular sinus rhythm and elevation of the blood pressure to normal (Urschel, H.C., Jr., Finney, J.W., Morales, A.R., Balla, G.A. and Mallams, J.T. Cardiac resuscitation with hydrogen peroxide. Abstract of the 38th Scientific Sessions. 1965; Suppl II, Vol. 31 & 32).

24.15 REGIONAL H₂O₂ FOR CLOSTRIDIA MYOSITIS

The following was excerpted or modified from: (Finney, J.W., Haberman, S., Race, G.J., Bala, G.A. and Mallams, J.T. Local and regional application of hydrogen peroxide in the control of clostridia myositis in rabbits. J Bacterio 1967; 93: 1430-1437).

The intra-arterial infusion of hydrogen peroxide has been used as a method for producing a hyperoxic environment in experimental animals for the treatment of experimentally induced clostridia myositis. Eighty-five rabbits were employed in this study; 43 were controls and 42 were experimental animals. In the experimental study, 21 animals were treated with hydrogen peroxide by each route of administration. In this group, **52.4% of the animals receiving the intra-arterial H₂O₂ infusion and 66.6% receiving intramuscular clysis with H₂O₂ survived. There were no survivors past 72 hours in the control group**.

The objective was to get the O₂ tension to the point that it was not conducive to the survival of the anaerobic organisms. This can be accomplished conveniently by three methods: 1) breathing oxygen at increased pressures; 2) the administration of hydrogen peroxide intra-arterially; or 3) the intramuscularly (im) administration of hydrogen peroxide in a physiological solution delivered directly to the invaded area.

It has been shown in vivo that the breakdown of hydrogen peroxide progresses at a sufficiently rapid rate to prevent any unacceptable side reactions, and that oxygen supplied in this fashion is in a form which is metabolically usable by the animal.

The animals treated intra-arterially with hydrogen peroxide were given 10 ml of 0.24% hydrogen peroxide which contained 0.25 mg of Priscoline delivered at 0.25 ml/min. the im clysis control and hydrogen peroxide-treated animals were given 10 ml of "Ionosol T" or 0.12% hydrogen peroxide at a rate of 0.5 ml/min.

There were no survivors past the 72 hour period in any of the control groups, whereas 52.4 and 66.6% of the animals survived in the intra-arterial and intra-muscular hydrogen peroxide groups, respectively. In addition, the majority of the animals expiring in the experimental group were lost within the first 24 hours, whereas the greatest animal loss in the control groups occurred between 24 and 48 hours.

It became evident during the study that the rate at which the spread of the disease was halted and at which the disease subsequently healed was more rapid than expected in the hydrogen peroxide-treated animals. (Balla, G.A., Finney, J.W., Aronoff, B.L., Byrd, D.L., Race, G.J., Mallams, J.T. and Davis, G. Use of intra-arterial hydrogen peroxide to promote wound. Part II. Wound healing, clinical aspects. Am J Surg 1964; 108: 625-629), (Finney, J. W., Balla, G.A., Collier, R.E., Wakley, J., Urschel, H.C. and Mallams, J.T. Differential localization of isotopes in tumors through the use of intra-arterial hydrogen peroxide. Part I. Basic Science. Am J Roentgenol Radium Therapy Nucl Med 1965; 94: 783-788), (Jay, B.W., Finney, J.W., Balla, G.A. and Mallams, J.T. The supersaturation of biologic fluids with oxygen by the decomposition of hydrogen peroxide. Tex Rept Biol Med 1964; 22: 106-109), (Mallams, J.T., Balla, G.A., Finney, J.W. and Aronoff, B.L. Regional oxygenation and irradiation. Head and neck. Arch Otolaryngology 1964; 79: 155-159).

**"Future's shape is sculpted by the
persistent kneading hands of
the impossible dreamer."**

R. M. Howes, M.D., Ph.D.

5/2/04

PART V - IMMUNE SYSTEM

27.4 MY INTERPRETATION AND CONCLUSION

The DS patients have significantly elevated levels of SOD and consequently, have lower levels of superoxide anion. SOD is one of the primary endogenous enzymatic antioxidants. Thus, having 3 times normal amounts, should produce 3 times the benefits, but it does not. The presence of 3 times the normal amount of SOD actually lowers the DS patient's RONS/excytomer levels to a deficiency state and "allows" the manifestations of premature aging, malignancy and diabetes. Also, since they have normal levels of catalase and glutathione peroxidase, they should also have low levels of H_2O_2. Because of these facts, **the oxy-moron's Free Radi-Crap Theory of aging and oxidative stress would predict that DS patients would have increased life spans and decreased disease such as, cancer and diabetes…..but they are wrong.** However, these observations and clinical manifestations in DS patients are consistent with my **Unified Theory** in that, deficient levels of RONS and excited states <u>allow</u> for the development of cancer, infections and a shortened life expectancy.

Admittedly, there have been studies on cultured cortical neurons form fetal Down's syndrome cases which exhibit a 2-3 fold higher intracellular level of ROS, when compared to age-matched normal brain cells but it is unclear what this fetal data means.

Since superoxide dismutase is over expressed in DS, the Free Radi-Crap theory suggests that it is possible that the oxidative stress may be involved in neuronal death in DS. While in vitro studies have shown increased sensitivity to oxidative stress of DS neurons, **two post-mortem studies in DS have shown no evidence of a pathogenic role of SOD or reactive oxygen species** (http://www.ds-health.com/abst/a0006.htm).

28 CHRONIC GRANULOMATOUS DISEASE

Chronic Granulomatous Disease (CGD) is a genetically determined (inherited) disease character-ized by an inability of the body's phagocytic cells to kill certain microorganisms. As a result of this defect in phagocytic cell killing, patients with CGD have an increased susceptibility to infections caused by certain bacteria and fungi and the development of tumorous lesions called granulomas.

Children with Chronic Granulomatous Disease (CGD) are usually healthy at birth. However, sometime **in their first few months or years of life, they develop recurrent infections,** infections that are difficult to treat, or infections that are caused by unusual organisms such as fungi. The infections may involve any organ system or tissue of the body, but the skin, lungs, lymph nodes, liver, or bones are the usual sites of infection. Infected lesions may have prolonged drainage, delayed healing and residual scarring.

Pneumonia is a recurrent and common problem in patients with CGD. Many of the lung infections are chronic.

28.1 BIOCHEMICAL DEFECT

CGD is a primary immunodeficiency disorder that results from the absence or malfunction of NADPH oxidase, which is normally expressed in neutrophils and other phagocytic leukocytes. The disorder is usually a result of defective cytochrome b function. **Granulocytes normally respond to the stimulus of phagocytosis with an oxidative respiratory burst. In patients with CGD, this response fails to occur, and as a result, reactive oxygen radicals (e.g., superoxide, hydrogen peroxide, hydroxyl radicals, singlet oxygen) are not formed.** In CGD, phagocytes can ingest bacteria normally but cannot kill them. The same abnormality is also present in eosinophils and mononuclear phagocytes.

Patients with CGD are susceptible to severe and recurrent infections due to catalase-positive organisms (which breaks down H_2O_2) and organisms resistant to oxidative killing. Catalase-negative bacteria, such as streptococci and pneumococci that have the capacity to generate hydrogen peroxide, are killed as they usually are, because they bring the H_2O_2 with them. The intracellular survival of ingested bacteria leads to the development of granulomata in the lymph nodes, skin, lungs, liver, gastrointestinal tract, and/or bones.

Some bacterial species, such as the **pneumococci and streptococcus, produce oxygen-containing compounds such as hydrogen peroxide.** When these bacteria are ingested by the phagocytic cells of patients with CGD, **the bacterium contributes its own hydrogen peroxide to the defective phagocytic cell. As a result, the defect is overcome, and the phagocytic cells can kill these organisms using the hydrogen peroxide contributed by the bacteria itself.** Thus, patients with CGD do not have an increased susceptibility to these organisms. They are only susceptible to organisms, such as staphylococci and fungi, which cannot produce hydrogen peroxide and other oxygen-containing compounds. These microbes cannot supply the missing chemical needed by the phagocytic cell for normal killing (at least H_2O_2). According to the Free Radi-crap theory of aging and oxidative stress, this RONS, namely H_2O_2, which they have repeatedly said is deadly, once again saves patient's lives and weakens their theory. Yet, **thousands of papers continue to demonize H_2O_2 (RONS) and leading organizations try to scare everyone away from its use by citing less than a handful of historical instances in which H_2O_2 caused untoward effects because of its having been used in powerful concentrations in the wrong places and for the wrong purposes.**

Patients with CGD have normal antibody production, normal T cell function, and a normal complement system, in short, the rest of their immune system is normal.

28.2 COMPLEXITY OF THE IMMUNE SYSTEM

In order for the immune system to kill a bug or a cancer cell, a series of complex reactions must occur and an immunodeficiency at any one of a number of steps can prevent the kill from taking place. Before RONS or O_2 excytomers can act on infections or cancer cells, and assuming that adequate levels of O_2 are present for the electron transport chain, bacteria and cancer cells are acted upon by a variety of opsonins, complement factors, etc. Clinically, **immunodeficiency syndromes are associated with increased susceptibility to infection, increased risk for certain cancers** and increased incidence of autoimmune disorders.

Types of infection provide clues as to the specific immunologic defect involved. Defects in humoral immunity tend to be associated with frequent bacterial infections while defects in cell-mediated immunity typically leads to infections by opportunistic organisms or intracellular pathogens such as viruses. Mucocutaneous candidiasis, pneumocystis pneumonia and herpes zoster infections are particularly common with T- lymphocyte disorders. Decreased complement levels or abnormalities in WBC function are associated with pyogenic infections similar to those seen in disorders of humoral immunity.

Patients with T Cell immunodeficiencies are prone to certain types of cancers, especially leukemias and lymphomas. The following generalities can be made.

Examples of Infectious Agents in Different Types of Immune Disorders

Pathogen Type	T-cell defect	B-cell defect	Granulocyte	Complement
Bacteria	Bacterial sepsis	Streptococci, Staphylococci, Haemophilus	Staphylococci, Pseudomonas	Neisseria, Other pyogenic bacteria
Viruses	CMV, Epstein-Barr, varicellai-zoster, chronic infections from respiratory and gastrointestinal viruses	Enterviral encephalitis (echovirus, coxsackievirus)		
Fungi and Parasites	Candida, pneumocystis	Giardiasis	Candida, Nocardia, Aspergillus	
Special Features	Aggressive diseases with opportunistic pathogens, failure to clear infections, Disseminated viral infections. Mucocutaneous candidiasis. Pneumocystis pneumonia.	Recurrent sinoplumonary infections, sepsis, chronic meningitis, chronic otitis		

Again, I need to emphasize that there are many points which can affect pathogen and/or cancer kill, even in the presence of adequate oxygen levels.

28.3 MY INTERPRETATION AND CONCLUSION

CGD patients represent one of the best models to study the importance of O_2^-/H_2O_2. In drastic and direct contrast to the Free Radi-Crap Theory of aging and oxidative stress, CGD patients demonstrate a direct dependence upon adequate levels of O_2^-/H_2O_2 and ROS to maintain normal health and to avoid infections.

O_2^-/H_2O_2 provided by the patient → no infections

H_2O_2 provided by the bacteria → no infections

No patient H_2O_2 → infections

Catalase in bacteria → infections

No patient NADPH oxidase → infections

This is about as direct of a **"relationship-revelation"** as nature can provide. Naturally, this is consistent with my **Unified Theory**. Peroxide or other oxidative agents, such as RONS and O_2 excytomers, are crucial for health and homeostasis. **CGD is a classic example of a chronic infection being caused by a deficiency of RONS and O_2 excytomers. Thus, this is in direct contrast to the Free Radi-Crap Theory of aging and oxidative stress. In actuality, more H_2O_2 and RONS would clear up the infections in CGD patients.**

At this juncture in my research, I was puzzled by the fact that my Unified Theory predicted that CGD patients would also have increased levels of tumors or cancerous growths but I could not find such examples in the literature. Thus, I went back to the basics and found a Dorland's Medical dictionary, 27th edition, definition of **tumor**, which it described as the following: 1. Swelling, one of the cardinal signs of inflammation 2. **A new growth of tissue in which the multiplication of cells is uncontrolled and progressive**; called also neoplasm.

Benign tumor - one that lacks the properties of invasion and metastasis and that is usually surrounded by a fibrous capsule; its cells also show a lesser degree of anaplasia than those of malignant tumors.

Malignant tumor - one that has the properties of invasion and metastasis and that shows a greater degree of anaplasia than do benign tumors.

Then, I was struck by the obviousness of the situation in that **the granulomata themselves are tumors and the CGD patients are full of them**. In fact, pyogenic granulomas and eosinophil granulomas are listed under "Benign oral cavity and oro- pharyngeal tumors." Further reading revealed that pyogenic granulomas are seen most often in children and pregnant women ("pregnancy tumor") and those taking the drugs Indinavir, Soriatane, Accutane and oral contraceptives. Although usually benign, on rare occasion a cancer can mimic a pyogenic granuloma. As many as half of those treated will recur and at times, multiple smaller pyogenic granuloma form following a treatment and are called "satellites" (**invasion**). It appears that pieces of pyogenic granuloma may spread through local blood vessels (**metastasis**). Pyogenic granuloma in pregnant women may go away after delivery on their own (**"spontaneous regression"**).

Specific cell types and varying degrees of anaplasia in granulomas has led to the concept of **"polyclonality."**

Then, I had added another plank to the platform of my **Unified Theory**.

29 PHOTODYNAMIC THERAPY (PDT) FOR CANCER

PDT will be covered in some detail because of the fact that it generates similar products, with similar chemical reactivity as the **Howes Singlet Oxygen Delivery system.**

29.1 WHAT IS PHOTODYNAMIC THERAPY (PDT)?

Although there are well over ten thousand published papers on PDT very few physicians other than specialists in Ophthalmology and Dermatology are familiar with either this type of treatment or with its underlying biochemical mode of action.

29.2 BASICS OF PDT

The basic elements of PDT are as simple as 1-2-3: Photosensitizer + Visible light + Oxygen = Tissue Response. The unique property of photosensitizers to selectively accumulate in malignant and dysplastic tissues is exploited in the treatment of malignancies.

Once the drugs are absorbed in place, the light is used to irradiate the tissues with a fixed frequency light source unique to each drug and disease. The drug absorbs the light, which stimulates the drug to destroy only the diseased tissues in which the drug has been absorbed.

The basic steps are as follows:

- Light activated drug is applied topically or injected or injected intravenously.
- Drug accumulates in the affected tissue.
- Low power light is delivered through the illuminating device and focused on the affected tissue.
- Light activates photo reactive drug, releasing agents that destroy only affected cells.

PDT selectively destroys tumors with a simple concept. The PDT agents, mainly porphrins and their derivatives, preferentially accumulate in neoplastic tissue. This occurs either from **selective up-take** or delayed elimination relative to normal tissue. When the photosensitizer is activated by a light source (laser or filament), the molecule absorbs the light energy. In this excited state it is extremely reactive and interacts with molecular oxygen to **produce highly reactive oxygen "singlet." In biological systems, singlet oxygen has a short lifetime of <0.04** μs **and has also been shown to have a short radius of action of <0.02** μm. (Moan, J. and Berg, K. The photodegradation of porphyrins n cells can be used to estimate the lifetime of singlet oxygen. Photochem Photobiol 1991; 53: 549-553).   This chemical moiety is highly cytotoxic. Since the agent is concentrated in the tumor and the light is directed at the mass, the resulting direct tumoricidal activity and microvascular damage, with associated thrombosis, destroys tumor cells. The result is inflammation and necrosis of the cancer. If the cancer is adjacent to a cavity or lumen (esophagus, bronchus, intestinal tract or bladder) the treated tissue sloughs away with the help of macrophages and there is normal healing and re-epithelialization of the affected site.

Since the PDT process is a "cold" photochemical process, **there is essentially no thermal damage to the tissues;** connective tissue (collagen and elastin) and vasculature are largely spared. Compared to surgery and conventional thermal Yag and argon laser treatment, there is much less damage and disruption of the underlying and adjacent normal tissue structures. Both the patient and clinician have much to benefit from this approach. Superficial treatments do not require sterile theatre conditions and can be delivered in an outpatient setting. There is little post-treatment discomfort and **the only significant side effect is residual photosensitivity (protection from direct sunlight is necessary for a period of time).**

29.3 METHOD OF ADMINISTRATION AND TREATMENT

PDT agents can be administered either systemically or topically. Following a period of time to allow the photosensitizer to accumulate in the target tissue, low intensity of the appropriate wavelength is directed into the tumor. The depth and effectiveness of the treatment is contingent upon several factors. Longer wavelengths of light achieve greater depths of penetration into the tissue; thus allowing more effective treatment of deeper tumors. Also, **the efficiency of converting light energy into tumoricidal reactive 'singlet' oxygen varies greatly between PDT agents**. Newer agents show higher efficiency in this regard. For example, the second-generation agent Temporfin is 100 times more efficient in creating 'singlets' compared to the older approved agent Photofrin. It also is more selectively concentrated in tumor cells and is activated at longer wavelength. All this will translate into improved treatment results for patients.

29.3.0 Photochemical Internalization

Cytosolic delivery of macromolecules is called photochemical internalization and this technique allows $^1O_2$ to oxidize biomolecules in the membranes of endosomes and lysosomes, resulting in the subsequent release of these contents into the cytosol (Selbo, P.K., Hogset, A., Prasmickaite, L. and Berg, K. Photochemical internalization: A novel drug delivery system. Tumour Bio 2002; 23(2): 103-112).

29.3.1 PDT Applications

At present photodynamic therapy is in use or under investigation for both oncology and nononcology areas of medicine and surgery.

The following material has been excerpted from or based upon a review paper by Dougherty, T.J., Gomer, C.J., Henderson, B.W., Jori, G., Kessel, D., Korbelik, M., Moan, J. and Peng, Q. Photodynamic Therapy J Natl Canc Inst 1998; 90(12): 889-905.

With PDT, the site of photodamage reflects the localization of the photosensitizer at the time of irradiation, due to the short migration or **diffusion range of singlet oxygen being <0.02 um.** Reports indicate that the **mitochondria were among the targets of photodamage** (Salet C. Hematoporphyrin and hematoporphyrin-derivative photosensitization of mitochondria. Biochimie 1986; 68: 865-868). Other sites of photodamage are the lysyl chlorin p6 for lysosomes, the monocationic porphyrin for membranes and the propylene monomer for mitochondria. Sensitizers that are not taken up by cells, e.g., uroporphyrin, are extremely inefficient even though some of them give a high photochemical yield of $^1O_2$. Moreover, since most PDT sensitizers do not accumulate in cell nuclei, PDT has generally a low potential of causing DNA damage, mutations, and carcinogenesis. Also, **long-term studies on phototherapy for hyperbilirubinemia have not shown untoward effects with this singlet oxygen generating system.** Sensitizers that localize in **mitochondria,** like Photofrin, or are produced in mitochondria, like 5-aminolevulmic acid (ALA)-induced protoporphyrin IX, are likely to induce **apoptosis**, while sensitizers localized in the **plasma membrane** are likely to cause **necrosis** during light exposure. The probability of cell inactivation per quantum of absorbed light is widely different among PDT sensitizers (Berg, K., Steen, H.B., Windelman, J.W. and Moan, J. Synergistic effects of photo activated tetra(4-sulfonatophenyl)porphine and nocodazole on microtubule assembly, accumulation of cells in mitosis and cell survival. J Photochem Photobiol B 1992; 13: 59-70). Thus, **the PDT system is much more difficult to predict and quantitate than the Howes Singlet Oxygen Delivery System.**

29.3.2 Initial PDT Damage

PDT damage to the plasma membrane can be observed within minutes after light exposure. This type of damage is manifested as swelling, bleb formation, shedding of vesicles containing plasma membrane marker enzymes, cytosolic and lysomal enzymes, reduction of active transport, depolarization of the plasma membrane, increased uptake of a photosensitizer, increased permeability to chromate and even to cytosolic enzymes like lactate dehydrogenase, inhibition of the activities of plasma membrane enzymes such as Na^+K^+-adenosine triphosphate (ATPase) and Mg^{2+}-ATPase, a rise in Ca^{2+}, up-and down-regulation of surface antigens, lipid peroxidation that may lead to protein cross linking, and damage to multidrug transporters.

PDT induces lipid peroxidation in cells as a detrimental action. **Phospholipid hydroperoxide glutathione peroxidase (PhGPx) provides significant protection against $^1O_2$ generated lipid peroxidation via removal of LOOH** and that its activity could contribute to the resistance of tumor cells to PDT (Wang, H.P., Qian, S.Y., Schafer, F.Q., Domann, F.E., Oberly, L.W. and Buettner, G.R. Phospholipid hydroperoxide glutathione peroxidase protects against single oxygen induced cell damage of photodynamic therapy. Free Radic Biol Med 2001; 30(8): 825-835).

29.3.3 Apoptosis and PDT

In 1991, investigators described an apoptotic response to PDT (Agarwal, M.L., Clay, M.E., Harvey, E.J., Evans, H.H., Antunez, A.R. and Oleinick, N.L. Photodynamic therapy induces rapid cell death by apoptosis in L5178Y mouse lymphoma cells. Cancer Res 1991; 51: 5993-5996). The end result of apoptosis is fragmentation of nuclear DNA and dissociation of the cell into membrane-bound particles that are engulfed by adjoining cells, minimizing release of inflammatory products, e.g., lysosomal enzymes. **Malignant cell types often exhibit an impaired ability to undergo apoptosis,** an effect associated with the ability to survive chemotherapy. Since a broad spectrum of clinical PDT responses is observed, PDT is effective against otherwise drug-resistant cell types.

The time required for initiation of apoptosis varies widely. Most cells, in response to inducing agents, go through a latency period, variable in duration, which **usually results in the death of greater than 80% of cell population in 1-3 days.** A novel feature of apoptosis after PDT is the rapidity of execution, as judged by the appearance of DNA ladders are early as 30 minutes after photodamage.

It is known that release of cytochrome c and other mitochondrial factors into the cytoplasm can trigger an apoptotic response, effects that can also be produced by enhanced mitochondrial permeability. Mitochondrial permeability is known to be involved in a pore transition that can be triggered by protoporphyrin (in the dark), and it is interesting to note that some other photosensitizing agents have a similar effect.

PDT-mediated oxidative stress induces a transient increase in the downstream early response genes c-fos, c-jun, c-myc, and egr-1 (Luna, M.C., Wong, S. and Gomer, C.J. Photodynamic therapy mediated induction or early response genes. Cancer Res 1994; 14: 315-321). The in vivo tumoricidal reaction after PDT is accompanied by a complex immune response.

The abnormal structure of tumor stroma characterized by a large interstitial space, a leaky vasculature, compromised lymphatic drainage, a high amount of newly synthesized collagen (that binds porphyrins), and a high amount of lipid (that has a high affinity for lipophilic dyes) also favors a preferential distribution of sensitizers. The interstitial fluid is the fluid surrounding the cells and localized between their plasma membranes and the vascular walls. **The pH value of interstitial fluid is lower and the content of lactic acid is higher in tumors than in most normal tissues. The intracellular pH, however, is identical or slightly higher in tumors than in** normal tissue (Gerweck, L.E. and Seetharaman, K. Cellular pH gradient in tumor versus normal tissue: Potential exploitation for the treatment of cancer. Cancer Res 1996; 56: 1194-1198).

It has been shown that tumor-associated macrophages in animal tumors take up large amounts of hematoporphyrin derivative (HPD) and Photofrin. Thus, tumor-associated macrophages play a role for the tumor-selective uptake of aggregated sensitizers.

29.3.4 PDT Tumor Destruction

The targets of PDT inside tumor cells include the microvasculature of the tumor bed as well as normal microvasculature, and the inflammatory and immune host system. **Vascular shutdown is clearly an important aspect of PDT** (Henderson, B.W. and Dougherty, T.J. How does photodynamic therapy work? Photochem Photobiol 1992; 55: 145-157). Studies in rodent tumor systems employing curative procedures with several photosensitizers showed direct photodynamic tumor cell kill to be less than 2 logs and in most cases less than 1 log, i.e., far short of the 6-8 log reduction required for tumor cure.

Availability of ground state oxygen within the tumor can dramatically influence and limit direct tumor cell kill. Two mechanisms can produce such limitations: the photochemical consumption of oxygen during the photodynamic process and the effects of PDT on the tissue microvasculature. The rates of $^1O_2$ generation and therefore tissue oxygen consumption/depletion are high when both tissue photosensitizer levels and the fluence rate of light are high (Zilberstein, J., Bromberg, A., Frantz, A., Rosenbach-Belkin, V., Kritzman, A. and Pfefermann, R., et al. Light-dependent oxygen consumption in bacterio-chlorophyll-serine-treated melanoma tumors: On-line determination using a tissue-inserted oxygen microsensor. Photochem Photobiol 1997; 65: 1012-1019).

Preliminary clinical studies at the Roswell Park Cancer Institute show oxygen depletion also occurring during PDT in patients. The kinetics for this depletion varied from very rapid (within seconds of light exposure) to slow (>10 minutes of light exposure) and to no effect at all in basal cell carcinoma lesions in patients undergoing Photofrin.

An important parameter influencing the rate of tissue oxygen consumption is photobleaching of the sensitizer because the reduction of sensitizer levels also reduces the rate of photochemical oxygen consumption. **Photobleaching can not occur with the Howes Singlet Oxygen Delivery System.** Also, the mechanisms underlying PDT vascular damage varies greatly with different photosensitizers.

Photofrin-PDT leads to vessel constriction, macromolecular vessel leakage, leukocyte adhesion and thrombus formation, all apparently linked to platelet activation and release of thromboxanes. PDT with certain phthalocyanines derivatives causes primarily vascular leakage, and PDT with mono-L-aspartyl chlorin e6 results in blood flow stasis primarily because of platelet aggregation. All of these effects may include components related to damage of the vascular endothelium. **Agents that inhibit nitric oxide synthase or scavenge nitric oxide appear to enhance tumor cures by enhancing PDT induced disruption of vascular perfusion.** Recent studies reveal important differences between PDT and effects on normal and tumor vasculature.

29.3.5 PDT Immunologic Effects

The curative properties of PDT arise from the death of cancer cells spared from the direct cytotoxic effect by a combination of oxidative stress-initiated secondary tumoricidal activities (Korbelik, M. Induction of tumor immunity by photodynamic therapy. J Clin Laser Med Surg 1996; 14: 329-334). Contrary to the contemporary prevailing concepts, these secondary effects are by no means limited to the ischemic death caused by the occlusion of tumor vasculature. Other events that are increasingly coming into focus are as follows: 1) **antitumor activity of inflammatory cells and 2) tumor-sensitized immune reaction.** They all can be elicited by phototoxic damage that is not necessarily lethal and bears an inflammatory impact.

Photodynamically induced changes in the plasma membrane and membranes of cellular organelles, which represent the most abundant damage with a majority of photosensitizers used for PDT, can trigger events with far-reaching consequences. **One process initiated at the membrane level involves signal transduction pathways**. These include enhanced expression of stress proteins and early response genes, activation of genes regulating the process of apoptotic cell death, and possibly the up-regulation of some cytokine genes. Due to their role in cell adhesion and antigen presentation, some of the PDT-induced stress proteins may participate in the development of inflammatory/immune responses manifested by this therapy.

The curative ability of photodynamic therapy (PDT) is severely compromised if treated tumors are growing in immunodeficient hosts. Reconstitution of severe combined immunodeficient (scid) mice with spherocyte from naïve immunologically intact BALB/c mice did not improve the response to Photofrin-based PDT of EMT 6 tumors growing in these animals. **PDT is a highly effective means of generating tumor-sensitized immune cells that can be recovered from lymphoid sites distant to the treated tumor at protracted time intervals after PDT, which asserts their immune memory character.** Treatment of tumors by PDT creates the conditions necessary for converting the inactive adoptively transferred pre-effector, tumor-sensitized immune cells into fully functional antitumor effector cells. Investigators found evidence for NK cell activation in PDT-treated Meth-A sarcomas (Korbelik, M. and Dougherty, G.J. Photodynamic therapy-mediated immune response against subcutaneous mouse tumors. Cancer Research 1999; 59: 1441-1446).

29.3.6 Memory Cell Activation

At least three major factors appear to be involved in the induction of a strong immune response against PDT-treated cancers. PDT-mediated oxidative stress triggers a variety of cellular signal transduction pathways (Dougherty, G.J., Gomer, C.J., Henderson, B.W., Jon, G., Kessel, D., Korbelik, M., Moan, J. and Peng, Q. Photodynamic therapy. J Natl Cancer Inst 1998; 90: 889-905). The Howes Singlet Oxygen Delivery System should likewise activate memory cells and a long term immune response.

PDT has been shown to activate nuclear factor-kB and AP-1, which in turn control the expression of various cytokines and other immunologically important genes. Among the cytokines whose expression has been reported to be modulated by PDT are IL-6, IL-10 and tumor necrosis factor-a.

Another important factor that contributes to the induction of PDT-mediated immune responses is the proinflammatory damage generated in cellular membranes and the vasculature of treated tumor and normal tissues. A dominant event in such PDT-induced inflammation is **rapid and massive invasion of activated inflammatory cells, including neutrophils/granulocytes, mast cells, and monocytes/macrophages, from the circulation to the PDT-treated site.** These cells appear to be the main contributors to the inflammation-primed immune development process associated with PDT (Korbelik, M. Induction of tumor immunity by photodynamic therapy. J Clin Laser Med Surg 1996; 14: 315-334).

The nature, rate and extent of tumor cell death induced by PDT may also play a crucial role in determining the generation of effective antitumor immune response. Large amounts of cellular debris are generated at a tumor site within a short time interval of PDT treatment. The particular nature of such material facilitates the uptake and presentation of putative tumor antigens by macrophages and dendritic cells recruited to the tumor site in response to PDT-induced inflammatory signals, **ensuring the recognition of tumor-specific epitopes by T-lymphocytes and their subsequent activation.**

It has been demonstrated that lymphoid populations are essential for preventing the regrowth of PDT-treated mouse EMT6 sarcomas.

29.3.7 Inflammation Induced by PDT

A strong inflammatory reaction is a central event in the mechanism of PDT-mediated tumor destruction. Differences in the nature and intensity of the inflammatory reaction between normal and cancerous tissues may contribute to the selectivity of PDT-induced tissue damage. **A major hallmark of the inflammatory process is the release of a wide variety of potent mediators, including vasoactive substances,** components of the complement and clotting cascades, acute phase proteins, proteinases, peroxidases, radicals, leukocyte chemoattractants, cytokines, growth factors, and other immunoregulators. Among cytokine, IL-6 mRNA and protein were found to be strongly enhanced in PDT treated mouse tumors, as well as in exposed spleen and skin. There is also evidence for PDT induced or up-regulated IL-1B, IL-2, tumor necrosis factor-a (TNF-a) and granulocyte colony-stimulating factor (G-CSF).

The inflammatory signaling after PDT initiates and supports the recruitment of leukocytes from the blood and amplifies their activity. **A massive regulated invasion of neutrophils, mast cells, and monocytes/macrophages during and after photodynamic light treatment has been documented in studies using rodent tumor models** (Krosi, G., Korbelik, M. and Dougherty, G.J. Induction of immune cell infiltration into murine SCCVII tumor by Photofrin-based photodynamic therapy. Br J Cancer 1995; 71: 549-555). These newly arrived nonspecific immune effector cells will outnumber resident cancer cells. Most notable is a rapid accumulation of large numbers of neutrophils.

The tumoricidal activity of monocytes/macrophages was found to be potentiated by PDT in vivo and in vitro. Macrophages were reported to release TNF-a following PDT treatment and to preferentially recognize PDT treated cancer cells as their targets. Degranulation of errant neutrophils liberates toxic oxygen radicals, myeloperoxidase, and lysosomal enzymes acting as a potent system for the breakdown of proteins and causing considerable damage to the affected tumor tissue.

Tumor sensitized lymphocytes can, under reduced tumor burden, eliminate small foci of viable cancer cells that have escaped other PDT mediated antitumor effects. Cancer immunity elicited by PDT has the attributes of an inflammation primed immune development process and bears similarities to the immune reaction induced by tumor inflammation caused by bacterial vaccines or some cytokines. Although the PDT treatment is localized to the tumor site, its effect can have systemic attributes due to the induction of an immune reaction. PDT generated tumor-sensitized lymphocytes can be recovered from distant lymphoid tissues (spleen, lymph nodes) at protracted times after light treatment. Therefore, these lymphocyte populations consist of immune memory cells. In contrast to most other cancer therapies, PDT can induce immunity, even against less immunogenic tumors (Canti, G., Lattuada, D., Nicolin, A., Taroni, P., Valentini, G. and Cubeddu, U. Antitumor immunity induced by photodynamic therapy and aluminum phthalocyanines and laser light. Anticancer Drugs 1994; 5: 443-447). This very important work indicates that **singlet oxygen induced apoptosis produces a long lasting immune response against tumors**. This should also apply to the **Howes Singlet Oxygen Delivery System. Generation of immune memory cells sensitized to PDT treated tumor**, suggests that PDT may be particularly suitable for a combined application with adoptive immunotherapy.

Inflammation is frequently accompanied by immunosuppressive effects, as is the case with PDT. The PDT-induced immunosuppression was detected primarily as a transient reduction in the delayed-type contact hypersensitivity response, which appears to be mediated by antigen nonspecific suppressor cells. (Lynch, D.H., Haddad, S., King, V.J., Ott, M.J., Straight, R.C. and Jolles, C.J. Systemic immunosuppression induced by photodynamic therapy (PDT) is adoptively transferred by macrophages. Photochem Photobiol 1989; 49: 453-458). Due to its inflammatory/immune character, PDT can be successfully combined with various immunotherapy protocols for achieving substantial gains in long-term tumor controls.

29.3.8 Oncology

PDT has significant potential in the management and treatment of malignant tumors. Photofrin, a 'first' generation agent, is approved for use in the palliation and treatment of lung, esophageal, gastric, gall bladder, cervical and bladder cancer in various countries throughout the world. Foscan, a 'second' generation photosensitizer, has been assigned FDA fast track designation for approval .5-ALA (aminolevulenic acid, a naturally occurring compound) has also recently been approved by the FDA for use in actinic pre-malignant skin lesions. In numerous studies, **ALA has been shown to be very successful in basal and squamous cell carcinoma of the skin** and other forms of cutaneous malignancy such as keratoses. A recent article in Lancet Oncology Vol, December 2000, by Colin Hopper stated: "Compared with standard approaches, PDT can achieve equivalent or greater efficacy in the treatment of many cancers, particularly in the head and neck and basal-cell carcinoma, with greatly reduced morbidity and disfigurement." The technique is relatively simple to perform, can commonly be carried out in outpatient clinics and is quite acceptable to patients. PDT is not confined to the treatment of small superficial tumors. It can be repeated to debulk large tumors progressively, and can also be applied through interstitial light delivery to large solid tumors with the use of fiber optic conduits. This same approach applies equally to the Howes Singlet Oxygen Delivery system.

PDT is currently approved in the palliation of locally advanced cancers and a few early-stage diseases. **It should now be included for first-line treatment in early malignant and premalignant disease, adjuvant therapy for surgery, and interstitial treatment of deep-seated tumors.**

PDT can be utilized before or after surgery, chemotherapy and/or ionizing radiation therapy. None of these other therapies are compromised by PDT and unlike the latter treatment, can be repeated many times with no resistance developing, minimal morbidity and better functional and cosmetic results. Excellent esthetic outcome with PDT makes it important in skin lesions and cancer of the head and neck where preserving function and respecting delicate underlying structures is critical. Procedures of the past were frequently quite disfiguring. Treatment of extensive areas of pleura and peritoneum can likewise be treated relatively easily, unlike radiation, which would result in unacceptable damage to surrounding tissues. The adjunctive use of PDT at the time of surgical removal of a primary tumor can be a valuable aid in the elimination of residual microscopic metastases. Today, innovative uses of interstitial light delivery (light is delivered by inserting fiber optic bundles through needles directed into the tumor mass under image guidance) have allowed a subcutaneous tumor 60 cubic centimeters to be successfully treated with Photofrin or other photosensitizers. Aside from care to avoid major blood vessels, this minimally invasive treatment is applicable to most areas of the body.

Barrett's esophagus and cervical dysplasia are examples of conditions associated with frequent progression to malignancy. **The incidence of esophageal cancer is increasing, presumably due to increased cases of esophageal reflux of acid.** PDT has been found in numerous studies to be a successful treatment for high-grade dysplasia of the esophagus and **Japan has already approved Photofrin for use in cervical dysplasia.**

29.3.9 Anemia and PDT

Anemia emphasizes the essential role of oxygen in PDT.

Some of the following material was excerpted or modified from: Golab, J., Olszewska, D., Mroz, P., Kozar, K., Kaminski, R., Jalili, A. and Jakobisiak, M. Erythropoietin restores the antitumor effectiveness of photodynamic therapy in mice with chemotherapy-induced anemia. Clinical Cancer Research 2002; 8: 1265-1270.

Introduction:

Anemia is a frequent complication of cancer occurring in up to 60% of patients (Henke, M. and Guttenberger, R. Erythropoietin in radiation oncology - a review. Oncology 2000; 58: 175-182). It may result from the malignant disease itself, accompanying infections or from chemotherapy administered to cancer patients or a combination of the two (Groopman, J.E. and Itri, M. Chemotherapy-induced anemia in adults: Incidence and treatment. J Natl Cancer Inst 1999; 91: 1616-1634). Anemia in cancer patients has a complex and generally negative impact on the disease. **The complications of anemia result from hypoxia of virtually all organs.** Moreover, patients with anemia have a poorer outcome of medical interventions including radiotherapy and chemotherapy (Obermair, A., Handisurya, A., Kaider, A., Sevelda, P., Kolbt, H. and Gitsch, G. The relationship of pretreatment serum hemoglobin level to the survival of epithelial ovarian carcinoma patients: A prospective review. Cancer (Philadelphia) 1998; 83: 726-731).

Several observations indicate that hypoxia influences the antitumor effectiveness of PDT. PDT involves the combination of visible light and photosensitizer. **Neither of the PDT components alone can induce antitumor effects, but when combined with oxygen they produce lethal cytotoxic agents (likely $^1O_2$) that can either directly kill tumor cells or destroy blood vessels within the tumor, thus contributing to the antitumor effects.** Because reactive oxygen species generated during PDT arise from the ground state oxygen it is apparent that oxygen availability is a rate-limiting factor influencing the effectiveness of treatment. Early observations indicate that **hypoxic or anoxic conditions almost completely reduce the antitumor effectiveness of PDT in vitro** (Henderson, B.W. and Fingar, V.H. Relationship of tumor hypoxia and response to photodynamic treatment in an experimental mouse model. Cancer Res 1987; 47: 3110-3114).

Tumor hypoxia is frequently considered a potential therapeutic problem because it renders solid tumors more resistant to ionizing radiation and may also confer decreased sensitivity to most anticancer drugs (Brown, J.M. The hypoxic cell: A target for selective cancer therapy - eighteenth Bruce F. Cain memorial award lecture. Cancer Res 1999; 59: 5863-5870).

Several studies indicated that the use of fractionated light delivery with either short- or long-term intervals significantly improves the efficacy of PDT by **allowing reoxygenation of tumor tissue during dark periods**. In other studies it was demonstrated that **hyperbaric oxygen can enhance the effects of PDT.**

Anemia correlates with a worsening of the tumor oxygenation status (Kelleher, D.K., Mathiensen, U., Thews, O. and Vaupel, P. Blood flow, oxygenation and bioenergetic status of tumors after erythropoietin treatment in normal and anemic rats. Cancer Res 1996; 56: 4728-4734).

29.3.10 Age-Related Macular Degeneration (AMD)

Age-related macular degeneration (AMD) is the leading cause of new cases of blindness in those over 50 rears of age in the developed world. **Choroidal neovascularization (CNV)** leads to hemorrhage and fibrosis in a number of ocular diseases including AMD. Conventional treatment utilized the Argon Laser to occlude the leaking vessels by thermal photocoagulation. The percentages of patients eligible for treatment however is limited since CVN may be too near the fovea to "safely" treat this sensitive area with heat. Other considerations and limited success have clearly shown thermal photocoagulation to be less than an ideal treatment. PDT treatment of the more aggressive forms of AMD, which cause 90% of the severe central vision loss, involves the IV injection of verteporfin followed by the application of non-thermal light at 692nm. The resulting selective thrombosis of new 'leaking' vessels is accomplished with minimal damage to the surrounding retina and choroids, since it is a cool procedure. **Treated lesions usually demonstrate closure of classic CNV within one-week post PDT.** This beneficial response is not associated with any additional central visual field defects and in some favorable groups the central visual field is actually increased. Due to partial reperfusion, usually patients need around five treatments over a two-year period. **This fact also demonstrates that the effects of PDT continue for prolonged periods of time and that the initial generation of the short lived reactant, singlet oxygen, acts as a signal for long term events**. This treatment is potentially beneficial only to patients who have early macular degeneration. Late stage AMD is associated with irreversible damage and fibrosis of the critical foveal function, obviating the need for early intervention.

29.3.11 Atherosclerotic Disease

Heart disease is a huge problem for global health because it strikes working-age people in developing countries and thereby hampers their economies. A close look at the populations of Russia, Brazil, India, China and South Africa calculates the number of productive years lost to heart disease as an indicator of economic cost. In total, the loss is 21 million productive years annually and it will climb to 34 million by 2030. Governments should do all they can to make sure **inexpensive drugs** to treat cardiovascular disease and arteriosclerosis are available. **India alone is losing a million people a year from its potential active work force.** Personally, I do not see the very profitable pharmaceutical industry address this problem with anything other than more unaffordable synthetics. Thus, **I feel that the Howes Singlet Oxygen Delivery System could be an inexpensive answer, in part, to the cardiovascular disease problem, especially to developing third world countries.**

The possible application of PDT in the treatment of atherosclerosis and the prevention of restenosis following balloon angioplasty is based on the observation that **atherosclerotic plaques take up higher concentrations of**

porphyrin than the normal vessel wall. The selectivity of uptake probably is associated with the high mitotic activity of smooth muscle cells in atheroma. Verteporfin, in animal studies, has shown the potential for treating atherosclerosis. The photosensitive agent selectively accumulates within the proliferating element of the plaque.

With light exposure, the generation of 'singlet' oxygen kills the foam cells that form the fibroelastic plaque. The lesion is debulked and necrotic tissue sloughs or is removed by phagocytosis. The potential of PDT in this area is only beginning to be seriously investigated with the primary agent being texaphrin.

The ability of PDT to destroy target tissues selectively is especially appealing for atherosclerotic plaque. Biotechnology has developed a new generation of selective photosensitizers and catheter-based technological advances in light delivery have allowed the introduction of PDT into the vasculature. The largest experience to date is with motexafin lutetium (Mlu, Antrin), an expanded porphyrin (texaphrin) that accumulates in plaque. **The combination of the motexafin lutetium and endovascular illumination, or Antrin phototherapy, has been shown to reduce plaque in animal models. Antrin phototherapy generates cytotoxic singlet oxygen that has been shown to induce apoptosis in macrophages and smooth muscle cells.** The safety, tolerability and preliminary efficacy of Antrin phototherapy has been assessed in phase I dose-ranging clinical trial in subject with coronary arteries undergoing stent implantation. The preliminary results suggest that **Antrin phototherapy is safe, well tolerated and nontraumatic** (Chou, T.M., Woodburn, K.W., Cheong, W.F., Lacy, S.A., Sudhir, K., Adelman, D.C. and Wahr, D. Photodynamic therapy: Applications in atherosclerotic vascular disease with motexfin lutetium. Catheter Cardiovasc Interv 2002; 57(3): 387-394).

PDT is successfully being used for vascular occlusion and thrombosis in intimal hyperplasia, restenosis, atherosclerotic plaques, corneal neovascularization and port-wine stains (Krammer, B., Vascular effects of photodynamic therapy. Anticancer Res 2001; 21(6B): 4271.7).

The Howes Singlet Oxygen Delivery System should be ideal for the removal of arterial plaque blockages, without surgical intervention or placement of stents. My system can be infused into the vascular system, such that the direction of blood flow carries the generated singlet oxygen over the plaque to dissolve it. Hemolysis could be avoided by decreasing concentrations of reagents and infusion rates, which would only extend the time needed to destroy foam cells and dissolve the blockage.

Phase I trials of photoangioplasty have been done.

29.3.12 PDT Bacteriocidal Effect

PDT has been shown to have significant bacteriocidal effects when laser power outputs are >6-mW (which have been used in physical therapy practice) are directed toward pathogenic or opportunistic bacteria previously treated with photosensitizing agents (DeSimone, N.A., Christiansen, C. and Dore, D. Bactericidal effect of 0.95-mW helium-neon and 5-mW indium-gallium-aluminum-phosphate laser irradiation at exposure times of 30, 60, and 120 seconds on photosensitized staphylococcus aureus and pseudomonas aerations in vitro. Phys Therapy 1999; 79(9): 839-849). The **mechanism of PDT-bacteriocidal action reportedly involves the formation of singlet oxygen and free radicals at the cell membrane.** The Howes Singlet Oxygen Delivery System should operate similarly and with increased efficiency.

This treatment of irradiating cells after sensitization to the light by a dye has been termed **"photochemotherapy"** and photodynamic therapy. The **term "photodynamic therapy" is often used to describe an anticancer treatment that involves laser irradiation after the systemic administration of a photosensitizing drug that is preferentially absorbed by the tumor.**

The mechanism of laser-induced cell destruction has important implications in clinical therapy. According to Karu, **exposing a cell to laser light causes acceleration of electron transfer in some areas of the respiratory chain** (Karu, T. Molecular mechanism of the therapeutic effect of low-intensity laser radiation. Laser in the Life Sciences 1988; 2(1): 53-74). At higher doses, this excitation energy is transferred to oxygen to form **singlet oxygen**. When cells are exposed without dye, **the flavins and cytochromes of the electron transport chain serve as photosensitizers.** The dyeing agents, which can absorb the radiation, bind to components of the cell and thereby enable more laser light to be absorbed. **Photodyes produce their cytotoxic effect at the cell membrane level in bacteria because their respiratory chain is located there.**

The interaction of laser light with eukaryotic cells is not well elucidated but is suspected to be more complicated. However, **the respiratory chain within the mitochondrial membrane would still be affected, and free radical and singlet oxygen production would cause cell death.** Therefore, information regarding the relative susceptibilities of the human and bacterial cell membranes, to the binding or absorption of the dye is needed to determine whether concomitant host cell killing would result. The results of the in vivo study by Meyer et al, which involved laser irradiation in rabbits, suggest that adjacent host tissue damage may not be a cause for concern. In this experiment, **small ulcers formed where the tissue has been treated, but they healed in approximately 2 weeks** (Meyer, M., Speight, P. and Bown, S.G. A study of the effects of photodynamic therapy on the normal tissues of the rabbit jaw. Br J Cancer 1993; 75: 299-306).

There could be many benefits in using this method of disinfecting pressure ulcers and wounds. First, killing is fast; therefore, both dye and laser exposure times would be minimal. Concern regarding the prospect of negative effects from dye itself would be minimized by the requirement of only small amounts of the dye. Second, **because free radical and singlet oxygen production are responsible for cell death, the development of resistant strains is highly unlikely** (Wilson, M. and Pratten, J. Sensitization of Staphylococcus aureus to killing by low-power laser light. J Antimicrob Chemother 1994; 33: 619-624). Finally, with this topical method, only the microbes in those areas exposed to dye and laser light would be subjected to killing. Thus, unlike with systemic treatments, normal flora elsewhere in the body would be spared.

An understanding of PDT gives immediate insight into the Howes Singlet Oxygen Delivery system because the end product/s appear to be the same. In other words, anything PDT can do, my system can do it better at a fraction of the cost and with increased accuracy.

The Howes Singlet Oxygen Delivery System offers these same bactericidal benefits and in a much more accurate and cost effective way. Importantly, it offers a means of treating and preventing wound infections without developing resistant bacterial strains.

29.3.13 Rheumatoid and Inflammatory Arthritis

Rheumatoid arthritis (RA) is a common chronic immunological disorder, characterized by a proliferative synovitis or inflammation of the joint surface tissue. At present, medical treatment is the mainstay of therapy for RA. Synovectomy is a treatment alternative for joints failing medical management but represents a serious step. PDT and PDT synovectomy are new treatment modalities for the removal of pathological synovial tissue and suppression of autoimmune inflammatory process. There are numerous potential considerations in the treatment of this complex and debilitating disease. Choice of sensitizers, dosage and timing of light delivery of the energizing light all require extensive investigation before the full beneficial potential of PDT for RA can be realized. Although **many investigators believe that ROS are causative for RA, they may ultimately prove to be curative.**

29.3.14 Psoriasis, Acne, Alopecia Areata, Portwine Stains and Hair Removal

Improvement in clinical appearance of psoriatic plaques and palmopustular psoriasis using PDT with hematoporphyrin (HpD) has been reported. Topical ALA with multiple UVA treatments improves psoriatic plaques in more than 50% of patients in 46% of the treated sites in a pilot study in 1995. The mechanism of action of PDT in psoriasis is not precisely known. **Results of PDT treatment are encouraging, because the treatment does not appear to be carcinogenic, unlike PUVA therapy.** Acne, alopecia areata, portwine stains and hair removal are the subject of current clinical investigations since they all, to some degree, show promise with PDT treatment.

29.4 CONCLUSION

In 1963 Kahn and Kasha identified singlet oxygen liberated by the hydrogen peroxide-hypochlorite reaction. Many studies have now shown that reaction with a variety of organic compounds gives the same products as those obtained via the photooxygenation method. The hydrogen peroxide-sodium hypochlorite reaction is the functional system in the Howes Singlet Oxygen Delivery System.

Photodynamic therapy (PDT) is a minimally invasive treatment with great promise in malignant disease, tumors, dermatologic lesions, age related macular degeneration and host of other chronic disease processes. Although it represents an entirely new modality of treatment, it remains surprisingly unfamiliar to many established physicians. However, **it holds great promise and it contributed a spark for my creative thinking to formulate my Unified Theory.**

29.5 SUMMARY

Photodynamic therapy (PDT), as the name implies, is the treatment of cancer by means of light. It is a non-invasive form of therapy that is less harmful to the body than radiation, or chemotherapy. The procedure involves injecting a photosensitive drug into the patient, which becomes concentrated in cancer cells within 48 to 72d hours post administration and it is this chemical which targets cancer cells with the effects of light. A beam of laser light is then focused on the tumor which kills the cancer cells and does little, if any, damage to normal cells. The technology has advanced in recent years with the introduction of small fiber-optic cables that direct the laser beam to tumors into remote areas of the body. **Photodynamic therapy is as close to a magic bullet as we can get to kill cancers close to the surface and it is the only thing that kills cancerous tissue and precancerous tissue, but does not harm the normal tissue** (Castellanos, P. and Fantry, G. Laser Light Therapy Seen as **"Magic Bullet"** for Treating Some Throat and Oral Cancers. University of Maryland Medical Center. Press Release: February 27, 2003). (Light Therapy Tackles Cancer. BBC News. Broadcast March 14, 2002). Actually, **I believe that my singlet oxygen delivery system is closer to a "magic bullet" because it does not require the laser or the photosensitizer, it can be elegantly regulated for accuracy and it has no tissue penetration limitations or side effects of the photosensitizer.**

Patients can receive other forms of treatment such as surgery, chemotherapy and irradiation along with photodynamic therapy. Also, PDT can be repeated as many times as necessary.

The photosensitive molecule has he ability to absorb light energy and undergoes an internal rearrangement of its electrons to a triplet state. The triplet state molecule slowly transfers its energy to molecular oxygen to form highly reactive electronically excited singlet molecular oxygen. **Singlet oxygen appears to kill cells primarily by its effect on the cellular structure known as the mitochondria.** The mitochondria are responsible for energy production in the cell, and singlet oxygen shuts down the formation of the energy molecule ATP, which in turn is required for the vital processes of protein and DNA synthesis.

The first sensitizer to have clinical applications was a derivative of a molecular entity known as porphyrin, found in hemoglobin and chlorophyll. The drug is known as porfimer sodium, with the trade name of Photofrin. The product is approved by the Food and Drug Administration in cases of non-small cell lung cancer when the tumors are located in the bronchial lining. This procedure has been shown to be very successful when the cancer is not too far advanced, and when surgery and radiotherapy are not indicated. **The FDA has also approved the use of Photofrin to treat esophageal cancer and precancerous skin cancer condition known as actinic keratosis** (HHS News. First Drug Device combined Treatment for Certain Pre-Cancerous Skin Lesions Approved. Press Release: Dec. 6, 1999).

Actinic keratosis (AK) are extremely common premalignant lesions occurring on chronically sun-exposed skin. They appear as rough, scaly erythematous patches with poorly defined borders. The prevalence increases with advancing age.

Actinic keratosis (AK) usually occur in fair skinned individuals over 45 years of age (skin type I or II). They rarely occur in type IV skin. The prevalence increases with advancing age. However, in Australia and in the southwestern U.S., younger people are affected more frequently.

Accurate figures on the prevalence and incidence are hard to obtain but Medical Industry Today estimates about 20 million cases occur worldwide. AK is the most common precursor lesion for squamous cell carcinoma (SCC) in whites. Approximately 5-20% of AKs will transform into SCC within 10-25 years but estimates go as high as 40%. The one year risk that AK lesion transform into SCC was estimated to 1.1% compared with the 10-year risk of 10.2%. By treating AKs the development of SCC can be prevented. Basal cell carcinoma is documented in about 2 million cases worldwide annually.

Clinical studies have shown that the PDT procedure is very promising in early-stage cancers of the mouth, throat, larynx and bladder.

A major **disadvantage** in the use of Photofrin is that the drug remains in the cells of the skin and eyes, so patients who are treated must avoid bright light for about six weeks. Also, Photofrin is excited by red light at a wavelength that can only penetrate tissue to a depth of a few millimeters, making it unsuitable for the treatment of deep-seated tumors, unless one uses fiber optics.

Second generation photosensitizers Meta-Tetrahydroxylphenylchlorine, known by the trade names of Foscan and Temporfin is chemically related to Photofrin, but has several advantages. It is excited at a longer wavelength, and achieves similar results to Photofrin at lower doses and short illumination times. After excitation, it stays a longer time in the triplet, **thus producing more cytotoxic singlet oxygen**. It also may be more selective between tumor cells and normal tissue. This product is currently in clinical trails for a large variety of cancers.

Studies with AML5 leukemia cells showed that cell kill correlated strongly with cumulative $^1O_2$ luminescence and **allowed direct estimation of the $^1O_2$ per cell required to achieve a specific level of cell kill** and also supported the validity and potential utility of $^1O_2$ luminescence as a dosimetric tool for PDT, as well as **confirming the likely role of $^1O_2$ in porphyrin-based PDT** (Niedre, M.J., Secord, A.J., Patterson, M.S. and Wilson, B.C. In vitro tests of the validity of singlet oxygen luminescence measurements as a dosimetric in photodynamic therapy. Cancer Res 2003; 63: 7986-7994). Thus, the **original work of Dougherty on $^1O_2$ was validated** (Weishaupt, K.R., Gomer, C.J. and Dougherty, T.J. Identification of singlet oxygen as the cytotoxic agent in photoactivation of a murine tumor. Cancer Res 1976, 36(7): 2326-2639). Additionally, studies show that **a strong inflammatory response can contribute substantially to local tumor control when the PDT regimen is suboptimal** and local inflammation does not appear critical for tumor control under optimal PDT treatment conditions (Henderson, B.W., Gollnick, S.O., Synder, J.W., Busch, T.M., Kousis, P.C., Cheney, R.T. and Morgan, J. Choice of oxygen-conserving treatment regimen determines the inflammatory response and outcome of photodynamic therapy of tumors. Cancer Res 2004, 64(6): 2120-2126).

I find this work to be very convincing of the role of $^1O_2$ and possibly of the role of inflammatory cells with their production of ROS.

Phthalocyanines are of interest as they absorb color at longer wavelengths. This could permit increased tissue penetration to be used on more advanced tumors. However, there are still problems in the purification and handling of these compounds that still need further study.

5-aminolevulinic acid (ALA) works by enhancing a natural process in the body. ALA is a metabolic precursor to protoporphyrin IX, which is a natural photosynthesizer. Normally, protoporphyrin levels in the body are kept low, due to control mechanisms that keep ALA levels low. By administering additional ALA, protoporphyrin IX levels can be built up to phototoxic levels. **The dynamics of this natural photosynthesizer are different than the synthetic drugs, in that therapeutic levels are reached 2-4 hours after ALA administration, and are depleted rapidly from the body**. This means that there is not a problem of prolonged photosensitivity of the skin and eyes. Also, the treatment **can be repeated** frequently without the risk of damage to normal tissue.

29.6 PROSPECTS

One of the problems with photodynamic therapy has been the requirement for adequate oxygen. As a tumor grows, it can become poorly vascularized, leading to low cellular concentrations of oxygen. Researchers at the Gray Cancer Institute have come across a possible solution to the problem with the use of the plant hormone auxin, or indole-3-acetic acid (Folkes, L. and Wardman, P. Enhancing the efficacy of photodynamic cancer therapy by radicals from plant auxin (indole-3-acetic acid). Cancer Res 2003; 63(4): 776-779 Onco Link). They administered auxin together with a photosensitizer in a laboratory mammalian cell culture under low oxygen concentration conditions. The auxin was oxidized into free radicals, which further broke down forming reactive cytotoxins. However, results are still pending in clinical trials.

Since little is known about interactions of photodynamic drugs with chemotherapeutic drugs, work is proceeding in this area (Zimmerman, A. et. al. Effects of chlorine-mediated photodynamic therapy combined with fluropyrimidines in vitro and in a patient. Cancer Chemother Pharmacol 2003; 51(2): 147-154). All in all, PDT is limited only by man's creativity and imagination and his willingness to pursue discovery.

"The metabolic rhythm of life, the harmony exhibited by proteins, sugars, lipids and nucleic acids and the diurnal anabolic cellular grind are prima facie evidence of the presence of heretofore undefined and unidentified powerfully precise primeval forces which have interacted to propel mankind's evolutionary launch."

R. M. Howes, M.D., Ph.D.

5/27/04

"The R. M. Howes, M.D., Ph.D. Tribute to the Living/Breathing Cell"

The living /breathing cell is a heterogeneous isothermal conglomerate, containing a dynamic commingled biochemical infrastructure, held rather precariously, yet intentionally, in a most meaningful spatial conformation by lipid interlinks utilizing weak non-covalent and co-valent forces, and capable of assimilating nutrients and processing data during energy production. Stretching the laws of thermodynamics, it maintains steady states of oxygen free radicals and electronic excitation states far from equilibrium.

The living/breathing cell is :

> **Self-sustaining**
> **Self-contained**
> **Self-adjusting**
> **Self-assembling**
> **Self-medicating**
> **Self-healing**
> **Self-replicating**

Self-mutilating
Self-mutating
Self-terminating

It is an anti-chaotic, anti-entropy living unit, one hundred trillionth of the whole man, which carries on to-and-fro cross talk within itself and throughout the whole, all for the sake of self-survival. As I grapple with its spiritual overtones, I am awe-struck by its biochemical beauty and inspired by its will to live and thus, to win.

The living /breathing cell is home to the savant of living matter and to the pundit of protoplasm.

"The metabolic rhythm of life, the harmony exhibited by proteins, sugars, lipids and nucleic acids and the diurnal anabolic cellular grind are prima facie evidence of the presence of heretofore undefined and unidentified powerfully precise primeval forces which have interacted to propel mankind's evolutionary launch."
R. M. Howes, M.D., Ph.D.

5/27/04

PART VI - SINGLET OXYGEN

30 HYPERICIN

30.1 BACKGROUND

The cytotoxic effects of photoactive chemicals were first recognized in cattle that had eaten a plant containing hypericin. Reportedly, **it had been observed that cattle that had consumed Hypericum perforatum and remained in direct sunlight became ill and would die; whereas, if the animal retreated to the shade of the barn, they would recover.**

Countless doses of hypericin have been safely taken by humans as an antidepressant for many years without any known harmful effects, including a lack of photosensitive reactions at these dosage levels. The daily dose if about 500mg of extract, which corresponds to a total dose of 1-2 mg of hypericin. Recent studies indicate that it may be hyperforin, not hypericin, that is responsible for the majority of the antidepressive effect.

Hypericin is a photochemical extracted from the St. John's Wort plant (Hypericum perforatum) and related species and has been shown to have potent, broad spectrum antimicrobial activity. Hypericin was found in 27 out of 36 evaluated Hypericum species and it is a perennial herb with golden yellow flowers (Kitanov, G.M. Hypericin and pseudohypericin in some Hypericum species. Biochem Syst Ecol 2001; 29: 171-178). This can only make one wonder why such a high concentration of a photosensitive compound is present and is so widely distributed within the species, unless it has an unknown beneficial effect.

Traditionally, a photosensitizer is a chemical compound that generates superoxide radicals in a Type I reaction or **singlet oxygen molecules in a Type II reaction in the presence of light and oxygen.** The Type I reaction may subsequently lead to the formation of hydrogen peroxide, **singlet oxygen** or hydroxyl radicals. **These reactive oxygen species or oxygen modifications are generally felt to be responsible for cellular death following photodynamic therapy (PDT),** even though there is a release of cytokines and other mediators of inflammation from treated cells. Nonetheless, **PDT is a method of treatment that combines minimal systemic toxicity with a highly selective photodynamic destruction of tumor cells.** Although PDT is ideal for the treatment for superficial skin lesions, it is also the subject of intense study for the treatment of early young cancer, bladder cancer, esophageal cancer, brain cancer, head and neck cancer and cancers of the eye and ovary. PDT is currently an accepted method used to treat skin cancer such as, basal and squamous cell carcinoma, Kaposi's sarcoma and T cell lymphoma.

30.1.1 Virucidal Activity

Hypericin is believed to be the most powerful photosensitizer found in nature. It is an aromatic polycyclic anthrone which is a class of colored or pigmented chemical substances which have **strong photosensitizing activity.** Hypericin produces a bright fluorescence and is a potent photosensitizing agent with a **high singlet oxygen quantum yield** (Ehrenberg, B., Anderson, J.L. and Foote, C.S. Kinetics and yield of singlet oxygen photosensitized by hypericin in organic and biological media. Photochem. Photobiol 1998; 68: 135-140), (Redmond, R.W. and Gamlin, J.N. A compilation of singlet oxygen yields from biologically relevant molecules. Photochem Photobiol 1990; 70: 391-475), and minimal dark toxicity (Jacobson, J.M., Feinman, L., Liebes, L., Ostrow, N., Tobia, A., Cabana, B.E., Lee, D., Spritzler, J. and Prince, A.M. Pharmacokinetics, safety and antiviral effects of hypericin, a derivative of St. John's wort plant, in patients with chronic hepatitis C virus infection. Antimicrob Agents Chemother 2001; 45: 517-524). In both in vitro and in vivo animal studies, low, **non-toxic doses of hypericin significantly inhibited the replication of several viruses, includ- ing HIV, influenza A, cytomegalovirus (CMV), Herpes simplex 1 and 2 (HSV-1 and HSV-2), and Epstein-Barr virus (EBV**).

St. John's Wort has **usually been used as an antidepressant** which may act as a monamine oxidase inhibitor (MAO). The psychotropic effects attributed to hypericin suggest that the pigment compound can cross the blood brain barrier. Its administration should be monitored by a physician but the levels found in most commercially available extracts of St. John's Wort generally are not sufficient to be theoretically effective against viral infections.

Quantity and quality of hypericin content in the plants varies according to geographical locale, climate, time of the day and time of the year. St. John's Wort contains dianthrone derivatives, mainly in the form of hypericin and pseu- dohypericin as well as flavonoids. Also present are small amounts of coumarins, phenolic carboxylic compounds, phloroglucinol derivatives, monoterpenes, sesquiterpenes, n-alkanes, n-alkanols, carotenoids, and beta-sitosterol. The roots contain zanthones.

In vitro and in vivo pre-clinical studies suggest that hypericin and pseudohypericin may have thera- peutic benefits for HIV infection and other retroviral diseases. The plant's **extract antibiotic and antiretroviral activity has been primarily attributed to hypericin** (Jayasuriya, H, et al. Antimicrobial and cytotoxic activity of rottlerin-type compounds from Hypericum Drummond, J Nat Prod 1989; 52(2): 325-31), (Valentine, F.T. Hypericin: A hex hydroxyl dimethyl-napthodiantrone with activity against HIV in vitro and against murine retroviruses in vivo, JAIDS 1991; 4(3): 317), (Hudson, J.B., et al. Antiviral activities of hypericin. Antiviral Research. 1991; 15(2): 101-112), (Kraus, G.A. Antiretroviral activity of synthetic hypericin and related analogues. Biochem and Biophy Research Comm 1990; 172(1): 149-153), (James, J.S. 1991 Hypericin Update. AIDS Treatment News #125). General hypericin data was reviewed by A. Y. Oubre in an article entitled, "Hypericin: the active ingredient in St. John's Wort" at www.lifelinknet.com web site.

30.1.2 Animal Studies

With in vitro and in vivo studies, both hypericin and pseudohypericin (extracted from Hypericum triquetifolium) had antiviral activity against several retroviruses (Meruelo, D., et al. Therapeutic agents with dramatic antiretrovi- ral activity and little toxicity at effective doses: Aromatic polycyclic diones hypericin and pseudohypericin. Proc. Natl Acad Sci USA. 1988; 85(14): 5230-5234). In one experiment, mice were simultaneously injected with low doses of the compounds and with Friend leukemia virus (FV). **This aggressive retrovirus normally causes rapid splenomegaly (swelling of the spleen) and acute erythroleukemia in mice. However, these symptoms were effectively suppressed by the addition of hypericin.** Splenomegaly had not occurred ten days after infection at the close of the study. No infectious virus could be recovered from the spleen. Also, vire- mia normally associated with FV was absent. **Mice treated with hypericin and pseudohypericin survived a much longer time than mice treated with toxic antiviral (N3dthd). Unlike most antiretroviral drugs, hypericin (given in a single dose of low concentration) was effective without being cytotoxic. Even when it was administered after viral infection had already started; it still inhibited the onset of disease.**

With in vitro studies, mouse cell lines were infected with radiation leukemia virus (Rad LV) and then incubated with hypericin. The activity of reverse transcriptase in these cells was suppressed through indirect mechanisms. In contrast to nucleoside analogues, polycyclic diones such as **hypericin interfere directly with the viral replica- tion cycle during stages in which virions are assembled or intact virions are shedded from immature cores.** Other **findings indicate that hypericin is able to inactivate virions and block viral release from infected cells by interacting with the cell membrane.**

Other investigations indicate that the antiviral effects of hypericin on murine cytomegalovirus (MCMV), Sindbus virus (SV) and HIV are enhanced by exposure to fluorescent light. Hypericin and to some degree, pseudohy- pericin, were effective against FV and HSV-1 when the viruses were first incubated with the compounds for one hour at 37⁰ C before mice were infected. Pre-incubation for one hour at 4⁰ C, however, produced no antiviral effects. The authors of this study (who are scientists at Lilly Research Laboratories) reported that hypericin and pseudohypericin were effective in vitro against enveloped viruses such as HSV and influenza when the cultures were pre-incubated with these agents at 37⁰ C. **They also correctly showed that hypericin and its analogue inhibit DNA and RNA viruses, but not viruses which lack a lipid envelope.**

30.1.3 Site of Activity

Hypericin and pseudohypericin had no effect on purified reverse transcriptase alone. They did not alter levels of intracellular viral mRNA. Instead, hypericin lowers the number of mature viral particles without suppressing intracellular levels of viral mRNA. The concentrations of viral antigens on the cell surface were also unaffected by hypericin. These findings, as a whole, imply that **the compounds interfere with viral assembly, budding, shedding or stability at the level of the cell membrane**. When hypericin was added to viral infected cell cultures, red fluorescence appeared to localized areas on the lipid surface membrane (Lavie, G., et al. Studies of the mechanisms of action of the antiretroviral agents hypericin and pseudohypericin. Proc Natl Acad Sci USA. 1989; 86(15): 5963-5967).

Cumulative studies demonstrate that PDT with hypericin inhibits protein kinase C (PKC) and other growth factor stimulated **protein kinases induces peroxidation** of membrane lipids, increases superoxide dismutase activity and decreases cellular glutathione levels, impairs mitochondria functions, cross-links the molten globule form of acetylcholinesterase, but not the native protein and causes photooxidation of lens alpha-crystalline.

Unlike nucleoside analogues, **polycyclic diones such as hypericin** have no effects on transcription, translation or transport of viral proteins to the cell membrane. They are not directly active against reverse transcriptase even though reverse transcriptase activity was reduced in infected cells that had first been incubated with hypericin. Cells treated with hypericin form immature or abnormally assembled cores. This indicates that hypericin may block the processing of gag-encoded precursor polypeptides. Hypericin, whether in the intracellular medium or bounded to the membrane, is thought to lower the activity of reverse transcriptase by interfering with protein synthesis.

Some investigators, however, propose that hypericin lyses the infectious virion by interacting directly with the viral envelope instead of disrupting gag-encoded precursor polyproteins or modifying other proteins. In any case, **the antiviral properties of hypericin appear to involve its interactions with the cell membrane or cell surface recognition sites** (Liebes, L., et al. A method for the quantitation of hypericin, an antiviral agent in biological fluids by high performance liquid chromatography. Analytical Biochem 1991; 195: 77-85). Such therapies may be able to block HIV-encoded protease located in the gag-pol region. Importantly, drugs of this type would not be toxic like AZT and other agents whose pharmacological actions are based on direct inhibition of reverse transcriptase.

The aromatic, ringed structure encircled by six phenolic hydroxy groups seems critical to the antiviral activity of the hypericin molecule. Quinone groups, which often have antiviral properties, also exert photodynamic effects. **Hypericin is thought to generate singlet oxygen. However, free radical quenchers can interfere with singlet oxygen reactions involving hypericin thereby reducing its antiviral properties.**

Hypericin has a unique molecular structure in which one-half of the molecule is hydrophilic (water loving) while the other half are hydrophobic (water repelling). The top, bottom and side (non-polar) of the hypericin molecule which contains the methyl groups are hydrophobic. It is thought that the molecule might bond to the outer surface of the cell membrane. Presumably, the hydrophobic side would be immersed in fat. **Singlet oxygen, though more reactive than triplet oxygen, binds with two electron targets, including, for example, the double bonds found in polyunsaturated fatty acids.** The hydrophilic sides, in contrast, could hydrogen-bond to the aqueous media (Gerhardt, J.J. and Fowkes, S.W. Hypericin Forefront. Palo Alto: MegaHealth Society 1991; 6(6): 1-5).

30.1.4 Light Activation

Light is required for the photosensitization of hypericin. **The compound absorbs light quanta and generates it in the form of singlet oxygen.** In so doing, hypericin triggers the photooxidation of cellular components, including, for example, the photohemolysis of red blood cells. The underlying mechanism of photodynamic reactions is not fully understood. It is thought to involve interactions between oxygen and light as well as sensitizing pigment which binds to the cell membrane (Duran, N. and Song, P. Hypericin and its photodynamic action. Photochem Photobio 1986; 43(6): 677-680).

In photodynamic reactions mediated by hypericin, singlet oxygen serves as the main oxidant. Singlet oxygen has strong affinity for pi electron-systems found in compounds such as polycyclic diones. The pi electrons, responsible for the photoactive properties of hypericin, absorb visible and ultraviolet light and then reemit it within the range of green and red light. Pi electrons therefore, seem to play a major role in the antiviral activity of hypericin.

The "impressive light-mediated antiviral activities" of hypericin have been shown in several studies. Sindbus virus (SV), for example, was 99% inhibited in the presence of light. In the dark, however, the antiviral effects of hypericin were reduced by more than two orders of magnitude. **On the exposure to light (650-700 nm.), hypericin undergoes Type II photosensitization in which singlet oxygen** and other reactive molecular species are produced. **Though not as destructive as free radicals (which are generated in Type I photosensitization, singlet oxygen could damage viral membranes**, thereby interfering with proteins and nucleic acids. Nonetheless, hypericin also has some degree of virucidal activity in the dark, though much less so than in light. It is thought that the antiviral effects produced in the absence of light take place through a different mode of action than light-mediated virucidal activity.

30.2 TUMORICIDAL ACTIVITY

Hypericin has created great interest as a tumoricidal agent due to its triplet quantum yield and its efficient generation of singlet oxygen and superoxide anions (Thomas, C., MacGill, R.S., Miller, G.C. and Pardini, R.S. Photoactivation of hypericin generates singlet oxygen in mitochondria and inhibits succinoxidase. Photochem Photobiol 1992; 55: 47-53). This hypericin-PDT reaction is thought to be oxygen-dependent and is supported by the fact that **hypericin does not exhibit photocytotoxicity under hypoxic conditions** (Thomas, C. and Pardini, R.S. Oxygen dependence of hypericin-induced photo toxicity to EMT6 mouse mammary carcinoma cells. Photochem Photobiol 1992; 55: 831-837), (Delaey, E.M., Vandenbogaerde, A.L., Merlevede, W.J. and de Witte, P.A.M. Photocytotoxicity of hypericin in oxic and hypoxic conditions. J. Photochem Photobiol B 2000; 56: 19-24), and it did not cause a mitochondrial inhibitory effect.

Repeatedly, studies have shown that singlet oxygen, which is generated via a Type II mechanism, has the major role with its tumoricidal photosensitive activity. Cancer cell studies indicate that hypericin accumulates in the membranes of the endoplasmic reticulum and the Golgi complex but seems to be excluded from mitochondria. This organelle distribution appears to be dependent on the cancer cell type (Vandenbogaerde, A.L., Cuveele, J.F., Proot, P., Himpens, B.E., Merlevede, W.J. and de Witte, P.A.M. Differential cytotoxic effects induced after photosensitization by hypericin. J Photochem Photobiol B 1997; 38: 136-142). Even though hypericin is excluded from the mitochondrion **it causes inhibition of mitochondrial succinoxidase, a decrease in the respiratory control ratio and a drop in the mitochondrial membrane potential** and it therefore appears to be a primary cellular site for photocytotoxicity.

30.2.1 Apoptosis and Necrosis

Cell death usually occurs by either apoptosis or necrosis. Cellular suicide or apoptosis is an orderly and regulated process; whereas, necrosis is less defined and is a more rapid form of cell death following physical or chemical damage. Cells undergoing apoptosis exhibit a quite distinct and profound set of coordinated structural changes that are characteristic of this process and independent from the death signal that originally induced them. The dying cell typically shrinks, widespread membrane blebbing occurs, followed by chromatin condensation and genomic DNA fragmentation. The cell further disassembles into membrane-enclosed vesicles called apoptotic bodies that are rapidly and cleanly ingested by neighboring cells and phagocytes. Therefore, **during apoptosis, the cellular content is never accessible to the immune system, thus, minimizing the occurrence of inflammatory reactions.** Necrosis is characterized by swelling of the entire cytoplasm and organelles which causes the plasma membrane to burst. **Since the cellular content is spilled extracellular, necrotic cell death evokes invariably an inflammatory response** (Fiers, W., Beyaert, R., Declercq, W. and Vandenabeele, P. More than one way to die: Apoptosis, necrosis and reactive oxygen damage. Oncogene 1999; 18: 7719-7730).

It now appears that each cell has its own innate capacity to trigger its own death when it is given the correct signal and it is known that malignant cells have an impaired ability to undergo apoptosis (Ellis, R.E., Yuan, J. and Horvitz, H.R., Mechanisms and functions of cell death. Ann. Rev Cell Biol 1991; 7: 663-689). It has been suggested **that hypericin-mediated PKC inhibition is the apoptotic triggering event** in same cells (Hamilton, H.B., Hinton, D.R., Law, R.E., Gopalakrishna, R., Zu, Y.Z., Chen, Z.H., Weiss, M.H. and Couldwell, W.T. Inhibition of cellular growth and induction of apoptosis in pituitary adenoma cell lines by the protein kinase inhibitor hypericin: Potential therapeutic application. J Neurosurg 1996; 85: 329-334). **Studies with hypericin PDT now show that many signaling pathways are involved in apoptosis of different cancer cell lines.** Different photosensitizers with different irradiation protocols and with different levels of oxygenation tend to complicate the interpretation of the data. However, **it is generally accepted that singlet oxygen, produced by the Type II reaction, is the agent responsible for cancer cell apoptosis or necrosis.**

Singlet oxygen site of origin is of importance because of its short half-life (<0.04 us) and because of its limited range of diffusion (Moan, J. and Berg, K. The photodegradation of porphyrins in cells can be used to estimate the lifetime of singlet oxygen. Photochem Photobiol 1991; 53: 549-553). **The photo-dynamic killing of cancer cells by hypericin-PDT is very efficient** but whether or not the cell dies from apoptosis or necrosis mechanisms and pathways is dependent upon cell type and a multitude of signaling events.

30.2.2 Pathway Complexities

The factors involved in both apoptotic and necrotic mechanisms of cell death have grown to stagger-ing levels of complexity, making data interpretation evermore difficult as the number of potential variables increases. This is readily exemplified by the following excerpts from a review in the current literature, (Agostinis, P., Vantieghem, A., Merlevede, W. and de Witte, P.A.M. Hypericin in cancer treatment: More light on the way. Internat J Biochem & Cell Biol 2002; 34(3): 221-241).

30.2.3 The Apoptotic Pathway in Hypericin-PDT

Burgeoning biochemical and genetic studies have firmly established the critical role of the caspase family of cyste-inyl proteases in the execution of the apoptotic program and revealed the existence of at least two major death pathways leading to their activation. The extrinsic pathway of caspase activation originates at the cell surface and is triggered by the binding of death ligands, including TNF-alpha (tumor necrosis factor-alpha), TRAIL (tumor ne-crosis factor-related apoptosis-inducing ligand) and Fas ligand (FasL)/CD95L, to their receptors. This event leads to receptor clustering and association of adapter proteins (e.g., Fas-associated death domain protein (FADD)) that recruit initiator caspases. The autocatalytic processing and activation of procaspase-8 initiates a caspase activation cascade leading to the downstream effector caspases (Ashkenazi, A. and Dixit, V.M. Apoptosis control by death and decoy receptors. Curr Opin Cell Biol 1999; 11: 255-260). Alternatively, caspases can be activated by an in-trinsic pathway, triggered by various environmental insults and developmental programs, which initiates inside the cell at the level of the mitochondria. This pathway is thought to be triggered by the release of cytochrome c and other apoptogenic proteins from the mitochondrial intermembrane space into the cytosol. Cytosolic cytochrome c acts as a cofactor in the formation of a complex with Apaf-1, procaspase-9, dATP/ATP (apoptosome) leading to the activation of caspase-9. **Active caspase-9 then leads to the activation of the executioner caspases and cell death commitment** (Green, D.R. and Reed, J.C. Mitochondria and apoptosis. Science 1998; 281: 1309-1312). Both pathways converge into the activation of effector caspases (e.g., caspase-3, -6 and -7) which, by cleaving several vital substrates, orchestrate the catabolic events that give rise to the characteristic phenotype of the apoptotic cells.

The processing of the pro-apoptotic Bcl-2 family member Bid, by mature caspase- 8 induces its transloca-tion to mitochondria where the C-terminal Bid fragment promotes cytochrome c release, thereby providing a positive amplification loop between the extrinsic and intrinsic pathway of caspase activation.

Mitochondrial damage has been recognized as one of the first events to occur in photosensitized cells and hence, it has been suggested to play a crucial role in the initiation of the apoptotic program by PDT. Consistently, photosensitization of human cervical carcinoma HeLa and rat/mouse T cell hybridoma (PC60) cell lines with hypericin was shown to result in the release of mitochondrial cytochrome c into the cytosol, followed by a sharp increase in the activity of procaspase-9/procaspase-3 and poly (ADP-ribose) polymerase (PARP) cleavage.

The view that hypericin-PDT activates the mitochondrial pathway of caspase activation is further reinforced by the findings that caspase3 directed peptide inhibitors as well as the specific over expression of X-linked inhibitor of apoptosis protein (XIAP0, a member of the IAP family of caspase inhibitors which preferentially suppresses the activation of caspase-9, -3 and -7 (Deveraux, Q.L. and Reed, J.C. IAP family proteins: Suppressors of apoptosis. Genes Dev 1999; 13: 239-252), significantly counteract the onset of apoptosis. In addition, since HeLa and PC60 cells stably over expressing the cytokine response modifier A (CrmA), a potent viral inhibitor of caspase-8 and -1, are fully susceptible to hypericin photokilling, we (Agostinis, et al.), concluded that signals triggered by the activation of death receptors are dispensable for the induction of apoptosis by hypericin-PDT. Consistently in these systems, no procaspase-8 activation/processing nor Bid cleavage, has been observed.

In many, if not all scenarios, **apoptosis is accompanied by loss of the mitochondrial membrane potential (MMP),** which is caused by a sudden increase in the permeability of the inner mitochondrial membrane to ions and solutes, a phenomenon called the **permeability transition (PT).** As a result of PT, the electrochemical gradient across the inner membrane is dissipated leading to uncoupling **of the respiratory chain**. PT is believed to be mediated by a cyclosporine A-sensitive opening of a mitochondrial mega channel, called **mitochondria permeability transition (MPT) pore**, whose protein composition is still obscure.

30.2.4 Hypericin-PDT-Induced Signaling Pathways Associated with Cell Survival

Recently, several signaling events were found to be associated with PDT-induced apoptosis. These include events involving alteration of regulatory enzymes, such as phospholipases, mitogen-activated protein kinase (MAPK), cyclin-dependent kinases and events involving the generation of second messengers such as PIP and ceramide. Relatively little is known about the induction of gene expression in response to PDT in general. It has, however, been established that **the oxidative stress generated by PDT is a transcriptional inducer of early response genes (c-fos, c-jun, c-myc, egr-1), and of gene associated with cytokine expression (IL-6 and IL-10) and stress responses, such as thermo-tolerance.**

Critical components of eukaryotic signal transduction pathways are protein kinases, and in particular the Ser/Thr MAPK, which are the central components of an evolutionarily well conserved module, typically composed of three kinases that establish a sequential activation pathway comprising of MAP kinase kinase kinase (MAPKKK), a MAP kinase kinase (MAPKK) and a MAPK. MAPK is found in all eukaryotic organisms and although they can regulate cytoplasmic targets, their ultimate role is to transmit extracellular signals to the nucleus where the transcription of specific genes is induced by phosphorylation and activation of transcription factors. Three distinct MAPK pathways have been exhaustively characterized in mammalian cells: the extracellular signal-regulated kinase (ERK) cascade, the c-Jun N-terminal kinase (JNK; also called the stress-activated protein kinase, SAPK0 cascade and the p38 MAP kinase cascade (Lewis, T.S., Shapiro, P.S. and Ahn, N.G. Signal transduction through MAP kinase cascades. Adv Cancer Res 1998; 74: 49-139). The ERK pathway typically transduces mitogenic signals whereas the NJK and p38 MAPK activation cascades are activated mainly in response to a variety of stress-stimuli. Although many stress-signals that cause JNK and p38 MAPK activation eventually lead to apoptosis, the physiological role of these kinases is highly variable and seems to depend on the kind of stress and on the cell type (Kyriakis, J.M. Making the connection: Coupling of stress-activated ERK/MAPK (extracellular-signal-regulate kinases/mitogen-activated protein kinase) core signaling modules to extracellular stimuli and biological responses. Biochem Soc Symp 1999; 64: 29-48).

In spite of the heightened interest in studying the importance of the MAPK for apoptosis, little is known concerning the potential involvement of these kinases in apoptosis induced by PDT.

The distribution data indicate that the PDT efficacy and potency of hypericin correlate well with the plasma concentrations rather than with the overall concentrations in the tumor. Significantly, a fluorescence microscopic study showed that complete to near complete tumor eradication is achieved only when high extravascular hypericin concentrations are present at the time of photoactivation (Chen, B., Zupko, I. and de Witte, P.A.M. Photodynamic therapy with hypericin in a mouse P388 tumor model: Vascular effects determine the efficacy. Int J Oncol 2001; 18: 737-742). It can therefore be assumed that **the antitumor effect of hypericin-PDT originates from the severe induced damage of the tumor vascular endothelial cells, resulting in the collapse of the entire microcirculation system**. Consequently, the persistent tumor ischemia contributes largely to the overall tumor ablation. Of interest, it could also be shown that **the tumor response to hypericin-PDT in anemic tumor-bearing mice is dramatically reduced, thereby proving the importance of oxygen as a mediator of the PDT effects**.

30.2.5 Conclusions

Hypericin-PDT is showing great promise in the treatment of basal and squamous cell carcinoma, recurrent mesothelioma, glioma, pituitary adenoma, bladder cancer, cutaneous T cell lymphoma, psoriasis and warts. Due to the fact that hypericin is not metabolized by mammalian cells (Vandenbogaerde, A.L., Delaey, E.M., Vantieghem, A.M., Himpens, B.E., Merlevede, W.J. and de Witte, P.A.M. Cytotoxicity and anti-proliferative effect of hypericin and derivatives after photosensitization. Photochem Photobiol 1998; 67: 119-125), and due to its fluorescence it is being investigated as a method to detect in situ neoplasms.

Hypericin is proving to be a powerful virucidal and tumoricidal agent which is likely operating via excited delta singlet molecular oxygen.

"Scare tactics of the oxy-morons have spawned a generation of oxy-phobes, who believe that ground state oxygen, itself, is a diabolical "toxin," which only acts as a catabolic cellular assassin."

R. M. Howes, M.D., Ph. D.

5/9/04

30.3 DIOXYGEN CHEMISTRY (TRIPLET OXYGEN)

The biochemical importance of oxygen is manifested as its role as the terminal acceptor of electrons, whose **reactions generate 95% of the energy requirements for aerobic life**. Nature has established a fundamental cycle whereby aerobic metabolism utilizes oxygen plus organic sugars to produce water and ATP. The plant kingdom utilized CO_2, water and sunlight to produce oxygen and ATP and thereby captures the light energy of the sun to maintain a steady-state concentration of oxygen while producing a continuous stream of ATP.

Oxygen is one of the few compounds that exists in a triplet state and in this ground state it has low reactivity. The periodic table shows other oxidizers, the chalcogens such as O, S, Se, Te, and the halogens, F, B, Cl, I, but they do not equal the suitability of oxygen. Fluorine is extremely reactive in attacking -C-H bonds, making it unsuitable as a controlled terminal oxidant. The less reactive halogens, chlorine and bromine unfortunately react with water to form hypochlorous and hypobromous acids, respectively. The other elements in the Groups VI and VII of the periodic table are poor oxidants.

Oxygen is an abundant gas which has a low solubility in water and a high solubility in non-polar, organic solvents such as CCl_4. Still, **oxygen provides a large free energy of combustion but it is kinetically inert and does not react spontaneously**. However, this poor reactivity is ultimately a very desirable property.

30.3.1 Singlet vs. Triplet States

Molecular oxygen is officially called **"dioxygen."** To distinguish the molecule from the atom. Dioxygen has 16 electrons and is a homonuclear diatomic with two unpaired electrons in its outer most valence orbits. Molecules with two electrons in the outer shell have them arranged in a number of different ways. If the electrons are in the same orbital, they must have opposite spins. There is only one magnetic moment derived from electrons in the same orbital and this is known as **the singlet state**. The first 14 electrons added fill the lowest seven levels and are all paired. The last two electrons enter the uppermost anti- bonding pair of levels. **These last two valence electrons are not paired and ground state oxygen molecule contains two unpaired electrons. It is a TRIPLET state molecule.**

With enough energy, normal triplet oxygen can be converted to singlet oxygen. When the energy involved is considered, a rule states that compounds in **one state can not react with compounds in another state.** In this case, the phrase "can not react," is really a statement of probability. Reactions between compounds in different states can occur, but only very slowly. **Photosynthetic pigments are capable of converting ground state triplet oxygen into the excited singlet state by the addition of 23 Kcal/mole.**

There are three ways in which the last two electrons can be installed or structured:

1. **Triplet or ground state oxygen** (unpaired electrons and thus, a **diradical**).
2. A species of singlet oxygen (**singlet delta state**), a relatively long lived and **gives off red light** when returning to triplet or ground state (paired electrons, **non-radical**).

3. A second species of singlet oxygen (**singlet sigma state**), very unstable and short lived. Triplet and singlet mean two and zero unpaired electrons, respectively. Sigma **gives off blue light** upon relaxation to ground state (paired electrons, **non-radical**).

Each arrangement has a different magnetic moment and all three have been detected and identified. **With energy addition, triplet oxygen can be converted to singlet oxygen. Hund's rule states that compounds in one state can not react with compounds in another state** (technically, that the probability of reactions between states is very low and rare). **When oxygen is in the singlet state, the reaction is said to be 1450-1500 times faster than with triplet state oxygen.** Some photosensitizing pigments are **chlorophyll, hematoporphyrin and flavin.** Some photosensitizing dyes are **methylene blue, rose Bengal, eosin, crystal violet and acridine orange.** Singlet oxygen is a high energy, electron-spin paired state of dioxygen that is approximately 1eV higher in energy than ground state triplet oxygen and is capable of oxidizing a number of biological molecules, including lipid and olefinic containing molecules in vitro.

30.3.2 Dioxygen Redox Reactions

Addition of the first electron to oxygen is very difficult requiring -0.6v and produces a product called the superoxide anion (O_2^{-}). Addition of two electrons results in closing this subshell and is a favorable reaction for a total free energy of 0.6v. The product is formally called the dianion of peroxide ($O_2^{=}$), which is readily protonated to yield H_2O_2. **The addition of more electrons requires that the electron occupy the antibonding sigma orbital and the molecule dissociates.**

Addition of the third electron is not difficult and the free energy is about 0.4v. The bond between the two oxygen atoms breaks and produces the oxide (or its protonated form, hydroxide) and **the hydroxyl radical (OH.) which is an extremely powerful oxidizing reagent** which simultaneously reacts with any carbon center in its vicinity. **The hydroxyl radical is deemed to be highly toxic and to be the agent responsible for the alleged toxicity of oxygen in many disease conditions.** The addition of the fourth electron forms water (H_2O) and **the overall reduction of oxygen to water is extremely favorable at 0.8 volts/electron or 3.2 volts for the overall four-electron process.**

The step **for the first addition of an electron to oxygen is the most difficult to implement because of the energetic barrier.** This fact explains oxygen's ground state stability and if it did not exist, **we would spontaneously combust!** In addition to the energy barrier which inhibits 1-electron reactions, there is a kinetic barrier which ensures that the energetically favorable two-electron reactions do not proceed.

For the reactions to be facile the **Law of Spin Conservation requires that there is no change in the total spin of the system as it passes from reactants to products** and because of oxygen's unusual spin, this constraint is difficult to meet. Therefore the 1-electron reduction of oxygen to superoxide is kinetically allowed but thermodynamically forbidden: the 2-electron reduction to peroxide is thermodynamically allowed but kinetically forbidden. Thus, **in the absence of catalysts (enzymes), oxygen is an unreactive molecule at physiological temperatures.**

30.3.3 Oxygen Factoids

Normally, oxygen exists as a bound pair of atoms or a diradical. Unbound oxygen is referred to as a **"singlet of oxygen,"** which is **to distinguish atomic or elemental oxygen from electronically excited molecular metastable singlet oxygen (singlet oxygen).** It is the bound gas which is an essential for human life, although it is reported that some small amounts of "singlets of oxygen" are also produced during normal metabolism. Please keep in mind the fact that ground state oxygen is relatively stable and unreactive and it is only when electrons are exchanged or have their spin or orbitals altered do we see the phenomenon of life manifested. Basically, stable atoms and molecules are not participating in life rendering energetics and atoms and molecules of non-change (stable) are more associated with conditions characteristic of "dead" or inanimate objects. **Living/breathing entities**

are products of "change:" changing energy potentials, changing electronic configurations, chang-ing membrane potentials, changes in proton osmosis, changing gene regulators, changing intra- and inter-cellular signaling, changing electron orbitals and changing numbers of valence electrons. It is these changes which burn the organic fuels to provide the energy of life. I submit that these changes sustain the life forces and these are the changes that are associated with free radicals, reactive oxygen species, active oxygen species, reactive oxygen metabolites, active oxygen intermediates and electronic excitation states. **Stable and non-changing electrons, atoms and molecules are the hallmark of states of death or of inanimate objects. Life is a state of change.**

Free radicals are defined as any species capable of independent existence (hence the term "free") that contains one or more unpaired electrons. **These highly maligned species are the ones that make life, as we know it, possible.** Yet, current literature is obsessed with the idea that, specifically, oxygen free radicals are the harbingers of all death and disease. Quite to the contrary, the **oxygen free radicals give us life.**

In fact, reactive oxygen species are now being found to be produced in many cells of the body on an ongoing ba-sis, at rates which were previously unappreciated. These **oxygen modifications (RONS/excytomers) are responsible for ever-increasing important cellular regulatory and signaling processes of normal me-tabolism and for controlling the cellular life cycle.** Thus, **free radical "leaks" seems naïve, at best and at worst, the oxidative stress theory appears out and out wrong.**

At the Nov. 21, 2003 meeting of the Society of Free Radical Biology and Medicine, Dr. Irwin Fridovich presented a glimpse into the evolution of the free radical hypothesis of chronic disease and aging (which I now, tongue and cheek, refer to as the free radi-crap theory of aging and oxidative stress). However, his prior graduate student, **Dr. Joe McCord, (Webb-Warring Institute,** University of Colorado), **discussed the shift in paradigm from viewing reactive oxygen species as cytotoxic species to their more subtle roles as second messen-gers or modulators of metabolic pathways.** He proposed that a physiological role of superoxide may be for the modulation of lipid peroxidation.

30.3.4 Oxygen Miscellaneous Factoids
(Referenced and Un-Referenced)

-Lungs have 300 million alveolar sacs.

-90% of cellular oxygen is consumed by the mitochondrial electron transport system.

-We consume approximately each day: 3.5 kg of oxygen,
of which, 2.8% (2-5%) forms free radicals

RMH Note: figures vary as to the % of free radical formation.

-It is like being irradiated at low levels all the time.

-Free radicals in vivo are in the pico molar range 10^{-12} (Lam).

-An adult uses the equivalent of 250 ml of pure O_2/min

15,000 ml/hr
360,000 ml/day or 360 liters of pure O_2/day
131,400,000/yr

-Only 1.5% O_2 is dissolved in plasma.

-Paramagnetic - unpaired electronic spins; O_2 has 2 unpaired electrons and they have the same spin state (direc-tion) and is a barrier to insertion of a pair of electrons. Therefore, O_2 has to have electrons added one at a time.

-Exercise increase O_2 consumption 10-20 fold to 35-70 ml/kg/min of which 2.5% forms free radicals, or 0.6 to 3.5 ml/kg/min free radicals produced in exercise.

-The electrons seem to escape at the ubiquinone-cytochrome c level (Sjodin, 1990).

-We breathe 10-20 liters/min of O_2 (air), 21% O_2.

- ATP anaerobic production requires almost 20-fold increases in glucose utilization compared to aerobic ATP production.

- **Numerous studies have shown that the degree of PMN bactericidal function is directly dependent on oxygen tensions.**

- Oxygen independent killing can occur with lysosomes, acidic vacuoles and lactoferrin, but they are less efficient and vary according to the organism.

- Aminoglycosides such as gentamicin, tobramycin, amikacin and netilmicin are **oxygen dependent** for antimicrobial activity. Sulfonamides antimicrobial effect is **potentially by hyperbaric oxygen.**

- There is no direct antimicrobial effect of enhanced O_2 on aerobic organisms. Indirect antimicrobial effects are related to improved PMN function in killing bacteria. **RMH Note: It is not ground state O_2, but rather RONS/ excytomers which do the killing.**

- Each cell contains hundreds of mitochondria, each contains thousands of mtDNA in the cytoplasm and is maternally inherited.

- Mitochondrial diseases commonly involve tissue with high energy requirements: heart, muscle, renal and endocrine systems.

-**Lung capacity decreases 5% with every decade of life.**

-At sea level, each breath is about 500 ml and contains about 21% O_2.

-Pressure at sea level is 760 mm Hg for air and partial pressure at sea level of O_2 is 160 mm Hg.

-Partial pressure of alveolar air is 100 mm Hg.

-Partial pressure of pulmonary arteries is 40 mm Hg.

-Thus, oxygen diffuses into venous blood to red cells and hemoglobin.

-Hgb leaving the lung is 98% saturated with O_2.

-Hgb in one liter of blood is about 200 ml, of which 50 ml (25%) is extracted each pass through the capillaries.

-A 60 kg man requires 200-250 ml of pure O_2 per minute.

-Human suffocation occurs at around 7% O_2.

-Johnson found in rabbits, that 0.01 volume of 0.12% H_2O_2 caused gas embolism and completely shut down capillary blood flow.

-100 ml of plasma at 100 mm Hg can hold only 0.3 ml of O_2.

-**Thus, a 60 kg adult has about 20 ml O_2 in their plasma.**

-Our body is at least 80% H_2O which is, which is 8/9 oxygen. Thus, we are composed of over 2/3 oxygen, twice as much as everything else in us combined.

- **O_2 is the most common free radical, having 2 unpaired electrons.**

- Oxygenation refers to increasing O_2 content and O_2 supply refers to the O_2 available.

-Oxygen and nitrous oxide are the only important biological molecules that exist in a triplet ground state.

-**O_2 concentration is 0.07 mM in living tissue.**

-A few puffs on a cigarette will reduce your oxygen absorbing capability by about 25%.

RMH Note: I believe that this oxygen reduction "allows" for development of a wide variety of diseases and cancer.

-A mitochondrion "breathes in," O_2 and pyruvic acid into the Kreb's cycle to produce ATP. When a mitochondrion "breathes out" it releases ATP, H_2O_2, and CO_2 into the cytoplasm. ATP is especially important to neurons because in a resting human about 40% of total energy consumption is used to operate the "pumps" that keep certain ions (e.g., Na^+, K^+), either inside or outside of the neurons to regulate their excitability. This is why the brain is so sensitive to damage by O_2 deprivation or reduction in ATP.

-The brain has about 100 billion cells (neurons), each connected to about 1000 other cells (this is probably a low estimate).

RMH Note: In the brain, O_2 is the energy source that produces and promotes consciousness. The brain is a "heavy breather" using 20% of the body's total O_2 intake.

-Normal tissue O_2 gradient is from 2-5% across a 400 mm distance from a blood supply. Tumor cells are hypoxic with cells adjacent to capillaries with an O_2 gradient of 2% and with cells located 200 mm from the nearest capillary have a mean O_2 concentration of 0.2%. Thus, tumors have increased lactic acid and other acids and it is an acidic environment.

-O_2 concentration is of the order of 0.07 mM in living tissue (Johan Moan, 2001).

-Mitochondrial O_2 partial pressure	0.5 mm Hg
-Tissue levels with hyperbaric O_2	1200 mm Hg
-Rabbit ear capillaries range	3-30 mm Hg
-Wounds range	30-50 mm Hg
-Chronic wounds range	5-20 mm Hg

RMH Note: My Unified Theory is supported by the fact that chronic wounds are associated with cancer. This is because the chronic wound does not have enough O_2 to kill bacteria and it certainly does not have enough O_2 with RONS to kill cancer cells.

-Molecular O_2 is the only homonuclear diatomic that has triplet spin multiplicity in its ground state ($^3\Sigma_g^-$).

- Oxygenation is usually exothermic and hence, can thermodynamically occur in every place on this planet. This means that organisms live under an oxidative environment.

- Aerobic respiration produces 686 kcal by complete oxidation of 1 mole glucose to CO_2 and H_2O; while fermentation releases only 47 kcal for conversion of 1 mole of glucose to lactate.

- O_2 is an absolute requirement for differentiation and it is more than an essential cofactor for aerobic metabolism.

-1 in 10^5 electrons (1:10,000) in respiratory transport chain is caught and produces $O_2^{.-}$.

-10^{12} O_2 molecules are consumed everyday.

-Skeletal muscle accounts for 20-30% of the total resting oxygen uptake and the brain takes 20%. **RMH Note: The incidence of skeletal muscle and brain cancer should therefore total 40% of the body cancer rate....but it does not.**

-Oxygen can be "our dangerous friend" (Passwater interview). **RMH Note: So could countless other compounds in deficiency or excess states.**

"The cell's intracellular cytoplasmic sea is an ocean of symphonic motion awash with incomprehensible complexity."

R. M. Howes, M.D., Ph.D.

1/24/04

30.4 H$_2$O$_2$ FACTOIDS

30.4.1 H$_2$O$_2$ and the Central Nervous System

Under normal physiological conditions, RONS are tightly regulated and can serve as cellular messengers (Topper, J.N., Cai, J., Falb, D. and Gimbrone, M.A., Jr. Identification of vascular endothelial genes differentially responsive to fluid mechanical stimuli: Cyclooxygenase-2, manganese superoxide dismutase and endothelial cell nitric oxide synthase are selectively upregulated by steady laminar shear stress. Proc Natl Acad Sci USA 1996; 93: 10417-10422), (Wung, B.S., Cheng, J.J., Chao, Y.J., Hsieh, H.J. and Wang, D.L. Modulation of Ras/Raf/extracellular signal-regulated kinase pathway by reactive oxygen species is involved in cyclic strain-induced early growth response-1 gene expression in endothelial cells. Circ Res 1999; 84: 804-812).

RONS have recently been implicated in a variety of redox-based signaling mechanisms that can mediate changes in neural plasticity including:

> **activation of oxidative stress-responsive transcription factors**
> **modulation of LTP induction**
> **and mediation of nonsynaptic communication between neurons and glia.**

In addition, **RONS have been implicated as modulators of synaptic transmission,** following demonstration that H$_2$O$_2$ can reversibly depress evoked population spikes in slices of guinea pig hippocampus.

Oxidative metabolism in brain tissue occurs in the mitochondria as in all cells. During the process of oxidative phosphorylation, a significant amount of O$_2$ consumed is diverted to from superoxide (**O$_2$·¯**), **which is the stoichiometric precursor of H$_2$O$_2$. The amount of H$_2$O$_2$ produced by brain mitochondria is up to 5% of the amount of O$_2$ consumed** (Arnaiz, S.L., Coronel, M.F. and Boveris, A. Nitric oxide, superoxide and hydrogen peroxide production in brain mitochondria after haloperidol treatment. Nitric Oxide 1999; 3: 235-243). Given that the rate of O$_2$ consumption in gray matter is 2-5 mmol/g tissue wet weight per minute; or 2-5mM (assuming 1 g = 1 mL), this would mean that **concentrations of up to 250 μM H$_2$O$_2$ could be generated every minute within brain neutrophils.** Because **the rate of O$_2$ consumption is roughly 10-fold higher in neurons than in glia**, however, this H$_2$O$_2$ would be produced predominantly in the neuronal compartment, which could lead to higher, intra-neuronal concentrations. Moreover, the presence of mitochondria within 250 nm of the synapse in **DA (dopamine)** terminals suggests that even higher levels could be reached in the restricted, intracellular compartment of a synaptic terminal. It is relevant to note, however, that such local increases are likely to be transient because H$_2$O$_2$ is membrane permeable and thus can readily leave the compartment in which it is produced.

In addition to mitochondrial sources, H$_2$O$_2$ will also be produced in DA terminals by **monoamine oxidase (MAO),** which is a metabolizing enzyme for DA. Importantly, **MAO is localized on the outer membrane of mitochondria**, which would further enhance H$_2$O$_2$ concentrations near DA synapses.

Actual concentration of H$_2$O$_2$ at a given location will depend not only on the activity of sources of H$_2$O$_2$ and the size of the compartment it enters, but also on the activity of the local antioxidant network. **In brain tissue,**

H_2O_2 levels are regulated largely by the intracellular enzyme, glutathione (GSH) peroxidase, and by endogenous catalase in peroxisomes. Importantly, the present results with exogenous catalase indicate that **cellular antioxidant regulation does not completely remove endogenously generated H_2O_2.** Rather these processes **appear to permit levels of H_2O_2 that are sufficient to exert modulatory actions.** The lack of effect of up to 10 mM exogenous H_2O_2 in elevated $[Ca^{2+}]$, however, indicates that H_2O_2-mediated effects are saturable; this is also consistent with the calculation that competing levels of endogenous H_2O_2 might be milli-molar. Indeed, the concentration of exogenous H_2O_2 used in the present studies (1.5 mM) is **within the range (1-3 mM) found to have biological effects in many other studies in the literature.**

Catalase is present in trace quantities in brain and is localized in peroxisomes, which in the brain are referred to as "microperoxisomes." **In contrast to glutathione peroxidase and catalase, which exhibit relatively low enzymatic activity in brain, superoxide dismutase is relatively abundant** (Sies, H. Oxidative Stress. Academic Press 1985; 388).

I believe that the above fact "that the antioxidant enzymes in the brain do not completely deplete H_2O_2 levels" is again evidence of the need for these RONS for normal brain function. According to the Free Radi-Crap theory, leaving steady state levels of H_2O_2 and extremely dangerous RONS would have disastrous consequences, especially a chain reaction involving lipid peroxidation, but ....under normal physiological conditions, that does not happen.

It was recently shown that H_2O_2 caused a decrease in ATP production, which interfered with stimulus secretion in pancreatic cells.

There is evidence in the literature to suggest that H_2O_2 application can cause membrane hyperpolarization mediated by an increased K^+ in some cell types, including CA1 pyramidal neurons, which could lead to a decrease in transmitter release.

Independent of the possible mechanisms by which H_2O_2 may act, the finding that H_2O_2 can inhibit transmitter release reveals a novel process by which synaptic transmission might be modulated physiologically (Chen, B.T., Avshalumov, M.V. and Rice, M.E. H_2O_2 is a novel, endogenous modulator of synaptic dopamine release. J Neurophysiol 2001; 85: 2468-2476).

I am amazed at the number of instances in which RONS/excytomers are acting as sensitive and crucial signaling and regulating agents in cellular metabolism.

30.4.2 Pancreatic Beta Cells and H_2O_2

The control of insulin secretion in the pancreatic beta cell depends on the precise tuning of glucose metabolism leading to signal transduction.

Type 1 diabetes, or insulin dependent diabetes mellitus, is an autoimmune disease characterized by altered function and beta cell death subsequent to exposure to inflammation products. During insulitis, macrophages infiltrate the islets of Langerhans and generate reactive oxygen species such as hydrogen peroxide (H_2O_2), which exert alleged deleterious actions on the beta cells and on mitochondrial oxidative metabolism. **Activated phagocytes can produce as much as 47 nmol of $H_2O_2/10^6$ cells within 30 minutes corresponding to a concentration of**

47 μM H_2O_2 in a diluted volume of 1 ml (Anderson, R. J Immunol Methods 1992; 155: 49-55). Nitric oxide (NO), another free radical precursor produced by macrophages, suppresses mitochondrial activity leading to a defective insulin release in response to nutrient secretagogues (Welsh, N., Eizirik, D.L., Bendtzen, K. and Sandler, S. Endocrinology 1991; 129: 3167-3173). Moreover, it has been shown that **NO damages islet cell DNA and mitochondrial DNA in beta cells.** In general, mitochondrial DNA is more sensitive to oxidative stress than nuclear DNA (Yakes, F.M. and Van Houten, B. Proc Natl Acad Sci USA 1997; 94: 514-519), (Beckman, K.B. and Ames, B.N. Physiol Rev 1998; 78: 547-581).

In cells, the mitochondrion is the main source of oxidants. Indeed, imperfect electron transport generates superoxide anions, which are spontaneously dismuted to H_2O_2. Thus, the mitochondria are pivotal in the control of insulin secretion, whereas at the same time generating reactive oxygen species in the cell mostly in the form of H_2O_2.

Of particular importance is the high sensitivity of pancreatic beta cells to oxidative stress. Moreover, the diabetic state is associated with increased oxidative stress and free radical damage (Yu, B.P. Physiol Rev 1994; 74: 139-162). In fact, **the expression of the H_2O_2-inactivating enzymes catalase and glutathione peroxidase in rat pancreatic islets is twenty times lower than in the liver** (Tiedge, M., Lortz, S., Drinkgern, J. and Lenizen, S. Diabetes 1997; 46: 1733-1742).

In mouse pancreatic beta cells, H_2O_2 hyperpolarizes the cell membrane coupled with an increase of cell membrane conductance (Krippeit-Drews, P., Lang, F., Haussinger, D. and Drews, G. Pflugers Arch Eur J Physiol 1994; 426: 552-554).

Moreover, it has recently been shown that H_2O_2:

> **increases intracellular Ca^{2+}**
> **decreases the ATP/ADP ratio**
> **and inhibits glucose-stimulated insulin secretion from isolated mouse islets** (Krippeit-Drews, P., Kramer, C., Welker, S., Lang, F., Ammon, H.P. and Drews, G. J Physiol (Lond) 1999; 514: 471-481).

The cells were exposed to **200 μM H_2O_2 which is a level seen during activation of phagocytes in vitro. The diabetogenic compound alloxan is known to generate H_2O_2 and free radicals** (Maechler, P., Jornot, L. and Wollheim, C.B. Hydrogen peroxide alters mitochondrial activation and insulin secretion in pancreatic beta cells. J Biol Chem 1999; 274: 27905-27913).

30.4.3 Peroxynitrite

Reactive oxygen and nitrogen species play a central role in the maintenance of vascular homeostasis and injury. Nitric oxide (NO)-dependent cell signaling, including endothelial-dependent relaxation, is modulated by both superoxide (O_2^{-}) and superoxide dismutase (SOD), the family of enzymes catalyzing the formation of hydrogen peroxide (H_2O_2) and molecular oxygen from O_2^{-}. Alterations in both the rates of formation and extents of scavenging of O_2^{-} have been implicated in vascular dysfunction seen in atherosclerosis, hypertension, diabetes and chronic nitrate tolerance as well as in postischemic myocardium. Increased rates of vascular production of O_2^{-} and H_2O_2 contribute to initiation of proinflammatory events, with transcriptional regulation of the gene expression of vascular cellular adhesion molecule-1 and moncyte chemotactic protein-1 sensitive to changes in cellular oxidant production as well as to modulation of cell signaling events. **Peroxynitrite (ONOO⁻), the diffusion-limited reaction product of O_2^{-} and NO, although limiting the bioavailability of NO, has been proposed to mediate many of the cytotoxic effects associated with NO because of the multiplicity of its reactions with cellular thiols, lipids, proteins and DNA.** In addition to its putative role in pathologic processes. ONOO⁻ may also serve a physiological function as a cell signaling molecule (Go, Y.M, Patel, R.P., Maland, M.C., Park, H., Beckman, J.S., Darley-Usmar, V.M. and Jo, H. Evidence for peroxynitrite as a signaling molecule in flow-dependent activation of c-Jun NH_2-terminal kinases. Am J Physiol 1999; 277: H1647-H1653).

Hydrogen peroxide at elevated pH can act both as a reductant and as an oxidant.

30.4.4 Hydrogen Peroxide Production

Because **of the rapid dismutation of O_2^{-} to H_2O_2 (spontaneous, 10^5 [mol/L]$^{-1}$ ·s^{-1}, SOD-catalyzed, 10^9 [mol/L]$^{-1}$ × s^{-1})**, endogenous rates of cellular H_2O_2 production can be used as an indirect measure of O_2^{-} formation, recognizing that such measurements will also reflect direct divalent reduction of molecular oxygen to H_2O_2. Intracellular steady state H_2O_2 can be estimated by aminotriazole-mediated catalase inactivation (Royall, J.A., Gwin,

P.D., Parks, D.A. and Freeman, B.A. Responses of vascular endothelial oxidant metabolism to lipopolysaccharide and tumor necrosis factor-*a* (TNF-*a*). Arch Biochem Biophys 1992; 294: 686-694).

H_2O_2 and O_2^- enzymatic production

Enzyme	Tissue	Location
Monoamine oxidase	Liver	Mitochondrial outer membrane
D-amino acid oxidase	Kidney	peroxisome
Glycolate oxidase	liver	peroxisome
Fatty acyl-CoA oxidase liver		peroxisome
L-Gulonolactone oxidase	liver	microsomal
Pyridoxamine-5'-phosphate	liver	cytosol
Diamine oxidase	placenta	
Thiol oxidase	kidney	plasma
Urate oxidase	liver	peroxisome
Xanthine oxidase	milk	
Sulfite oxidase	liver	mitochondria
Xanthine oxidase	neutrophil	specific granules
Aldehyde oxidase		

Copper containing oxidases that produce H_2O_2:

Cytochrome oxidase
Laccase
Ferroxidase I

30.4.5 Cautions in Measurements of RONS

It is apparent that no single technique will accurately reflect quantitative rates of formation of a particular RONS/ excytomers under all circumstances; i.e., when measuring free radical and oxidizing species in vascular cells and tissues, one size will not fit all. Because of the often overlapping capacity of reactive oxygen and nitrogen species to chemically react with detector molecules, **robust conclusions concerning rates of formation of reactive species will be markedly enhanced when a multifaceted approach is used.** With the provided mechanisms of reaction for reactive species and the detector molecules used in a particular assay system and the recognition and accounting for potentially significant side reactions, experimentalists should be able to more reliably use detection methods yielding data that accurately reflect cell and tissue conditions (Tarpey, M.M. and Fridovich, I. Methods of detection of vascular reactive species nitric oxide, superoxide, hydrogen peroxide and peroxynitrite. Circ Res 2001; 89: 224-236).

30.4.6 Hydrogen Peroxide Miscellaneous Factoids (Referenced and Un-Referenced)

-Microsomes produce 80% of the H_2O_2 in vivo in 100% O_2 (Jamieson et al. 1973).

-Peroxisomes produce H_2O_2, but not O_2^- (Chance et al. 1979).

-Sugars, glucose, mannose and deoxy sugars auto-oxidize to produce H_2O_2 (Lam).

-H_2O_2 production is 8.1% total O_2 consumed (liver cell) mitochondria.

-H_2O_2 production is 5.3% total O_2 consumed (liver cell) peroxisomes.

-Thus, a total of 13.4% H_2O_2 production in liver cell (Oxygen Paradox, page 93).

-Fibroblast proliferation was reduced 50-60% by SOD and 80-90% with catalase, like occurred with HeLa cells, human ovarian cells and human melanoma cells (O_2 Paradox, page 428). **RMH Note: These authors seem surprised to find O_2^- and H_2O_2 released from varied cell types; however, any aerobic cell should be capable of O_2^- and H_2O_2 production due to oxidative phosphorylation and electron transport chain.**

-Low concentrations of O_2^- or H_2O_2 (10nM - 1mM) can stimulate growth responses in hamster and rate fibroblasts, mouse epidermal cells, mouse osteoclastic cells and human primary fibroblasts, HeLa cells and human amnion cells (O_2 Paradox, page 430).

-H_2O_2 stimulates c-fos and c-jun and early growth response 1 transcription (ERG1) and activation of DNA binding of NF-Kappa B. Therefore, cell growth signal transduction pathways (i.e., kinases and transcription factors) may depend on their redox status (O_2 Paradox, page 430).

-**5 μM H_2O_2 is non-toxic** (O_2 Paradox, page 574).

- Over 6,000 articles have been written on I.V. use of H_2O_2.

- William Campbell Douglas M.D. states in his book, "Into The Light", that a H_2O_2 I.V. drip relieves even severe emphysema.

- Antibodies react with O_2 to produce H_2O_2.

- **H_2O_2 has a constant cellular concentration of 10^{-9}-10^{-7} M. (figures vary)**

- **H_2O_2 is regulated by catalase at concentrations higher than 10^{-7}-10^{-6} M in the entire cell** (membranes easily diffuse H_2O_2).

- Antimycin A (a site 2 inhibitor) increases H_2O_2 generation and utilizes almost all O_2 consumed to produce H_2O_2; whereas, rotenone (a site 1 inhibitor) reduces H_2O_2 production.

- **Any mitochondrial substrate incorporated in the respiratory chain through NADH or ubiquinone, will generate H_2O_2. Thus, H_2O_2 generation is a physiologic event under aerobic conditions.**

- The main sites for H_2O_2 and O_2^- production are the :

    1. NADH-ubiquinone-reductase (complex I)
    2. ubiquinol-cytochrome c-reductase (complex III)
    Both have ubiquinone as a common component.

In addition to H_2O_2 and O_2^-, other species are generated such as .OH and $^1O_2$, depending on the primary production of H_2O_2 and O_2^-. Many of these species may be intermediates.

- **All aqueous systems that produce O_2^- will produce H_2O_2 by dismutation.**

- **H_2O_2 is involved in any metabolic pathway which utilizes oxidases, peroxidases, cyclo-oxygenases, lipoxygenases, myeloperoxidase, catalase, etc.**

- IV H_2O_2 : 30% diluted to 15% with sterile distilled water. Pass through a 0.22 mm Millipore medium flow filter, store in 100 ml sterile container, refrigerate. Add ¼ ml of 15% H_2O_2 to 100 ml D5W solution for IV this produces a 0.0375% H_2O_2 D5W solution for infusion.

- Father Richard Willhelm called H_2O_2 "God's given immune system."

- Ozone + Blood → H_2O_2.

-**At physiological pH the peroxy radical is protonated to form H_2O_2.**

-Low H_2O_2 levels inhibit cyclooxyengenase and is a key step in PGE_2 (prostaglandin) synthesis.

- Insulin stimulates H_2O_2 production in fat cells and **H_2O_2 acts as a secondary messenger for insulin.** .OH mediates the induction of diabetes in mice by alloxan.

- H_2O_2 autoxidize oxyhemoglobin to form methemoglobin to produce O_2^{-}.

-H_2O_2 inactivates SOD.

-Glucose oxidase plus O_2 produces H_2O_2.

-H_2O_2 is weakly acidic with pKa = 11.7 (Ka of 2.4×10^{-12})

-H_2O_2 has weak O-O bond, unstable, bond dissociation energy with only 51 kcal/mol. Energy from photons can break H_2O_2 O-O bond.

-H_2O_2 consequences:

1. hexose monophosphate shunt activation
2. glutathione redox cycle activation
3. oxidation of intracellular sulfhydryls
4. decreased intracellular ATP
5. DNA damage
6. loss of NAD^+
7. Poly (ADP-ribose) polymerase activation
8. increased free Ca^{++}
9. cytoskeleton alterations
10. plasma membrane alterations
11. inhibition of glycolysis

-H_2O_2 and O_2^{-} are in steady state in pico and nano molar range and H_2O_2 concentration can be as high as 25 μM.

-Oxidized proteins and nucleic acids exists in cells at all times.

-Post mitotic neurons (brain cells cannot regenerate), **the brain is prone to oxidation because:** 1) it has high amounts of easily peroxidizable 20:4 and 22:6 fatty acids; 2) it is not particularly enriched with antioxidant enzymes or with vitamin E; 3) certain regions of the brain (especially in humans), contain lots of Fe (iron). Brain homogenates rapidly peroxidize at 37 degrees but it is blocked by an iron ligate or dopamine.

- In RONS studies, we must take into account male vs. female; old vs. young; brain vs. heart vs. liver vs. muscle; skeletal muscle vs. cardiac muscle; rat vs. mouse vs. man; intracellular levels vs. extracellular, plasma, mitochondrial, peroxisome, etc.

-HOCl oxidizes 100 x greater than O_2^{-} or H_2O_2.

"The electron never rests.
Nonetheless, oxygen occasionally naps,
until enlivened by an
electron-volt jolt."

R. M. Howes, M.D., Ph.D.

7/11/04

30.5 SINGLET OXYGEN $^1\Delta_G O_2$ FACTOIDS

Since oxygen is ubiquitous and efficiently quenches electronically excited states, $^1O_2$ is likely to be formed following irradiation in countless situations and involved in various chemical and biological process as well as in several disease processes.

Another physical method for $^1O_2$ production is microwave or radio frequency discharge that generates up to 10% concentration of singlet oxygen ($^1\Delta_g$) in an oxygen atmosphere.

30.5.0 Ultrasonic Irradiation and $^1O_2$

Ultrasound-imaging devices are now being placed in shopping malls and for $200 a pregnant mother can get a sonographic snapshot of her fetus. However, there may be risks. The FDA has released a statement that it does not know if repeatedly sending high doses of energy across a mother's womb is harmful. Ultrasonic waves are the same ones that are used to break up kidney stones and studies have shown that even low levels can produce physical effects in tissue, including jarring vibrations and increases in temperature. **I feel that it needs to be pointed out that ultrasonic waves has been shown to generate RONS, such as $O_2^{\cdot-}$ and $^1O_2$, upon ultrasonic irradiation of sensitizers (e.g., porphyrins, chlorins, methylene-blue, fluorescein, acridine derivatives, rhodamines and tetracyclines).** This is analogous to PDT and has been used to treat tumors and it is reported that it affects only tumorous tissue and not normal cells. Please keep in mind the fact that fetal tissue act like tumorous or cancerous tissue. Thus, in the presence of photosensitizers, it is possible to generate RONS by ultrasonic irradiation (Patent No. US4971991: Physiological function enhancing agents activated by ultrasonic waves for the treatment of tumors).

30.5.1 $^1O_2$ Scavengers

Scavengers can inhibit a reaction dependent of $^1O_2$. For example, **azide** acting as a physical scavenger reacts with $^1O_2$ to give a reactive azide radical, $N_3^- + {}^1O_2 \rightarrow N_3^{\cdot} + O_2$.

Other $^1O_2$ scavengers include:

> **carotene**
> **ascorbate**
> **thiols**
> **and histidine act as chemical scavengers.**

The reactions of $^1O_2$ often involve carbon-carbon double bond, which are present in many biological molecules, such as **carotene, chlorophyll and unsaturated fatty acids.**

With acceptors such as cis dienes or aromatic hydrocarbons, $^1O_2$ **can react as good dienophile.**

Singlet oxygen can also react with electron rich systems, in which carbon-carbon double bonds have adjacent electron donating atoms **(nitrogen, sulfur).** In these reactions, an oxetane type adduct is formed. These dioxetanes may be unstable and decompose to give carbonyl compounds.

30.5.2 Quenching of $^1O_2$

The quenching of singlet oxygen involves the deactivation of the excited state of molecule. Deactivation can be accomplished by either physical or chemical quenching. **Physical quenching leads only to the deactivation of singlet oxygen to its ground state with no oxygen consumption or product formation.** In **chemical quenching, by contrast, singlet oxygen reacts with quencher R to produce RO_2.**

Two major mechanisms of $^1O_2$ quenching are known:

> **energy transfer**
> **and charge transfer** quenching (Zhao, L. Singlet oxygen. Free Radical and   Radiation Biology Graduate Program Unv of Iowa 2001; 77: 222).

Thousands of reactions of singlet oxygen have been studied.

The quenching of $^1O_2$ involves the deactivation of the excited singlet states of oxygen molecule. It may be either physical or chemical quenching. Chemical quenching is that in which $^1O_2$ reacts with quencher (Q) to give product QO_2. Physical quenching leads only to the deactivation of $^1O_2$ to its ground state with no oxygen consumption or product formation.

Schafer et al. reported that $^1O_2$ can be quenched by:

> **water**
> **lipids**
> **nucleic acids**
> **polyunsaturated fatty acids**
> **and other small molecules.**

Two major mechanisms of $^1O_2$ are known. They are energy transfer and charge transfer quenching.

30.5.3 Energy Transfer Quenching

This mechanism of quenching is the reverse of reaction by which $^1O_2$ is formed.

Other quenchers like dyes, metal complex and other compounds with very extensive conjugated systems may also involve this mechanism of quenching.

30.5.4 Charge Transfer Quenching

This mechanism involves the interaction of the electron deficient $^1O_2$ with electron donors.

$$D + {}^1O_2 \ll [\,D\text{---}O_2{}^{.-}\,]^1 \ll [\,D^+ \text{---} O_2{}^{.-}\,]^3 \ll D + {}^3O_2$$

Since $^1O_2$ acts as an electron acceptor, easily oxidizable compounds prove to be the best quenchers.

Some $^1O_2$ quenchers have no specificity for $^1O_2$ and will often lead to secondary excited molecules (e.g., carotenoids, vitamin E, and azide).

Compounds quenching $^1O_2$ by the charge transfer mechanism include:

> amines
> phenols
> metal complexes
> sulfides
> iodide
> azide
> superoxide anion
> **and similar electron rich compounds. Recently, Hessler et al., used humic substances** (HSs) to quench $^1O_2$. The efficiency of $^1O_2$ quenching depends on the origin of the HS sample.

Solution $^1O_2$ quenching rate constants of metal chelates can be found in Singlet Oxygen Reactions with Organic compounds & Polymers, edited by B. Ranby and J. F. Rabek, John Wiley & Sons, A Wiley-Interscience Publication, 1978, pages 96-99.

Singlet Oxygen Production

Several methods are available for the generation of $^1O_2$.

30.5.5 Chemical Methods for $^1O_2$ Production

Hydrogen peroxide reacting with sodium hypochlorite can produce $^1O_2$. The biological meaning of this reaction is that hypochlorite can be produced by the enzyme called myeloperoxidase during phagocytosis (Halliwell, B. and Gutteridge, J.M.C. Free Radical in Biology and Medicine. 1982; Second Edition, Clarwindon Press, Oxford).

$$H_2O_2 + Na^+OCl^- \rightarrow {}^1O_2 + NaCl + H_2O$$

Solid adducts formed between the **triaryl phosphite and ozone at low temperature decompose to release** $^1O_2$ (Ameta, S.C., Punjabi, P.B., Chobisa, C.S., Mangal, N. and Bhardwaj, R. Singlet molecular oxygen. Asian J Chem Rev 1990; 1(2): 106-124).

Superoxide ion O_2^- is another potential source of $^1O_2$, since loss of an electron of appropriate spin could produce ground state molecular oxygen or $^1O_2$.

Generation of $^1O_2$ by peroxidase-catalyzed reactions:

> Chloroperoxidase
> Lactoperoxidase
> Horseradish peroxidase
> Prostaglandin hydroperoxidase

30.5.6 $^1O_2$ Reactions

Singlet oxygen can interact with other molecules in two ways. One is that $^1O_2$ may combine with other molecules chemically. Another is that $^1O_2$ may transfer its excitation energy to other molecules.

30.5.7 Alder-Ene Type Reaction

This reaction occurs when $^1O_2$ reacts with a compound with one double bond. This reaction is also called Schenck reaction or "ene" reaction. They involve either a six-centered transition state typical of the classical reaction, a peroxide of closed related intermediate or a biradical intermeidate.

30.5.8 Diels-Alder Reaction

With acceptors such as cis dienes or aromatic hydrocarbons, $^1O_2$ appears to behave as a good dienophile.

Reaction with Electron Rich Systems

Singlet oxygen may react with double bonds which have electron donating atoms such as nitrogen and sulphur. In this reaction, an oxetane type adduct is formed. These dioxetanes may be unstable and decompose to give carbonyl fragments. Decomposition of dioxetane is sometimes accompanied by chemiluminescence.

Based on in vitro studies, singlet oxygen can react with **DNA, carotene, tryptophan, methionine, cystine, histidine and NADPH**. $^1O_2$ can oxidize these amino acids and thus damage proteins. **Histidine has the highest second order rate constant for reaction with $^1O_2$.** Oxidative destruction of histidine is the major cause of destruction of many enzymes.

30.5.9 $^1O_2$ Biological Reactions

Singlet oxygen is involved in many biological areas such as: (based on in vitro studies)

> **dye sensitized photo oxygenation**
> **erythrocyte dysfunction associated with G6PD deficiency**
> **membrane destructive process**
> **phagocytosis**
> **photoaging**
> **metabolic hydroxylation**
> **age related changes of the lens**
> **carcinogenesis**
> **signaling transduction pathway**
> the **activation of transcription factor AP-2**
> and **cellular signaling cascades comprising the activation of c-Jun-N-terminal kinases (JNK/SAPK) and NF-kappa B system.**

Singlet oxygen can also **induce oxidative DNA base damage, in vitro,** and may have dramatic effects on eukaryotic gene expression. The toxicity of $^1O_2$ is cell line-dependent. The greater the protein content of cells, the more they are protected against membrane damage. The cell size correlates inversely with the ability of cells to cope with a given flux of $^1O_2$.

Human catalase can be oxidized by $^1O_2$ in myeloid leukemia cells. Catalases are oxidized by $^1O_2$ giving rise to more acidic conformers detected in zymurgies after electrophoresis in polyacrylamide gels. This shift in catalase mobility can be indicative of $^1O_2$ production in vivo.

Stief et al., reported that singlet oxygen can inactivate:

> **fibrinogen**
> **factor V**
> **factor VIII**
> **factor X**
> **and platelet aggregation of human blood, suggesting that singlet oxygen is an anti-thrombotic agent.** (Steif, T.W., Kurz, J., Doss, M.O. and Fareed, J. Singlet oxygen inactivates factor V, factor VIII, factor, X and platelet aggregation of human blood. Thrombosis Research 2000; 97(6): 473-480).

Singlet oxygen produced by photodynamic action can **inactivate the mitochondrial permeability transition pore.** The most likely targets for $^1O_2$ are **critical histidine molecules** that undergo degradation. Tatsuzawa, et al., reported that singlet oxygen **can inactivate bacterial respiratory chain enzymes.** Exposure of wild-type E. coli to $^1O_2$ causes a significant loss of E. coli viability, due to inactivation of membrane respiratory chain enzymes by $^1O_2$, **suggesting that singlet oxygen produced by phagocytic leukocytes is a major bactericidal oxidant in the phagosome** (Luo, J. Singlet oxygen. Free Radical and Radiation Biology Program. Univ of Iowa 2001; 77: 222).

The importance of O_2^- and H_2O_2 production for polymorphonuclear leukocytes (PMN) bactericidal activity is well known and a lack of production of O_2^- and H_2O_2 by PMNs, from patients with chromic granulomatous disease, results in an increased susceptibility to life-threatening bacterial infections. **The amount of $O_2(^1\Delta_g)$ produced by phagocytically stimulated PMNs was calculated to be 11.3 ± 4.9 nmol of $O_2(^1\Delta_g)/1.25 \times 10^6$ cells.** Low dose PMA co-stimulation increased the production of $O_2(^1\Delta_g)$ to 14.1 ± 4.1 nmol/1.25 × 10^6 cells. Averaged together these amounts **represent approximately 19 ± 5.0% of the total oxygen consumed by PMNs** in response to DPA- and perylene-coated beads (Steinbeck, M.J., Khan, A.U. and Karnovsky, M.J. Intracellular singlet oxygen generation by phagocytosing neutrophils in response to particles coated with a chemical trap. J Biol Chem 1992; 267: 13425-13433).

Singlet oxygen ($^1\Delta_g$) is a highly reactive, diffusing and long-lived electronically excited state of molecular oxygen (Wilson and Hastings, 1970; Khan and Kasha, 1970; Browne and Ogryzlo, 1965; Corey and Taylor, 1964; Foote and Wexler, 1964).

Highly efficient mechanisms for $^1O_2$ generation exist that involve:

> **photosensitization of the ground triplet state of oxygen ($^3\Sigma_g$)**
> **electron transfer from O_2^-**
> **thermal dissociation of endoperoxides**
> **and chemical reactions involving H_2O_2 and hypohalites.**

30.6 $O_2(^1\Delta_g)$ IN THE RESPIRATORY BURST

The work of Steinbeck, et al., is the first reported evidence that PMNs produce a measurable amount of $O_2(^1\Delta_g)$ and that the MPO/H_2O_2/Cl⁻ system, in the presence of phagolysosome concentrations of H_2O_2, generates $O_2(^1\Delta_g)$.

The involvement of $O_2(^1\Delta_g)$ in the respiratory burst of PMNs was suggested some time ago, based on the emission of light by PMNs during phagocytosis (Allen, R.C., Stejernholm, R.L. and Steele, R.H. Biochem Biophys Res Commun 1972; 47: 679-684), (Allen, R.C. Biochem Biophys Res Commun 1975; 63: 675-683). They proposed that the MPO/H_2O_2/Cl⁻ system might be a source of $O_2(^1\Delta_g)$ generation in phagocytically stimulated PMNs. This suggestion was based on the early work of Khan and Kasha (1963), that established the production of $O_2(^1\Delta_g)$ in a chemical reaction between H_2O_2 and HOCl (Khan and Kasha, 1970). It has been suspected previously that the poor yield of $O_2(^1\Delta_g)$ by this system could be the result of product inactivation of the MPO (Kanofsky, J.R., Wright, J., Miles-Richardson, G.E. and Tauber, A.I. J Clin Invest 1984; 74: 1489-1495). It has only been reported recently that quantities of the substrate H_2O_2 above 100 µM can also lead to the inactivation of MPO at pH 7.5 and that the physiological concentration of H_2O_2 in the phagolysosome in probably less than 100 mM. This data merely indicates that very high levels, of any compound or agent, including H_2O_2, can have deleterious effects.

Allen (1975) postulated that O_2 produced during dismutation could be in the singlet excited state ($^1\Delta_g$). The generation of H_2O_2 and $O_2(^1\Delta_g)$ by the direct interaction of two molecules of $O_2^{\cdot-}$ is summarized:

$$O_2^{\cdot-} + O_2^{\cdot-} + 2H^+ \rightarrow H_2O_2 + O_2(^1\Delta_g)$$

The suggestion by Allen was based on a proposal by Khan (1970) that an electron transfer reaction between two molecules of $O_2^{\cdot-}$ could lead to the formation of electronically excited $O_2(^1\Delta_g)$. **It was later verified that $O_2(^1\Delta_g)$ was produced in a H_2O-induced dismutation reaction** (Khan, A.U. J Am Chem Soc 1981; 103: 6516-6517), (Corey, E.J., Mehrotra, M.M. and Khan, A.U. Biochem Biophys Res Commun 1987; 145: 842-846). It is therefore possible that the dismutation of $O_2^{\cdot-}$ produced by the phagocytically stimulated PMNs, plays a direct role in the production of $O_2(^1\Delta_g)$. At the same time, production of **large amounts of $O_2^{\cdot-}$ would limit the amount of $O_2(^1\Delta_g)$, since it is an efficient quencher of $O_2(^1\Delta_g)$, when present at high concentrations** (Khan, 1978).

Based on chemical product and luminescence sensitization studies using potassium superoxide, it was proposed that SOD protects the host system by preventing the generation of the highly reactive, long-lived, diffusible, singlet oxygen molecule $O_2(^1\Delta_g)$ from superoxide anion. Spectroscopic evidence has established the generation of singlet oxygen in the water-induced dismutation of superoxide anions and in the electron transfer reactions of superoxide anion with metal redox systems (Khan, A.U. and Kasha, M. Singlet molecular oxygen in the Haber-Weiss reaction. Proc Natl Acad Sci 1994; 91: 12365-12367).

30.7 ELECTRON TRANSFER REACTION MECHANISMS IN $O_2^{\cdot-}$ TO $^1O_2$ CONVERSION

To interpret these results, 3 possible reactions were proposed as a source of singlet oxygen:

Haber-Weiss: $O_2^{\cdot-}$ + H_2O_2 ➔ $^1O_2(^1\Delta_g)$ + OH + OH^-

Electron transfer: OH + $O_2^{\cdot-}$ ➔ $^1O_2(^1\Delta_g)$ + OH^-

Dismutation: $2H^+$ + $2O_2^{\cdot-}$ ➔ $^1O_2(^1\Delta_g)$ + H_2O_2

The hydroxyl radical, $\cdot$OH, is postulated to be only a short-lived transient intermediate. It is so highly reactive that in the biological milieu, it will either react at a diffusion-controlled rate in an unselective way with practically any cell constituent or **possibly abstract an electron from another superoxide anion reducing $\cdot$OH to OH^- and generating a singlet oxygen molecule. The superoxide anion can act both as an efficient generator an efficient quencher of singlet oxygen, via electron transfer.** Thus, superoxide anion is expected to be an efficient generator of singlet oxygen only over a narrow concentration range. In addition, **H_2O is also a highly efficient quencher of singlet oxygen,** consistent with the observed weak [H_2O]-induced singlet oxygen emission. In addition, electron transfer processes are very solvent-sensitive. The observed decreased intensity of singlet oxygen emission in acetonitrile solution compared with that in carbon tetrachloride solution may reflect this, as well as the fact that singlet oxygen has a much shorter lifetime in CH_2CN than in CCl_4. These quenching processes in which the singlet dioxygen is deexcited to ground-state triplet dioxygen can be summarized as follows:

Electron transfer: $O_2^{\cdot-}(^2\Pi)$ + $^1O_2(^1\Delta_g)$ ➔ $^3O_2(^3\Sigma_g^-)$ + $O_2^{\cdot-}(^2\Pi)$

Solvent quenching: $^1O_2(^1\Delta_g)$ + solvent ➔ $^3O_2(^3\Sigma_g^-)$ + solvent

Khan and Kasha conclude that these results strongly support the interpretation that the chemical reactivity of superoxide-generating enzymes could depend on the evolution of singlet molecular oxygen. The high reactivity of this species toward biological components is well documented. That singlet oxygen could be the prime oxidative agent should not be surprising. In recent reports, Steinbeck et al., observed **that 19 ± 5% of the total oxygen consumed in a respiratory burst by the polymorphonuclear leukocytes is converted to singlet oxygen inside the phagolysosome when these white blood cells are phagocytically stimulated.** Macrophages, on the other hand, generate singlet oxygen extracellularly when stimulated. **Singlet oxygen thus appears to be a key component also in the oxidation reactions of the host defense and immune system.**

30.8 Miscellaneous Singlet Oxygen Factoids

-$^1O_2$ and .OH are known to react directly with DNA or DNA components (O_2 Paradox, page 150). **RMH Note: Others argue that singlet oxygen does not readily react with DNA if it is added extracellularly.**

- **DNA oxidation by $^1O_2$ can give rise to G ➔ T transversions.**

-$^1O_2$ mainly causes in vitro damage to proteins (tryptophan, tyrosine, cysteine and histidine residues).

-**In tissue, $^1O_2$ has a lifetime of 0.01 μs.**

-Millions of jaundiced babies have been successfully treated with $^1O_2$ generating phototherapy with no known damaging long term effects. Thus, I feel that this illustrates the rather "harmless' and beneficial nature of $^1O_2$.

-$O_2^{\cdot-}$ is much more cellular damaging than $^1O_2$.

-$^1O_2$ in vivo lifetime is 0.03-0.18 ms.

-$^1O_2$ is only a minor product of the respiratory burst of phagocytes, with limited ability to produce breakage in isolated DNA, it might add to DNA strand breaks (Mutation Research, 1992; 265: 256).

-**Chemiexcitation:** $^1O_2$ can be generated in a dark reaction enzymatically by peroxidases or lipoxygenases or by reaction of H_2O_2 with HOCl or peroxynitrite, thermodecomposition of dioxetanes or respiratory burst of phagocytes.

-It appears that intracellular, not extracellular, $^1O_2$ elicits gene activation and expression (Biochemistry of Oxidative Stress).

-Fungi use $^1O_2$ to damage protective membranes, so they can enter cells.

-Plants use $^1O_2$ to kill insects or injure mammals that feed on them.

-$^1O_2$ quenchers - $^1O_2$ reacts a thousand times greater than triplet ground state O_2.

-Photosensitizers, i.e., phytin pigments, FD&C red No.3, may convert O_2 to $^1O_2$.

- A lifetime of 10^{-9} -10^{-10} seconds for an excited state is enough time for 10-100 collisions.

-Khan and Kasha, 1964, confirmed the existence of $^1O_2$ when they assigned strong red emission bands from the reaction between hypochlorite with H_2O_2 to produce $^1O_2$ (Khan, A.U. and Kasha, M.J. J am Chem Soc 1964; 86: 3879).

-**$^1O_2$ generation by three techniques:**

1. **Chemical generation** - physical - chemistry aspects; Frimer, A.A. Ed., CRC Press, Boca Raton, FL 1985; Vol. 1).
   $H_2O_2 + CLO- \rightarrow {}^1O_2 + Cl- + H_2O$
   This give very high concentrations of $^1O_2$ and a bright "dimol' chemiluminescence emission at 635 nm and 703 nm due to the reaction of 2 delta $^1O_2$ molecules.

2. **Gas phase discharge** - in the gas phase, an electric discharge (usually **microwave radiation at 2450 Hz**), is used to excite O_2 to delta $^1O_2$ in high yields (Rosenthal, I. In Singlet Oxygen, 1985; Frimer, A.A. Ed., CRC Press, Boca Raton, FL 1985; Vol. 1, Physical-Chemical Aspects; p 13).

3. **Photosensitization**

-Xanthine oxidase plus H_2O_2 produces $^1O_2$.

-Bucky balls C60 and C70 are powerful photosensitizers for production of $^1O_2$.

-$^1O_2$ reacts 1000 times faster than $^3O_2$.

30.9 SUPEROXIDE MISCELLANEOUS FACTOIDS

-3% of total hemoglobin forms $O_2^{\cdot-}$ (Free Radical Vet Paper).

-If $O_2^{\cdot-}$ were stable, O_2 cellular utilization would produce 5 μmol l^{-1} intracellular $O_2^{\cdot-}$ per second (O_2 toxicity, Fridovich).

-During the respiratory burst, 70-90% of the O_2 → $O_2^{\cdot-}$ (Barbior, B.M., 1978).

-Molecules that undergo auto-oxidation catecholamines, hemoglobin, myoglobin, reduced cytochrome c, thiol, Fe^{++} produce $O_2^{\cdot-}$

-Organelles known to produce $O_2^{\cdot-}$ are mitochondria, chloroplasts, microsomes, peroxisomes, nuclei (Asada & Kiso, 1973).

-Cigarette smoke - 100 trillion free radicals per puff.

-$O_2^{\cdot-}$ has lifetime of 60 ms in apolar media

-$O_2^{\cdot-}$ has lifetime of 3 ms in H_2O

-$O_2^{\cdot-}$ is intrinsically unstable in protic solvents such as water, but at higher pH, the more stable it becomes. At neutral pH, it is stable enough to oxidize polyphenols, thiols, ascorbate, catecholamines, leukoflavins, tetrahydro-proteins and sulfite and can rapidly inactivate aconitase and similar [4Fe-4S]-containing dehydratases.

-$O_2^{\cdot-}$ is a vasoconstrictive mediator after experimental angioplasty (O_2 Paradox, page 242).

-$O_2^{\cdot-}$ is relatively impermeable to membranes. **RMH Note: Others say that it is relatively permeable.**

-$O_2^{\cdot-}$ is quite non-reactive in aqueous medium and **can permeate cell membranes**, probably thru anion channels (O_2 Paradox, page 235).

-Collagen and $O_2^{\cdot-}$ cause collagen degradation, which attracts chemo-attractants and activators of PMNs (O_2 Paradox, Page 205).

-Guanyl cyclase in smooth muscle endothelium is inhibited by $O_2^{\cdot-}$ and activated by $NO^{\cdot}$ (O_2 Paradox, page 235).

-**$O_2^{\cdot-}$ probably cannot attack DNA (O_2 Paradox, page 351).**

-Influenza virus infection leads to $O_2^{\cdot-}$ production by lung epithelial cells, partly due to increased activity of O_2 generating xanthine oxidase. HIV similarly takes control of the cells redox status (O_2 Paradox, page 389).

- $O_2^{\cdot-}$ **can be formed enzymatically** by flavoprotein dehdydrogenases and more importantly **non-enzymatically** by autoxidation of ferridoxins, hydroquinones, thiols and reduced hemoproteins (Fridovich).

-The stationary stage concentration of $O_2^{\cdot-}$ is maintained by SOD at 10^{-11} M in cytosol and 10^{-10} M in mitochondrial matrix.

- Semiquinones, present in cigarette smoke, can bind and interchelate with DNA generating $O_2^{\cdot-}$ and H_2O_2 in situ. **Active O_2 species are responsible for ~70% of all DNA strand breaks in radiation-induced carcinogenesis. (Dr. C.W. Lam)**

- Sugars, such as glucose, mannose and deoxy sugars autoxidize to produce H_2O_2. (Lam)

Simple sugars can also autoxidize under physiological conditions to produce O_2^- that may enhance the oxidation and crosslinking of various proteins and is implicated in microangiographic complications in diabetes mellitus. (Lam)

- Neither O_2^- nor H_2O_2 can directly react with DNA but both can be reduced in the Fenton reaction and produce .OH.

- O_2^- can release iron (Fe++) from ferritin.

-Oxyhemoglobin slowly releases O_2^- to form methemoglobin, which can not bind and transport O_2. This occurs in 1 in 1000 cycles of O_2 binding and release but it is estimated that **3% of hemoglobin releases O_2^-. RMH Note: This represents another huge source of O_2^-, H_2O_2 and $^1O_2$.**

-Activated phagocytic cells, such as monocytes, neutrophils, eosinophils and macrophages generate O_2^-. These terms are used interchangeably: stimulated, activated, induced, elicited, upregulated, etc.

-O_2^- inactivates catalase and glutathione peroxidase and epinephrine oxidation. **RMH Note: Thus, O_2^- blocks the breakdown of H_2O_2.**

- Based on O_2^- generation in vitro in the mitochondria and microsomes of rat lungs and livers, **the formation rate of ROS is estimated to be 50 nmol/g of tissue per min or about 10^{11} radicals/cell/day** (Free Radicals in Aging, Yu).

-**O_2^- at physiological pH has a pK of 4.8 and it can readily pass through membranes on the anion channels.**

-**One mitochondrion (rat liver) produces 3×10^7 O_2^-/day.**

-Low concentrations of O_2^- or H_2O_2 (10 nM - 1 mM) can stimulate hamster and rat fibroblast growth.

"In searching for the road of truth, for the Free Radical theory of Aging and Oxidative stress, I found that it was riddled with gaping paradoxical potholes of contradiction, which rendered it impassable.
In fact, I found that this avenue to enlightenment had been completely blockaded by bricks of biochemistry.
The theory had been distributed and taught from a passage in the Great Book of Medical Mythology, along with phlogistin, spontaneous generation, thymic hypertrophy and hormone replacement therapy."

R. M. Howes, M.D., Ph.D.
7/18/04

32.20 MY CONCLUSIONS ON AGING AND FREE RADICALS...

"In searching for the road of truth, for the Free Radical theory of Aging and Oxidative stress, I found that it was riddled with gaping paradoxical potholes of contradiction,
which rendered it impassable.
"In fact, I found that this avenue to enlightenment
had been completely blockaded
by bricks of biochemical knowledge.
The theory had been distributed and taught from
a passage in the Great Book of
Medical Mythology, along with phlogistin,
spontaneous generation, thymic hypertrophy
and hormone replacement therapy."

R. M. Howes, M.D., Ph.D.

5/8/04

Dr. Denham **Harman's free radical theory of aging has been hailed** as the following:

- "The biggest advance since the discovery of germs," said Richard A. Passwater, Ph.D.
- It ranks with Galileo's invention of the telescope
- Newton's discovery of gravity
- Einstein's theory of relativity
- The best understood and most widely accepted explanation of the aging process
- "He deserves the Nobel Prize," said Dr. Donald Ingram, acting chief of the laboratory of experimental gerontology at the National Institute of Aging in Baltimore.

With all due respect, I believe that the free radical theory of aging is wrong, even though over 50 million Americans consume antioxidant supplements on a daily basis, because of false promises of reversing aging and guarantees of avoiding any one of 100 allegedly free-radical-caused diseases. Estimates for 2004 indicate that 30% of Americans take dietary supplements (figures vary) and it has grown to a $19 billion annual industry.

32.21 BACKGROUND

I feel that it is important to remember the following significant facts:

1. Free radicals are essential to life.
2. All energy in aerobic cells require free radical reactions.
3. It takes a free radical to stop a free radical.
4. Many, if not all, antioxidants can also serve as pro-oxidants.
5. All evidence implicating oxygen free radicals as a cause of disease is circumstantial.
6. Not everything called free radicals are free radicals.
7. Not all free radicals are fleeting and some are quite stable.
8. Not all free radicals are ripping electrons and some radicals are relatively non-reactive and basically stable, depending upon their chemical surroundings.
9. In vitro studies can not be extrapolated directly to the living/breathing cell.
10. The concept of "oxidative stress" serves no useful purpose unless we look at all other compounds and elements in the same biased way.
11. We should, thus, consider "reductive stress" or "antioxidant stress."
12. There are hundreds of theories of aging and combinations thereof, many of which hold up to scrutiny far better than the free radical theory of aging.
13. Rationally, there is no single cause of aging, because it is such a   m u l t i f a c t o r i a l phenomenon.
14. The cell is an unbelievably complex dynamic entity which is normally capable of self sufficiency, including the ability to reproduce itself.
15. Intracellular biochemical interactions are unbelievably complex.
16. Intracellular biochemical "cross talk" is unbelievably complex.
17. It is rare, if not impossible, for a singular chemical event to occur in the living/breathing cell, as opposed to situational in vitro experiments.
18. In vitro conditions give a bright investigator the power and the latitude to produce nearly any desirable artifactual result.
19. Since free radical reactions are constantly occurring in living cells, they can readily be associated with countless parameters to which they may or may not have a causal relationship.
20. Attempting to link and implicate non-causal parameters, for the purpose of promoting flawed theories, is tantamount to scientific fraud.
21. There is a growing awareness that antioxidants can be harmful or even deadly.
22. Humans have the ability of self-cure and it is frequently based on free radicals and products of oxidation (RONS/excytomers) (EMODs).
23. Many of our current medical practices are likely working against our ability for self-cure, as has been the case throughout the history of medicine.
24. It is extremely difficult to measure RONS/excytomers in vivo, if at all and more than one form of measurement should always be used.
25. Inter-conversion of RONS and excytomers makes it very difficult, if not impossible, to determine which RONS/excytomer(s) were present, when they were present and in what amounts.

32.22 IN AN INTERVIEW BETWEEN DR. HARMAN AND DR. PASSWATER, COMMENTS WERE AS FOLLOWS:

Passwater: When you conceived the free radical theory of aging, virtually no one was looking at the role of free radicals in biological systems, let alone in the aging process. When exactly did you conceive the concept?

Harman: In the first part of November, 1954.

Passwater: Why did you become interested in the aging process?

Harman: I guess I was always curious about it, but my interest in aging was sparked in December, 1945 by an article in a popular magazine that my wife had called to my attention. The article, "Tomorrow you may be younger," was written by William Laurence, science editor of the New York Times. It was concerned with the research of Dr. Alexander Bogomolets (a Russian gerontologist), of the Institute of Gerontology in Kiev, Russia, on an "antireticular-cytoxic serum." The article was from The Ladies Home Journal.

Harman: **The theory was first published on July 14, 1955** as a University of California Radiation Laboratory report titled, "Aging: A theory based on free radical and radiation chemistry," and as a journal article a year later in the Journal of Gerontology. The first talk, "Aging: The theory based on free radical and radiation chemistry with application to cancer and atherosclerosis," was presented on February 6, 1956 at a Donner Laboratory Seminar.

Harman: Free radical reactions are implicated in 50 disorders. These "free radical diseases" include cancer, heart attacks, strokes, rheumatoid arthritis, cataracts and Alzheimer's disease — the major cause of admission to nursing homes. The list keeps growing.

Passwater: I would not be surprised if the list eventually exceeds 80 diseases. **(RMH Note: The list now exceeds 100 diseases. This hyperbolic "let's jump on the band wagon" behavior, serves only to dilute the importance of reliably collected data in this area).** Before your free radical theory, it was just germs and aging — and aging was some unknown thing. Now we have disease pathology that we can follow. I'm still thinking about how you were reading when the theory fell into place in your mind. Please tell us more about that experience.

Harman: It's a common experience to work for a day on a problem, say in chemistry or physics, and to finally give up and go to bed. Then after going to bed and not even trying to think about the problem, and just before dropping off to sleep, the answer comes to you — it just pops into your head. When it happens, you know it is correct **(RMH Note: This is a good story but the facts must be scientifically verified, which has not been done).** All the pieces fall together. **RMH Note: Actually, the pieces have fallen all over the place.** This was essentially what happened with the aging problem except that it took over four months of intense and frustrating effort to arrive at the solution.

Harman: Decreasing caloric consumption can indeed increase maximum life span. Decreasing the caloric intake of rats decreased body weight and oxygen consumption by 40 percent, and increased maximum life span by 49 percent. I believe these effects are caused by the lowered oxygen utilization; one to three percent of the oxygen we use is diverted to superoxide radical and hydrogen peroxide. In essence, by decreasing caloric intake we decrease our exposure to internal radiation. **RMH Note: Many studies contradict these statements and show either no change or even an increase in oxygen consumption.**

Passwater: Dr. Harman, in Part I, you mentioned that eating less food reduces oxygen consumption and the load on the mitochondria. There is good evidence that calorie restriction — cutting calorie intake by 30% or so while maintaining high micronutrient levels slows aging. Calorie restriction seems to lower the levels of undesirable sugar-damaged proteins called Advanced Glycosylation End-products (AGE).

Harman: Yes. These products are formed by the **Maillard reaction**. Interest in the deleterious effects of glucose (blood sugar) in diabetes focused attention on this reaction, now an active area of research. The Maillard reaction is initiated by glycation, a reversible non-enzymatic reaction between reducing sugars such as glucose and ribose, and primary amino groups on proteins to form Schiff bases (a class of derivatives of the condensation of aldehydes or ketones with primary amines): these can form **Amadori (rearrangement) compounds.** The Amadori compounds slowly — over months or years — form a heterogeneous group of irreversible compounds by oxidation, condensation, rearrangements and elimination reactions collectively called **AGE**. Free radical reactions are involved in the slow peroxidation reactions.

(RMH Note: Unfortunately, neither Drs. Harman nor Passwater mention the fact that reducing sugars start the biochemical process of AGE compound formation and oxidation occurs subsequent to these reduction reactions).

Passwater: What supplements do you take?

Harman: I take 200 milligrams of vitamin E per day; ten milligrams of coenzyme Q-10 with each meal; one yeast tablet containing 50 micrograms of selenium twice a day and I also take one multivitamin tablet.

There are other things involved in living a long life. These include keeping your weight down at a level compatible with a sense of well-being, getting a moderate amount of exercise, little or no smoking, and minimal alcohol. There is nothing new about these suggestions; they have come down to us from our ancestors. RMH Note: This is, in my opinion, the most brilliant of Dr. Harman's many statements over many decades, Fortunately, his work has stimulated considerable experimentation and great interest in the area of free radicals in biological systems.

32.23 NON-SCIENCE/NON-SENSE

Unfortunately, the free radical theory of aging led to frenzied and far-flung theories of cellular sabotage by oxygen's cellular assassins, as is illustrated by current quotes as follows: (but please do not believe this non-science/non-sense).

- A list of the causes of free radicals would include virtually every toxic substance known. A list of the effects of free radicals would also be long, encompassing all of the common diseases afflicting humans.
- The damage referred to in the phrase damage theory is caused by free radicals. Free radicals, the rogues' gallery of biochemistry, are highly charged, rapidly moving molecular fragments that harm healthy cells. The more free radicals present, the more damage they cause, and the more the aging process speeds up as a result.
- In their reckless quest for electrons, free radical do a lot of structural damage to healthy cells. Injured cells can't function properly and may even die.
- The cell membrane is a pushover for free radical attack because it is composed primarily of easily oxidized fatty acids. Like tiny but powerful bullets, highly charged free radical particles rip into the cell membrane, literally puncturing holes in it.
- Free radicals can even bang their way through the protective membrane surrounding the nucleus, gaining access to the DNA molecules housed inside. If free radicals happen to break the DNA molecules in order to snatch electrons, the cell dies, or loses its ability to replicate, or replicates abnormally - a process known as mutation. Mutation can give rise to the collections of abnormal cells that we know as cancer.
- But cancer isn't the only health problem for which free radicals are responsible. Cumulative free radical damage contributes to all sorts of organ - and tissue-specific disease, including allergies, Alzheimer's disease, arthritis, atherosclerosis (hardening and clogging of the arteries), cancer, cataracts, infections, macular degeneration, multiple sclerosis and Parkinson's disease. In fact, researchers now agree that most common ailments, including virtually all chronic degenerative diseases, are either caused directly by or are closely associated with free radical damage.

The above is exactly the kind of scientific nonsense to which I object so strongly. The simple facts are as follows:

32.24 FREE RADICAL COMMON SENSE

- We are constantly generating exponential numbers of free radicals.
- We have indigenous antioxidant enzyme systems to elegantly control free radicals within the body. In fact, I see no reason that these antioxidant systems could not also get out of "whack" and result in a ROS/excytomer deficiency. To my knowledge, this scenario has never heretofore been discussed in detail, as I have done in UTOPIA.
- Without oxygen we die.
- Without free radicals to perpetuate electron transport, we die.
- The nutrients of our foods generate free radicals.
- Free radicals are a major part of the oxidative killing of bacteria.
- Free radicals are a major part of the oxidative killing of fungi.
- Free radicals are a major part of the oxidative killing of viruses.
- Free radicals are a major part of the oxidative killing of parasites.
- Free radicals are a major part of the oxidative killing of pro-neoplasia.
- Free radicals are a major part of the oxidative killing of cancer.
- Free radicals are an integral part of maintaining good health.
- Free radicals are not "just harmful waste products of oxidative metabolism."
- Free radicals are crucial signaling molecules within and between cells.
- Free radicals are essentials in regulating natural cellular death (apoptosis).
- Oxygen is the greatest ally of all aerobic life.
- Oxygen metabolism, at most, is only a small part of the aging phenomenon.
- Synthetic antioxidants and supplements can be harmful or deadly.
- Antioxidants can increase rates of cancer.
- Antioxidants can increase rates of arteriosclerosis.
- Antioxidants can worsen infections.
- Singlet oxygen can kill cancer.
- Singlet oxygen can kill bacteria.
- Singlet oxygen can kill fungi.
- Singlet oxygen can kill viruses.
- Singlet oxygen can kill parasites.
- Singlet oxygen can kill pro-neoplasia.
- Hydrogen peroxide can kill cancer.
- Hydrogen peroxide can kill bacteria.
- Hydrogen peroxide can kill fungi.
- Hydrogen peroxide can kill viruses.
- Hydrogen peroxide can kill parasites.
- Hydrogen peroxide can kill pro-neoplasia.
- Singlet oxygen can dissolve arteriosclerotic plaques.
- Hydrogen peroxide can dissolve arteriosclerotic plaques.
- Singlet oxygen is a crucial signaling molecule within and between cells.
- Hydrogen peroxide is a crucial signaling molecule within and between cells.

- Hydrogen peroxide can resuscitate an ischemic heart.

And I could go on and on but **hopefully, you get the point**. The point being that today's **free radical phobia** is unjustified and is distorting the true biochemical purpose of these agents, which are generated in steady state levels by all aerobic cells. As a physician, surgeon and biochemist, **I am continually impressed with the precision and wisdom exhibited by a living/breathing cell**. To me, it is inconceivable that such a miraculous living, internal combustion machine would have evolved with such a prominent error (i.e., the lethal oxidative generation of free radicals by a "leak") within the primary pathway of energy production, which is necessary to maintain its very existence.

This is precisely why, with all due respect, that I refer with such tongue-in-cheek terms to Dr. Harman's and Ames' concepts as the Free Radi-Crap Theory of aging and oxidative stress and to its oxy-moronic supporters.

32.25 UNPROVEN ANTI-AGING PRODUCTS

Many of today's 21st century snake oil salesmen are hawking all sorts of anti-aging products such as the following:

Deprenyl	Selenium
Human Growth Hormone	Procaine (GH3 and KH3)
DHEA	DMAE
Melatonin	Centrophenoxine
Acetyl-L-Carnitine	Aminoguanidine
Coenzyme Q10	Hydergine
Alpha Lipoic Acid	Piracetam
Cysteine and Procysteine	Vinpocetin
NADH	Chromium Picolinate
Lycopene	Dilantin (Phyenytoin) and Phenformin
Vitamin E	Picamilon
Vitamin B5 (Pantothenic Acid	Pregnenolone
Vitamin B6 (Pyridoxine)	Pyritinol
Synthetic Antioxidants	
BHT, 2-MEA, NDGA,	
Ethoxyquin	Testosterone
Levodopa (L-Dopa	Estrogen and Progesterone

A cursory review of the alleged increases in human lifespan by only seven of the above agents, **should result in a lifespan of about 250 years based on their claims....but it doesn't.**

Also, it is important to keep in mind the fact that the U.S. Food and Drug Administration does not require products that are sold as dietary supplements to undergo the rigorous tests of safety effectiveness that medicines must pass before they can be sold to the public. Thus, **dietary supplements and vitamins have no guidelines for dosage, purity or potency and no warnings as regards side effects or drug interactions.**

32.26 AGING, BODY SIZE AND METABOLIC RATES

A major component of free radical aging is a correlation between larger animals (with slower metabolic rates) and smaller animals (with faster metabolic rates). The metabolic rates supposedly indicates the rate of free radical formation within a respective species. There are so many exceptions to this aspect of the theory, that it is nearly ludicrous.

In answering the question how long do they live, Reader's Digest Book of Facts provides the following:

Most animals die through violence, disease or accident, not through old age. Because of this, the maximum lifespan of animals in the wild are not known with any certainty. Actually, in nature few animals live much longer than humans.

The list below has the longest lifespans, in years for a number of animals.

152	Marion's tortoise	50	Lobster
100	Deep-sea clam (up to 220)	48	Cow
90	Killer whale	47	Splendor Beetle
90	Blue whale	38	Bats
90	Fin whale	35	Domestic pigeon
81	Elephant (Asian)	24	Domestic cat
80	Freshwater oyster	29	Dog (Labrador)
80	Cockatoo	28	Sheep
70	Condor	18	Goat
62	Ostrich	10	Golden hamster
62	Horse	10	Hummingbird
59	Chimpanzee	6	House mouse
50	Termite	0.2	Housefly
42	Goldfish		

Birds live three times longer than mammals of equivalent size. They have the same metabolic rate and size as a rat yet a pigeon lives 30 years compared to the rat's four. A bird has 5-7 times the metabolic potential of a non-primate mammal. **The humming bird can have a heart beat as fast as 1000 beats per minute and can consume up to 500,000 liters of O_2/kg and still live for 10 years.** This type of metabolism led Gustavo Barja, University of Madrid, to study mitochondrial H_2O_2 production in pigeons and rats. He found that pigeon mitochondria produced 1/3 as much H_2O_2 as rat mitochondria under similar conditions. He surmised that the proportion of O_2 converted into free radicals in pigeons is only 10% that of rats. Thus, birds needed less antioxidants than rats, since they produced considerably less free radicals. However, I feel that the jury is still out on this research.

I see little, if any, trend in the comparative life spans of a blue whale and a clam or an elephant and a cockatoo or an oyster. In short, I believe that the Free Radi-Crap theory of aging has little, if any, validity on the basis of metabolic rates.

James Goss, University of Pittsburgh, answered the question, "Why do different animals have different length of lifespans?" on the MadSci Network as follows:

While there are some general rules that can be applied to maximum lifespan, they are not concrete and there is much variance from theoretically predicted lifespan to observed lifespan among species. We usually think of aging and senescence when we think of maximum lifespan. But the concept of aging and what constitutes aging has been hotly debated over the years. **There is no agreement as to why we age in the first place.** You have to remember that most individual organisms never reach a point in the wild when they start to show signs of senescence (I will define senescence as the decline of physiological function over time). However, almost all organisms show signs of aging, with the possible exception of some single-celled organisms.

One of the first global generalities we can assign to maximum lifespan is the correlation between fecundity and longevity. **Basically, the more offspring an individual of a species is capable of producing, the shorter the maximum lifespan of that species**. Evolutionarily speaking, two basic reproductive methods have evolved to increase the likelihood that an individual will contribute their genes to the next generation. The first is called prodigal (or r-selected, where r is the mathematical symbol for the rate of population increase) and is associated with high fecundity and high mortality. The second is called prudent (or K-selected, where K is the mathematical symbol for the carrying capacity of the environment) and is associated with small numbers of offspring coupled with lower mortality. These differences are obvious when one compares flies to humans. The common housefly only lives for a few days but on average lays 120 eggs. In a given year there will be an average of 7 generations of houseflies born. If you had a fly in your house in January that laid its eggs and if all the subsequent generations survived at the end of the year there would be 5,598,720,000,000 flies in your home! A fly has a lot of offspring but doesn't stick around too long to make sure they live. The vast number of flies born will ensure some will live. Humans on the other hand give birth to relatively few babies during their lifetime but spend a lot of energy making sure each offspring survives. This correlation between reproduction and lifespan is obvious when we discuss organisms as different as flies and humans but it generally holds true for more related animals. If we look at only mammals this correlation between fecundity and lifespan also holds true (dogs and cats can have several litters of multiple offspring and they rarely live more than two decades) there is a correlation between the age of the animal when it is first capable of reproducing (reaches sexual maturity) and its maximum lifespan. The longer the developmental period (that time between birth and sexual maturity) the longer lived the animal is. Of all animals, humans have the longest developmental period and are among the longest lived of all animals.

RMH Note: there is considerable variation in the nurturing time or development period for animals according to World Features Syndicate. Please note that these facts argue against the currently popular "grand mother hypothesis."

How long they stay with their moms:

1. Male elephants stay with mom 12 years
2. Zebras stay 2 years
3. Baby chimps stay 3 years
4. Female African wild dogs stay 3 years
5. Cheetahs stay 18-20 months
6. Female lions stay their entire lives

Another correlation with lifespan is body size. Generally speaking, the larger the animal and the larger its brain, the longer lived. This is generally believed to be the result of the metabolic rate and is best exemplified in mammals. Small mammals have a large surface area compared to their weight and lose body heat a greater rate than a large animal. In order to maintain their body temperature they have a higher metabolic rate (i.e., they burn food faster). This tends to "burn out" their bodies quicker. Incidentally, if warm-blooded animals are raised in cold environments they have a shorter lifespan because their metabolic rate is higher; cold-blooded animals show the opposite affect. One of the major exceptions to the body size rule are humans. Humans have a much longer lifespan than their body size should allow (we should live about as long as most pigs). This lead to the idea that brain size must be just as important as body size. **Generally, the greater the brain/body size ratio, the longer lived the animal. Humans have the biggest brain to body size ratio and live a long time (accepted maximum is about 122 years).**

Lastly, there appears to be a correlation with lifespan and the number of hazards in an animal's normal environmental niche; the more hazardous the environment, the shorter the maximal lifespan. This may be due to the necessity of reaching sexual maturity quicker in these animals to ensure their reproduction.

RMH Note: Keep in mind that the brain is the organ which has the highest utilization of oxygen in the body. Consequently, it produces one of the highest levels of RONS/excytomers and it is correlated with longer lifespans.....just the opposite of what would be predicted by the Free Radi-Crap theory.

Over the past few years, discoveries have overturned many previous theories of aging. Generally, it is now believed that aging and life span are under genetic control, which in turn controls hormones, metabolic rate, oxidative rates, etc.

Current thinking is revising the common idea that advancing age inevitably leads to extreme deterioration. It is also said that animals get "more unsaturated" as they age. I feel that this is related to the fact that lipids with double bonds act as chemical sinks for RONS/excytomers, which produces a deficiency state of RONS/excytomers, which is associated with disease manifestation and aging.

The annual conference of the World Cancer Research Fund International and the American Institute for Cancer Research (AICR) recommend 14 habits to prevent chronic disease. Suggestions include: exercising daily; gaining no more that 11 pounds after age 18; eating five or more vegetables and fruit's a day; avoiding tobacco; limiting alcohol, red meat, fat and salt. I feel that this may also be good advise to prevent premature aging.

RMH Note:
Things That We Know:
All living things will die.

Dead things do not return to life, in the form in which they died.

The life span of the may fly is 24 hours.

The life span of the tortoise is 100 years.

What role does oxidative stress play in their aging?

In spite of increasing environmental pollutants, a decreasing ozone layer and increasing radiation, the human life span is increasing.

Despite living in a world of excessive external and internal sources of free radicals, the life span is increasing.

Whether one exercises, avoids fats, avoids cooked meats, or lives a healthy life style, we all live to about the same age. We may be in better health, but these activities, basically, do not extend the lifespan.

People who eat more fruits and vegetables are healthier, likely, because they eat less cooked food or because of the peroxide content of fresh foods.

People who exercise are healthier, even though they drastically increase their intake of oxygen by 10-20 fold.

Life forms kill and consume other life forms to sustain themselves.

Life forms are driven to increase the number of life forms like themselves.

Please remember the French proverb, which says, **"Forty is the old age of youth. Fifty is the youth of old age."**

32.27 AGING IS ALWAYS THERE

Just as my thinking on cancer changed, I am currently changing my thinking regarding aging. It is commonly believed that we are in a state of good health through the second and third decades of life and then aging hits us. This is analogous to the situation with cancer, in that we were thought to be in a cancer-free state, and then, rather suddenly, we get cancer; when, in fact, cancer was always present. It is only certain circumstances which "allow" cancer to manifest itself. Similarly, aging is always there from the moment we are born, until the time of our death. For example, an 8 month child looks older than an 8 hour old child and an 80 year old looks older than an 8 year old. In other words, aging is a continual, gradual process. It is always there. We can see its effects. I believe that the physiological and biochemical changes, which accompany aging, are creating the circumstances which "allow" for aging to occur.

**"Singlet oxygen is spawned from the erotic mating
ritual between stately hydrogen peroxide
and perky hypochlorite. From this molecular
true romance, is born the excited singlet
love-child, which, within micro-seconds,
rises to be a great leader
of electrons."**

R. M. Howes, M.D., Ph.D.
5/26/04

**"Out of the compacted, fertile soil of controversy, will sprout
the rose of the Howes Unified Theory, which will blossom
above the specious weeds of the Free Radical
Theory of Aging and Oxidative Stress."**

R. M. Howes, M.D., Ph.D.
5/26/04

PART VIII - SELECTIVE BOOK REVIEWS

PART IX - OXYGEN PHYSIOLOGY

38.20   OXYGEN FACTS AND MY UNIFIED THEORY

It is unwise to be too sure of one's own wisdom. It is healthy to be reminded that the strongest might weaken and the wisest might err.

Mahatma Gandhi (1869-1948)

My Unified Theory states that body areas that have high metabolic rates, utilizing high oxygen consumption and more importantly, generating high levels of reactive oxygen species and electronic excitation states (RONS/excytomers) are predictably going to have less cancer than areas which have low oxygen consumption levels and consequent low levels of reactive oxygen species or electronic states which would kill germs, invaders or cancer. I believe that this is analogous to that which is seen in spontaneous regression of cancer following an infection (respiratory burst) and that which is seen with photodynamic therapy ($^1O_2$). Furthermore, **I believe that I have duplicated the body's mechanism for the killing of cancer with my singlet oxygen method, utilizing hydrogen peroxide, deuterium peroxide and sodium hypochlorite. My system parallels that of the action of photodynamic therapy (singlet oxygen) and is consistent with the neutrophil response in cases of spontaneous regression (the respiratory burst production of H_2O_2 and HOCl, thus leading to the formation of $^1O_2$).**

Oxygen, in one of its many forms (oxygen modifications or derivatives RONS), constantly protects us from being overtaken by infective threats, which are always on or in our bodies, and keeps cancer development from occurring by the mutations which are constantly being formed within all of our aerobic cells. **Oxygen is central to our existence and the maintenance of a condition of good health.**

A clearer understanding of general oxygen considerations is necessary to follow the logic of my **Unified Theory**. One interesting application of this concept was to consider the metabolism of the heart and its oxygen needs. My **Unified Theory** would predict that the heart's cardiac muscle, composed of mitochondria-dense myocytes, and which has a high rate of oxygen consumption for its energy needs, would have very low rates of tumor or cancer formation. Keep in mind that the widely accepted Free Radi-Crap theory of aging and oxidative stress states that this high production of reactive oxygen species and electronic excitation states should have devastating effects upon cardiac muscle. Consequently, **according to the Free Radical theory the heart should have one of the highest rates of malignant changes in the body; but, it doesn't.** Again, literature research supported my theory, in that heart muscle tumors or cancer are very rare and that cardiac muscle does have a very high oxygen utilization rate.

With all due respect, the highly revered theory of oxidative stress will be referred to as "**the oxy-moronic theory or better yet, the Free Radi-Crap theory**" and its acolytes will appropriately, and not pejoratively, be referred to as "**oxy-morons**." With all due respect, this approach makes **Dr. Denham Harman the**

Father of all oxy-morons. We should all move past the intellectual impasse called oxidative stress. Also, the free radical theory of aging and oxidative stress will be referred to as "The Free Radi-Crap Theory of Aging and Oxidative stress." Paradigms which are proven incorrect are of value in that they can give rise to better paradigms.

The influence of Dr. Harman has added confusion to medical and scientific investigations for the past half century. His theory of oxidative balance and oxidative stress has not been proven by the scientific method, over decades of study that has produced thousands upon thousands of published papers. In fact, it has been disproven many times. Many of these studies have yielded repeated **contradictions, unpredictable results, negative results, diametrically opposed results and "paradoxes."** Nonetheless, investigators have continued to attempt to apply this erroneous concept and attempts have been made to **force the data to fit the flawed theory**. Basically, this is because the free radical/oxidative stress theory is wrong. There is no more of an oxidative stress in the body than there is an antioxidant stress, a sodium stress, a nitrogen stress, a thyroxin stress, a chloride stress, a glucose stress, an iron stress, etc. **Oxygen metabolism should be viewed as any other metabolic process in which variations from a homeostatic state produces illness or disease.** Furthermore, we should keep in mind the almost mystical salutary role of oxygen. As a matter of fact, oxygen is the crucial cardinal molecular ingredient of sustenance in the living/breathing cell and in all aerobiotic processes. **If the cell isn't breathing, it isn't living, and to live it has to breathe oxygen.**

As a matter of fact, all creatures are constantly consuming oxygen and all surface plant life is constantly producing oxygen. The waters of the ocean and the atmosphere have seasonal breathing cycles of oxygen and all of the creatures within the ocean act as either consumers or generators of oxygen, excluding the flora and fauna around thermal vents. **It is as if the entire surface of the earth is an oxygen cycling entity. This is exemplified by the photosynthesis/respiration cycle between plant and animal life forms.**

The literature is replete with references to the normal process of oxygen metabolism, in which oxygen is reduced to water, whereby it is stated that during the reduction of oxygen, certain reactive oxygen species **"leak"** from the electron transport chain. Reports indicate that the size of the "leak" varies anywhere from 1-5%, but usually it is considered to be between 3-5% of the total amount of oxygen that is consumed in the production of ATP, oxidative phosphorylation and the electron transport chain. These "leaked" oxygen species are accused of allegedly producing over 100 different diseases. Yet, **countless studies have failed to prove a causal relationship between these "leaked" oxygen species and any of these disease states**. The marketers of products to counteract, trap or eliminate these "leaked" oxygen species have a thriving multi-billion dollar industry that is based on an erroneous theory, namely, the free radical theory of aging and oxidative stress. **The vitamin and supplement sales business is a $19 billion industry.** That represents a lot of motivation to perpetuate a flawed theory. Alarmed by this marketing trend, **scientists studying aging have issued a position statement containing this warning: no currently marketed intervention—none—has yet been proved to slow, stop or reverse human aging, and some can be downright dangerous. Further, scientists, other than myself, have acknowledged that without free radicals, we are dead.**

I can hardly imagine that nature and evolution would design a cell, which usually functions flawlessly over a lifetime, which can approach 100 years, with such a glaring defect. In fact, **nature has formed an organelle, the peroxisome, specifically for the production of additional H_2O_2 subsequent to fatty acid oxidation, which is supposed to be a dastardly devastating and deadly substance.** How could nature and/or evolution be so stupid? Fortunately, a few other investigators are beginning to realize that **these oxygen modifications are, indeed, purposeful and serve in many signaling and triggering points during normal oxidative metabolism, cellular replication and cellular apoptosis.** Most scientists are now familiar with the important role of an oxygen (nitrative) modification called nitric oxide (NO), which normally has a significant and beneficial role in blood pressure regulation, vessel dilation and cell death and **which can act as either a prooxidant or an antioxidant.**

In fact, the production of these "leaked" oxygen species is an essential component of all aerobic cells for establishing a healthy condition and it does so by keeping bacteria, viruses, fungi, parasites and cancer at bay and under control. **If one were to assume that modified oxygen does not keep bacteria, viruses, fungi,** parasites and cancer cells in continual abeyance, then an important query here is: **"What does keep disease and infection at bay during the many years of a normal life span?"** I submit that the non-oxidative defense mechanisms of proteolytic, enzymatic and acid digestion are too slow to accommodate the ever present, humongous homeostatic needs of the living/breathing cell. However, oxygen modifications having pico-, nano-, micro- and milli-second half- lives are capable of doing the job. Many of these oxygen modifications are continuously present in all of our aerobic cells in steady state exponential numbers, ready and waiting to do their job and doing so on a continual basis. **Each aerobic cell utilizes 10^{13} molecules of oxygen per day. Multiply this figure times 75-100 trillion cells and that calculates out to a lot of oxygen used each day by a 70 kg man, of which 3-5% is oxygen free radicals.** Superoxide is the predominant radical formed and it is thought that it is rapidly converted into H_2O_2 by either spontaneous or enzymatic dismutation. **I do not believe for a minute, that the body generates these large quantities of hydrogen peroxide (H_2O_2) through a "mistake."** All of the cells of our body normally automatically maintain a state of homeostasis and good health. We consciously have very little to do with it. It is, indeed, rather miraculous.

Terms such as reactive oxygen and/or nitrogen species (RONS), metabolites and intermediates become confusing and grouping of oxygen into free radicals or non-free radicals adds to this confusion. **Each oxygen modification should be viewed as a distinct entity with its own reactivities and properties.** Each has differing kinetics, electron conformations, bonding strengths, reactivities, diffusion rates, etc. Since oxygen is the central player, all other forms of it should be referred to as **"oxygen modifications"** or **"modified oxygen"** and **should be dealt with on an individual and specifically named basis** (i.e., superoxide anion, hydrogen peroxide, hydroxyl radical, singlet oxygen ($^1O_2$), peroxyl radical, nitric oxide, peroxynitrite radical, hypochlorous acid, etc.). Throwing all of these oxygen modifications into one large and meaningless group is naïve at best and misleading at worst. We must consider each of these species with the chemical sophistication which they deserve and **avoid the erroneous, lazy thinking of the past century.**

38.30 MILIEU INTERIEUR

The 19ᵗʰ century French physiologist, Claude Bernard, introduced the term "milieu interieur" which means the "environment within." Bernard was convinced that the body's and the cell's internal environments were of the utmost importance in maintaining health and homeostasis. **Louis Pasteur, the father of the Germ Theory of Disease, reportedly said on his deathbed that, "Bernard was right, the germ in nothing — the milieu is everything."** In other words, the germ itself is only a pathogen if the internal environment <u>allows</u> it to express its pathogenic potential. Otherwise, it is just a bug. **I believe that the integrity of the milieu interieur is markedly dependent on adequate levels of oxygen,** with the all important subsequent production of oxygen modifications, to keep invaders in abeyance and keep mutagenically altered cells from becoming overt cancer. In that sense, the milieu interieur is of utmost importance to prevent infection by countless germs within the body and to stop the development of thousands of DNA alterations which occur every day in every aerobic cell in the body.

To amplify this concept, we usually tend to think that we are in a state of health and we are invaded by germs that make us sick. When in fact, the germs are always present and illness is only manifested when we become in a "run-down condition." We need to be aware that **we are constantly potentially infected and that we are constantly on the verge of allowing mutagenic changes to become full blown cancers**. We remain in a state of health only by the grace of oxygen modifications (RONS/excytomers) which keep bacteria, viruses, fungi, parasites and cancer at bay.

The first and most obvious change occurring with the death of an animal or a person is that it stops breathing, it no longer has its constant supply of life-giving oxygen to sustain it and protect it. Immediately, the bacteria on its surface and the germs within it, being to furiously replicate, to the extent that within a few days, the entire body is decomposed by these runaway bugs. Had this same animal or person been immediately placed on a heart-lung machine at the moment of death, thereby maintaining a supply of oxygen to the cells, this consumption by germs would not have occurred. Obviously, **countless biochemical changes are triggered by death, including the loss of an energy source**, but this extreme scenario dramatically illustrates the significance of a functional oxygen system in maintaining the healthful status of the "milieu interieur."

Investigators can call oxygen whatever they want, from a killer to the ultimate enemy within, but it is abundantly apparent that **oxygen is our singular greatest ally.**

Maintaining the body's natural health does not occur by serendipity or accident and neither does the production of the altered states of oxygen by the electron transport chain. This is one of the most basic pathways for maintaining the body's health. I firmly believe that these "leaked" oxygen species are essential agents of overall oxygen metabolism. I will term this the **"Requisite Oxygen Pathway for Electron Escape" (ROPEE)** which has evolved over the last 2.5 billion years.

38.40   REQUISITE SUPEROXIDE VALIDATED PEROXIDE PATHWAY (RSVP PATHWAY)

Actually, because of the fact that superoxide is rapidly converted to hydrogen peroxide, I feel that this "leak" is more logically an **intentional pathway for peroxide production, which I will refer to as the "Requisite Superoxide Validated Peroxide Pathway (RSVP Pathway).** This is the cell's self-sustaining, innate pathway whereby the electron transport chain produces modifications of oxygen, which are automatically there to protect us and not to harm us. **Please keep in mind the wisdom of Paracelsus, in that anything in an over abundance can be harmful, just as a deficiency of any essential can be damaging. Yes, size matters (size of the dose).**

"Dosis sola venenum facit", which roughly translates as "only the dosage makes the poison." Paracelsus (1493-1541) sought out an education that was unobtainable from a curriculum of scholastic disputations on Aristotle, Galen and Avicenna: "One cannot manage with books written over two centuries ago. Patients are your textbooks, the sickbed is your study." Also, he disapproved of the professional code that separated the physician and surgeon, and he denounced physicians as being in league with apothecaries to profit from ignorance and poly-pharmacy.

The magnificent inner workings of the cell are occurring at mind-boggling speeds, with exponential numbers of reactants and are doing so without our conscious input. **In fact, it seems that electrons, atoms and molecules may possess an innate intelligence higher than that of the entire organism.** Frequently, it is the conscious actions of the organism that gets it into dangerous situations and/or trouble. The living/breathing cell is far too beautiful to have perpetual "leaks" of exponential numbers of reactive oxygen species wreaking constant havoc on the fragile intracellular organelles and the cytoplasmic chemical components. In this instance, I believe that the test tube interpretation and extrapolation to the living cell have led to disastrous inaccuracies. In fact, **I believe that normally it is the deficiency or absence of these "leaked" oxygen species that leads or predisposes us to disease states, not their presence.   However, an overabundance of anything, including oxygen modifications, can prove to be harmful.**

Stated another way, a deficiency state of RONS does not induce a bacterium to cause an infection, nor does it cause a pre-cancerous cell to become a cancer but it "allows" the bacterium or the precancerous cell to "fulfill" its programmed destiny, if all other circumstances are favorable for it to do so.

38.50 KEY CELLULAR FACTORS AFFECTING O$_2$ LEVELS

The final concentration or production of oxygen modifications (RONS/excytomers) at the cellular level is dependent upon a multitude of factors such as:

atmospheric oxygen content
atmospheric humidity
atmospheric temperature
physiological condition of the patient
respiratory ability
oxygen uptake
oxygen consumption
respiratory vascular integrity
condition of the alveoli
hemoglobin levels
iron levels
red blood cell concentrations
integrity of the cardiovascular system
all aspects of heart function
all aspects of pulmonary function
all aspects of the oxygen carrying capacity of the blood
all factors relating to release of oxygen at the cellular level
integrity of the electron transport chain and the complexes and enzymes of oxidative phosphorylation, etc.

All of these variables must be taken into account to access an organism's ability to ward off infections and cancer.

38.60 AGING AND OXYGEN

According to Cecil's Textbook of Medicine, 2004, 22nd Edition, page 107,

"The most characteristic change in the chest wall with advancing age is stiffening. Not only do cartilages thicken and calcify, but also spinal ligaments and joints become stiffer. The primary internal change in the lungs is the loss of the elastic recoil. The result is a modest expansion of the chest wall with the appearance of a mild barrel chest. Although resting lung mechanics do not seem to change in any major way, **the loss of maximum breathing capacity declines by approximately 40%. At the alveolar level, the capacity to exchange oxygen and carbon dioxide decreases by approximately 50% between ages 30 and 65 years.** Although these changes are not noticeable at rest, individuals experience fatigue or shortness of breath when the respiratory system is under stress (e.g., during exercise or major illness). Pulmonary reflexes, such as coughing and cilial function, decrease, predisposing elderly individuals to the pooling of secretions and to aspiration pneumonia." Thus, **I believe that it is not an over abundance of oxygen that is responsible for the many changes and diseases associated with aging but it is more directly related to an oxygen deficiency**. Obviously, a deficiency of ground state oxygen will lead to deficiency states of RONS/excytomers.

"All of these changes do not produce substantial abnormalities in resting oxygen saturation, but **they produce a steady decline in arterial $_PO_2$. The arterial $_PO_2$ of many individuals older than age 80 is about 70 to 75 mm Hg.** As with other age-related physiologic findings, these changes do not interfere with function under resting conditions but dramatically affect survival during severe respiratory illness."

According to my **Unified Theory**, the decreased oxygen levels associated with aging are, in part, explanatory for the many diseases associated with aging including cardiovascular disease, cancer and diabetes. Also, the fact that oxygen consumption decreases with age tends to argue against the free radical theory of aging which would imply that oxygen free radicals and oxygen consumption would be increasing with age as opposed to decreasing. This aspect of aging is never discussed in the literature concerning aging. Additionally, one should consider the high frequency of anemia in elderly patients and its impact on oxygen uptake, transport and distribution at the cellular level. This also is in direct opposition to the erroneous free radical theory of aging.

Droge presents a limited discussion of free radicals and aging and states that, "The published data do not allow us to distinguish whether these age-related changes result from an age-related accumulation of oxidative damage or from an age-related increase in ROS production per unit time." (Droge, W. Free radicals in the physiological control of cell function. Physiol Rev Vol. 82, No. 1, Jan. 2002, pp. 47-95).   He mentions a study which examined rat skeletal muscle and **revealed a significant age-related increase in the H_2O_2 scavenging enzymes catalase and glutathione peroxidase**. I believe that these enzymatic changes would result in a RONS/excytomer deficiency state, which would be consistent with the degenerative changes seen with increasing age and my Unified Theory. Droge also points out that **the aging process in the elderly is remarkably slow, indicating that even the elderly have adopted a nearly steady state of redox homeostasis.**

Further, Droge cautions that, "Although it may be a plausible and attractive paradigm to postulate that aging related changes in the thiol/disulfide redox state and the changes in gene expression profiles are direct consequences of an age-related increase in the rate of ROS production, **this cause-and-effect relationship remains to be proven."** He states that the replicative life span in vitro is not an inherent property of somatic cells but is determined, at least in part, by the redox state of the micro-environment.

38.70 ANEMIA

One of the ways anemia increases mortality is by influencing treatment efficacy. Anemia influences responses to radiation therapy because it limits the oxygen-transporting capacity of the blood and consequently tissue oxygenation. Thus, **anemia can contribute to tumor hypoxia, which makes solid tumors resistant to sparsely ionizing radiation and some forms of chemotherapy** (Vaupel, P., Kelleher, D.K. and Hockel, M. Oxygen status of malignant tumors: Pathogenesis of hypoxia and significance for tumor therapy. Semin Oncol 2001; 28(suppl): 29-35).

Many factors contribute to cancer related anemia, some associated with the progression of cancer and others associated with cancer therapy. Factors likely to increase the risk of anemia include the type, state and duration of disease; treatment regimen and intensity; presence of infection; and the need for surgical intervention. (Mercadante, S., Gebbia, V. and Marrazzo, A., et al. Anemia in cancer: Pathophysiology and treatment. Cancer Treat Rev. 2000; 26: 303-311).

Hypoxia also influences the number of cells destroyed following therapy by modulating the proliferation and cell cycle position of tumor cells. In contrast, well-oxygenated tumors have a greater chance of being controlled. (Brizel, D.M., Dodge, R.K. and Clough, R.W., et al. Oxygenation of head and neck cancer: Changes during radiotherapy and impact on treatment outcome. Radiother Oncol 1999; 53: 113-117). **Many studies have documented the association between anemia and poor outcome in cancers of the head and neck, respiratory tract, pelvis and genitourinary organs.** (Kumar, P. Tumor hypoxia and anemia: impact on the efficacy of radiation therapy. Semin Hematol 2000; 37(suppl 6): 4-8).

Pretreatment anemia has been identified in more than 40 studies as an adverse prognosticator in patients receiving radiotherapy or chemoradiation for solid tumors. (Shasha, D. The negative impact of anemia on radiotherapy and chemoradiation outcomes. Semin Hematol 2000; 38(suppl 7): 8-15).

It becomes readily apparent that oxygen levels are of key importance in keeping cancer in abeyance under normal circumstances, during chemotherapy, during irradiation and with photodynamic therapy (PDT). Without adequate ground state oxygen levels, the ROS and electronic excitation states that are needed to kill cancer are insufficient and restoring them to normal levels allows for adequate cancer killing activity.

Results indicate that anemia can negatively influence the therapeutic effectiveness of PDT. For optimal antitumor response, anemia should be corrected before PDT procedure. (Jakub, G., Dominika, O., Pawe, M., Katarzyna, K., Rafa, K., Alimad, J. and Marek, J. Erythropoietin Restores the antitumor effectiveness of photodynamic therapy in mice with chemotherapy-induced anemia. Clin Can Res 2002; 8: 1265-1270).

The underlying anemia affects these treatment modalities as follows:

- anemia symptoms are caused by decreased oxygen content of the arterial blood

- it causes cellular hypoxia

- some symptoms are due to compensatory responses of the cardiovascular and respiratory systems as they respond to tissue hypoxia

- cardiovascular compensation

- tachycardia (increased heart rate) causing increased cardiac output, dilation of microvasculature

- respiratory compensation

- increased alveolar minute ventilation caused by increased respiratory rate and/or tidal volume

- symptoms of inadequate compensation

- dizziness, fatigue at rest, reduced exercise tolerance, rapid bounding pulse, renal malfunction, heart failure

My point here is to emphasize the complex set of physiological and biochemical reactions that are necessary to produce and maintain adequate tissue oxygenation. The fact that all of **the body's efforts are designed to be compensated in such a way as to maintain normal oxygen levels**, underscores the importance of my **Unified Theory** and its intentional evolutionary development.

38.80 OXYGEN TRANSPORT

For adequate oxygen transport:

- there must be adequate amount of oxygen in arterial blood to provide adequate oxygen to the cells throughout the body, or cellular hypoxia results
- movement of oxygen for inspired air to hemoglobin (Hb) in the alveolar capillaries
- the partial pressure difference between the air in the alveoli and deoxygenated blood in the alveolar capillaries drives the diffusion of oxygen across the alveolocapillary membrane into the capillary blood
- the oxygen dissolves in the plasma, and this dissolved oxygen in the plasma determines the partial pressure of oxygen in the capillary blood
- as the partial pressure of oxygen in alveolar capillaries rises, the oxygen diffuses across the red blood cell (RBC) membrane and attaches to hemoglobin
- this continues until hemoglobin is saturated with oxygen (O_2) and the partial pressure of oxygen in the alveolar capillary equals the partial pressure of oxygen in the alveolar air

The oxyhemoglobin dissociation curve is important because:

- Hb binds with O_2 in the alveolar capillaries forming oxyhemoglobin

- pulse oximeter values (O_2 sats measurements) are the % saturation of Hb with O_2 (% oxyhemoglobin)

- the plot of the % saturation of Hb with oxygen against the partial pressure of oxygen in the blood results in an S shaped curve called the oxyhemoglobin dissociation curve

- if the PaO_2 (partial pressure of O_2 in arterial blood) is 60 mmHg or above, Hb is virtually 100% saturated with O_2

- the normal PaO_2 is 80 mmHg or greater

- the normal Hb saturation in arterial blood is 95% or higher

- after the PaO_2 falls below 60 mmHg, the decrease in Hb saturation is very rapid

- at times the actual PaO_2 in arterial blood is measured since it is more accurate than the results obtained from a pulse oximeter

38.90 NORMAL O_2 CONTENT OF BLOOD

The oxygen content of the blood is as follows:

- normally, ~20 ml of oxygen is contained in 100 ml of arterial blood (100ml O_2/dL arterial blood)
- O_2 is not very soluble in plasma, so only 0.3ml of O_2 is dissolved in 100ml of arterial blood
- the remaining 19.7 ml of O_2 is bound to Hb
- factors influencing the O_2 content of blood
- hemoglobin concentration
- % Hb saturated with O_2
- partial pressure of O_2 in arterial blood
- so, measuring % oxyhemoglobin allows you to monitor O_2 content of arterial blood
- as % oxyhemoglobin decreases, the O_2 content of arterial blood decreases
- as the O_2 content of arterial blood decreases, there is less oxygen available for delivery to tissues, and cellular hypoxia results

Much of the following general data was excerpted or modified from the work of Richard Klabunde, Ph.D. www.cvphysiology.com.

39 HEART FUNCTION

The primary function of the heart is to impart energy to blood in order to generate and sustain an arterial blood pressure necessary to provide adequate perfusion of organs with oxygen rich blood. The heart achieves this by contracting its muscular walls around a closed chamber to generate sufficient pressure to propel blood from the cardiac chamber (e.g., left ventricle), through the aortic valve and into the aorta, which leads to the remainder of the body.

Each time the heart beats, a volume of blood is ejected from the left ventricle. This stroke volume (SV), times the number of beats per minute (heart rate, HR), equals the cardiac output (CO).

$$CO = SV \cdot HR$$

Therefore, changes in either stroke volume or heart rate will alter cardiac output, unless the heart rate gets so fast that it can no longer fill adequately.

39.1 OXYGEN DELIVERY

Materials in this section have been summarized from Law, R. and Bukwirwa, The Physiology of Oxygen Delivery. Physiology 1999; 10(3): 1-2.

Introduction

In order to survive, humans have to be able to extract oxygen from the atmosphere and transport it to their cells where it is utilized for essential metabolic processes. Some cells can produce energy without oxygen (anaerobic metabolism) for a short time, although it is inefficient. Other organs (e.g. brain) are made up of cells that can only make the energy necessary for survival in the presence of a continual supply of oxygen (aerobic metabolism). **Tissues differ in their ability to withstand anoxia (lack of oxygen). The brain and the heart are the most sensitive.** Initially, a lack of oxygen affects organ function but with time, irreversible damage is done (within minutes in the case of the brain) and revival is impossible. **Heart attacks, myocardial infarction, angina and strokes are all about deficiencies of oxygen**.

39.2 OXYGEN TRANSPORT FROM AIR TO TISSUES

Oxygen is transported from the air that we breathe to each cell in the body. **Every aerobic cell must have an adequate and continual supply of oxygen.** In general, gases move from an area of high concentration (pressure) to areas of low concentration (pressure). If there is a mixture of gases in a container, the pressure of each gas (partial pressure) is equal to the pressure that each gas would produce if it occupied the container alone.

39.2.1 Atmosphere to Alveolus

The air (atmosphere) around us has a total pressure of 760 mmHg (1 atmosphere of pressure = 760 mmHg = 101kPa= 15 lbs/sq. in). Air is made of 21% oxygen, 78% nitrogen and small quantities of CO_2, argon and helium. The pressure exerted by the main two gases individually, when added together, equals the total surrounding pressure or atmospheric pressure. **The pressure of oxygen (PO_2) of dry air at sea level is therefore 159 mmHg** (21/100 x 760 = 159). However, by the time the inspired air reaches the trachea it has been warmed and humidified by the upper respiratory tract. The humidity is formed by water vapor which as a gas exerts a pressure. **At 37 degrees Celsius the water vapor pressure in the trachea is 47 mmHg.** Taking the water vapor pressure into account, **the PO_2 in the trachea when breathing air is (760 - 47) x 21/100 = 150 mmHg.** By the time oxygen has reached **the alveoli the PO_2 has fallen to about 100 mmHg.** This is because the PO_2 of the gas in the alveoli (PAO_2) is a balance between two processes: the removal of oxygen by the pulmonary capillaries and its continual supply by alveolar ventilation (breathing).

39.2.2 Alveolus to Blood

Blood returning to the heart from the tissues has a low PO2 (40 mmHg) and travels to the lungs via the pulmonary arteries. The pulmonary arteries form pulmonary capillaries, which surround alveoli. **Oxygen diffuses (moves through the membrane separating the air and the blood) from the high pressure in the alveoli (100 mmHg) to the area of lower pressure of the blood in the pulmonary capillaries (40 mmHg).** After oxygenation, blood moves into the pulmonary veins which return to the left side of the heart to be pumped to the systemic tissues. In a 'perfect lung' the PO_2 of pulmonary venous blood would be equal to the PO_2 in the alveolus. Three factors may cause the PO_2 in the pulmonary veins to be less than the PAO_2: ventilation/perfusion mismatch, shunt and slow diffusion. The transfer of oxygen up to this point is based on pressure differentials.

39.2.3 Ventilation/Perfusion Mismatch

In a 'perfect lung' all alveoli would receive an equal share of alveolar ventilation and the pulmonary capillaries that surround different alveoli would receive an equal share of cardiac output, i.e., ventilation and perfusion would be perfectly matched. Diseased lungs may have marked mismatch between ventilation and perfusion. This is to be considered in cases of asthma, bronchiectasis, emphysema, pneumonia, tuberculosis of the lung, etc. Some alveoli are relatively over ventilated while others are relatively over-perfused (the most extreme form of this is a shunt where blood flows past alveoli with no gas exchange taking place. Well ventilated alveoli (high PO_2 in capillary blood) cannot make up for the oxygen not transferred in the under ventilated alveoli with a low PO_2 in the capillary blood. This is because there is a maximum amount of oxygen which can combine with hemoglobin. The pulmonary venous blood (mixture of pulmonary capillary blood from all alveoli) will therefore have a lower PO_2 than the PO_2 in the alveoli (PAO_2). **Even normal lungs have some degree of ventilation/perfusion mismatch, the upper zones are relatively over ventilated while the lower zones are relatively over-perfused and under ventilated.**

Shunting occurs when deoxygenated venous blood from the body passes unventilated alveoli to enter the pulmonary veins and the systemic arterial system with an unchanged PO_2 (40 mmHg). Atelectasis (collapsed alveoli), consolidation of the lung, pulmonary edema or small airway closure will cause shunting.

39.2.4 Diffusion

Oxygen diffuses from the alveolus to the capillary until the PO_2 in the capillary is equal to that in the alveolus. **This process is normally complete by the time the blood has passed about one third of the way along the pulmonary capillary.** In the normal lung, the diffusion of oxygen into the blood is very rapid and is complete, even if the cardiac out put is increased (exercise) and the blood spends less time in contact with the alveolus. This may not happened when the alveolar capillary network is abnormal (Pulmonary disease). However, **the ability of the lung to compensate is great** and problems caused by poor gas diffusion are a rare cause of hypoxia, except with disease such as alveolar fibrosis. In order to decrease the detrimental effect that shunt and ventilation/perfusion mismatch have on oxygenation, the blood vessels in the lung are adapted to vasoconstrict and therefore reduce blood flow to areas which are under ventilated. This is termed **hypoxic pulmonary vasoconstriction** and reduces the effect of shunt. Oxygen delivery can be a complicated process in various disease states.

39.2.5 Oxygen Carriage by the Blood

Oxygen is carried in the blood in two forms. Most is carried combined with hemoglobin but there is a very small amount dissolved in the plasma. Each gram of hemoglobin can carry 1.31 ml of oxygen when it is fully saturated. Therefore, **every liter of blood with a Hb concentration of 15 g/dl can carry about 200 mls of oxygen when fully saturated** (occupied).

If the PO_2 of oxygen in arterial blood (PAO_2) is increased significantly (by breathing 100% oxygen) then a small amount of extra oxygen will dissolve in the plasma (at a rate of 0.003 ml O_2/100 ml of blood / mmHg PO_2) but there will normally be no significant increase in the amount carried by hemoglobin, which is already >95% saturated with oxygen. When considering the adequacy of oxygen delivery to the tissues, three factors need to be taken into account, hemoglobin concentration, cardiac output and oxygenation. Each step is important and can affect the amount of oxygen ultimately delivered to the tissue.

39.3 Oxygen Cascade

Oxygen moves down the pressure or concentration gradient from a relatively high level in air, to the levels in the respiratory tract and then alveolar gas, the arterial blood, capillaries and finally the cell. **The pO_2 reaches the lowest level (4-20 mmHg) in the mitochondria** (structures in cells responsible for energy production). This decrease in $_pO_2$ from air to the mitochondrion is known as the **oxygen cascade** and the size of any one step in the cascade may be increased under pathological circumstances and may result in hypoxia. **Hypoxia at the mitochondrial level is of most importance.**

39.4 OXYGEN DELIVERY

The quantity of oxygen made available to the body in one minute is known as the oxygen delivery and is equal to the cardiac output x the arterial oxygen content, i.e., 5000 ml blood / min x 200 ml O_2/1000 ml blood = 1000 ml O_2/min.

Oxygen delivery (mls O_2/min) = Cardiac output (liters/min) x Hb concentration (g/liter) x 1.31 (mls O_2/g Hb) x % saturation.

39.5 OXYGEN CONSUMPTION

Approximately **250 ml of oxygen are used every minute by a conscious resting person** (oxygen consumption) and therefore about 25% of the arterial oxygen is used every minute. The **hemoglobin in mixed venous blood is about 70% saturated** (95% less 25%).

In general, there is more oxygen delivered to the cells of the body than they actually use. If the free radical/oxidation theory of "all things bad for the body come from oxygen," then **it appears that evolution and nature were totally wrong by bringing in such high quantities of such a harmful agent into the body.** However, we now know of nature's wisdom in that oxygen is constantly needed and in short intervals of deficiency states, it is critical to have it available, especially for the brain and the heart. When oxygen consumption is high (e.g., during exercise) the increased oxygen requirements are usually provided by an increased cardiac output. However, **a low cardiac output, a low hemoglobin concentration (anemia) or a low hemoglobin O_2 saturation will result in an inadequate delivery of oxygen, unless a compensatory change occurs in one of the other factors.** Alternatively, if oxygen delivery falls relative to oxygen consumption the tissues extract more oxygen from the hemoglobin (the saturation of mixed venous blood falls below 70%). Again, this emphasizes the importance of an adequate and constant oxygen supply to the tissues.

39.6 OXYGEN STORES

In spite of the great importance of oxygen, **the stores of oxygen in the body are small and would be unable to sustain life for more than a few minutes**. If breathing ceases, oxygen stores are limited to the oxygen in the lung and in the blood. The amount of oxygen in the blood depends on the blood volume and hemoglobin concentration. The amount of oxygen in the lung is dependent on the lung volume at functional residual capacity (FRC) and the alveolar concentration of oxygen. The FRC is the volume of air (about 3 liters in an adult) that is present in the lungs at the end of a normal expiration, i.e., when the elastic recoil of the lung is balanced by the relaxed chest wall and diaphragm. While breathing air the total stores (oxygen in blood and lungs) are small and because the major component of this store is the oxygen bound to hemoglobin, only a small part of these stores can be released without an unacceptable reduction in PaO_2 **(when hemoglobin is 50% saturated with oxygen the PaO_2 will have fallen to 26 mmHg)**. Breathing 100% oxygen causes a large increase in the total stores as the FRC fills with oxygen.

The major component of the store is now in the lung and 80% of this oxygen can be used without any reduction in hemoglobin saturation (PaO_2 still about 100 mmHg). This is the reason why pre-oxygenation is so effective.

Principle stores of oxygen in the body

	While breathing AIR	While breathing 100% O_2
In the lungs (FRC)	**450 ml**	**3000 ml**
In the blood	850 ml	950 ml
Dissolved or bound		
In tissues (FRC)	250 ml	300 ml
Total	1550 ml	4250 ml

If a PaO_2 falls to less than 60 mmHg the aortic and carotid body chemoreceptors respond by causing hyperventilation and increasing cardiac output through the sympathetic nervous system stimulation. This normal protective response to hypoxia is reduced by anesthetic drugs and this effect extends into the post-operative period.

Anesthesia causes a 15% reduction in metabolic rate and therefore a reduction in oxygen requirements. Artificial ventilation causes a further 6% reduction in oxygen requirements as the work of breathing is removed. **Anesthetic agents do not affect the carriage of oxygen by hemoglobin.**

39.6.1 Crisis Management

Oxygen is of such importance that it essential for crisis management. When managing emergencies during anesthesia consideration should **always be given to the immediate administration of 100% oxygen** while the cause is found and rectified. It is the most appropriate treatment for acute deterioration in cardiorespiratory function.

Problems associated with 100% oxygen administration

It has been suggested that high concentrations of oxygen (90-100%) administered to patients for a prolonged period (several days) may cause pulmonary damage. **There is little evidence to support this and should never**

prevent its use in treating severe hypoxia. In fact, astronauts frequently live under high oxygen concentrations, including 100%, for prolonged periods without adverse effects. Additionally, I know of individual physicians who claim great benefits to the prolonged administration, for a month or more, of 100% oxygen.

However, high concentrations of oxygen will encourage collapse of alveoli with low ventilation/perfusion ratios. Oxygen is rapidly and completely absorbed from these alveoli, and when it is the only gas being given, these under ventilated alveoli collapse. When air and oxygen is used, the nitrogen present is absorbed more slowly and prevents the alveolus from collapsing.

39.7 OXYGEN CONSUMPTION: OVERALL CONSIDERATIONS

Oxygen consumption and oxygen demand are frequently used interchangeably but they are not equivalent. Organs with high oxidative requirements, such as the heart, logically have a high demand for oxygen and therefore have a relatively high oxygen consumption. Myocardial oxygen consumption (MVO_2) is required to synthesize and re-generate ATP that is utilized by membrane transport mechanisms and which serves as an energy source for 90% of cellular functions. Two such ATP requiring enzymes are the sodium/potassium ATPase pump and by myocyte contraction and relaxation (e.g. myosin ATPase).

Below is listed the comparative MVO_2 values for oxygen consumption of the heart at different levels of activity:

Cardiac State	MVO_2 (ml O_2/min.-100g)
Arrested heart	2
Resting heart rate	8
Heavy exercise	70

Below, the oxygen consumption (ml O_2/min.-100 g) for other organs is:

Organ	O_2 Consumption (ml O_2/min.-100g)
Brain	3
Kidney	5
Skin	0.2
Resting muscle	1
Contracting muscle (skeletal muscle)	50

As can be seen in the above chart, and as would be predicted by my **Unified Theory**, the skin has the lowest oxygen consumption rate and it is commonly known to have the highest rate of cancer formation. Again, this is consistent with my overall **Unified Theory** and reactive oxygen species and excited state function and reactivities.

Additionally, the above chart shows that skeletal muscle has the next highest level of oxygen consumption, compared to the heart, and according to my **Unified Theory,** it should and does have a low incidence of malignancies. Again, the oxidative stress theory teaches that the high production of reactive oxygen species and electronic excitation states should be destroying the skeletal muscle and doing irreparable damage to the rest of the body; but, it doesn't. In fact, quite the contrary happens as the result of exercise. Repeated studies show that exercise is good for us.

According to Marco E. Cabrena, Ph.D. as presented in "Metabolic Processes in Cardiac & Skeletal Muscle.":

39.7.1
Contributions to Standard Metabolic Rate (SMR)

{ 70 kg; 250 mL O_2/min}

Relative Sizes (mass, kg)			Contributions to SMR		
• Liver	2%	(1.4)	Liver	20%	50mL/min
• GI Tract	2%	(1.4)	GI Tract	5%	12.5
• Kidney	0.5%	(0.35)	Kidney	6%	15
• Lungs	1%	(0.7)	Lungs	1%	2.5
• Brain	2%	(1.4)	Brain	20%	50
• Heart	0.5%	(0.35)	Heart	10%	25
• Muscle	42%	(~30)	Muscle	25%	62.5
• Rest	50%	(35)	Rest	13%	32.5

Physiological function can be broken down into a series of biochemical events which generally take place intracellularly. The sum of these biochemical events is responsible for homeostasis. **Individual cells exhibit homeostasis, as does a tissue, organ system and intact organism.** (Northrop, RB Endogenous and Exogenous Regulation and Control of Physiological Systems, 1999).

39.7.2
Specific Rates of Blood Flow

(Flow rate / mass; mL min^{-1} kg^{-1})

- Liver and GI Tract   ~500 (3rd)
- Kidney   3500 (1st)
- Brain   500 (3rd)
- Heart   700 (2nd)
- Skeletal Muscle   30
- Rest of the Tissues   20

39.7.3
Specific Rates of O_2 Consumption

(Metabolism / mass; mL O_2 min^{-1} kg^{-1})

- Liver   35 (3rd)
- GI Tract   8
- Kidney   40 (2nd)
- Lungs   3
- Brain   35 (3rd)
- Heart   70 (1st)
- Skeletal Muscle   2
- Rest of the Tissues   1

39.7.4
Cerebral Blood Flow (CBF)

- CBF Value: 750 mL/min; 500 mL min-1 kg-1
- Maintenance of blood flow to the brain is critical
- The brain is protected from changes in systemic blood pressure under a wide variety of circumstances
- Cerebral blood flow remains constant for systemic pressure changes in the range of 60- 150 mmHg (Autoregulation)
- Blood flow to local brain regions is controlled by local factors

39.7.5
Coronary Blood Flow

- Resting coronary blood flow in a human is ~225 - 250 ml/min (4% - 5% CO)
- During exercise, there is a:
  a) 4x - 7x? CO against a higher arterial pressure
  b) ? 6x - 9x ? in work output requiring a
  c) 3 x - 4x ? in myocardial blood flow
  d) increased oxygen extraction and
  e) increased efficiency of cardiac utilization of energy

39.7.6
Muscle Blood Flow

Conditions	Muscle Blood Flow
• Resting	30 - 36 ml min-1 kg-1 (1.0 L/min)
• Maximal Exercise	900 ml min-1 kg-1 (27.0 L/min)

- It constitutes most of the soft tissue mass in the body
- The body contains ~600 muscles

40 APPLICATION OF MY UNIFIED THEORY

40.1 SKIN CANCER

Skin cancer is the most common form of cancer in the United States. The three major types of skin cancer are the highly curable basal cell and squamous cell carcinomas and the more serious malignant melanoma. The two most prevalent forms of **non-melanoma skin cancer (NMSC) are basal cell carcinoma (BCC) and squamous cell carcinoma (SCC)**. The American Cancer Society estimates that during 2003, about 1 million new cases of basal cell or squamous cell carcinoma and about 54,200 new cases of malignant melanoma will be diagnosed. It is also expected that skin cancer will claim the lives of approximately 9,800 Americans.

Basal and squamous cell carcinomas have an excellent prognosis, but persons diagnosed with non-melanoma skin cancer are at higher risk for developing additional skin cancers. Melanoma accounts for approximately three fourths of all skin cancer deaths. (Hall, H.I., Miller, D.R. and Rogers, J.D. et al,: Update on the incidence and mortality from melanoma in the United States. J Am Acad Dermatol 1999; 40(1): 35-42).

Exposure to sunlight is the main environmental etiologic cause of NMSC and it is generally accepted that solar-derived ultraviolet radiation (UVR) induces damage to keratinocyte DNA and causes **attenuation of cutaneous immune function** and is the main pathogenic factor in tumor production in BCC and SCC (Preston D.S. and Stern R.S. Non-melanoma cancers of the skin. N Engl J Med 1992; 327: 1649-1662).

Basal Cell Carcinoma

Other risk factors for BCC include genetic predisposition expressed as skin type 1 (always burns, never tans), red/blond hair, and blue/green eyes and patients with a history of BCC. The most common clinical types of BCC are nodular and superficial. Nodular BCCs (nBCCs) appear mostly on the head and neck and account for about 45% to 60% of all BCCs and the rest tend to be superficial (sBCCs), occurring on the trunk and extremities. Other types of BCC, including morphea-form, infiltrative, basosquamous, and cystic, occur less frequently. Current therapies include cryotherapy, curettage, electrodessication, excision and Moh's micrographic surgery.

I feel it is because of the very low oxygen consumption level of skin, that it has such a propensity to develop cancer. This is because its level of oxidative metabolism is generating low levels of reactive oxygen species and electronic excitation states, which are needed to kill the cancer cells. In fact, oxygen delivery to the outermost layer of the skin is so critical that very low levels of oxygen are actually absorbed by the skin from the air. **These critically low levels of oxygen may be the primary reason that the cells of the skin have the highest rate of malignant transformations of any cells of the body.**

Previous investigators have pointed out the fact that one of the major risk factors for developing skin cancer is the presence of light colored skin. It has been further pointed out that black skinned individuals have a very low incidence of skin cancer. The major difference between these two types of skin coloring is that light skinned individuals reflect sunlight, whereas, black skinned individuals absorb sunlight. The absorbance of ultraviolet light from the sun would produce additional reactive oxygen species and electronic excitation states within black skin, by photodynamic mechanisms. This approach also explains the overall lack of skin cancer in black skinned individuals, who in general, have higher overall cancer rates than do light skinned individuals. I explain this overall difference in light and dark skin as being attributable to the fact that **African Americans have consistently lower normal levels of white blood cells.** Thus, they have less generalized cancer killing ability than Caucasians. My explanation eliminates one more of the popular paradoxes.

40.2 IMMUNOSUPPRESSION AND SKIN CANCER

As a byproduct of immunosuppression, liver transplant recipients experience a high incidence of skin cancer. **Skin cancer is the most common malignancy arising in the postransplantation setting.** Multiple factors contribute to the high risk for cutaneous carcinoma in immunosuppressed organ-transplant recipients. Skin cancer is a significant medical and surgical problem for organ-transplant recipients. With prolonged allograft function and patient survival, the majority of solid-organ **transplant recipients will eventually develop skin cancer.** Although squamous cell carcinoma is the most common cutaneous malignancy in this population, basal cell carcinoma, melanoma, and Kaposi's sarcoma, as well as uncommon skin malignancies; may occur. **Highly susceptible patients may develop hundreds of squamous cell carcinomas,** which may be life threatening. (Otley, C.C. and Pittelkow, M.R. Skin cancer in liver transplant recipients. Liver Transplantation 2003; 6(3): 253-262).

Skin cancer is also the most common malignancy occurring in kidney transplant recipients (KTR). A recent study confirms the high incidence of non-melanoma skin cancer among KTRs in a Mediterranean population with occupational sun exposure and the patient's age at the time of transplantation being the main risk factor.

According to my **Unified Theory**, I interpret the fact that the skin is the predominant site of malignancies in immunosuppressed patients, to be due to the fact that **the skin has such a low oxygen consumption rate and consequently generates low levels of reactive oxygen species and electronic excitation states (RONS /excytomers).** This is consistent with the fact that other organs or tissue with higher oxygen consumption rates, are not more frequently seen as the site of malignancies in immunosuppressed patients. In short, the skin has the least capability to defend itself against cancer development and it is therefore more vulnerable than other sites with higher levels of reactive oxygen species and electronic excitation states.

Immunosuppressed renal and heart transplant patients have an increased incidence of NMSC (Euvrard, s., Kanitakis, J. and Pouteil-Noble, C., et al. Comparative epidemiologic study of premalignant and malignant epithelial cutaneous lesions developing after kidney and heart transplantation. J am Acad Dermatol 1995; 33: 222-229). In an Australian study, the cumulative incidence of developing skin cancer in renal transplant patients **increased progressively from 7% after 1 year of immunosuppression to 45% after 11 years and to as high at 70% after 20 years of immunosuppression**. In a number of studies of renal transplant patients, an increase risk of developing both SCC and BCC has been reported; however, patients are more at risk of developing SCC than BCC. In the immunosuppressed organ transplant patient, the ratio of SC to BCC is approximately 3:1, which is in stark contrast to the 0.25:1 ratio in the general population. This patient group therefore has a significantly higher risk of developing the disease than the general population. In one small study of six patients, the **cessation of immunosuppressive therapy was shown to lead to a deceleration of cutaneous carcinogenesis,** further exemplifying the role of the immune response in the pathogenesis of NMSC. (Otley, C.C., Coliron, B.M., Stasko, T. and Goldman, G.D. Decreased skin cancer after cessation of therapy with transplant-associated immunosuppression. Arch Dermatol 2001; 137: 459-463). **This is an extremely important study model of cancer causation and cessation and figures prominently in my Unified Theory.**

A paper by Gaspari, et al. (Gaspari, A.A. and Sauder, D.N. Immunotherapy of basal cell carcinoma: Evolving approaches. Am Soc Dermatol Surg 2003; 29: 1027-1034), discusses current concepts of the relationships between immunosuppression and development of NMSC. The impact of immunosuppression on the development of NMSC

Previous epidemiologic studies have suggested that sunscreen use is associated with an increased risk of melanoma skin cancer. (Drolet, B.A. and Conner M.J. Sunscreens and the prevention of ultraviolet radiation-induced skin cancer. J Dermatol Surg Oncol 1992; 18(7): 571-576), (Autier P., Dore, J.F. and Cattaruzza, M.S. et al.: Sunscreen use, wearing clothes, and number of nevi in 6- to 7- year old European children. European Organization for Research and Treatment of Cancer Melanoma Cooperative Group. J Natl Cancer Inst 1998; 90(24): 1873-1880).

The difficulties of establishing a dose-response relationship for skin cancer and UV light have been pointed out by others. A study [Am J Epidemiol 1996; 144: 1034-1040] published by Australian scientists states that:

> In any white-skinned populations, routine monitoring of the most common [skin] cancers...is difficult; and this is particularly so in high-risk populations...

> Although it is accepted that solar radiation causes skin cancer, there is a paucity of quantitative evidence regarding the relation in humans. Indeed, in epidemiologic studies, characteristics associated with a sun-sensitive complexion appear to be more strongly linked to the occurrence of skin cancer than sun exposure itself. This is partly due to the **difficulty in measuring the received dose of solar ultraviolet radiation**, the salient component of sunlight. Even for chronic sun exposure, which traditionally has been linked with skin cancer since the nineteenth century, epidemiologic studies show no greater than a doubling of risk relative to minimal levels of sun exposure.

Also, **skin cancer such as melanoma, usually occurs in areas of the body not routinely exposed to direct sunlight**.

is highlighted by the **increased incidence of BCC and other NMSCs in HIV-positive patients.** (Smith, K.J., Skelton, H.G., Yager, J. Angritt, P. and Wagner, K.F. cutaneous neoplasms in a military population of HIV-1-positive patients: Military medical consortium for the advancement of retroviral research. J Am Acad Dermatol 1993; 29: 400-406). The major risk factors for developing skin cancer have been found to be the same for this subset of patients as for the general population: fair skin, a positive family history and sun exposure.

The role of the cutaneous immune system in the development of BCC is also implicated by the observation that UVR, the main etiologic factor for BCC, has profound effects on both the local and systemic immune system. (Kondo, S. and Sauder, D.N. Keratinocyte-derived cytokines and UVB-induced immunosuppression. J Dermatol 1995; 22: 888-893). The effect of UVR on the immune system has been investigated by analyzing one aspect of immune function: cutaneous delayed-type hypersensitivity.

One mechanism that is thought to mediate the immunosuppressive effect of UVR is alterations to Langerhans cells (LCs), as UVR impairs their ability to present antigens to Th1 lymphocytes. UV radiation also stimulates keratinocyte to produce certain cytokines, including tumor necrosis factor (TNF) and Interleukins (IL)-10, which promote the development of suppressor T cells.

Generally, the immune response to BCC lesions is not adequate to clear these tumors; however, **both the innate and acquired immune pathways are thought to play a role in skin cancer immunosurveillance**. As cell-mediated immunity depends on direct interactions between T-lymphocytes and professional antigen-presenting cells that process and present tumor-associated antigens, it is thought that this arm of acquired immunity is critical for BCC regression. Cytotoxic T-lymphocytes also require the assistance of T helper cells, which can be divided into T helper 1 (Th-1, interferon-γ [IFN-γ] producing) cells and T helper 2 (Th-2, IL-4, IL-5, IL-6 producing) cells, each with a distinct profile of cytokine secretion. Both **CD4+ T-lymphocytes (cytokine secreting cells)** and the **CD8+ T-lymphocytes (cytotoxic effector cells)** are necessary for tumor regression in most tumor model systems, including skin cancer.

In BCCs, very few CD4+ helper lymphocytes are observed invading the tumor stroma or the tumor islands, indicating that the cell-mediated immune response to the tumor is limited. However, **spontaneous regression of BCC lesions is a recognized phenomenon and does occur relatively frequently**. In Curson and Weedon's study, (Curson, C. and Weedon, D. Spontaneous regression in basal cell carcinomas. J Cutan Pathol 1979; 6: 432-437), **approximately 20% of BCC lesions were actively in regression or had shown evidence of regression at some time**. It is thought that the cell-mediated immune response contributes to the spontaneous regression of BCCs, as infiltrates of large numbers of activated CD3+ and CD4+ T-cells have been observed in regressing BCC lesions compared with nonregressing tumors. (Hunt, M.J., Halliday, G.M., Weedon, D., Cooke, B.E. and Barneston, R.S. Regression in basal cell carcinomas: An immunohistochemical analysis. Br J Dermatol 1994; 130: 1-8). It has been proposed that the CD4+ cells might bring about tumor destruction via the secretion of various cytokines. In a study by Wong et al. (Wong, D.A., Bishop, G.A., Lowes, M.A., Cooke, B., Barneston, R.S. and Halliday, G.M. Cytokine profiles in spontaneously regressing basal cell carcinomas. Br J Dermatol 2000; 143: 91-98), in which the level of cytokines in regressing and nonregressing BCC tumors was analyzed, **a significant increase in the level of IFN-γ was demonstrated in regressing BCCs.** Increased in IL-2 and TNF were also reported, and the authors concluded that their findings support a role for Th-1-type cytokines in mediating spontaneous regression of BCCs.

40.3 A STORY OF THE OLD WEST (JUST ANOTHER SILLY METAPHOR)

My Tombstone Metaphor:

Neo-cancer (bad hombres) -normal cells containing mutations from oxidative metabolism

Sheriff and deputies -steady state levels of reactive oxygen species and electronic excitation states

Tombstone -a potential site of cancer

Hired guns -assassins (cells of the respiratory burst, PMN's, macrophages, neutrophils, etc.)

Telegraph -cytokines

The cancerous mutations, which are constantly occurring within our aerobic cells, will be referred to as "neo-cancer" and it is normally kept at bay by the reactive oxygen species and electronic states, which are being constantly produced within all of our aerobic cells ("young guns"). I will use the analogy of an old Western town, such as Tombstone (a site for potential cancer destruction) and there are always present some bad hombres (neo-cancers) . Normally, the Sheriff (steady state levels of reactive oxygen species and electronic excitation states) can control these hombres with the assistance of his deputies (young guns, O_2^-, H_2O_2, $^1O_2$, HOCl, etc.). However, there are times when the Sheriff or the deputies will be incapacitated, absent or dead, in which case, the hombres can have a destructive run of the town, to the extent of over running it and destroying it. If, however, the Sheriff and his deputies believe that they can not handle these bad guys, they keep in touch, by telegraph (cytokines), with some "hired guns" (mercenaries, assassins) who they can call in to kill the out-of-control hombres (fully developed and dividing cancer cells). The hired guns quickly ferret out the hombres and kill them. At times, some members of the hombre's gang may flee to another distant area (metastasis) to try to start trouble there.

On some occasions, the reputation and dastardly deeds of the hombres have preceded them and because of their nefarious acts elsewhere, hired guns are waiting to kill them upon sight (spontaneous regression following an infection or an immune response). At other times, if the Sheriff and his deputies are ill or incapacitated (immunosuppression), the hombres may temporarily take over, but when the Sheriff and his deputies return, they defeat and control the hombres (the effect of removing an immunosuppressing drug or removing hormonal stimulation of a cancer).

There are also occasions when the federal marshal (photosensitizer) comes into Tombstone and shares the light of his knowledge with the Sheriff and his deputies, about the presence of and the identity of the bad hombres, such that they can be rounded up and killed, while protecting the innocent citizens (selectivity).

The Sheriff and his deputies carry a variety of weapons such as a Winchester rifle, a derringer and their favorite weapon, the Colt 45 (refers to oxidative and non-oxidative cidal agents). However, The Colt 45 (the sheriff's favorite weapon) only shoots **silver bullets (singlet oxygen).**

**"Persistence transforms the weakling acorn
into the mighty oak of the informed, which can withstand
the wicked winds of ignorance
throughout a storm of discovery
and a vortex of controversy."**

R. M. Howes, M.D., Ph.D.

5/3/04

41 EXERCISE

Cells with high levels of aerobic activity, such as cardiac myocytes, hepatocytes, renal proximal tubule cells and neurons, the mitochondria occupy up to a quarter of the volume of the cytoplasm (Lemasters, J.J. and Nieminen A-L, Mitochondria in Pathogenesis, Kluwer Academic/Plenum Publishers, 2001 pg. 21). The Free Radi-Crap theory would predict that these organs would have the highest incidence of cancer in the body, but they do not.

Just as with all other areas of oxygen free radicals and oxidative stress, the **literature is filled with contradictions** and one can choose selected support for almost any point of view. Obviously, this weakens the validity of the entire field of research which usually attempts to demonstrate the alleged harmful and deadly effects of oxygen free radicals and oxidative stress. More important, perhaps, is the fact that exercise biochemistry basically, in and of itself, refutes the free radical/oxidation theory. Nonetheless, the persistence of biased investigators keeps this outdated theory limping along and in the headlines.

Because of the vast array of conflicting data, as it relates to individual athlete supplement recommendations, physicians and patients must proceed with caution. By far, the best recommendation is to eat fresh fruits and vegetables on a daily basis. Unsubstantiated claims have filled books, journals, articles, newspapers and magazines advertisements heralding the incredulous benefits of antioxidants in enhancing exercise performance, preventing serious illnesses and even stopping or reversing aging. These wild claims are unsupported by randomized clinical trials and in vivo data analysis.

It still remains unknown whether increased free radical production is an unwanted consequence of exercise that promotes further inflammation and tissue damage, or if the body regulates oxidant production to control inflammation and repair. (Tidall, J.G. Inflammatory cell response to acute muscle injury. Med Sci Sports Exerc 1995; 27(7): 1022-1032). Resistance exercise may also increase free radical production, although the evidence is less convincing. (McBride, J.M., Kraemer, W.J. and Triplett-McBride, T. et al. The effect of resistance exercise on free radical production. Med Sci Sports Exerc 1998; 30(1): 67-72). Oxygen consumption increases up to 20 times greater than the resting level, resulting in an elevated flow of oxygen through the mitochondrial electron transport chain. Superoxide radical may leak from this pathway and be reduced to hydrogen peroxide by mitochondrial SOD. Cytosolic SOD is also available to perform this function.

Considerable debate surrounds the issue of whether the rate of adaptation of skeletal muscle O_2 consumption (QO_2) at the onset of exercise is limited by the inertia of intrinsic cellular metabolic signals and enzyme activation or the availability of O_2 to the mitochondria, as determined by an extrinsic inertia of convective and diffusive O_2 transport mechanisms. A review of biochemical evidence suggests that a given respiratory rate is a function of the net drive of phosphorylation potential and redox potential and cellular mitochondrial PO_2 ($PmitoO_2$). (Tschakovsky, M.E. and Hughson, R.L. Interaction of factors determining oxygen uptake at the onset of exercise. J Appl Physiol 1999; 86: 1101-1113).

Physiological functional capacity (PFC) is defined as the ability to perform the physical tasks of daily life and the ease with which these tasks can be performed. A progressive reduction in maximal O_2 consumption (VO_2max) appears to be the primary physiological mechanism associated with declines in endurance running performance with advancing age, along with a reduction in the exercise velocity at lactate threshold. (Tanaka, H and Seals, D.R. Invited review: Dynamic exercise performance in masters athletes: Insight into the effects of primary human aging on physiological functional capacity. J Apply Physiol 2003; 95: 2152-2162).

Exercise requires energy, which is obtained through the increased flow of electrons in the mitochondrial respiratory chain leading to **increased formation of O_2^- and H_2O_2** and increased formation of ATP. Exercise exhausts the ATP pool, leading to high levels of ADP triggering ADP catabolism and conversion of xanthine dehydrogenase to xanthine oxidase. Xanthine oxidase in turn produces O_2^-. Oxidative stress should result in damage to lipids, proteins, and DNA. The biological markers for lipid peroxidation are malondialdehyde (MDA) (thiobarbituric acid reactive products) or ethane and pentane in the exhaled breath. In addition, a more direct way of measuring lipid peroxidation is by chemiluminescence measurement of lipid hydroperoxides (Frei, B., Yamamoto, Y., Nicolas, D. and Ames, B.N. Evaluation of a isoluminal chemiluminescence assay for the detection of hydroperoxides in human blood plasma. Anal Biochem 1988; 175: 120). DNA damage is assessed by measuring its change in migration in the single cell electrophoresis assay (SCG) or by formation of 8-OHdG..

Most studies indicate **an increase in RONS which is associated with exercise. Superoxide anion and hydrogen peroxide are chemically not very reactive**, but can theoretically be converted to the highly reactive .OH radical by an iron-catalyzed reaction. As a rule, **exercise increases loosely bound iron and therefore increases oxidative stress**. Thus, exercise should be harmful but it is not. Individuals who do not exercise have much lower levels of loosely bound iron ions.

Following exercise, tissue damage and local inflammation are observed after running or cycling with leukocytosis and leukocyte activation (Forster, N.K., Martyn, J.B., Rangno, R.E., Hogg, J.C. and Pardy, R.L. Leukocytosis of exercise: Role of cardiac output and catecholamines. J Appl Physiol 1986; 61: 2218). **During exercise, the total number of leukocytes increase proportional to the duration of the exercise** (Schaefer, R.A., Kokoi, K., Heidland, A. and Plass, R. Jogger's leukocytes. N Engl J Med 1987; 316: 223). It has been said that **the response of polymorphonuclear (PMN) leukocytes to physical exercise is similar to their response to infection. Oxygen consumption always increases with exercise.** These facts are supportive of my **Unified Theory,** in that oxygen consumption is increased, PMN numbers are increased, production of RONS and electronic excitation states are increased and this process has a cumulative beneficial effect on the body. It's that simple.

I feel compelled to remind you that the free radical/oxidation theory predicts that this sequence of events would lead to one's early demise….but it doesn't.

Vigorous **exercise over a lifetime increases the amount of mitochondria** (Davies, K.J.A., Packer, L. and Brooks, G.A. Biochemical adaptation of mitochondria, muscle, and whole-animal respiration to endurance training. Arch Biochem Biophys 1981; 209: 539), (mitochondrial volume) in muscle and these mitochondria may better withstand the onslaught of ROMs during exercise, but **the fact remains that exercise increases oxidative stress.** Vigorous exercise increases the amount of ethane and pentane, and MDA and 8-OHdG formation. **The antioxidant defenses never completely compensate for the increased formation of RONS during exhaustive exercise** (Eberhardt, M.K. Reactive oxygen metabolites chemistry and medical consequences. 2000; 386).

41.0.1 A Paradoxical Antioxidant

Here we go with another **"paradox"** because of the erroneous concept of oxidative balance, oxidative stress and the free radical/oxidation theory. Dr. David Leaf and Dr. Peter Glassman discuss this in their book entitled, **"The Oxidative Balance"** Emis, Inc. 2000, **(selective book review).**

Exercise, according to Leaf, Glassman and many others, is a "paradoxical" antioxidant. Although **it is almost universally agreed that exercise is good for the body, it also creates much more oxidative stress than occurs at rest. RMH Note: the production of large amounts of damaging and harmful reactive oxygen species and free radicals is the bedrock upon which the theory of oxidative stress is built. This huge factor of inconsistency, alone, should refute and put to rest the fallacious free radical/oxidative theory. However, its followers are willing to overlook this gigantic "paradox."** They say that while any one episode of exercise increases oxidative stress, long-term exercise, when performed correctly, is the most powerful determinant of beneficial oxidative balance. Regular exercise literally changes the body's oxidative zone so powerfully that it overwhelms any downside to activity. **RMH Note: The prodigious amounts of reactive oxygen species and free radicals produced by strenuous exercise should have killed you with any one of the 100 diseases attributed to oxidative stress, but instead, it is universally accepted that exercise makes you healthier. It does so because of the augmented production of oxygen modifications, which are needed to protect against diseases, infections and cancer. Each bout of moderate exercise is equivalent to getting a dose of an anti-infective or anti-cancer drug.**

During exercise, the body's greater energy demands require an increase of oxygen to the muscles. The higher the energy needs, the greater the oxygen flux; and the greater the oxygen flux, the higher the formation of free radicals in muscle cells. In fact, **high-intensity exercise generates almost 1000 times more free radicals than are generated at rest. (RMH Note: If one were to double the rate of ingestion of a known harmful agent, that acts with linearity, then it should reduce their life span by one half. At that rate, strenuous exercise would likely kill you on the spot.....but, it doesn't.).**

They say that exercise is one of the most powerful known pro-oxidants. **RMH Note: It is definitely the most powerful pro-oxidants known.** They claim that regular aerobic exercise has powerful antioxidants effects but the degree of the induction of antioxidant enzymes is controversial.

Exercise increases oxygen needs, as more oxygen is required to help burn fats for energy. **More oxygen equals more free-radicals in the short term**. Regular exercise, though, improves oxidative balance. **RMH Note: Any time you are increasing oxygen consumption and the burning of oxygen in the manufacture of ATP, you have to produce proportionately more reactive oxygen species and free radicals. In short, if you want more energy from more ATP for exercise, then you are going to get more ROS and free radicals. Period!**

They say that the amount of oxygen used during exercise can be expressed in **metabolic equivalents**, known as METs. **One MET equals the amount of oxygen used at rest**. A five-MET level means that five times the amount of at-rest oxygen is being used, i.e., five times the amount of oxygen is fluxing through the mitochondria and causing oxidative stress.

Five METs is the level of oxygen required by most people for walking at a moderate pace. However, for extremely preconditioned individuals (e.g., patients with severe heart disease), five METs can be the peak exercise level.

For individuals whose usual peak exercise capacity is approximately five METs, oxidative stress begins to worsen significantly at approximately three METs. For healthier, conditioned persons, peak exercise level is approximately 12 METs and oxidative stress begins to worsen at about seven METs.

Deconditioned people have little exercise tolerance. Their peak potential, measured in metabolic equivalents, or METs, is about half that of those who exercise moderately.

At low levels of work intensity, the amounts of oxygen used, or MET levels, are similar for both conditioned and deconditioned persons but that, at higher levels of work, conditioned persons use less oxygen. While these differences do not appear to be large, **a lifetime of increased oxygen use raises cumulative oxidative stress substantially. RMH Note: Yes, and it is good for you, which is diametrically opposed to the theory of oxidative stress but is consistent with and supportive of my Unified Theory.**

This phenomenon might be interpreted to mean that deconditioned people should avoid exercise to protect themselves from oxidative stress. A healthy, fit person has a greater ceiling of peak exercise and can enjoy a more productive and active life. **RMH Note: This is due to the wide spread benefits of modified oxygen, as explained in my Unified Theory. This has little, if anything, to do with METs or LATs or any other such thing which can be thrown in to confuse the issue.**

Table 1 - Oxygen Flux (METs) During Common Household Tasks

Task	METs	
	Deconditioned	Physically Fit
Washing dishes	2.3	2.0
Scrubbing pots	2.3	2.0
Ironing clothes	2.3	2.0
Unpacking groceries	2.5	2.5
Sweeping	3.0	2.5
Vacuuming	3.0	3.0
Changing a bed	3.5	3.0
Mopping	4.0	3.5

Exercise limit for most severely deconditioned people = approximately 5 METs

Leisure bicycling	Cannot do	6.0
Dancing	Cannot do	6.0
Jogging	Cannot do	7.0
Running	Cannot do	9.0

Exercise limit for most active people = 12 METs

Fit people require less oxygen to do the same work as their unfit counterparts. **However, anytime you are burning more oxygen, you are creating proportionately more oxygen free radicals.**

Exercise actually optimizes oxidative balance in three ways. First, regular exercise decreases baseline oxidative stress levels. In a study by Dr. Leaf, the baseline oxidative stress levels of preconditioned persons fell by 70 percent after they completed a 12-week program of regular aerobic training. Thus, the level of oxidative stress during daily activity is far lower in persons who engage in regular exercise. Simply put, fit people need less energy to do the same physical tasks as unfit people; and lower energy requirements translate into fewer fatty acids that burn up and, thus, less oxygen that is required for energy production. Lower oxygen flux produces lower levels of free radical formation.

These guys sound like politicians trying to "spin" their point of view. **RMH Note: Simply put, any increase in the production of reactive oxygen species or free radicals, according to the theory of oxidative stress, is theoretically dreadfully harmful to you….but, it isn't. Actually, exercise with its horrid 1000 times increase of reactive oxygen species and free radicals, is, predictably (by my Unified Theory), quite good for you.**

They say that regular exercise benefits oxidative balance in three ways. **RMH Note: Regular exercise benefit's the body in countless ways by giving it the equivalent of a mini-injection of modified oxygen RONS with each exercise session.** The first benefit is to decrease baseline, or resting, levels of free radical production.

The second benefit of regular exercise is that it raises peak exercise capacity. A deconditioned person has oxidative stress at three METs, and a conditioned person at seven. **RMH Note: This still means that a conditioned person is using seven times his resting rate of oxygen consumption and according to the theory of oxidative stress, is consequently, producing seven times as many reactive oxygen species and free radicals and is injuring his body seven times as fast as normal and is doing seven times the normal damage and is causing a seven times greater rate in causing 100 different diseases. Nevertheless, as we all know, that is not the case.** These levels correspond to the point at which metabolism switches from aerobic to anaerobic during exercise.

Aerobic metabolism utilizes oxygen in energy production, while anaerobic metabolism does not. While this might sound helpful in reducing free radical formation, **anaerobic metabolism is inefficient and, in fact, causes more oxidative stress when the body eventually catches up to its oxygen "debt."** Moreover, with anaerobic metabolism, lactic acid (produced when muscles crave energy but cannot get enough oxygen to sustain its production) forms and requires additional energy to be cleared away.

The transition between aerobic and anaerobic metabolism is known as the **lactic acidosis threshold (LAT).** At LAT, the muscles find an alternative energy source that, unfortunately, is far less efficient than the usual oxygen, fat, and glucose mixture. The result is a painful, burning sensation.

In terms of oxidative stress, LAT is the point at which free radical production accelerates dramatically. **RMH Note: What free radicals of glycolysis? There is no oxygen in anaerobic metabolism, consequently, there can be no reactive oxygen species or oxygen free radicals. Likely, they are referring to the oxygen metabolized to pay off the oxygen debt.** Energy production is far more efficient below than above LAT. Regular aerobic exercise raises LAT, reducing oxidative stress at a given level of exertion.

Ironically, the potential for raising LAT and peak exercise levels is greater for deconditioned individuals. In a sense, the less conditioned people are physically, the more they stand to gain from regular exercise because they require less intense training than highly fit people in order to improve exercise capacity.

This second benefit of regular exercise raises the lactic acid threshold, or LAT, the point at which free radical formation increases dramatically. **Many investigators state that the formation of lactic acid actually takes more energy via aerobic metabolism to get rid of the lactic acid.**

Muscles consist of two main kinds of fibers, Types I and II. Type I, slow twitch, fibers are primarily used for sustained activities (e.g., walking or long distance running). Type II, fast-twitch, fibers are more important for the sudden bursts of power needed in weight lifting or sprinting. Aerobic exercise training increases Type I fibers, which are packed with mitochondria and, thus, are efficient in making energy from fat combustion. Greater efficiency means fewer free radicals. **RMH Note: More mitochondria means more oxidative metabolism, which means more reactive oxygen species and free radicals, not fewer free radicals.**

They say that besides being an antioxidant advantage, aerobic exercise also increases the internal antioxidant systems of these muscles. For example, in exercise trained animals, researchers have noted higher levels of glutathione and superoxide dismutase in Type I muscle fibers. **RMH Note: Yes, but is it increased 1000 times? Also these increased levels of antioxidants are usually transient and temporary.**

Thus, they say that the paradox is resolved. **RMH Note: The paradox is not resolved by the theory of oxidative stress and the exercise effect is exactly the opposite of what it would have predicted. However, my Unified Theory solves the paradox and it is supported by the observations on exercise.** Exercise itself is a prooxidant. The take-home message is that regular even low-level, exercise is critical for optimizing oxidative states and health. **RMH Note: The take-home message is, once again, that the oxidative stress theory is wrong. The oxy-morons just don't get it.**

Skeletal muscle mass decreases with advancing age. Whether this reduced muscle mass is a result of an age-associated decrease in activity or a change in muscle function is unclear. However, **the age-dependent decline of muscle mass is associated with reduced aerobic capacity and muscle strength.** As the age of humans exceeds 75 years, the decline in exercise capacity is accelerated (Jette, A.M. et al. The Framingham disability study. II. Physical disability among the aging. Am J Public Health 1981; 71: 1211). They say that in oxidative stress conditions, higher levels of oxygen radicals are produced, exceeding the cellular antioxidant defense system, resulting in the peroxidation of polyunsaturated fatty acids (PUFA) in membrane structures. **Lipid peroxidation also releases reactive free radicals and toxic aldehydes,** which then can completely inactivate enzymes and other cell components (Halliwell, B., Oxidants and human disease; some new concepts. FASEB J 1987; 1: 358). Prolonged sub maximal exercise has been demonstrated to result in elevated whole body (indicated by increased exhaled pentane, but not ethane) and skeletal muscle levels of lipid peroxidation byproducts. **These studies seem to indicate that the greatly increased oxygen consumption (up to a 100-fold increase in skeletal muscle) of exercise produces superoxide radicals which are associated with a host of deleterious effects.** I submit that the cardiovascular response to exercise reflects the increased need for oxygen transport and utilization associated with the raised metabolic rate. **However, studies consistently demonstrate the beneficial effects of exercise as opposed to the harmful and damaging effects that are predicted by the theory of oxidative stress.**

However, events such as marathons or the Iron Man competition, can predispose participants to increased viral infections and possibly to cancer. I will discuss this in the section on exercise and immunity.

Local stores of glycogen and fat are the energy sources for continuous regeneration of ATP during exercise that requires molecular oxygen as an electron acceptor for the oxidation process in the critic acid cycle and in the electron transport chain of mitochondria. Molecular oxygen contains two unpaired electrons which, through reduction with four electrons and hydrogen ions, forms water. This process occurs in the mitochondria, with cytochrome oxidase as the final catalyst.

During intensive exercise, due to probable loss of cytochrome oxidase activity (which is speculative), the level of molecular oxygen that is required to be reduced through four-electron reduction exceeds the muscle mitochondrial respiratory capacity. This condition leads to the univalent reduction of molecular oxygen through semiquinones, an alternative electron acceptor in the inner mitochondria membrane, and generates superoxide radicals (Boveris, A., Cadenas, E. and Stoppani, A.O.K. Role of ubiquinone in mitochondria generation of hydrogen peroxide. Biochem J 1976; 156: 435). (Gollnick, P.D., Bertocci, L.A., Kelso, T.B., Witt, E.H. and Hodgson, D.R. The effect of high intensity exercise on the respiratory capacity of skeletal muscle. Eur J Physiol 1990; 415: 407). **Using electron paramagnetic resonance (EPR) and electron spin resonance (ESR), evidence is still lacking that free radicals produced during exercise are the consequence of damage or that the higher concentrations were the cause of damage. There are no conclusions as to whether the increase in radicals associated with exercise is primary or secondary to the exercise-induced damage.**

Reactive oxygen species are generated during ischemia/hypoxia and subsequent reperfusion/reoxygenation. In this process, ATP is depleted and intracellular calcium is increased, leading to cellular necrosis, which is known as the "oxygen paradox." **RMH Note: Every time the data rebuts the free radical/oxidation theory, they call it a paradox, when, in fact, it is a rejection of the theory. The theory just does not hold up to testing.** The method that is presently accepted for the generation of free radicals through hypoxia and reoxygenation is that, during hypoxia, xanthine is formed from the degradation of ATP, and, during the reoxygenation upon the mild proteolysis, xanthine dehydrogenase is converted to xanthine oxidase, which then generates oxygen radicals and uric acid from xanthine (McCord, J.M. Oxygen-derived free radicals in postischemic tissue injury. N Engl J Med 1985; 312: 159).

Following exercise, infiltration of neutrophils and phagocytic cells in exercised muscles has been observed in animals and humans (Jones, D.A., Newsham, D.J., Round, J.M. and Tolfree, S.E.J. Experimental human muscle damage, morphological changes in relation to other indices of damage. J Physiol 1986; 375: 435). Activation of chemotactic factors by superoxide radical , similar to early manifestation of acute phase response in infection, has been suggested to occur following exercise (Petrone, W.F., English, D.K., Wong, K. and McCord, J.M. Free radicals and inflammation: Superoxide dependent chemotactic factor in plasma. Proc Natl Acad Sci USA 1980; 77: 1159). **Products of lipoxygenase pathway in muscle are chemotactic for immune cells.** Several studies have also demonstrated that, following exercise, immune complements are activated, which is an initial event in the inflammatory response. This process is then followed by the mobilization and activation of neutrophils, production of acute phase proteins and accumulation of monocytes and macrophages at the site of injury (Cannon, J.G. and Kluger, M.J. Endogenous pyrogen activity in human plasma after exercise. Science 1983; 220: 617). **This is the same response as is seen in the adipocytes of obese patients and will be discussed in the section on obesity.**

Neutrophils contain several enzymes, such as myeloperoxidase and nicotinamide-adenine dinucleotide phosphate (reduced) (NADPH) oxidase, that generate radicals such as NO., HO., H_2O_2, and hypochlorous acid. Neutrophils and monocytes release superoxide anions and degradative enzymes, such as elastase and lysozyme, that further break down muscle to be phagocytosed by macrophages and monocytes, and this will be followed by the production of growth factors for new muscle fiber regeneration. As a part of the inflammatory response, **activated neutrophils and macrophages produced both superoxide anions and hydrogen peroxide** at the site of damaged muscle, which, in turn, is directly responsible for the disruption of phospholipid bilayer and lipid peroxidation (Kokot, K., Schaefer, R.M., Teschiner, M., Plass, G.U.R. and Heidland, A. Activation of leukocytes during prolonged physical exercise. Adv Exp Med Biol 1988; 240: 57).

It is theorized that because of the increased rates of generation of oxygen radicals, the body has developed protective antioxidant enzymes such as, catalase and glutathione peroxidase. **Catalase is predominantly located in peroxisomes, whereas GSH-Px, as well as glutathione tripeptide, are found in mitochondria and cytosol.** Animal studies demonstrated that exercise training and exhaustive exercise increased SOD activity in skeletal and heart muscle (Jenkin, R.R. Free radical chemistry: Relationship in exercise. Sports Med 1988; 5: 156), (Higuchi, M., Cartier, L.J., Chen, M. and Holloszy, J.O. Superoxide dismutase and catalase in skeletal muscle: Adaptive response to exercise. J Gerentol 1985; 40: 281). Other studies reported an increase in Cu-Zn SOD activity in human skeletal muscle after training (Jenkin, R.R., Friendland, R. and Howald, H. The relationship of oxygen uptake to superoxide dismutase and catalase in human skeletal muscle. Int J Sports Med 1984; 5: 11). **In contrast, some investigators found that total SOD activity was not affected by either acute or chronic exercise** (Alessio, H.M. and Goldfarb, A.H. Lipid peroxidation and scavenger enzymes during exercise: Adaptive response to training. J Appl Physiol 1988; 64: 1333), (Alessio, H.M., Goldfarb, A.H. and Cutler, R.G. MDA content increases in fast and slow-twitch skeletal muscle with intensity of exercise in a rat. Am J Physiol 1988; 255: C874).

Just as indicated above, there is considerable inconsistency in the data. Results of many studies show opposites in terms of antioxidant effects, damage produced by oxygen free radicals and induction of antioxidant enzymes. However, **a few clear conclusions can be drawn: 1) oxygen consumption is dramatically increased during exercise; 2) increased oxygen metabolism leads to increased production of reactive oxygen species and free radicals; 3) exercise has an overall beneficial effect on many systems within the body; 4) once again, the data clearly shows that the theory of oxidative stress is wrong; 5) exercise improves immune function and 6) exercise increase muscle mass and its oxidative capacity.** I firmly believe that the increase in reactive oxygen species and electronic excitation states, from both the microsomal and mitochondria systems, are directly responsible for the salutary effects of exercise. This is **supportive of my Unified Theory.**

Inconsistent, is the only way to describe data regarding the influence of vitamins and antioxidant supplements in regards to exercise.

41.1   EXERCISE AND CANCER

RMH Note: To set the record straight, exercise helps to stabilize and to reverse many of the se-quelae of cancer therapy, which is consistent with my Unified Theory and diametrically opposed to the Free Radi-Crap theory of aging and oxidative stress, which states that exercise with its increased levels of reactive oxygen species and free radicals are the cause of cancer and over 100 diseases.

During exercise, the heart pumps increased volumes of blood to supply oxygen and nutrients and to remove carbon dioxide and metabolic wastes; the respiratory system handles an increased workload, exchanging oxygen and carbon dioxide between the blood and the atmosphere. The nervous system and various hormones have important roles as well, integrating the body's response to exercise and regulating the metabolic changes that occur in muscle and other tissues (Microsoft Encarta Encyclopedia 99. Microsoft Corp). Exercise appears to **influence host defense against both viral infection and cancer.** Exercise also causes the **release of several cytokines involved in resistance to tumors,** which may also influence the activity of cytotoxic cells.

Moreover, stress influences resistance to tumor growth and some stress hormones released during exercise such as **corticosteroids or catecholamines can modulate the ability of immune cells to kill tumor cells** (Mackinnon, LT. Advance in exercise immunology. Champaign, IL: Human Kinetics, 1999). Thus, it can be postulated that exercise may influence host defense against tumor growth via directly or indirectly modulating the activity of cytotoxic cells. Most research in this area has focused on natural killer (NK) cells, with relatively less attention given to the effects of exercise on cytotoxic T-lymphocytes and monocytes cytotoxicity.

The decline in functional capacity experienced by 1/3 or more of cancer patients, regardless of the stages of the disease, can be attributed to hypokinetic conditions developed from prolonged physical inactivity. This hypokinetic condition may cause the reduction in the efficiency of the energy systems (metabolic pathways) that may lower the assimilation of energy substrates by the body that are essential for the daily task performance. In addition, the hypokinetic condition may have some effects on hormone levels that could lead to further homeostatic unbalance. These modifications that may occur due to physical inactivity could lead to a malfunctioning of many systems within the body, which can also be correlated to high levels of fatigue experienced by the patient.

Numerous studies have suggested that exercise, including light to moderate intensities, has many benefits for people with cancer (Courneya, K.S. and Friedenreich, C.M. 1999, Physical exercise and quality of life following cancer diagnosis: a literature review. Annuals of Behavioral Medicine 21(2): 171-179), (Derman, W.E., Coleman, K.L. and Noakes, T.D. Effects of exercise training in patients with cancer who have undergone chemotherapy, abstracted. Medicine of Science and Sports and Exercise 1999; 31(5): S368), (Durack, E.P. and Lilly, P.C. The application of an exercise and wellness program for cancer patients: A two-year follow-up survey with prostate, leukemia and general carcinoma. Journal of Strength and Conditioning 1998; 12(1): 3-6), (Durack, E.P., Lilly, P.C. and Hackworth, J.L. Physical and psychosocial responses to exercise in cancer patients: A two-year follow-up survey with prostate, leukemia and general carcinoma. J Exerc Physiol (online) 2000; Accessed March 6, 2001 http://www.css.edu/users/tboone2/asep/jan12b.htm), (Mock, V., Ropka, M.E., Rhodes, V.A., Pickett, M., Grimm, P.M., McDaniel, R., Lin, E.M., Allocca, P., Dienemann, J.A., Halsfield-Wolfe, M.E., Stewart, K.J. and McCorkle, R. Establishing mechanisms to conduct multi-institutional research-fatigue in patients with cancer: An exercise intervention. Oncology of Nursing Forum   1998; 25(8): 1391-1397), (Schultz, K.H., Szlovak, C. and Schultz, H.

Implementation and evaluation of an ambulatory exercise therapy based rehabilitation program for breast cancer patients. Medical Psychology 1998; 48: 398-407). Some of the **benefits of exercise include**: increases in cardiovascular, pulmonary and muscular functioning produced by regular exercise result in **improved oxygen consumption**, stroke volume, cardiac output, visualization of muscles, lymphatic circulations, metabolic rate, muscle tone, strength, coordination and balance (Smith, S. Physical exercise as an oncology nursing intervention to enhance quality of life. Oncology Nursing Forum 1996; 23(5): 771-778). During cancer treatment, chemotherapy, radiation and surgery can cause lasting effects to various biological systems. The benefits of exercise for the systems of cardiovascular, pulmonary, musculoskeletal and endocrine are discussed briefly below.

Exercise has been suggested by many researchers as a rehabilitative solution for energy loss in cancer patients. **Defined as rhythmic contraction and relaxation of large muscle groups over an extended period of time, aerobic exercises have been shown to improve physical capabilities in cancer patients** (Dimeo, F.C., Rumberger, B. and Keul, J. Aerobic exercise as therapy for cancer fatigue. Medicine and Science in Sports and Exercise 1998; 30: 475-478). In a study conducted by Dimeo et al. the most significant results of the study was that the patients experienced a clear reduction of fatigue and could carry out normal daily activities without limitations.

More often than not, **cancer patients are not as active during and after treatment as they were before treatment**, or even diagnosis. Reductions in activity cause muscle atrophy, changes in muscle properties, and reductions in bone density. Muscle atrophy and reduced bone density lead to diminished musculoskeletal strength and performance, and contribute to an increased risk for bone fractures and musculoskeletal injuries (American College of Sports Medicine: ACSM's Resource Manual for Guidelines for Exercise Testing and Prescription, 3rd Edition, Baltimore, MD: Williams & Wilkins Publishing Co., 1998). Musculoskeletal atrophy and changes in muscle properties contribute to declines in cardiovascular efficiency. Declines in cardiac efficiency are reflected in increased heart rate and blood pressure at rest and with sub-maximal exercise. Reductions in cardiovascular efficiency combined with elevations in cholesterol levels and decreases in HDL levels from inactivity contribute to an increased cardiovascular risk profile (American College of Sports Medicine: ACSM's Guidelines for Exercise Testing and Prescription, 6th Edition, Baltimore, MD: Williams & Wilkins Publishing Co., 2000). **I believe that the decreases cardio-pulmonary function and activity, leads to reduced oxygen consumption.**

Declines in pulmonary function that result from inactivity may include a dulled ventilatory response, diminished airflow and respiratory muscle function and impairments in gas exchange from ventilation/perfusion mismatches, shunting and declines in diffusion that predispose people to respiratory disease such as pneumonia (American College of Sports Medicine: ACSM's Resource Manual for Guidelines for Exercise Testing and Prescription, 3rd Edition, Baltimore, MD: Williams & Wilkins Publishing Co., 1998). **I believe that any factor that results in the ultimate reduction of reactive oxygen species or electronic excitation states of oxygen (RONS/ excytomers), predisposes to infections and cancer.**

Some initial clinical concerns about exercise in cancer patients include: a) the potential immunosuppressive effects of vigorous exercise, b) the increase likelihood of pathological bone fractures arising from compromised bone integrity, c) possible worsening of cardiotoxicity from chemotherapy and/or radiation, d) severe pain, nausea and fatigue that may be intensified by physical exercise, and e) the inability and/or unwillingness of cancer patients to tolerate exercise given their weakened physical and emotional condition (Courneya, K.S., Mackey, J.R. and Jones, L.W. Coping with cancer: can exercise help? The Physician and Sports Medicine 2000; 28(5): 49-73). **Despite all of these concerns, there is a growing body of evidence that shows how exercise can benefit cancer patients.**

41.2 CAN EXERCISE HELP REVERSE THE EFFECTS OF CANCER TREATMENT?

Cardiovascular benefits of exercise for cancer patients were shown to be evident in patients that had no signs of impaired cardiac function before cancer treatment (Dimeo, F.C., Tilmann, M.H.M., Bertz, H., Kanz, L., Mertelsmann, R. and Keul, J. Aerobic exercise in the rehabilitation of cancer patients after high dose chemotherapy and autologous peripheral stem cell transplantation. Cancer 1997; 79(9): 1717-1722). In this study, no patients in the training group developed clinical signs of cardiotoxicity during the two months after chemotherapy. For women with breast cancer, a fitness program that included aerobic exercise would decrease the risk of developing cardiovascular disease and osteoporosis (Mock, V., Burke, M.B., Sheehan, P., Creaton, E.M., Winningham, M.L., McKenney-Tedder, S., Schwager, L.P. and Liebman, M. A nursing rehabilitation program for women with breast cancer receiving adjuvant chemotherapy. Oncology Nursing Forum 1994; 21: 899-908). Because treatment for breast cancer often results in a decrease in natural or exogenous sources of estrogen, these women face a greater risk of developing cardiovascular disease and osteoporosis.

Cancer treatment has been shown in some cases to be harmful to the cardiovascular system. **RMH Note: This effect decreases the body's ability to distribute oxygen to the organs and tissue, which is needed for both normal metabolism and for fighting cancerous cells with modified oxygen molecules.** The heart in a cancer patient becomes less efficient in pumping blood to organs and tissues, therefore compromising the ability to perform daily activities and reaching high levels of fatigue. Exercise can promote cardiovascular training again throughout aerobic activities, allowing the heart to become more efficient in supplying blood to the body, and lowering the levels of fatigue experienced by the patient.

Pulmonary benefits from exercise in regards to the damage done by the cancer treatment is related to improvements in the lung volume, decreased work of breathing and better ability for gas exchange. Athletic performance can be measured through many physiological variables observed in exercise training. However, most pulmonary function measures do not apply for this performance prediction. No substantial relationship appears between athletic performance and vital capacity, total lung capacity or forced expiratory volume (Hayward, R. Cardiopulmonary physiology: The physiological response at rest and during exercise. Greely, CO: UNC, 1999). The most useful adaptation is probably an increase in the endurance capacity of respiratory muscles. When the respiratory muscles become trained due to exercise, the patient would experience a relief of the heavy breathing due to the fact that energy expenditure by these muscles would be lowered. Also, **a more efficient gas exchange ratio would proportionate a more effective oxygen distribution to the systems throughout the body.**

Given the fact that alveoli of a cancer patient are diminished in number, and compromised by alveolar septa's thickening, (**RMH Note: These effects would decrease oxygen delivery to the body and would benefit cancer survival or growth and not benefit the patient),** the exercise effects on the cancer patient pulmonary system is not known. One hypothesis is that the alveoli regenerate due to a supposed increase in blood supply to this organ, however the septa's thickening does not seem likely to be reversible.

The side effects of cancer treated on the musculoskeletal system have demonstrated physiological improvements from exercise interventions. The loss in lean body mass that is reported during cancer treatment is still not well explained. This reduction in skeletal muscle could be attributed to surgery reduction, treatment depletions and inactivity during recovery. This loss is muscle may be responsible for the exertion of higher energy needed to produce enough contractile forces required during energy performance or during sitting or standing (Dimeo, F.C., Rumberger, B. and Keul, J. Aerobic exercise as therapy for cancer fatigue. Medicine and Science in Sports and Exercise 1998; 30: 475-478), (Reich, P.R. and Metcalf, J.E. The facts about chemotherapy: A guide for cancer patients and their families. Mount Vernon, NY: Consumer Reports Book, 1991). Exercise may stimulate various benefits to the musculoskeletal system. Such benefits include the development of new healthy cells that will replace the healthy cells that died from the cancer treatment. This process has been shown to give patients the strength gains needed to perform daily activities, more motivation and energy and improvement in the overall quality of life.

The endocrine system appears to be a biological system that suffers severe consequences in regards to cancer treatments (mainly radiation). For example, the decreased production of hormones **thyroxin and triiodothyronine have biological effects on oxygen consumption,** the central and peripheral nervous system, skeletal and cardiac muscle, carbohydrate and cholesterol metabolism, and growth and development (Yarbro, C.H., Frogge, M.H., Goodman, M. and Groenwald, S.L. Cancer Nursing: Principles and Practices, 5th Edition. Sudbury, MA: Jones and Barlett Publishers, 2000). Also, alterations in metabolism can potentially lead to future heart complications. Heart complications can occur because of the increased amount of cholesterol due to the decreased carbohydrate metabolism.

Exercise interventions may have an important role in returning hormone levels back to pre-cancer levels. Exercise may stimulate release of hormones that may have been suppressed, as well as helping to increase the metabolic pathways efficiency that was compromised by cancer. All of these alterations that may occur with exercise interventions could potentially help cancer patients to improve their activities and functional capacities. Improvements in metabolism, fluid balance, **oxygen transportation** and central and peripheral nervous system functioning would create an overall homeostasis. This homeostasis would possibly give the patient an overall feeling of wellness.

Exercise is likely one of the most potent interventions for cancer patients, but with this also comes risks. Not all exercises are created equal. To be effective and safe, exercise should be prescribed, and include five criteria: 1) Status of the individual, 2) Type of exercise, 3) Intensity of exercise, 4) Frequency of exercise, and 5) Anaerobic and aerobic exercise training should be an integral component in the lifestyle of people fighting through or recovering from cancer.

Because the latency period of some late toxicities is many years after completion of treatment, the consequences of permanent tissue damage across the lifespan are unknown. **Exercise could possibly be a link physiologically that slows or even reverses the effects of chemotherapy, radiation therapy and surgery**. More investigations still need to occur in the area of exercise as rehabilitation for cancer patients. Regardless, **all the findings of the research up to now have shown that moderate exercise is beneficial for the cancer patients (cardiovascular, pulmonary, musculoskeletal and endocrine systems included).**

Fatigue is one of the most prevalent symptoms associated with cancer therapy, and yet fatigue is the least understood. Clinically knowing that exercise has helped alleviate some or all of the feelings of fatigue in cancer patients, bodes well for future research in this area in the years to come.

41.3 EXERCISE AND IMMUNITY

41.4 INTRODUCTION

Exercise serves as a study model for susceptibility to infections and neoplasia. The following material has been excerpted from and based on an article by Shepard et al (Shepard, R.J. and Pang P.N. Exercise, immunity and susceptibility to infection: A J-shaped relationship? The Physician and Sports Medicine 1999; 27(6).

Regular, moderate exercise enhances function and attenuates immune disturbances associated with acute exercise or with a single bout of vigorous exercise. Vigorous exercise may temporarily reduce resistance to viral infection. It is presently recommended that persons who have systemic symptoms should avoid competition and heavy training.

Some exercise physiologists have postulated a J-shaped relationship between physical activity and susceptibility to viral infection. According to this hypothesis, regular **moderate physical activity enhances immune responses**, reducing susceptibility to the common cold (Nieman, D.C. Exercise infection and immunity. Int J Sports Med 1994, 15: S131-S141), (Peters-Futre, E.M. Vitamin C, neutrophil function and upper respiratory tract infection risk in distance runners: The missing link? Exerc Immunol Rev 1997; 3: 32-52), and certain cancers (Shepard, R.J. and Futcher, R. Physical activity and cancer: How may protection be maximized? Crit Rev Oncogen 1997; 8(2-3): 219-272). In contrast, excessive exercise, such as an **ultramarathon or a period of very heavy conditioning, suppresses immunity** for several hours to a week or longer, creating a brief period of vulnerability when the risk of upper respiratory tract infections (URTIs) — and possibly of cancer — is increased (Shepard, R.J. Physical activity, training and the immune response. Carmel, IN, Cooper Publications Group, 1997).

Many viruses and carcinogens are suspended as droplets in inspired air. Most viruses remain in suspension until they reach the bronchi. Particles are then cleared from the throat by swallowing or expectoration. Susceptibility to viruses is increased after a marathon run but not after a 20- to 30-km run, which probably has an almost equal impact on physical barriers such as mucus, tracheal cilia, coughing, etc. It thus seems unlikely that impairment of physical defense mechanisms is a major cause of increased susceptibility to URTI in heavy exercisers.

The immediate biologic reaction to infection is an acute inflammation. Local increases in blood flow and vascular permeability facilitate the migration of various leukocytes and plasma proteins into the affected region of the body.

Immediate mechanisms that counter viral infections and destroy fully developed neoplastic cells include the actions of natural killer (NK) cells, phagocytes and the immunoglobulin A (IgA) present in nasal and bronchial mucus. The NK cells can lyse virally infected host cells and tumor cells in the absence of major-histocompatibility-complex (MHC) proteins and cytokine messengers, although their action is enhanced by various cytokines (particularly interferon [IFN] -gamma). **In contrast, cytotoxic T-cells act only if an antigen is presented to them by a macrophage that has attacked the invading microorganism or tumor cell and processed its surface proteins.**

Acute exercise (a single bout of intense exercise) temporarily decreases the activity of several of the immune systems cellular components. **Particularly important are the decreases in CD4+ (T helper) cell counts and NK cell counts.** CD4+ cells interact with macrophages and B-cells. Cytokines are secreted by the macrophages (after antigen response), increase the cytokine production of CD4+ cells, and augment the activity of NK cells. Thus, a reduction in CD4+ cells can suppress the proliferative response and may reduce NK cell activity. NK cell counts initially rise with vigorous exercise but temporarily drop below normal levels afterward. In addition, **acute exercise may raise the number of CD8+ (T suppressor) cells**, causing a decrease of CD4+/CD8+ ratio, an important indicator of immunity. Although **exercise often increases neutrophil counts, phagocytic activity and the oxidative burst that kills bacteria may decrease**. The effect of acute exercise on **macrophages is mixed; cell counts increase with exercise, but heavy exercise reduces their function and response to inflammation**. I feel that this results in the increased production of reactive oxygen species and excitation states. **Affecting the number and/or function of the microphages will, in turn, affect the levels of RONS/excytomers.**

The phagocytes ingest viral particles, destroying them with potent enzymes and chemicals, especially RONS and excited states. Soluble elements such as **complement and acute-phase protein play a supportive role, attracting phagocytes to the infected region** and rendering viral particles more vulnerable to lysis. Specific antibodies, such as IgA, also contribute to early protection, by either preventing the virus from penetrating the endothelial cell membrane or by opsonizing the viral particle (a process of ingestion that facilitates phagocytosis).

The main biologic defense against infections develops more slowly. A complex sequence of events includes macrocytic phagocytosis of the infecting organism or abnormal cell; killing by lysozymes and/or oxidizing agents; processing of the abnormal surface proteins and their presentation to T-cells in association with MHC-restricted protein; and the secretion of cytokines such as Interleukins (IL)-1 and IFN-alpha. Proliferation of specific cytotoxic lymphocytes peaks about 7 days after initial triggering of the immune response. **B-cells, antibodies and complement also act against certain viruses and tumor cells.**

The main basis for any exercise-induced change in susceptibility to URTIs and neoplasms seems to be a modulation of either the nonspecific or specific biologic defense mechanisms. The effects of exercise on these mechanisms offer some support for the J-curve hypothesis, because regular moderate exercise appears to enhance these mechanisms, whereas very heavy exercise of intensive training appears to weaken them. Both cellular and humoral changes may contribute to the transient depression of immune function.

Table I. Physical and Biologic Defenses Against Viral Infection and Neoplastic Cells

41.5.1 Physical Mechanisms

Filtration mechanisms of the nose
Expectoration of particles trapped in nasal and bronchial mucus
Integrity of endothelial membrane

41.5.2 Biologic Mechanisms

Cellular

NK cells and cytotoxic lymphocytes: Lyse infected or abnormal cells

Phagocytes: Ingest foreign cells; present foreign protein to CD4+ cells

Humoral

Interferons: Enhance NK cell activity; inhibit viral replication, inhibit or destroy tumor cells

Tumor necrosis factor: Inhibit or destroy tumor cells

Specific antibodies: Prevent membrane penetration by virus; opsonized virus or abnormal cell

Complement and acute-phase protein: Attract phagocytes to affected tissue; increase susceptibility of virus and abnormal cells to lysis

41.5.3 Natural Killer (NK) cells

Acute exercise induces a substantial, immediate intensity-dependent increase in circulating NK cell count, usually with a matching rise of NK cytolytic activity. The response **can be mimicked by physiologic doses of catecholamines** given at rest (norepinephrine for moderate exercise and epinephrine for more intensive activity).

In theory, the increase in circulating NK cell numbers and cytolytic activity should augment resistance to viral infections and tumor cells. However, the increase usually persists only as long as exercise continues — too brief a time to have any clinical importance. Moreover, if exercise continues for several hours, the NK cell count and cytolytic activity gradually return toward baseline. However, **each increase of NK cells acts like a "dose of a therapeutic agent" in helping prevent infections and cancer, just as occurs with macrophages.**

Immediately following vigorous, but not moderate, exercise, NK cell counts and cytolytic activity usually drop substantially below normal values, but resting function is often restored within a few hours, leaving only a very brief window of opportunity for viruses and neoplastic cells. It is difficult to reconcile a 2- to 3-hour reduction of NK-cell activity with the reported 2- to 6-fold increase in the incidence of URTIs in the weeks following participation in a marathon or ultra marathon run. **Common sense tells us that these extremes are deleterious and should be avoided.**

If athletes were to develop a similar prolonged depression of NK cell function, a substantial increase in their risk of viral illnesses might be anticipated. Possible explanations of the suppression of NK cell activity following vigorous exercise have included a lack of IL-2 and an accumulation of **prostaglandins (PG).** Various prostaglandins are released by tissue microtrauma, and these substances could inhibit NK cell cytotoxic activity (Pedersen, B.K., Tvede, N. and Hansen, F.R., et al. Modulation of natural killer cell activity in peripheral blood by physical exercise. Scand J Immunol 1998; 27(6): 673-678), although attempts to restore normal function by use of indomethacin have not always been successful.

The resting NK cell count is increased by repeated bouts of moderate exercise. This could explain why immune defenses are sometimes enhanced in habitual exercisers.

41.5.3 Macrophages

The activated macrophage is important to early immune defenses as an initial phagocytic agent, an antigen-presenting cell, and an initial source of lymphocyte-stimulating cytokines. Cell counts are increased by exercise, but normal values are restored within several hours of ceasing physical activity. Moderate exercise increases the cytostatic activity of macrophages, apparently because their production of tumor necrosis factor (TNF) is increased, but **very heavy exercise reduces macrophage function** (Woods, J.A., Davis, J.M. and Mayer, E.P. et al. Effects of exercise on macrophage activation for antitumor cytotoxicity. J Appl Physiol 1994; 79(3): 748-755). Moderate training has little effect on macrophage function, but heavy training reduces macrophage response to inflammation. **Macrophage activity is down-regulated by PGE2,** whether the PG is generated by muscle microtrauma or a tumor. **Again, this will affect levels of RONS/excytomers.**

41.5.4 T-Cells

Any decrease in **CD4+ (T helper)** cell count limits the output of cytokines that activate NK and T-cells and stimulate the proliferation and maturation of B-cells. An appropriate CD4+/CD8+ (T-helpers/T-suppressors) cell ratio of 1.5 or greater is thus important to immune defenses. Both heavy exercise and excessive training can cause this ratio to decrease.

41.5.5 Proliferative Response

Lymphocyte proliferation, stimulated by CD4+ cell-released IL-2, offers the main long-term defense against both viral infections and neoplastic cells. Heavy physical activity or rigorous training reduces this proliferative response. This reduction sometimes persists for several hours, contributing to the window of opportunity for viruses and neoplastic cells. On the other hand, moderate training reduces the depression of proliferation induced by any single bout of heavy exercise (Verde, T.J., Thomas, S.G. and Moore, R.W. et al. Immune responses and increased training of the athlete. J Appl Physiol 1992;73(4): 1494-1499). **This emphasizes the fact that all infections and neoplastic events are controlled by the same RONS and excited state generating system.**

41.5.6 Neutrophil Impairment

Secondary bacterial infections can complicate and prolong URTIs. Circulating neutrophil counts often increase dramatically during and for some hours following exercise, but this does not necessarily increase resistance to secondary infection, since phagocytic activity may simultaneously decrease (Lotzerich, H., Wilczkowiak, I-U. and Stein, N. et al. Influence of training and completion on the phagocyte activity of athletes. Int J. Sports Med 1997; 18(1): S111). **Intensive training may decrease the oxidative burst** associated with bacterial killing in isolated neutrophils, but, again, the athlete's susceptibility is not necessarily affected (Mackinnon, L.T. Immunity in athletes. Int J Sports Med 1997; 18(1): S62-S68). **We must distinguish between in vitro conditions, from what is occurring in the living/breathing cell.**

41.5.7 Cytokines

Exercise increases production of the cytokine IL-1, and resting levels of this substance may also be augmented by training. IL-1 has a direct cytotoxic effect. **It also stimulates T-cells to produce increased amounts of IL-1 and IL-2**, augmenting the cytotoxicity of NK and **lymphokine-activated killer (LAK) cells.**

IL-2 has an indirect effect on the immune defenses, stimulating the function of NK, LAK and T-cells. In vitro studies suggest that exercise decreases free levels of IL-2, possibly by increasing the proportion of lymphocytes that express IL-2 receptors.

41.5.8 Interferons Slow Viral Replication

They also alter the surface properties of NK cells and macrophages, with resultant increases in lytic activity. Moderate training may increase IFN production, but the output of IFN-alpha is unchanged by several weeks of exhaustive training.

41.5.9 TNF-Alpha is Produced by Monocyte

It is cytotoxic, stimulating the activity of macrophages and T- and B-cells. It also contributes significantly to muscle-wasting in cancer. **TNF-B is produced by active T- cells. It is both cytostatic and cytotoxic against tumor cells**. Acute exercise increases TNF output, but the effect of training is as yet unknown.

41.5.10 Immunoglobulins

Moderate exercise does not change the concentration of salivary IgA or serum IgG. In contrast, very vigorous exercise decreases IgA concentrations in both saliva and nasal washings. One report found low concentrations for 18 hours following a 31-km race. **Moderate training increases salivary IgA, but concentrations fall progressively with rigorous training**. Partial recovery is seen during precompetitive tapering. Top competitors also show minor decreases in serum IgG concentrations during peak training.

Other Humoral Factors

Acute exercise induces increased concentrations of the main acute-phase protein, C-reactive protein; however, the tissue injury associated with heavy training may lead to decreases in resting levels of both serum complement and C-reactive protein.

Overall Immune Responsiveness

The response to vaccines provides one measure of overall immune responsiveness. **In the first few days after participation in an Ironman triathlon, there was a reduced response to tetanus and diphtheria toxoid, as well as to purified pneumococci polysaccharide**. This is consistent with other data indicating a period of increased vulnerability following overly severe exercise.

Experimental Data

Animal observations suggest that excessive and/or stressful exercise weakens most resistance and increases the virulence of certain viruses; mortality rises and the time to death is shortened. Human experimental studies have evaluated only moderate exercise, which has little effect on either the likelihood of developing infection or its duration and severity after nasal installation of respiratory viruses.

41.6 MODERATE EXERCISE

Moderate exercise has little influence on the risk of URTI in young adults (Nieman, D.C., Nehlsen-Cannarella, S.L. and Markoff, P.A. et al. The effects of moderate exercise training on natural killer cells and acute upper respiratory tract infections. Int J Sports Med 1990; 11(6): 467-473). It was noted that 45 minutes of exercise five times per week at 60% of the heart rate reserve reduced the duration of respiratory symptoms but did not affect the incidence of URTI in 25- to 45- year-old women. **Any benefit of regular physical activity is more obvious in seniors** (Karper, W. B. and Boschen, M.B. Effects of exercise on acute respiratory tract infections and related symptoms: Moderate exercise may boost an elder's natural defenses against common illnesses. Geriatr Nurs 1993; 14(1): 15-18), (Nieman, D.C., Henson, D.A. and Gusewitch, G. et al. Physical activity and immune function in elderly women. Med Sci Sports Exerc 1993; 25(7): 823-831), perhaps because they begin an investigation with poor immune function and a low level of physical activity. Among 67- to 85-year-old women, the incidence of URTIs was lowest in a highly conditioned subgroup, intermediate in a subgroup of regular walkers and highest in calisthenic and sedentary control subgroups.

41.7 HEAVY EXERCISE

In another study, factors that increased runners' risk of respiratory infection over a 12-month period included running more than 15km per week, living alone and having a low body mass index. Runners who ran more than 97 km per week were twice as likely to develop URTIs as those who ran less than 32 km per week, even after adjustment for confounding variables. In a survey, about 76% of masters athletes considered themselves less vulnerable to colds than their sedentary colleagues and only 1.5% thought they were more vulnerable. Nevertheless, 16% of these athletes thought they became more susceptible when their training reached 70 to 80 km per week.

Among Australian elite athletes, the periods of heaviest training are associated with reduced salivary IgA concentrations and an increased susceptibility to URTIs. The incidence of respiratory infections is also increased by heavy military training. **However, some elite athletes — cross-country skiers, gymnasts, oarsmen, swimmers and wrestlers — develop URTIs no more frequently than sedentary people. Presumably, susceptibility depends on the type and volume of training.**

Current evidence is not yet sufficient to demonstrate a clear J-shaped relationship between the exercise volume and immune function. A similar pattern has been inferred for susceptibility to neoplasms, but here the data are even more limited.

41.8 NUTRITION

Clinical malnutrition is a well-recognized cause of impaired immune function. Most athletes show only small deficiencies of essential nutrients. Nevertheless, they may lack the glutamine needed for lymphocyte proliferation (Nesholme, E.A. Biochemical mechanisms to explain immunosuppression in well-trained and overtrained athletes. Int J Sports Med 1994; 15(3): S152-S147). Deficiencies in arginine, L-Carnitine, essential fatty acids, vitamin B6, folic acid, vitamin E and trace elements may also contribute to reduced immune function in athletes (Shepard, R.J. and Shek, P.N. Immunological hazards from nutritional imbalance in athletes. Exerc Immunol Rev 1998; 4: 22-48).

41.9 MUSCLE MICROTRAUMA

Cumulative microtrauma from exercise causes local and systemic acute-phase reactions. In the short term, the resulting release of **C-reactive protein (CRP)** stimulates monocyte phagocytosis. However, the migration of leukocytes to injured muscle may reduce immune function in other parts of the body, and the generation of oxidant free radicals during the repair process may suppress immune function in a manner analogous to clinical sepsis (Northoff, H., Enkel, S. and Weinstock, C. Exercise, injury and immune function. Exerc Immunol Rev 1995; 1: 1-25). Perhaps for this reason, antioxidants such as vitamin C reduce the risk of exercise-induced infections. Personally, **I feel that the ingestion of any antioxidants, while in an immunocompromised condition, is potentially harmful, in that it further decreases the RONS and excited states necessary to ward off infections and cancer.**

41.10 REDUCED STRESS

Psychological and environmental stress can interact with heavy training. A recent report (Bailey, D.M., Davies, B. and Romer, L. et al. Implications of moderate altitude training for sea-level endurance in elite distance runners. Eur J Appl Physiol 1998; 78(4): 360-368), **noted that the incidence of upper respiratory and gastrointestinal infections in elite runners who trained for 4 weeks at moderate altitudes (1,500 to 2,000 m) was increased 50% relative to training at sea level.**

Even though countless studies have attested to the benefits of exercise, and for whatever its worth, Thompson, et al., estimated the risk of sudden death in jogging to be seven times that in more sedentary activities (Thompson, P.D., Funk, E.J., Carleton, R.A. and Sturner, W.Q. Incidence of death during jogging in Rhode Island from 1975 through 1980. JAMA 1980; 247: 2535).

This fact supports my Unified Theory, in that any condition which potentially reduces the production of RONS and excited states also increases the chances of infection and cancer development. **In short, one can say that moderate exercise is good for you and excessive exercise is harmful.**

"Learned authors bombastically state
that horrid oxygen radicals
wreak devastation and havoc upon defenseless **DNA**,
unprotected proteins, helpless unsaturated
lipids and sugars slowly self-destruct under oxygen's fatal influence.
Lethal oxygen joins hands with its demonic
iron brethren and ushers out the hydroxyl
radical hit man, who is adept at killing
all in his path.Yet,
life endures and thrives.
Now, you prophets of oxidative doom,smile,
take a deep oxygen-breath and
go forth and prosper."

R. M. Howes, M.D., Ph.D.

6/11/04

"The nobility of oxygen has been smothered by
the suffocating smog emitted from heaps of decaying
pseudoscientific publications."

R. M. Howes, M.D., Ph.D.

5/10/04

"Sham medicine" is a thriving financial empire.

PART X - O$_2$ STUDY MODELS

44.5 ADDITIONAL SMOKING FACTS

According to the National Cancer Institute half of all cancers in the USA are caused by:

- **Smoking** - 35% of all cancers are related to smoking
  Obesity - 15% of all cancers in men and 20% of all cancers in women are related to obesity. The number is higher for women because fat cells make estrogen and exposure to large amounts of estrogen can promote cancer.

Dr. Jay Brooks, Jr. Oncologist at Oschner Clinic, says the following: **One out of every 3 persons in this country will have cancer at sometime in their lives.** Cancer is a disease of the aging."

Cigarette tar contains over 5,000 different compounds, including nicotine, polycyclic aromatic hydrocarbons, nitro amines, **phenols and polyphenols (which are claimed to have high antioxidant capability)**. Still, many investigators focus only on ROS as being culpable agents.

Subcutaneous wound-tissue oxygen (PsqO$_2$) tension in eight volunteers fell rapidly and significantly in response to smoking and remained low for 30 to 50 minutes. Sham "smoking" had no effect. These data suggest that a typical "pack-per-day" smoker experiences tissue hypoxia during a significant portion of each day. The degree of hypoxia found in thee subjects has been associated with poor wound healing in animal and human studies. The onset and duration of tissue **hypoxia** paralleled the well established plasma pharmacokinetics of nicotine. This suggests that peripheral vasoconstriction, induced by the adrenergic effects of nicotine, may contribute to the observed decrease in PsqO$_2$. (Jensen, J.A., Goodson, W.H., Hopf, H.W. and Hunt, T.K. Cigarette smoking decreases tissue oxygen. 1991; 126(9): 1131-1134).

In a study to determine whether **peripheral arterial occlusive disease (PAOD)** patients who smoked had more severe Claudication pain, reduced peripheral circulation and poorer cardiopulmonary measurements at peak exercise than nonsmoking patients, the smoking group had more severe Claudication pain, as maximal pain occurred 1:37 mins sooner during exercise ($p<0.05$), and the pain took 2:21 mins longer to subside ($p<0.01$) compared to the nonsmoking group. Additionally, at peak exercise **the smoking group had a lower oxygen uptake** (12.8 +/- 2.6 vs. 13.9 +/- 2.4 ml/kg/min, $p<0.01$), a higher ventilation (31.7 +/- 0.2 vs. 27.9 +/- 7.1 liters/min, $p<0.05$), and a higher oximeter electrode power (409 +/- 55 vs. 385 +/- 37 mW, $p<0.01$) than the nonsmoking group. Differences between the groups persisted ($p<0.05$) after adjusting for resting ankle/brachial systolic pressure index (ABI). It is concluded that cigarette smokers with PAOD had more severe Claudication pain, reduced peripheral circulation and poorer cardiopulmonary measurements at peak exercise than nonsmoking patients. (Gardner, A.W. The effect of cigarette smoking on exercise capacity in patients with intermittent Claudication. Vasc Med 1996; 1(3): 181-186).

Studies show that cigarette smoking does not seem to be associated with increased apneic activity during sleep. However, **it is associated with a decrease in nocturnal oxygen saturation.** (Casasola, G.G., Alvarez-Salia, J.L., Marques, J.A., Sanchez-Alarcos, J.M., Tashkin, D.P. and Espinos, D. Cigarette smoking behavior and respiratory alterations during sleep in a healthy population. Sleep Breath 2002; 6(1): 19-24).

An estimated 18% to 20% of pregnant women smoke throughout their pregnancies. Smoking is associated with multiple complications in pregnancy. Studies have confirmed that **smoking increases the rate of low birth weight babies, premature babies, spontaneous abortions, stillbirths, neonatal death, abruption placentae, placenta previa, bleeding during pregnancy, prolonged rupture of membranes and impaired development of the infant.** This can be attributed to several factors such as the **vasoconstriction** of placenta blood flow by nicotine, **elevated fetal carboxyhaemoglobin** and catecholamines levels, **fetal tissue hypoxia,** reduced delivery of nutrients to the fetus, and increased heart rate and blood pressure. **I believe that the various manifestations of oxygen deficiency is crucial in the development of many problem and disease states associated with smoking for both the mother and the fetus.**

Maternal smoking accounts for 21% to 39% of all low birth weight babies (less than 2500 g) in the USA. This effect is probably **secondary to fetal hypoxia**. This is quite disturbing as low birth weight is the single most important determinant of neonatal and infant morbidity and mortality. Maternal smoking is the most important factor for intrauterine growth retardation.

Furthermore, **smoking women are at greater risk of spontaneous abortion of chromosomally normal conceptions**. Women smoking 10 or more cigarettes per day have 46% greater odds of aborting, while women smoking more than 20 cigarettes per day have 61% greater odds of aborting than nonsmoking women. The risk of congenital defect in the children of smoking women is 1.7 to 2.3 times greater than that of nonsmoking women.

Smoking is also a known risk factor for infant mortality. Infant mortality per 1000 subjects adjusted for age, parity, education and marital status were 15.1 for nonsmoking whites, 18.8 for whites smoking one pack of cigarettes per day, and 23.3 for whites smoking more than one pack per day. **The infant mortality rates per 1000 subjects for blacks were much higher, 26.0 for nonsmoking mothers**, 32.4 for one pack per day, and 39.9 for more than one pack per day. Children of smokers are more likely to die from sudden infant death syndrome.

The fetus suffers chronic hypoxia stress as a consequence of smoking and is evidenced by elevated hematocrits. (Bush, P.G., Mayhew, T.M., Abramovich, D.R., Aggett, P.J., Burke, M.D. and Page, K.R. Maternal cigarette smoking and oxygen diffusion across placenta. Placenta 2000; 21(8): 824-833).

44.6 CARBON MONOXIDE

The smoke of one cigarette contains the poisonous gases of approximately **4,000 chemicals** including nicotine (an addictive drug known to cause **vasoconstriction),** carbon monoxide (an **oxygen displacing** chemical), benzene (a potent carcinogen), ammonia and formaldehyde. **Average human O_2 consumption is 3.5 ml O_2/kg body wt./min. and this is the first normal parameter to be affected by cigarette smoke.**

Carbon monoxide (CO) is both colorless and odorless and the first sign of severe poisoning is loss of consciousness, which is followed by death if there is additional inhalation of CO. CO interferes at two levels with O_2 metabolism in that it interferes with transport of O_2 by red cells in the blood (by the formation of carboxyhaemoglobin, which substantially reduces the ability of the red cell to carry O_2) and also by blocking essential biochemical reactions in cells. Brain damage is a common feature of survivors of CO poisoning. In normal CO unexposed people, levels below 1% are found. Non-smokers, exposed to concentrations in the air of 25-50 ppm might be expected to show carboxyhaemoglobin levels of 2-3% after several hours. **Smokers may have levels of HbCO 4% to as high as 15%, depending upon the amount smoked.** Two organs that are crucially dependent upon high rate of O_2 consumption are the heart and the brain and may be more likely to be impaired by CO.

Well conducted studies have shown that levels of carboxyhaemoglobin as low as 3-4% shorten the duration of exercise needed to induce changes in the electrocardiogram record and induce angina pain. Small changes have been detected at levels as low as 2%. It has been suggested that the increased risk of hardening of the arteries, arteriosclerosis, in cigarette smoke is due to their raised levels of carboxyhaemoglobin.

Studies of brain function have shown subtle changes when carboxyhaemoglobin levels exceed about 5% and levels of 15-25% have caused delays in behavioral development and impaired brain function in animals. **The decreased birth weight of babies born to mothers who smoke has been attributed to transfer of CO across the placenta and a consequent reduced fetal O_2 supply,** especially when levels exceed 5%, which would be attained as a result of prolonged exposure to 30 ppm of CO (Defra, UK - Environmental Protection - Air Quality). **I feel that CO plays a prominent role in the damage produced by smoke both by its presence and by its direct effects on O_2 transport and by blocking its ability to metabolically generate ROS and excited states.**

44.7 CONCLUSION

In view of the fact that smoking causes generalized increases in cancer, arteriosclerosis, decreased wound healing, difficulty in combating infections and premature aging, I believe that this profile is one which is manifested as a result of a generalized oxygen deficiency. Obviously, if **lower levels of oxygen are in the blood, then one would expect lower levels of O_2 to be converted to O_2^- and the subsequent generation of excited states which help keep disease conditions at bay.** However, in their absence, we see a full spectrum of the effects of oxygen deficiency.

In all of the discussions for correction of the harmful effects of smoking, I have yet to see the issue of lowered levels of O_2 considered as an option. I have only seen discussions of the potential harmful effects of oxygen radicals. **I believe that vasoconstriction, carboxyhaemoglobin (HbCO) and generalized and long lasting hypoxemia play a major role in the harmful consequences of smoking.** Likely, this group of patients will be harmed by the ingestion of supplemental antioxidants, since they are already in a deficit ROS and excited state condition. In fact, my Unified Theory explains the fact that beta-carotene supplementation increases cancer in smokers. Although the smoking model is a very complex one, I believe that my **Unified Theory** explains the model *in toto,* better than any of the alternatives.

45 DNA DAMAGE BY IRON/HYDROGEN PEROXIDE

45.1 H_2O_2 Background

Repeatedly, we see the literature state that the Fenton reaction is responsible for DNA mutations and that this reaction produces products that are identical to those produced by ionizing radiation. However, the energetics of these two processes are quite different and would not be expected to be identical. Ionizing radiation involves energies much greater than those of the intracellular Fenton reaction, which must have to occur in the immediate vicinity of DNA, lest it will react with whatever is closest to the hydroxyl radical. In fact, because of the extremely short half life of the .OH radical and it subsequent short diffusion distance, only if it is generated in the immediate proximity of DNA is it going to be harmful to DNA.

45.2 Howes' Harmful Hydroxyl/Hydrogen Peroxide Pathway.

I envision a much more plausible fate for the .OH radicals whereby they recombine with themselves to produce H_2O_2, and in doing so, the cell has converted a very harmful substance into a needed cellular signaling device of low reactivity and with the ability to diffuse for great distances. I will dub this the 4H-P pathway : **H**owes' **H**armful **H**ydroxyl/**H**ydrogen **P**eroxide pathway.

Some of the following materials were excerptedor fodified from: Halliwell, B., Clement, M.V. and Long, L.H., Hydrogen peroxide in the human body. FEBS Lett 2000; 486: 10-13.

H_2O_2 is a pale blue covalent liquid which readily traverses membranes by unknown pathways (Halliwell, B. and Gutteridge, J.M.C. Free Radicals in Biology and Medicine, 1999, 3rd Ed. Clarendon Press, Oxford). Chemically, **H_2O_2 is poorly reactive in the absence of transition metal ions and it can act as a mild oxidizing or as a mild reducing agent. It does not oxidize most biological molecules readily, including lipids, DNA and proteins**, unless the proteins have hyper-reactive thiol groups or methionine residues. Its supposed danger comes from its ready conversion to the highly reactive .OH, by either exposure to ultraviolet light

$H_2O_2 \rightarrow \rightarrow$ ultraviolet light$\rightarrow \rightarrow$ 2OH.

or by the interaction with a wide range of transition metal ions such as iron

$Fe^{+2} + H_2O_2 \rightarrow$ intermediate complexes (ferryl??) $\rightarrow Fe^{+3} + OH. + OH-$

Reportedly, H_2O_2 can liberate iron from heme proteins in vitro.

Reports have described levels of **H_2O_2 over 50 μM as being cytotoxic** for a wide range of plants and animal cells in vitro, but is dependent upon many factors such as, pH, media used, cell type used, length of exposure, etc. **Paradoxically**, acatalasemia in humans appears to produce no significant phenotype, nor does "knockout" of glutathione peroxidase in mice except under conditions of "abnormally high oxidative stress." **As you can imagine, I do not consider this paradoxical at all because this what my Unified Theory would have predicted,** which is contrary to the Free radical theory.

45.3 LOW H_2O_2 REACTIVITY

Levels of H_2O_2 at or below 20-50 μM have limited cytotoxicity to many cell types.

Growing data demonstrates the signaling ability of H_2O_2 and it was first shown to activate NFkB and later many other functions have seen found for H_2O_2 including modulation of the inflammatory process by:

    up-regulating expression of adhesion molecules
    controlling cell proliferation or apoptosis
    and modulating platelet aggregation.

Consequently, attempts at elimination of all H_2O_2 generated in vivo can be dangerous and probably deadly.

H_2O_2 is produced in vivo by:

    superoxide dismutase
    glycollate oxidase
    monamine oxidase
    and peroxisomal beta-oxidation of fatty acids

Transgenic mice lacking mitochondrial SOD suffer severe pulmonary and neurological damage. Some say that this indicates the toxicity of O_2^- and the need for its removal; however, **I believe that it may indicate the need to convert O_2^- to H_2O_2 so it can fulfill its signaling roles. Mitochondria in most tissues, other than cardiac and muscle, have limited capacity to remove H_2O_2, in that they generate substantial amounts in vitro and likely in vivo.**

Although mitochondria contain glutathione peroxidase and thioredoxin-linked peroxidase activities, the efficiency of these enzymes in removing **H_2O_2** is uncertain **given the ease with which mitochondria release H_2O_2.** (Kwong, L.K. and Sohal, R.S., Arch Biochem Biophys 1998 350: 118-126), (Chow, C.K., Ibrahim, W., Wei, Z. and Chan, A.C. Free Radic Biol Med 1999; 27: 580-587), (Braidot, E., Petrissa, E., Vicunello, A. and Macri, F. FEBS Lett 1999; 451: 347-350).

It is believed that all human cells are exposed to H_2O_2 and likely at all times.

45.4 H_2O_2 DISTRIBUTION

Several beverages commonly drunk by humans can **contain H_2O_2 at concentrations above 100 μM, including green and black tea and especially instant coffee**. Oral bacteria also produce H_2O_2.

The cells lining the respiratory system, in common with the oral and esophageal epithelium, are exposed to high O_2 concentrations (21%) as compared with most other body tissues. **Hydrogen peroxide is present in exhaled air of humans** and rats, although it is uncertain whether this H_2O_2 originates from oral bacteria, phagocytes (e.g., alveolar macrophages, neutrophils in the oral cavity, or neutrophils recruited to the lungs in inflammatory lung diseases) or other lung cells. Amounts of exhaled H_2O_2 appear greater in subjects with inflammatory lung diseases and in cigarette smokers. Nevertheless, **H_2O_2 is present in the air exhaled by healthy human subjects**.

Substantial quantities of **H_2O_2, at concentrations sometimes exceeding 100 μM, can be detected in freshly voided human urine, even in babies**. The simplest way of demonstrating its presence is to place urine into an oxygen electrode, and inject catalase through the cap. A 'spike' of O_2 release results as the H_2O_2 present is decomposed by catalase (Long, L.H., Evans, P.J. and Halliwell, B. Biochem Biophys Res Commun 1999; 262: 605-609).

The H_2O_2 detected in human urine appears to arise, at least in part, by $O_2^{\cdot-}$dependent autoxidation of urinary molecules, some of which originate from diet. **Traces of superoxide dismutase are present in urine**: this enzyme, as well as the acidic pH of urine, should facilitate both enzymic and non-enzymic dismutation of $O_2^{\cdot-}$ to H_2O_2. The pO_2 of urine within the bladder is below that of ambient air and so the rate of H_2O_2 generation in urine may well increase upon voiding. Nevertheless, the high levels of H_2O_2 that can be detected in some urine samples strongly suggest that at least some H_2O_2 generation occurs within the bladder. Indeed, **H_2O_2 has been detected in urine sampled by catheterization**. Hydrogen peroxide has an antibacterial effect and it may be that its presence at high levels in urine could be advantageous in diminishing infections of the bladder and urinary tract.

There are suggestions that H_2O_2 is involved in modulation of renal function (Nath, K.A., Grande, J., Croatt, A., Haugen, J., Kim, Y. and Rosenberg, M.E. Kidney Int 1998; 53: 367-381). Another possibility is that excretion of H_2O_2 represents a metabolic mechanism for controlling its levels in the human body. If so, measurement of urinary H_2O_2 levels may represent a valuable tool for assessment of 'oxidative stress,' since H_2O_2 can be measured rapidly and simply. This suggested route of H_2O_2 elimination by excretion is perhaps analogous to **certain fish, which appear to dispose of H_2O_2 by excreting it through their gills** (Wilhelm-Filho, D., Gonzalez-Flecha, B. and Boveris, A. Braz J Med Biol Res 1994; 27: 2879-2882).

Some **studies have claimed substantial levels of H_2O_2 (up to ~ 35 μM) in human blood plasma** (Varma, S.D. and Devamanoharan, P.S. Free Radic Res Commun 1991; 14: 125-131), (Lacy, F., O'Connor, D.T. and Schmid-Schonbein, G.W. J Hypertens 1998; 16: 291-303), (Deskur, E., Przywarska, I., Dylewicz, P., Szczesniak, L., Rychlewski, T., Wil, M. and Wysocki, H. Int J Cardiol 1998; 67: 219-224), but others have claimed levels to be very low, at or close to zero (Frei, B., Yamamoto, Y., Niclas, D. and Amers, B.N. Anal Biochem 1998; 175: 120-130). The latter data seem more credible, since H_2O_2 added to human plasma disappears rapidly. However, keep in mind that steady state levels can be present at all times. In part, it is degraded by the traces of catalase present, but H_2O_2 can also react with heme proteins, ascorbate and protein-SH groups. In vivo, H_2O_2 generated in plasma could also diffuse into erythrocytes, white cells, endothelial cells and platelets for metabolism. However, the studies in Varma, et al, Lacy, et al, and Deskur et al could be interpreted to suggest that H_2O_2 can be detected at high levels in plasma under assay conditions in which its removal is prevented. This implies that **human plasma may be continuously generating H_2O_2.** One enzyme involved in this process, at least under pathological conditions, appears to be xanthine oxidase. Levels of circulating and endothelium-bound xanthine oxidase are increased as a result of tissue injury.

The presence of **H_2O_2, at widely varying levels (in some cases, 100 μM or more), has been reported in human and other animal aqueous and vitreous humors.** The explanation might be essentially the same as that advanced above to account for the conflicting data reported for blood plasma, i.e., that ocular fluids constantly generate H_2O_2. The origin of this H_2O_2 is uncertain, but oxidation of glutathione or ascorbate is one possibility.

Hydrogen peroxide appears to be a ubiquitous molecule. We exhale it, excrete it and take it in from diet. It can be detected in drinking water, rain water and sea water (Halliwell, B, Clement, M.V. and Long, L.H. Hydrogen peroxide in the human body. FEBS Lett 2000; 486: 10-13).

46 SOD, NO, PEROXYNITRITE AND SUPEROXIDE ANION

Some of the following materials were excerpted or modified from: Beckman, J., the ABC's of the reactions between nitric oxide, superoxide, peroxynitrite and superoxide dismutase. Sunrise Free Radical School, Oxygen 1999. Joe.Beckman@ccc.uab.edu

Because of the high affinity for reaction between nitric oxide and superoxide to form peroxynitrite, SOD has considerable competition in vivo. In the 1980s the Haber-Weiss reaction was the accepted explanation for how O_2^- was toxic in vivo but it is no longer valid in vivo because the reduction step with O_2^- is slow and can be substituted by other reductants such as ascorbate. Sources of catalytic iron in vivo are uncertain and many form of chelated iron do not catalyze this reaction. The reaction of H_2O_2 with iron is slow, the hydroxyl radical has an extremely short diffusion distance and its toxicity is still far from clear. Many cells can produce NO as a signaling molecule and inflammatory cells can produce micromolar amounts.

NO is not a very reactive molecule nor is it highly toxic (Brunelli, D., Crow, J.P. and Beckman, J.S. The comparative toxicity of nitric oxide and peroxynitrite to E. coli. Arch Biochem Biophys 1995; 316: 327-334), (Beckman, J.S. The physiological and pathological chemistry of nitric oxide, in Nitric Oxide: Principles and Actions J.R. Lancaster, Ed. 1996, Academic Press. P. 1-82). NO is comparable in reactivity to ground state oxygen and similarly becomes toxic by conversion to much stronger oxidizers.

NO reactivity:

- NO is as unreactive as O_2
- NO is chain terminating by reacting with .N=O + .O=O.
- Binds to metals (nitrosylation)
- Most physiological actions are due to cGMP
- More NO than O2.- and metals in vivo
- Diffusion-limited reaction of radicals with NO
- All tissues are exposed to NO
- Novel products of unknown action

NO reacts at near diffusion limited rates with most free radicals, and thus, is a major participant in free radical injury.

The unpaired "radical" electrons on nitric oxide and superoxide combine to form a stable bond to produce peroxynitrite anion. **Peroxynitrite anion is not a free radical and is stable in alkaline solution of the solid state for years. It has a pKa of 6.8 and can decay to produce hydroxyl radical and nitrogen dioxide, two potent and strong oxidants.** It also reacts with carbon dioxide to produce nitrogen dioxide and bicarbonate radical. Peroxynitrite is also directly reactive with selective targets in vivo with extraordinarily rapid rates and thus can be relatively specific in the targets in inactivates. Examples include the rapid inactivation of tyrosine phosphates and with zinc thiolates.

The biological chemistry of peroxynitrite is in part determined by its conformation. Quantum mechanics dictates that superoxide and nitric oxide combine to form peroxynitrite only in the cis conformation. The unusual geometric stability of peroxynitrite allows it to diffuse significant distances on a cellular scale and to effectively find cellular targets that are particularly reactive with peroxynitrite.

U.T.O.P.I.A.

Oxygen is only 200-250 mM in air-saturated solutions and rapidly depleted.

Investigators have suggested **that the ratio of superoxide to nitric oxide determines pro- versus antioxidant effects.** In cells, the competition between NO and SOD is the critical ratio.

NO and SOD:

"overwhelms antioxidant defenses…"
"tenuous balance of O_2^- and NO…"
The ratio of NO to SOD is critical

Aerobic cells generally contain enormous concentrations of superoxide dismutase. It is a major fraction of cellular protein. Rae et al. indicate that yeast cells contain 10 mM SOD. These defenses are not easily overwhelmed.

Human CuZn SOD (% of total protein)
(Hartz et al. Clin Chem Acta 1973; 36: 125-132)

Cerebral grey-matter	0.37%
Liver	0.47%
Cardiac Muscle	0.18%
Lung	0.05%
Renal Cortex	0.19%
Renal Medulla	0.13%

Beckman says that the concentration of Cu, Zn SOD is a billion times greater than the concentration of superoxide itself, but at first glance, that is hard to believe .

However, when the concentration of SOD is increased to 10 mM, then the concentration of superoxide drops into the low picomolar range. **Then the reverse reactions become significant. A significant fraction of SOD becomes deoxidized by molecular oxygen to form superoxide. Even hydrogen peroxide tends to be converted back to superoxide by the reverse reaction.**

Czapski and Goldstein (Czapski, G. and Goldstein, S. The uniqueness of superoxide dismutase (SOD) - why cannot most copper compounds substitute SOD in vivo? Free Rad Res Comms 1988; 4(4): 225-229), pointed out the importance of minimizing the rate of reoxidation in SOD. **This reoxidation must also be considered with low molecular weight mimics of SOD.** To be effective as a superoxide scavenger, SOD is constrained by the following:

Constraints on SOD:

Reoxidation must be slow
Minimize reduction by intracellular ascorbate
Must hold copper tightly
Minimize reaction with peroxynitrite

Loss of Zinc affects these properties

The ALS (amyotrophic lateral sclerosis) mutants have a reduced affinity for zinc and we believe the altered redox activity of zinc deficient SOD is most likely to be the culprit in causing ALS.

The reoxidation of SOD is generally a significant problem because superoxide will be quickly recaptured by the high concentrations of SOD unless something can compete with the SOD. **For something to be a significant target of superoxide, it must be able to react fast enough and be present in high enough concentration to compete with micromolar concentrations of SOD. The biological molecule that meets these requirements in nitric oxide.** It reacts significantly faster with superoxide and can be produced in micromolar concentrations.

ABC's of NO, O$_2$, O$_2$.-, H$_2$O$_2$, ONOO- & SOD

- The slow reverse reoxidation of SOD is significant in vivo.
- Hydrogen peroxide reacts with oxidized SOD to generate superoxide and reduced SOD.
- Nitric oxide competes better than predicted with SOD to form peroxynitrite.
- Loss of Zinc from SOD turns even wild-type SOD into an oxidant that is also a toxic agent for motor neurons.

Some of the following materials were excerpted from: Henle, E.S. and Linn, S. Formation, Prevention and Repair of DNA Damage by Iron/Hydrogen Peroxide. J Biol Chem 1997; 272(31): 10995-19098.

The oxidative potential of atmospheric oxygen $^3\sum$g (O$_2$) is maintained by the non-alignment of electron spins and **aerobic life is based upon harnessing energy via the catalytic spin pairing of triplet oxygen by the electron transport chain** (Babcock, G.T. and Wikstrom, M. Nature 1992; 356: 301-309). Catabolic oxidases such as xanthine oxidase, anabolic processes such as nucleoside reduction and defense processes such as phagocytosis also produce oxygen radicals. In fact, contrary to commonly reported statements, **RONS are produced throughout the cell and not just in the mitochondrion.**

46.1 THE FENTON REACTION

Most transition metals have more than one oxidation state besides the ground state and their valence electrons may be unpaired, allowing **one-electron redox reactions**. As such, **transition metals can react with H_2O_2 to produce ·OH and related oxidants**. In 1894, Fenton (Fenton, H.J.H. J Chem Soc (London) 1894; 65: 899-910), described the oxidation of tartaric acid by Fe^{2+} and H_2O_2 and the stoichiometry of Fe^{2+} and H_2O_2 consumption was subsequently shown to be consistent with that of Reaction 5. **This is the infamous reaction (hydroxyl radical formation), which is always referred to when invoking damage from RONS, and likely deservedly so but the reactants are so fast, that they react at the site of their generation. This would require that the hydroxyl radical be generated by reaction of a transition metal and hydrogen peroxide on or at a DNA molecule for damage to occur and it would have to remain uncorrected. However, please look at reaction 6, in which no hydroxyl radical is formed and this is another reaction which is not discussed.**

Therefore, **after 100 years, the basic nature of the Fenton oxidants(s) is still undefined** so that ".OH" may be regarded as a symbol representing the stoichiometric equivalent of the univalent oxidation agents produced by the Fenton reaction. However, it is clear that whatever the oxidant, **hydroxylations and hydrogen abstractions are the two most common modifications of organic substrates by Fenton oxidants** (Henle, E.S., Luo, Y., Gassman, W. and Lann, S. J Biol Chem 1996; 271: 21177-21186).

Although it is rarely discussed, it is noteworthy that **H_2O_2 can also react with Fe^{3+} to form $O_2^{·-}$**, presumably via Reaction 8, and that if H_2O_2 is in excess, the Fe^{2+} which is thus formed can subsequently generate reactive oxygen species via the Fenton reaction.

(1)

$$O_2 \xrightarrow{e^-} O_2^{·-} \xrightarrow{e^-, 2H^+} H_2O_2$$
$$(0.32\ V) \qquad\qquad (0.94V)$$

$$\xrightarrow{e^-, H^+} .OH + H_2O \xrightarrow{e^-, H^+} 2H_2O$$
$$(0.32V) \qquad\qquad (2.31\ V)$$

(2)
$$2O_2^{·-} + 2H^+ \longrightarrow O_2 + H_2O_2$$

(3)
$$O_2^{·-} + Fe^{3+} \longrightarrow Fe^2 + O_2$$

(4)
$$[4Fe - 4S]^{2+} + O_2^{·-} + 2H^+ \longrightarrow [3Fe - 4S]^+ + H_2O_2 + Fe^{2+}$$

(5)
$$Fe^{2+} + H^+ + H_2O_2 \longrightarrow Fe^{3+} + .OH + H_2O$$

(6)
$$Fe^{2+} + H_2O_2 \longrightarrow FeO^{2+} + H_2O$$

(7)
$$FeO^{2+} + H^+ \rightarrow\rightarrow FeOH^{3+} \rightarrow Fe^{3+} + .OH$$

(8)
$$Fe^{3+} + H_2O_2 \rightarrow\rightarrow (FeOOH^{2+} + H^+) \rightarrow Fe^{2+} + 2H^+ + O_2^{.-}$$

(9)
$$H_2O_2 + Cl- \rightarrow\rightarrow OCl- + H_2O$$

(10)
$$H_2O_2 + OCl- \rightarrow\rightarrow {}^1O_2 + H_2O + Cl-$$

(11)
$$NO. + O_2 \rightarrow\rightarrow ONOO-$$

(12)
$$DNA. + Fe^{3+} \rightarrow\rightarrow DNA_{ox} + Fe^{2+} + H^+$$

(13)
$$DNA. + O_2 \rightarrow\rightarrow DNA\text{-}O_2.$$

(14)
$$DNA\text{-}O_2. + Fe^{2+} + H^+ \rightarrow\rightarrow DNA\text{-}O_2H + Fe^{3+}$$

(15)
$$2H_2O_2 \rightarrow\rightarrow 2H_2O + O_2$$

(16)
$$H_2O_2 + 2RH \rightarrow\rightarrow 2H_2O + 2 R_{ox}$$

I include these reactions to emphasize the point that the interaction of the RONS and excited states (excytomers) are complex and likely, in most physiological situations, there will be **an admixture of dynamic reactants** present and not just singular species (RONS). Also, please remember that because of their fleeting life times, their presence or participation can be very difficult to prove, if at all. **My main point is that we only hear about the reaction of H$_2$O$_2$ with transition metals causing the formation of the notorious hydroxyl radical, but that is not always the case.**

46.2 ANOTHER VIEW

Triplet ground state oxygen ($^3O_2$)   **.O-O.**

Singlet oxygen ($^1O_2$)   **O-O:**

Superoxide anion   **.O-O:**

Peroxyl radical   **.O-O:H**

Hydrogen Peroxide (H_2O_2)   **H:O-O:H**

Hydroxyl Radical   **H:O.**

Hydroxyl ion   **H:O:**

Water   **H:O:H**

$$^3O_2 \xrightarrow{\text{+23 Kcal}} {}^1O_2$$

$$^3O_2 \xrightarrow{\text{+7.6 Kcal}} O_2{}^{\cdot -}$$

$$O_2{}^{\cdot -} \xrightarrow{\text{-21.7 Kcal}} H_2O_2$$

$$H_2O_2 \xrightarrow{\text{-8.8 Kcal}} .OH$$

$$.OH \xrightarrow{\text{-53.7 Kcal}} H_2O$$

The first step with an electron addition to oxygen to form superoxide is **endothermic** but **subsequent reductions are exothermic**.

Superoxide can act as either an oxidant or a reductant; it can oxidize:
> Sulphur
> ascorbic acid
> NADPH

it can reduce:
> Cytochrome c
> Metal ions

Superoxide dismutase (SOD) was first isolated in 1938 by Mann and Keilis and was thought to be a copper storage protein until its catalytic function was discovered in 1969 by McCord and Fridovitch.

46.3 CELLULAR ORGANIZATION AND COMPARTMENTALIZATION

The major eukaryotic cellular organelles:

NUCLEUS : envelope, chromatin, nucleolus, nucleoplasm
MITOCHONDRIA : peri-mitochondrial space, cristae, matrix
CHLOROPLAST : peri-chloroplast space, hyaloids, stroma
RIBOSOME : small unit, large unit, polysomes
ENDOPLASMIC RETICULUM : smooth and rough
GOLGI BODY : sided - cis and trans; end membrane pathway
LYSOSOME : hydrolytic enzymes
MICROBODIES : peroxisome and glyoxysomes
CENTROSOME : centriole, basal body, flagella, cilia
CYTOSKELETON : microfilaments, microtubules, intermediate filaments
INTRACELLULAR JUNCTIONS : tight junctions, desmosomes, gap junctions, plasmodesmata
PLANT CELL VACUOLE
CELL MEMBRANE

EUKARYOTIC: cell plan of multi-cellular organisms, eukaryotes (eukarya) include the fungi, algae, protozoa, slime molds and all plants and animals; contain many internal membrane bounded organelles...

   organelle - a subcell part that has a distinct metabolic function

U.T.O.P.I.A.

Seven characteristics of Eucaryotes:

> nucleus - single greatest step in evolution of higher animals
>> genes in "chromosomes" [colored bodies…made of DNA + protein]
>> contains more DNA (1000 x more) than prokaryotes
>
> presence of organelles - significant internal compartmentalization of function
> presence of flexible cell walls (allows phagocytosis)
> presence of cytoskeleton (provides framework to be larger)
> reproduce sexually
>
> usually larger - cell volume 10x > than bacteria - size 5.0 to 20 μm diameter
> extensive internal membranes

H_2O_2 readily permeates membranes and is not compartmentalized in the cell. I question how nature could evolve such an alleged harmful agent and give it free range of the cell. **I believe it is obvious that it is natures' unparalleled wisdom that allows for high level steady states of H_2O_2 production and its unfettered access to all cellular compartments.** Numerous enzymes (peroxidases) use H_2O_2 as a substrate in oxidation reactions involving the synthesis of complex organic molecules.

The reaction of ROS and excytomers with organic substrates are complex, even in vitro with homogenous solutions, but in biological systems, such as the living/breathing cell, many complexities arise due to the surface properties of membranes, electrical charges, binding properties of macromolecules, and compartmentalization of enzymes, substrates and catalysts. **The inherent heterogeneity of the intracellular environment requires consideration of the immediate site of any and all RONS and excytomer reactions.** No one is denying that oxidation of proteins, lipids and nucleic acids can occur in vivo but one must be very circumspect at directly extrapolating in vitro results to the living/breathing cell.

H_2O_2 and $O_2^{\cdot-}$ may participate in the production of singlet oxygen and peroxynitrite. The generation of these species may be concurrent with reactions involving iron and under some circumstances they might be important contributors to H_2O_2 toxicity. **There is considerable debate concerning the toxicity of singlet oxygen and peroxynitrite.**

Singlet dioxygen is not spin-restricted from oxidizing organic compounds as is triplet state oxygen. I believe that this is a most important observation and each of the so called RONS need to be evaluated on the basis of its specific reactivity and not erroneously lumped into a meaningless broad category such as "reactive oxygen species.".

Hypochlorite produced by the reaction of Cl- with H_2O_2 might react with H_2O_2 to generate singlet oxygen. Reaction 9 is facilitated by **chloroperoxidase, which generates singlet oxygen from H_2O_2 and chloride in vitro and singlet oxygen is produced in neutrophils, which contain abundant H_2O_2 and chloroperoxidases** (Steinbeck, M.J., Khan, A.U. and Karnovsky, M.J. J Biol Chem 1992; 267: 13425-13433). At low pH, HOCl can oxidize $O_2^{\cdot-}$ or Fe2+ to form a strong oxidant, presumably ·OH.

$O_2^{\cdot-}$ reacts rapidly with nitric oxide to form peroxynitrite anion (Reaction 11), the protonated form of which, peroxynitrite acid (pk_a = 6.7), reacts well with biological molecules. Alternatively, **ONOO⁻ might form singlet oxygen from H_2O_2** (Di Mascio, P., Bechara, E.J., Medeiros, M.H., Briviba, K. and Sies, H. FEBS Lett 1994; 355: 287-289). Consequently, NO· production by nitric oxide synthases may render cells vulnerable to superoxide-mediated damage. However, I need to point out that **this is a controversial reaction and more recent papers doubt this source of $^1O_2$.**

434

46.4 ALLEGED DNA DAMAGE BY FENTON OXIDANTS

Reportedly, the role of the hydroxyl radical is analogous to the "spark" that starts a fire. The basis for the hydroxyl's extreme reactivity in lipid systems is that at very low concentrations it initiates a chain reaction **involving triplet ground state oxygen, the most abundant form of oxygen in the cell.** The lipid hydroperoxide (ROOH) is unstable in the presence of iron or other metal catalysts because ROOH will participate in a Fenton reaction leading to the formation of reactive alkoxyl radicals:

$$ROOH + Fe^{2+} \longrightarrow OH- + RO. + Fe^{3+}$$

Among the degradation products of ROOH are aldehydes, such as malondialdehyde and hydrocarbons such as ethane and ethylene, which are commonly used measured end products of lipid peroxidation.

A substantial portion of H_2O_2 lethality involves DNA damage by oxidants generated from iron-mediated Fenton reactions. It would appear that NADH can drive the process by replenishing Fe^{2+} from Fe^{3+} in bacteria and in vitro. Moreover, NADH enhances iron-DNA association.

Damage by Fenton oxidants may occur at the DNA bases or sugars. Sugar damage is initiated by hydrogen abstraction from one of the deoxyribose carbons and the predominant consequence is eventual strand breakage and base release. Degradation of the base will produce numerous products, including 8-hydroxyguanine, hydroxymethyl urea, urea, thiamine glycol, thiamine and adenine ring-opened and -saturated products. The principle cause of single strand breaks is oxidation of the sugar moiety by the hydroxyl radical. **In vitro neither H_2O_2 alone nor $O_2^{\cdot-}$ cause strand breaks under physiological conditions and thus their toxicity is the result of Fenton reactions. I feel that this is a most important observation in that it indicates the harmless nature of H_2O_2 in the absence of transition metals.** However, if a bound metal is reduced by a small diffusible molecule, such as NADPH or $O_2^{\cdot-}$, it will react with H_2O_2 to form .OH which then oxidizes an adjacent sugar or base causing breakage of the DNA chain. Even though DNA is effective in binding metals, it appears that it can be damaged secondarily by them.

The spectrum of damages due to iron/H_2O_2 is quite similar to (but not congruent with) that caused by ionizing radiation (Luo, Y., Henle, E.S. and Linn, S. J Biol Chem 1996; 271: 21167-21176). Once again, **this data indicates the fact that H_2O_2 damage is different than that produced by radiation.**

One source of the difference between products formed by Fenton oxidants versus ionizing radiation could be the participation of iron ions directly in product formation.

8-oxo-Gua is also the object of much study because of its highly mutagenic nature (it base pairs relatively well with adenine) and the relative ease of its isolation and quantitation. **I must remind you that reactions in the test tube may not reflect reactions in the biochemical heterogeneity of the cell.**

46.5 CELLULAR SOURCES OF ROS

46.5.1 Chloroplast

In plants, the chloroplasts have four sites that can activate oxygen but I will keep our discussion primarily focused on higher animals with eukaryotic cells.

46.5.2 Mitochondria

Most O_2 is consumed by the cytochrome oxidase and electron transport system involving the 4 electron transfer to O_2 with the release of water. **This system is believed to be the main source of RONS, which I have discussed elsewhere in detail.**

46.5.3 Endoplasmic Reticulum

Various oxidative processes, including oxidation, hydroxylations, dealkylations, deaminations, dehalogenation and denaturation, occur on the smooth endoplasmic reticulum. Mixed function oxygenases that contain a heme moiety add an oxygen atom into an organic substrate using NADPH as the electron donor, as seen with cytochrome P450. In the 1970s, **Dr. Richard H. Steele and I were the first to describe the generation of $^1O_2$ from a cytochrome P450 system.** Activation of O_2 is essential for xenobiotic and drug detoxifications. Obviously, superoxide is likely produced by this same system, which requires less free energy for formation.

46.5.4 Peroxisomes (Microbodies)

Peroxisomes and glyoxysomes are organelles with a single membrane that compartmentalizes enzymes involved in the beta-oxidation of fatty acids, and the glyoxylic acid cycle including glyocolate oxidase, catalase and various peroxidases. **Glycolate oxidase produces H_2O_2 and xanthine oxidase, urate oxidase and NADH oxidase generate O_2^- as a consequence of metabolism of xanthine to uric acid.** Another interesting fact is that peroxisomes can reportedly self-replicate. I can not help but wonder if this is prion-type activity.

46.5.5 Plasma Membranes

A superoxide-generating NADPH oxidase activity has been identified in the plasmolemma enriched fractions and these lipoproteins may produce O_2^- by the redox cycling of certain quinones or nitrogenous compounds in plant roots. **Leukocytes contain an NADH oxidase on the outer membrane surface which is activated in response to a foreign agent, generating O_2^- that initiates oxidative reactions that destroy the potential pathogen.**

Remember that NADPH oxidase, which generates O_2^-, is located in all 3 layers of the aorta, which again indicates the widespread generation of RONS/excytomers. Thus, **not only is the potential to generate RONS through out the cell but it is widespread through out tissues and organs.**

46.6 REMOVING FENTON OXIDANTS

The fidelity of the metabolic redox reactions and the sequestering of iron in ferritin and transferrin generally minimize the burden from reactive oxygen species. Moreover, compartmentalization of free iron and superoxide and the impediment for iron binding to DNA by histones diminish the occurrence of Fenton reaction on DNA. I feel that this fact is of extreme importance because of the total number of transitions that can theoretically participate in the Fenton type reaction to yield the hydroxyl radical. **If these metals were not accounted for in the cell, it would be rapidly catastrophic to its viability.**

Catalase does not appear to be nearly so important as SOD judging from the weak phenotypes of cells that lack it and persons with **acatalasemia** (Eaton, J.W. and Ma, M. The metabolic and molecular bases of inherited disease. Scriver, C.R., Beaudet, A.L., Sly, W.S. and Valle, D. Eds 7th Ed McGraw-Hill, Inc., New York 1995; 2371-2388). In fact, **in contrast to the dire predictions of the Free Radi-Crap theory of aging and oxidative stress, acatalasemia patients live relatively normal lives.**

In eukaryotes, glutathione peroxidases are found in the mitochondria, cytoplasm and peroxisomes. These enzymes, especially the selenium glutathione peroxidase, are more effective in removing H_2O_2 than catalase. Peroxidases are less specific than catalase and can also reduce organic hydroperoxides that can react in Fenton-like reactions. Oxidized glutathione is reduced by NADPH-dependent glutathione reductase, an auxiliary enzyme for this antioxidant function.

The relative levels of SOD, catalase and glutathione peroxidase are important. For instance, **an increase in SOD would deplete the cell of superoxide but would increase H_2O_2 production**, which might be deleterious unless sufficient catalase and/or glutathione peroxidase were available. Likewise, excess glutathione peroxidase could unnecessarily deplete glutathione and/or NADPH reserves even though sufficient catalase was present. I feel that **these facts are frequently over looked or not considered in discussions concerning effects of various enzymatic and non-enzymatic antioxidants.**

My review of the genetic models of alterations of enzymes, involved in the regulation of RONS, is **a land mine of confusion.** However, in general, **excesses in enzymes which decrease RONS levels of H_2O_2 or $O_2^{\cdot-}$, did not result in the absence of disease or prevent aging.** Additionally, genetic conditions which had a deficit or absence of enzymes to deactivate ROS levels of H_2O_2 or $O_2^{\cdot-}$, were not plagued with the 100 diseases attributed to RONS damage. In fact, in patients such as Swiss type acatalasemia, live a relatively normal life and reach a normal life span. There was little support for the Free Radi-Crap theory.

In support of my Unified Theory, a study utilizing L1210 **murine leukemia cells showed that these cells are killed by $O_2^{\cdot-}$ and H_2O_2 and addition of acatalasemia red cells also resulted in kill of the L1210 cells** (Agar, N.S., Sadrzadeh, S.M., Hallaway, P.E. and Eaton, P.E. Erythrocyte catalase. A somatic oxidant defense? 1986; 77(1): 319-321).

Furthermore, a study in patients with cardiovascular disease, showed an inverse relationship with glutathione peroxidase **but no relationship to superoxide dismutase activity** (Blankenberg, S., Rupprecht, H.J., Torzewski, M., Tiret, L., Smieja, M., Cambiem. F., Meyer, J., Lackner, K.J. Glutathione peroxidase 1 activity and cardiovascular events in patients with coronary artery disease. 2003; 349(17): 1587-1589).

Eukaryotes also contain a **thiol-specific antioxidant enzyme** that acts as a thiol-dependent peroxidase, at least at low H_2O_2 concentrations (~50 uM). At high concentrations of H_2O_2 (~10 mM), thiol-specific antioxidant enzyme is reported to protect DNA against damage by thiol/metal-catalyzed oxidation; however, this protection does not appear to be mediated by the peroxidase activity.

The only effective means of detoxification of .OH is to scavenge it non-enzymatically. Histones and the compact structure of chromatin protect the DNA by this means (Milligan, J.R., Auguilera, J.A. and Ward, J.F. Radiat Res 1993; 133: 158-162). However, **I must ask what protects mRNA on its long journey from the nucleus to the ribosomes and the endoplasmic reticulum, where it can be sniped at by a wide variety of ROS?**

As yet, an enzymatic apparatus for singlet oxygen removal has not been detected; rather the cell appears to employ scavengers such as carotenoids (Sies, H. and Stahl, W. Am J Clin Nutr 1995; 62(6): 1315-1321).

46.7 DNA REPAIR

O_2^-, H_2O_2 and iron may interfere in this "chemical restitution," and sulfhydryls may in fact exacerbate DNA damage by iron/H_2O_2 (Held, K.D., Sylvester, F.C., Hopcia, K.L. and Bigalow, J.E. Radiat Res 1996; 145: 542-553).

46.7.1 Caspases, H_2O_2 and Apoptosis

Some of the following materials were excerpted from the website: http://www.med.nus.edu.gs/phys/Hyp_Drug.htm

Cross talk between caspases and mitochondria during drug-induced tumor cell death - function of a permissive intracellular milieu:

Recent evidence has highlighted the pivotal role of intracellular cysteine proteases (caspases) and mitochondrial-derived apoptogenic factors, such as cytochrome C and AIF, during apoptotic execution. We hypothesize that if the interplay between caspases and mitochondria determine the fate of tumor cells during chemotherapy, then it is logical to identify compounds that directly target these effector components of the death pathway. In this regard, we have shown that the cytosolic release of cytochrome C could occur in the absence of a drop in the transmembrane potential of the mitochondria and without the induction of the mitochondrial permeability transition. Secondly, we demonstrated that the mere release of cytochrome C in the absence of efficient caspase activation was not sufficient for effective induction of drug-induced apoptosis. We identified mitochondrial hydrogen peroxide, in addition to cytochrome C release, and downstream induction of cytosolic acidification as critical effector mechanism(s) that determine the efficacy of anticancer therapy. These findings have substantially added to our knowledge of the signaling mechanism(s) operative in tumor cells, in particular the role of mitochondria in the execution phase.

Regulation of apoptotic signaling by intracellular reactive oxygen species - The concept of "Reductive Stress-Induced Apoptosis":

An increase in the intracellular generation of reactive oxygen species (ROS) such as superoxide ($O_2.-$) and hydrogen peroxide (H_2O_2) or a defect in the antioxidant defense system renders the cells oxidatively stressed, a state harmful for cell survival. However, recent evidence has added a newer dimension to the effects of elevated intracellular ROS by demonstrating **that a pro-oxidant state amplifies cell proliferation**, either by via direct stimulation of cell division and activation of transcription or indirectly by inhibiting the execution of the cell death signal. These findings seem to tie up well with the observations that certain cell types, in particular **tumor cells, constitutively generate ROS that function as autocrine growth stimulation signals**. We are working on the premise that sustained elevation of intracellular $O_2.-$ in tumor cells could contribute to drug resistance by inhibiting the execution of the death signal. Indeed, in our recent reports, we have shown that pharmacological or endogenous inhibition of intracellular $O_2.-$ production enhances tumor cell sensitivity to drug-induced apoptosis. On the contrary, an increase in intracellular $O_2.-$ inhibits apoptosis via a direct or indirect effect on caspase activation pathways. We hypothesize that the divergent signaling by ROS is a function of their absolute intracellular concentration and the critical balance between $O_2.-$ and H_2O_2. It is when the cellular generation of $O_2.-$ and H_2O_2 is excessive, that cells succumb to this stress by either activating apoptosis, or undergo necrosis. The critical determinant between survival and apoptotic or necrotic cell death, we believe may be the cytosolic pH, downstream of ROS production. According to our model, **survival is favored with a mild sustainable increase in intracellular O₂.- that maintains cytosolic pH in the alkaline range. Apoptosis**, on the other hand is a function of intracellular H₂O₂ production accompanied by reduction of the intracellular milieu, and more importantly **a decrease in O₂.- level and cytosolic acidification**. Thus, in order to differentiate necrotic from apoptotic stress, we propose to refer to the mechanism of apoptosis induced by an increase in ROS production as **"reductive stress"** as opposed to the term "oxidative stress", which should appropriately be used for ROS-induced necrosis.

46.7.2 Apoptosis and ¹O₂

Ultraviolet A (UVA) irradiation is effectively used to treat patients with atopic dermatitis and other T cell mediated, inflammatory skin disease. In the present study, successful phototherapy of atopic dermatitis was found to result from UVA radiation-induced apoptosis in skin-infiltrating T helper cells, leading to T cell depletion from eczematous skin. In vitro, UVA radiation-induced human T helper cell apoptosis was mediated through the FAS/FAS-ligand system, which was activated in irradiated T-cells as a consequence of singlet oxygen generation. These studies demonstrate that **singlet oxygen is a potent trigger for the induction of human T-cell apoptosis.** They also identify **singlet oxygen generation as fundamental mechanism of action operative in phototherapy** (Morita, A., Werfel, T., Stege, H., Ahrens, C., Karmann, K., Grewe, M., Grether-Beck, S., Ruzicka, T., Kapp, A., Klotz, L., Sies, H. and Krutmann, J. Evidence that singlet oxygen-induced human T helper cell apoptosis is the basic mechanism of ultraviolet-A radiation phototherapy. J Exp Med 1997; 186: 1763-1768).

Studies were conducted to clarify the cytocidal effect of combination therapy consisting of administration of acridine orange (AO), which is a photosensitizer, and radiation therapy using in vitro and in vivo mouse osteosarcoma models. The results revealed that AO combined with low-dose X-ray irradiation of about 1-5 Gy had a strong cytocidal effect on the cultured mouse osteosarcoma cells regardless of their chemosensitivity, and that this combination therapy inhibit growth of the in vivo mouse osteosarcoma by induction of tumor necrosis. This effect was inhibited by L-histidine, but not by mannitol. These findings suggested that **AO might be excited by X-rays and kill osteosarcoma cells through the release of singlet oxygen** (Hashiguchi, S., Kusuzaki, K., Murata, H., Takeshita, H., Hashiba, M., Nishimura, T., Ashihara, T. and Hirasawa, Y. Acridine orange excited by low-dose radiation has a strong cytocidal effect on mouse osteosarcoma. Oncology 2002; 62: 85-93).

Studies by Moussavi-Harami, et al. indicate that acridine orange (AO) has been used to sensitize mouse osteosarcoma cells to low dose radiation. It has suggested AO excitation by radiation causes release of singlet oxygen, which is toxic to living cells (Kusuzaki, et al. Total tumor cell elimination with minimum damage to normal tissue in musculoskeletal sarcomas following photodynamic therapy with acridine orange. Oncology 2000; 59: 174-180). The aim of the present study is to determine if addition of AO can similarly sensitize chondrosarcoma cells to low-dose radiation.

Photodynamic therapy (PDT) involves use of a localized photosensitizer that is excited by light to cause damage and subsequent cell death. PDT is an encouraging new technique used in treatment of bladder, esophageal and lung cancers s well as in nonmalignant diseases. AO is a cell-permeable, fluorescent dye that interacts with DNA and RNA of living cells by intercalation or electrostatic attraction. Long exposures to AO (about 24 hours) cause mitotic arrest in normal chondrocytes in cell culture. AO is used in histochemistry for diagnosis, classification and prognosis of neoplasms and has been experimentally used in PDT of superficial tumors such as bladder, gastric and epithelial cancers because of its nature as a photosensitizing agent. Recent results published have demonstrated that AO can be excited to low-dose X-ray as well as visible light, making it feasible for use in deep structures of the body (Hashiguch, et al. Acridine orange excited by low-dose radiation has a strong cytocidal effect on mouse osteosarcoma. Oncology 202; 62: 85-93).

Results of our in vitro study demonstrate that a treatment regiment of AO and low-dose radiation was effective in eliminating or stopping division of the CS cells. In cells cultures treated with AO and 3 or 5Gy, there were many single cells and small colonies. This is an indication that the cells did not necessarily die as a result of the treatment but were incapable of cell division.

46.7.3 $^1O_2$ Does Not Break DNA Strands

The capacity of a photodynamic and chemical source of singlet molecular oxygen to cause DNA strand breakage at pH 7.8 was compared in the following systems: 1) dissolved rose Bengal plus light (400-660 nm), 2) a novel water-soluable naphthalene-derived endoperoxide showing temperature-dependent singlet oxygen release, in the absence of light. Comparatively large fluxes of singlet oxygen generated by the endoperoxide completely failed to produce DNA strand breaks. Studies conclude that, **although singlet oxygen seems to play a role in DNA strand breakage by rose Bengal plus light, singlet oxygen per se is very inefficient if not completely incapable of causing DNA strand breakage** (Nieuwint, A.W., Aubry, J.M., Arwert, F., Kortbeek, H., Hertzberg, S. and Joenje, H. Inability of chemical generated singlet oxygen to break the DNA backbone. Free Rad Res Comm 1985; 1(1): 1-9).

A naphthalene endoperoxide was used as a non-photochemical source of singlet oxygen ($^1O_2$) to examine some interactions between this reactive oxygen species and DNA. No evidence for $^1O_2$-induced interstrand cross linking was obtained. The capacity of $^1O_2$ to generate strand breaks in single-stranded (ss) and double-stranded (ds) DNA was investigated by sucrose gradient centrifugation analysis of bacteriophage phi X174 DNA. **Studies infer that $^1O_2$-induced inactivation of phi X174 DNA is not due to DNA backbone breakage nor to interstrand crosslinking, but rather to some form of damage to the base of sugar moiety of the DNA, the exact nature of which remains to be elucidated** (Lafleur, M.V., Nieuwint, A.W., Aubry, J.M., Kortbeek, H., Arwert, F. and Joenje, H. DNA damage by chemically generated singlet oxygen. Free Rad Res Comm 1987; 2(4-6): 343-350).

Ultraviolet (UV) A-1 (340-400 mm) radiation is highly effective in inducing apoptosis in skin-infiltrating T-cells and thereby exerts beneficial effects in patients with T-cell-mediated skin diseases. This in vitro study, reported that malignant and normal T-cells differ in their susceptibility toward UVA-1 radiation-induced apoptosis. It has been shown that UVA-1 radiation-induced T-cell apoptosis is initiated through the generation of singlet oxygen. This is in agreement with the present observation **that stimulation of unpredicted cells with a singlet oxygen-generating system induced apoptosis in malignant cells to a greater extent than in normal cells.** Moreover, down regulation of FAS surface expression in malignant T-cells was associated with the inhibition of UVA-1 radiation/singlet oxygen-induced apoptosis in these cells.

Studies indicate that the susceptibility of human T-cells toward UVA-1 radiation-induced apoptosis is related to the availability of caspases such as caspase-3 and that strategies directed at upregulating caspase levels will increase the efficacy of UVA-1 phototherapy (Yamauchi, R., Morita, A., Yasuda, Y., Grether-Beck, S., Klotz, L., Tasuji, T. and Krutmann, J. Different susceptibility of malignant versus nonmalignant human T-cells toward ultraviolet A-1 radiation-induced apoptosis. J of Invest Derm 2004; 122: 477-483).

46.8 CONCLUSION

By being mutagenic (in vitro), reactive oxygen species have been implicated in cancer and other degenerative disease. However, **p53-dependent apoptosis seems to be mediated by reactive oxygen species, so these agents have diametrical effects; they cause undesirable cellular alterations but also prevent undesirable consequences of DNA damage by helping to eliminate damaged cells.** This is another example of an important beneficial effect of ROS.

47 OXYGEN AND WOUND HEALING

I have been a student of wound healing for over 3 decades (Howes, R.M. and Hoopes, J. E. Current concepts of wound healing, Clinics in Plastic Surgery 1977; 4(20: 177-179), (Howes, R. M., Steele, R.H. and Hoopes, J.E. The role of electronic excitation states in collagen biosynthesis. Persp Biol Med 1977; 20(4): 539-544). In 1977, I had predicted that electronic excitation state biochemistry would be applied to wound healing within a decade. Dr. Robert O. Becker fulfilled this prophecy with his work on bone healing, which he wrote about extensively in his book, The Body Electric: Electromagnetism and the Foundation of Life. By R.O. Becker and G. Selden, William Morrow and Co., 1985. Further, Becker writes, "An infinitesimal electric field (0.025 volts/cm) pulsation at 10 hertz dramatically restored normal patterns to most of the biological measurements. Wever concluded that this frequency in the micro-pulsations of the earth's electromagnetic field was the prime timer of biocycles. The results have since been confirmed in guinea pigs and mice. In light of this work, the fact that 10 hertz is also the dominant (alpha) frequency of the EEG in all animals becomes another significant bit of evidence that **every creature is hooked up to the earth electromagnetically, through its DC system.**" Another interesting point by Becker relates to the fact that all organic compounds exist in two forms (isomers), which are either dextrarotary (D) or levoratory (L), depending upon its refraction of light. **All living things consist of either D or L forms, depending on the species, but never both.**

Becker points out that all matter, living and nonliving, is ultimately an electromagnetic phenomenon. He also mentions that as long-distance communications have used shorter and shorter wave length radio waves, that **we are in sea of energies life has never before experienced and the results of which are currently unknown**. Also, studies on rat brains subjected to microwaves at two levels, at half and also slightly more than the U.S. safety standard of 10,000 microwatts: "The results suggest **that microwave exposure inhibits electron transport chain function in brain mitochondria and results in decreased energy levels in the brain.**"

ELF (extremely low frequency) and electromagnetic waves appear to affect our immune systems and decrease the body's natural abilities to fight infections. Also, evidence has been found that **an electric field only slightly stronger than earth's background stimulated growth of all bacteria tested and increased their resistance to antibiotics.**

Electromagnetic energy is likely to also affect cell division and Winters **exposed human cancer cells to 60-hertz electromagnetic fields for just 24 hours and found a 6-fold increase in their growth rate 7-10 days later.** In the last few years, more reliable epidemiological studies have appeared, showing increased rates of cancer and birth defects among people exposed to higher-than-average levels of electromagnetic energy. **I suspect that this observation will also be subject to non-linearity, as has been seen with radiation hormesis.**

Mankind has managed to heal its wounds in spite of man's many frequently illogical and damaging interventions. Collagen biochemistry plays a primary role in wound healing by contributing significantly to the ultimate tensile strength of the healed wound. Previously, I have discussed the relationship between collagen and platelet aggregation, proline hydroxylation, microsomal mixed function oxidations and electronic excitation states of singlet oxygen. **My past studies have shown that human diploid fibroblasts will produce a chemiluminescence which is indicative of the presence of $^1O_2$.** The presence of $^1O_2$ placed the fibroblast in new and higher energetic levels that those available by ATP. Past studies on formation of hydroxy proline revealed a requirement for atmospheric oxygen, iron and alpha-ketoglutarate. Other studies have shown that the hydroxyl moiety of collagen is derived from molecular oxygen and not from water. Considering the similarities between substrate oxidations effected by hepatic microsomes, by $^1O_2$ and by in vitro and in vivo proline hydroxylation, we proposed that these reactions were going through a common intermediate of O_2^- and $^1O_2$ and that this represented the long sought after "active oxygen." Recent data of 2004 supports our initial proposal.

Dr. Albert Szent-Gyorgii once wrote, "Biology is the science of the improbable," and this holds true for the study of wound healing. Slow or chronic wound healing is a major medical and economic problem with patient care today. Insights into its mechanisms which might correct or accelerate the process could have dramatic consequences. Wound healing is also tied to oxygen metabolism.

Some of the following materials were excerpted from: Youn, B.A. **Oxygen and its role in wound healing** at the website http://www.etcbiomedical.com/hbo_two.htm.

47.1 ATP

According to some, oxygen has two major functions (I feel that it has countless functions) in cellular metabolism, the most important of which is the electron transfer oxidase system which is responsible for approximately 90% of the total oxygen consumption. This pathway produces high energy phosphate bonds in the form of ATP which is the general source of biological energy. The second category is oxygen's role in the many oxidative reactions such as the mixed function oxidase, cytochrome P-450 system, hydroxylases and oxidases. These compounds are very important in the metabolism of drugs and other metabolic intermediates. **Greater than 90% of the energy utilized in cellular metabolism is derived from oxidation of glucose to carbon dioxide, water and high energy phosphate products in the form of ATP.** Since **there are no significant stores of ATP, oxygen utilization must be an ongoing process to maintain cellular function.** In the event that oxygen is deprived to the tissues an alternative anaerobic pathway exists which converts glucose to pyretic acid and lactic acid in a much less efficient mode of energy production. **The anaerobic pathway requires almost a twentyfold increase in glucose utilization to provide the same amount of high energy phosphate bonds**, and in addition, the by-products of this pathway are free hydrogen ions which produce or cause a significant metabolic acidosis. This alternative pathway is incapable of providing sufficient ATP for cellular maintenance let alone the increased requirements during the stress or injury and repair. In evolving an efficient aerobic pathway, we have become critically dependent on adequate oxygen delivery to maintain cellular metabolism. Additionally, I feel that the glycolytic pathway does not afford the cell the opportunity to generate ROS and excytomers, which is much to its detriment.

47.2 Collagen

Early in the repair of wounds, fibroblasts begin to migrate, divide and produce **collagen** which is an essential matrix for wound healing,. In order to promote fibroblast proliferation and the production of collagen, **oxygen must be present in sufficient quantities.**

Oxygen is incorporated by two amino acids, **proline and lysine**, in collagen chain synthesis. **Collagen cannot be synthesized by the fibroblast unless adequate amounts of both proline and lysine are hydroxylated with oxygen.** Synthesis requires one atom of oxygen for every three amino acids in sequence. Oxygen is also required in increased amounts during the repair process to provide energy for protein synthesis.

47.3 Neovascularity

Macrophages release angiogenesis factor which is a potent stimuli for endothelial cell activity. The formation of new blind end capillary buds with single red cells begins. This process is extremely delicate to mechanical forces, **oxygen level**, blood volume and nutrients. Neovascularization also depends on the fibroblasts on the leading edge of the wound laying down collagen as the scaffolding for repair. Comprised states such as diabetes, atherosclerotic diseases and irradiation impair normal angiogenesis (Knighton, D.R., Hunt, T.K. and Schevenstuhl, H. et al. Oxygen tension regulates the expression of angiogenesis factor by macrophages. Science 1983; 221: 1283-1285), and may lead to chronic wounds.

47.4 PMNs

By definition, a wound disrupts the normal skin barrier which is the first line of defense against invading microorganisms. In wounds, **one of the first lines of defense are migrating polymorphonuclear cells (PMNs) which locate, identify, phagocytize, kill and digest microorganisms. Polymorphonuclear cells require oxygen to kill organism by producing superoxide, hydrogen peroxide, singlet oxygen and other products via the respiratory burst** (Babior, B.M. Oxygen dependent microbial killing by phagocytes. N Engl J Med 1974; 298: 659-668, 721-726). The PMN is protected by detoxifying free radicals with superoxide dismutase, catalase and glutathione. **It has been shown in numerous studies that the degree of polymorphonuclear cell function in killing of bacteria is directly dependent on oxygen tension** (DeChatelet, L.R. Oxidative bactericidal mechanisms of polymorphonuclear leukocytes. J Infect Dis 1975; 131: 295-303), (Hohn, D.C. Oxygen and leukocyte microbial killing. Davis, J.C., Hunt, T.K. Eds. Hyperbaric Oxygen Therapy, Bethesday, Undersea Med Soc 1977; 101-110).

47.5 Oxygen Cascade

There exists a significant gradient from the partial pressure of oxygen in the ambient air to that available immediately to the tissues on a cellular level. I have pointed this out in the primer section on oxygen physiology. **This gradient, or reduction in partial pressures, is also known as the oxygen cascade.** This is a progressive decline in the partial pressures of oxygen from the air we breath through alveolar gas, blood, major arteries, capillaries, tissue diffusion and finally, to what is immediately available at the mitochondrial level. **The largest gradient is from arterial to tissue and mitochondrial. The mitochondria may function at partial pressures as low as 0.5 mmHg.** Tissue injury produces two major problems involving oxygen delivery and metabolism: 1) injury disrupts the normal delicate capillary network, thereby reducing the effectual oxygen delivery to the injured tissues, and 2) injured tissues have an overall increase in metabolic rate and demand for oxygen utilization.

47.6 Bacteria and Oxygen

Oxygen is important to the PMN for oxygen dependent bacterial killing. Aerobic organisms are oxygen dependent for survival although most are facultative and can survive in relative hypoxic environments. **Oxygen is directly lethal to strict anaerobic bacteria because of the organisms inability to detoxify oxygen radicals.** Oxygen enhanced environments have been shown to be bactericidal for most clostridia species and inhibit alpha toxin release. Hyperbaric oxygen has been shown to be a beneficial adjunct to therapy in Bacteroides fragilis, Fusobacterium infections and nonclostridial anaerobic infections (Schreiner, A. Hyperbaric oxygen therapy in bactericides infections. Acta Chir Scand 1974; 140: 73-76).

Hyperbaric oxygen, tissue levels may approach 1200 mmHg, in which increased production of superoxide, peroxide and other oxygen radicals occurs, however, some organisms adapt by producing increased levels of superoxide dismutase. There is no direct antibacterial effect of enhanced oxygen on aerobic organisms. Indirect antibactericidal effects are related to improved PMN function in killing bacteria. **Results with hyperbaric oxygen is similar to that obtained by the Baylor investigators using intra-arterial H$_2$O$_2$.**

47.7 Oxygen and Antibiotics

Aminoglycosides such as gentamicin, tobramycin, alizarin and netilmicin are oxygen dependent for their antimicrobial activity. The effect of oxygen has been studied in vivo and in vitro using Pseudomonas treated with tobramycin and controls grown aerobically and anaerobically. The aerobic grown Pseudomonas controls had a 51% increase in colonies compared to the tobramycin treated. **Vancomycin is another antibiotic that does not kill microorganisms well under low oxygen tensions. Sulfonamides antimicrobial**

effect is potentiated in hyperbaric oxygen. Similarly, many of the chemotherapeutic drugs are oxygen dependent.

47.8 Wound Oxygen Levels

Chronic wounds have been studied with implanted polygraphic oxygen electrodes and found to be hypoxic with levels of 5 to 20 mmHg compared to control values of 30 to 50 mmHg. This is a very important point. The Free Radi-Crap theory states that chronic wounds induce cancer by the over-production of ROS, whereas in reality, these chromic wounds have an oxygen deficiency state and the body could likely kill the infecting pathogen if adequate levels of oxygen were available and it would also kill pro-neoplastic cells.

47.9 CONCLUSION

Supplemental oxygen has been shown to enhance healing dependent on dose and frequency, however, excessive or continuous oxygen may impair the normal healing process. Some period hypoxia in conjunction with other stimuli (including lactate and other intermediates) is necessary to promote the healing process. In a normal host, despite a large wound with definite hypoxia, healing will occur as long as factors such as nutrients, blood flow and immune function remain adequate to allow regeneration of capillaries and restoration of nutrient delivery. A delicate balance exists between one of the major stimuli to healing hypoxia and the **paradoxical** need for oxygen for wound repair. **In situations where oxygen delivery is impaired chronic non-healing wounds may develop.**

In summary, oxygen is essential for maintaining cellular integrity, function and repair when tissues are injured. Oxygen not only plays an important role in energy metabolism, but also is very important in polymorphonuclear cell function, neovascularization, fibroblast proliferation and collagen deposition. **Again, I point out that oxygen is not our enemy but is our greatest ally.**

There is evidence to suggest that oxygen may indeed be a very important rate limiting step in wound healing. Larger wounds may have significantly increased metabolic demands, and larger areas of compromised microvascular oxygen delivery limiting the healing process. In a normal host healing may be delayed, but may eventually occur as progressive microcapillary neovascularization ensues and oxygen delivery is restored. It is the problem patient with either compromised oxygen delivery or enhanced oxygen utilization where **their oxygen supply never meets their oxygen demands and a chronic wound situation develops.**

48 DNA METHYLATION

Some of the following materials were excerpted from: Scientists probe shutting down cancer cells by awakening silenced genes. Tracy Hampton, JAMA 2004; 291(19): 2301-2305).

48.1 CANCER IS NOT A CERTAINTY

Scientists have discovered many cases in which mutations in the DNA sequence - such as point mutations or deletions -alter gene expression and set the stage for cancer. However, as I have discussed, the data with identical twins demonstrates that a mutation is expressed with a varying frequency.

Scientists strive to decipher which genetic changes can make cells cancerous and they are also discovering that not all such changes involve mutations that alter the DNA sequence. Rather, some are a result of **"epigenetic" modifications, heritable changes in gene function that occur without any mutation in gene sequence.** In other words, **not everything in the cell dances to the tune played by DNA.**

At the annual American Association for Cancer Research Conference in Orlando in late March, 2004, experts spoke of ongoing investigations into the epigenetic aspects of cancer development and how this field might contribute to the detection and treatment of cancer.

All of this is of importance because of the frequently quoted data involving 8-OHd-Guanine, which is a product of DNA reaction with RONS and thus supposedly invariably leads to overt cancer. However, even in unrepaired DNA, this may not be the case.

48.2 MUTED BY METHYLATION

Although each somatic cell in the body has the same genetic material, different cell types express different combinations of genes. To ensure a cell can perform its particular functions, it is essential that the appropriate genes are active when needed, while the others remain mute. In a given cell, regulatory proteins bind to segments of DNA and control which neighboring genes on the chromosome are expressed. **Some proteins recognize and bind to DNA sequences via methyl (CH$_3$) groups attached to DNA's cytosine bases.** Enzymes called CAN-methyl-transferases act in this way to prevent nearby gene expression.

This is perfectly normal within most cells - in fact, it is crucial for maintaining a cell's function, and in females, it is important for silencing genes to inactivate one X chromosome in each cell of the body. But it is far from normal in cells that turn cancerous. Research has shown that **in many cancer cells, inappropriate methylation, or hypermethylation, shuts off expression of tumor suppressor genes** - genes that encode proteins that safeguard against uncontrolled cell growth (Hum Mol Genet 2001; 10: 687-692). This data further erodes the Free Radi-Crap theory, especially as it relates to cancer causation.

"Among the changes that occur in cancer cell is methylation of regions around the 'start' sites of genes that ought to be free of DNA methylation in normal cells," said Steve Baylin, M.D., of Johns Hopkins University, in Baltimore. "There's a whole host of genes across the chromosomes that have all had silencing in genes due to hypermethylation, which are potentially extremely important to cancer," he added.

DNA methylation patterns are heritable, so when a cell divides and its chromosomes are replicated, sequences that are methylated in the parent cell will be methylated in parent cell will be methylated in progeny cells as well. **"This is really equivalent to essentially a [gene] deletion,"** said David Sidranksy, M.D., of Johns Hopkins University.

The discovery that aberrant methylation can lead to clonal tumor cell growth suggests that the phenomenon could be an attractive target for cancer treatment, said Peter Jones, Ph.D., of the University of Southern California, in Los Angeles. "We think of methylated DNA as being a locked door," Jones said. "What we'd like to do therapeutically is try to break the lock and open the door and switch the gene back on again." **Unlike a genetic mutation, methylation is a reversible phenomenon.**

48.3 TREATMENT POSSIBILITIES

Research also has shown that hypermethylated DNA can be detected in serum, sputum and urine samples of patients, suggesting that methylation may one day provide the key to quick, noninvasive cancer diagnostic tests in the clinic.

A number of demethylation agents, which are all analogs of the nucleoside deoxycytidine, inhibit cancer cell growth both in vitro and in animal models. Four have been tested clinically: 5-azacytidine, 5-aza-2'-deoxycitidine (decitabine), 1-B-Darabinofuranosyl-5-azacytosine (fazarabine), and dihydro-5-azacytidine. The first two showed some efficacy for treating leukemia but had little effect against solid tumors. Furthermore, these compounds exhibit some toxicity and are unstable and require fresh preparation and administration by injection. Trails with the latter two agents were stopped due to lack of efficacy (Ann Oncol 2002; 13: 1699-1716).

Zebularine does in fact seem to show some level of selectivity in the sense that it preferentially activates genes in cancer cells relative to normal cells," said Jones. However, I must point out that **the Howes Singlet Oxygen Delivery System does have selectivity.**

49 RADIATION, HORMESIS, RONS, CANCER AND AGING

Dr. Robert J. Cihak states that **many vitamins and minerals have been known to promote health in small doses and cause diseases in high doses for some time. Accumulating evidence indicates that ionizing radiation and other agents also interact with biological systems in similar fashion.** The phenomenon is called **"hormesis."** Hormesis is now being considered as a general biological phenomenon (Gerber, L.M., Williams, G.C. and Gray, S.J. The nutrient-toxin dosage continuum in human evolution and modern health. The Quarterly Rev Biol 1999; 74(3): 273-289). The following article of Bernard L. Cohen, Ph.D. was originally published in the Medical Sentinel 2000; 5(4): 128-131.

Radiation protection regulators often claim that they try to err on the side of caution. But in doing so, regulators in the past have ignored the evidence of hormesis in response to ionizing radiation. **To look at only the bad effects of radiation and be blind to the good effects is comparable to banning penicillin based on the fact that penicillin can kill by anaphylaxis while ignoring lives saved by the substance.**

In addition to harming peoples health, public health policies based on incomplete evaluation of scientific evidence harms the reputation of science in the mind of the public. Service and the public reputation of science advance only when all pertinent evidence is considered. - Robert J. Cihak, M.D., Editorial Board Member

49.1 BACKGROUND

In the past, the cancer risk from low level radiation (LLR) has been estimated by use of a **linear-no threshold hypothesis (LNT).** This hypothesis assumes that a single particle of radiation interacting with a single DNA molecule can initiate a cancer; if the assumption were correct, the number of initiating events would be proportional to the number of particles of radiation, and hence to the radiation dose, LNT is frequently extrapolated to doses as low as 1/10,000 of those for which there is direct evidence of cancer induction by radiation. This extrapolation is the origin of the commonly used expression "no level of radiation is safe" and the consequent public fear of LLR. This article explores some of the scientific evidence bearing on this hypothesis.

Recent discoveries show that DNA damage events occur all the time in our bodies, due to natural metabolic processes. **Each human cell averages more than 200,000 damage events every day.** Reparative biochemical mechanisms continually repair this damage. Double-strand breaks (DSB) in DNA are more significant and occur much less frequently.

The hypothesis most favorable for LNT is that double-strand breaks (DSB) are the cancer initiators. **An average cell experiences about 200 spontaneous DSB per year, whereas 10 cSv (10 rem) of radiation gives the average cell only 4 DSB** (Pollycove, M. Human biology, epidemiology and low dose ionizing radiation. Presentation to NCRP, Bethesda, MD, Feb 17, 1998). Thus, a hypothetical lifetime exposure of 10cSv (10 rem)/year increases cancer initiating events by only 2% (4/200), however, LNT predicts that it should increase cancer risk by more than 150%. (10/rem/yr is about 50 times greater than the average annual human background radiation exposure).

49.2 BIOLOGICAL DEFENSE
MECHANISMS (BDM)

One problem with the rationale for LNT is that it does not consider the role of biological defense mechanisms (BDM) which prevent each of the trillions of potentially cancer initiating events each human experiences every year from developing into a fatal cancer. Likewise, I believe that this is also true for the oxygenic studies for cancer causation. Another problem is **the abundant evidence that LLR stimulates BDM** (UNSCEAR (United Nations Scientific Committee on Effects of Atomic Radiation), Report to the General Assembly, Annex B: Adaptive Response, United Nations, New York, 1994); this fact implies that LLR should prevent development of cancer. We cite here a few examples. Current evidence indicates that cancers are initiated by genetic damage in a cell nucleus. Chromosome aberrations are one type of widely studied genetic damage. **In both in vitro and in vivo experiments on various type cells, exposure to LLR substantially reduces the number of chromosome aberrations from subsequent exposure to large radiation doses; this effect is ascribed to stimulated production of repair enzymes by the LLR.**

Mutations are another type of genetic damage; **prior LLR also reduces induction of specific detectable gene mutations in cells later exposed to high level radiation --- both in vitro** (Kelsey, K.T., Memisoglu, A., Frenkel, A. and Liber, H.L. Human lymphocytes exposed to low doses of X-rays are less susceptible to radiation induced mutagenesis. Mutat Res 1991; 263: 197-201), **and in vivo** (Fritz-Niggli, H. and Schaeppi-Buechi, C. Adaptive response to dominant lethality of mature and immature oocytes of D. Melanogaster to low doses of ionizing radiation: Effects in repair-proficient and repair deficient strains. Int J Radiat Biol 1991; 59: 175-184).

Perhaps more directly relevant, exposures to LLR can reduce the rate of subsequent spontaneous neoplastic transformation in cells by 3-fold or more (Azzam, E.I., de Toledo, S.M., Raaphorst, G.P. and Mitchel, R.E.J. Low dose ionizing radiation decrease the frequency of neoplastic transformation to a level below spontaneous rate in C3H 10T½ cells. Radiat Res 1996; 146: 369-373).

LLR stimulates the immune system, an important contributor to BDM. Direct observation of repair of DNA base damage has shown that a gamma radiation dose of 25 cSv (25 rem) 4 hours before a 200 cSv (200 rem) dose, reduced the time for 50% lesion removal from 100 minutes to 50 minutes. In other words, DNA lesions healed more quickly if an initial, stimulating radiation dose was given.

Since exposure to low level radiation stimulates BDM, this healing effect must be added to the harmful effect of cancer initiations hypothesized by LNT, effectively reducing the total risk predictions based on LNT alone. If the healing effects of stimulated BDM are larger than the carcinogenic effects hypothesized by LNT in the low dose region, the net effect of LLR is to protect against cancer; this is called "hormesis."

The IARC (International Agency for Research on Cancer), study covered **95,673** monitored radiation workers in U.S., U.K. and Canada. For all cancers except leukemia, there were 3,930 deaths but no excess over the number expected. The risk is reported as -.0007/cSv; there is surely no support for LNT here. **These radiation doses were spread out over time in contrast with the instantaneous exposure experienced by the A-bomb**

survivors. Such long-term exposure is more relevant in establishing population and public health radiation exposure guidelines.

Powerful evidence against LNT is also found in studies of bone cancers among those exposed by ingested radium. Evans' elaborate analysis essentially demonstrates threshold behavior. Such a threshold behavior is also strongly supported with much better statistics in studies of radioactivity injected into animals.

49.3   DEPENDENCE OF LATENT PERIOD ON DOSE

A substantial body of data, both on animals on humans, indicates that the latent period between carcinogenic radiation exposure and cancer death increases with decreasing exposure. For low exposures, the theoretical latent period exceeds the normal lifespan, so no actual cancers develop. This latency effect alone, even in the absence of all considerations discussed previously, would invalidate LNT for LLR.

49.4 BENEFICIAL EFFECTS OF LOW DOSES OF RADIATION

The following materials were excerpted from an article by Jerry Cuttler and a summary by Ron Mitchel:

Mitchel, Senior Scientist in the Radiation Biology and Health Physics Branch at Chalk River Laboratories, and three co-workers have just published an outstanding paper in the journal Radiation Research. It presents convincing evidence that a single radiation dose of 10 or 100 milli-Gray (mGy) (1 or 10 rad) cobalt-60 gamma rays to cancer-prone, radiation-sensitive young (~50 day) mice **delays cancer death substantially**. The dose of 10 or 100 mGy is approximately 4 or 40 times the average natural radiation dose in a year, but it was delivered at 0.5 mGy per minute.

The research employed genetically modified Trp53+/- mice whose cells lack the cancer-fighting gene Trp53 in one of their two chromosomes. Such mice get cancer in middle age instead of old age, as would happen in normal mice (Trp53+/- ones). Not only are Trp53+/- mice cancer prone, they are also radiation sensitive. Such mice do serve as a model for cancer-prone and radiation-sensitive people who would be part of a workforce.

Normal mice have a mean lifespan of 578 +/- 138 days (1.6 +/- 0.4 y). Exposure to the large dose of 4 Gy (400 rad) at a high dose rate results in a lifespan loss of 125 days or 22% of their normal life. In comparison, Trp53+/- mice with a lifespan of 375 +/- 103 days (1.0 y), when exposed to 4 Gy, have their life reduced by 148 days or 40%. So Trp53+/- mice are therefore more sensitive than normal mice to a high dose.

Hormesis is an adaptive response of living organisms to low levels of chemical, biological or radiological stress or damage - a modest overcompensation to a disruption - resulting in improved fitness. Observations of this reproducible phenomenon (**low-dose stimulation and high-dose inhibition) have been widely reported in the scientific biomedical literature since for many and form the basis for all immunology treatment**. This is the basis for immunization programs. Despite the growing body of evidence for adaptive response to low-level radiation, epidemiological (population) studies are generally inconclusive. The reason given is that the dose-response is lost against the "noise" of background cancer incidence. Public and occupational health policies, which rely on such studies, therefore revert to the Linear-No-Threshold (LNT) hypothesis. Unfortunately, interpretation of the LNT hypothesis, implies proof of a negative health effect at any level of radiation exposure, has contributed **societal radiophobia and anti-nuclear propaganda**. This Chalk River paper reports on quality research carried out on radiation-sensitive animals and demonstrates that a low-dose or radiation, while neither increasing the average lifespan nor reducing the frequency of tumor initiation in the sample population, **did provide protection against spontaneous cancer by delaying death due to cancer**. This and other related research suggest the need to reconsider the conventional "ever lower is better" criterion for low-dose radiation limits in favor of criteria which consider the beneficial effects of radiation at low-dose levels. Such a policy shift would also enable the possible use of low-dose radiation therapy in many important medical applications (Mitchel, R.E., Jackson, J.S., Morrison, D.P. and Carlisle, S.M. Low doses of radiation increase the latency of spontaneous lymphomas and spinal osteosarcoma in cancer-prone, radiation-sensitive Trp53 heterozygous mice. Radiat Res 2003; 159(3): 320-327) . Note: One Gray (Gy) is one joule of radiation energy per kilogram of animal mass.

T. Don Luckey states (Radiation Hormesis Overview, RPM, July/August 1999; 16(4): 22-34), that there is evidence of health benefits and longer average lifespan following low-dose radiation which should replace fear, "all radiation is harmful," and "the perception of harm" as the basis for action in the 21st century. **Hormesis is the excitation, or stimulation, by small doses of any agent in any system. Large doses inhibit. "Low-dose" is defined as any dose between ambient levels of radiation and the threshold that marks the boundary between biopositive and bionegative effects.** That threshold negates the "linear no threshold" (LNT) paradigm. This overview summarizes almost **3000 reports** on stimulation by low-dose irradiation. Hormesis with ionizing radiation presented evidence of increased vigor in plants, bacteria, invertebrates and vertebrates. Most physiologic reactions in living cells are stimulated by low doses of ionizing radiation. This evidence of radiogenic metabolism (metabolism promoted by ionizing radiation) includes enzyme induction, photosynthesis, respiration and growth. **Radiation hormesis in immunity decreases infection** and premature death in radiation exposed populations. **Increased immune competence is a major factor in the increased average lifespan of populations exposed to low-dose irradiation. I believe that this argues in favor of increased levels of RONS and O$_2$ excytomers.** During the past decade statistically significant evidence showed that **whole body exposures of humans to low-doses of ionizing radiation decreased total cancer mortality rates**. This is based on information compiled from **7 million person-years** of exposed and control workers in nuclear shipyard and atomic bomb plants in Canada, Great Britain and the United States. Other human experiences with unusual exposures confirm radiation hormesis in cancer mortality. A variety of external sources are beneficial. **Internal sources (plutonium, radium and radon) are also effective.** The conclusions have both personal and national significance. Ionizing radiation is a benign environmental agent at background levels. We live with a subclinical deficiency of ionizing radiation. Low-doses of ionizing radiation significantly decrease premature cancer death. Health benefits should replace risk and death as the guide for safe exposures to ionizing radiation. Safe supplementation with ionizing radiation would provide a new plateau of health.

It has been said that low dose irradiation could be used for "prevention" of cancer, infectious diseases and to increase the life span (J Nucl Med 2001; 42(9): 26N-37N).

49.5 HIGH DOSE RADIATION CAUSES CANCER

Some of the following materials were excerpted from "Low-dose ionizing radiation, human biology and non-linearity" by Myron Pollycove, M.D.

The best scientific evidence of human radiation effects initially came from epidemiologic studies of atomic bomb survivors in Hiroshima and Nagasaki. While no evidence of genetic effects has been found, these studies showed a roughly linear relationship between the induction of cancer and extremely high dose-rate single high doses of atomic bomb radiation. This was consistent with the knowledge that ionizing radiation can damage DNA in linear proportion to high-dose exposures and so produce gene mutations known to be associated with cancer. **In the absence of comparable low dose effects it was prudent to propose tentatively the no threshold hypothesis that extrapolates linearly from effects observed at very high doses to the same effects at very low doses.** It was accepted in 1959 by the International Commission on Radiological Protection (ICRP) and afterwards adopted by national radiation protection organizations to guide regulations for the protection of occupationally exposed workers and the public.

This hypothesis that all radiation is harmful in linear proportion to the dose, is the principle used for collective dose calculations of the number of deaths produced by any radiation, natural or generated, no matter how small. The National Council of Radiation Protection and Measurements Report 121, "Principles and Application of Collective Dose in Radiation Protection," summarizes the basis for adherence to linearity of radiation health effects.

There are exceptions to this general rule of no threshold, including the induction of bone tumors in both laboratory animals and in some human studies due to incorporated radio nuclides, where there is clearly evidence for an apparent threshold.

Genetic effects may result from a gene mutation, or a chromosome aberration. The activation of a dominant acting oncogene is frequently associated with leukemias and lymphomas, while the loss of suppressor genes appears to be more frequently associated with solid tumors. Please remember that a genetic defect may not necessarily be expressed phenotypically.

In the September issue of Radiology, 2004, it was reported **that people who pay for whole body radiation with X-ray scans in hopes of finding cancer at its earliest stages, may be raising their overall risk of cancer.** The radiation dose from a full-body CT scan is comparable to the doses received by some of the atomic-bomb survivors from Hiroshima and Nagasaki, where there is clear evidence of increases cancer risk. The dose from a single full-body CT scan is only slightly lower than the mean dose experienced by some atomic bomb survivors and is nearly 100 times that of a typical screening mammogram.

49.6 LOW DOSE RADIATION
DECREASES CANCER

For several decades increased longevity and decreased cancer mortality have been reported in populations exposed to high background radiation. Established radiation protection authorities consider such observations to be spurious or inconclusive because of unreliable public health data or undetermined confounding factors such as pollution of air, water and food, smoking, income, education, medical care, population density and other socioeconomic variables. Recently, however, **several epidemiologic statistically significant controlled studies have demonstrated that exposure to low or intermediate levels of radiation are associated with positive health effects**.

Dr. Zbigniew Jawarowski past chairman of UNSCEAR, in his current review of hormesis cites recent data showing hormetic effects in humans from the former Soviet Union (Jawarowski, Z. Beneficial radiation. Nukleonika 1995; 40: 3-12). After radiation exposure from a thermal explosion in 1957, 7852 persons living in 22 villages in the Eastern Urals were divided into three exposure groups averaging 49.6 cGy, 12.0 cGy and 4.0 cGy and followed for 30 years. **Tumor related mortality was 28%, 39% and 27% lower in the 49.6 cGy, 12.0 cGy and 4.0 cGy groups, respectively, than in the no irradiated control population in the same region**. In the 49.6 cGy and 12.0 cGy groups the difference from the controls was statistically significant. Epidemiologic studies showing beneficial effects of low doses of radiation in atomic bomb survivors and other populations were reviewed by Sohei Kondo, Professor of Radiation Biology, Atomic Energy Research Institute, Kinki University, Osaka, Japan. **Included are the apparently beneficial effects of low doses of external gamma rays on the lifespan of radium-dial painters and the significantly low mortality form cancers at all sites of residents of Misasa, an urban area with radon spas, than residents of the suburbs of Misas**a.

These beneficial effects are consistent with the findings of B.L. Cohen, Professor of Physics, University of Pittsburgh, that relate the incidence of lung cancer to radon exposure in nearly 90% of the population of the United States (Cohen, B.L. Test of the linear no-threshold theory of radiation carcinogenesis in the low dose, low dose rate region. Health Phys 1995; 68: 157-174). The 1601 counties selected for adequate permanence of residence provide extremely high-power statistical analysis. After applying the BEIR IV correction for variations in smoking frequency.

The thirteen year US Nuclear Shipyard Workers study of the health effects of low-dose radiation was performed by the Johns Hopkins Department of Epidemiology, School of Public Health and Hygiene, reported to the Department of Energy in 1991 (Matanoski, G.M. Health effects of low-level radiation in the shipyard workers final report. Report No. DOE DE-AC02-79 EV10095. Washington US Department of Energy, 1991) and reported in UNSCEAR 1994. Professor Arthur C. Upton, who concurrently chaired the NAS BEIR V Committee on "Health Effects to Low Levels of Ionizing Radiation," chaired the Technical Advisory Panel that advised on the research and reviewed the results.

The results of this study contradict the conclusions of the BEIR V report that small amounts of radiation have risk - the LNT hypothesis. From the database of almost **700,000 shipyard workers**, including 108,000 nuclear workers, three closely matched study groups were selected, consisting of 28,542 nuclear workers with working lifetime doses +/- 5 mSv (many received doses well in excess of 50 mSv), 10,462 nuclear workers with doses +/- 5 mSv and 33,352 non-nuclear workers. Deaths in each of the groups were classified as due to: all causes, leukemia, lymphatic and hematopoietic cancers, mesothelioma and lung cancer. **The results demonstrated a statistically**

significant decrease in the standardized mortality ratio for the two groups of nuclear workers for "death from all causes" compared with the non-nuclear workers. For the +/- 5 mSv group of nuclear workers, the highly significant risk decrement to 0.76 standard deviations below 1.00, of the standard mortality ratio for death from all causes is inconsistent with the LNT hypothesis and dose do not appear to be explainable by the healthy worker effect. "The non-nuclear workers and the nuclear workers were similarly selected for employment, were afforded the same health care thereafter, and performed the identical type of work, except for exposure to "Co gamma radiation, with a similar medial age of entry into employment of about 34 years. **This provides evidence with extremely high statistical power that low levels of ionizing radiation are associated with risk decrements (hormesis).**

Nevertheless, Professor Arthur C. Upton and others consider the three-country low-dose radiation and cancer study of Cardis, et al. (Cardis, E., et al. Effects of low doses and low dose rates of external ionizing radiation: Cancer mortality among nuclear industry workers in three countries. Radia Res 1995; 142: 117-132), to be the best occupational study of nuclear workers. This study concluded, "There was no evidence of an association between radiation dose and mortality from all causes or from all cancers.

The Canadian Breast Cancer Fluoroscopy Study (Miller, A.B., Howe, G.R., Sherman, G.J., Lindsay, J.P., Yaffe, M.J., Dinner, P.J., Risch, H.A. and Preston, D.L. Mortality from breast cancer after irradiation during fluoroscopic examination in patients being treated for tuberculosis. N Eng J Med 1989; 321: 1285-1289), reports the observations of the mortality from breast cancer in a cohort of **31,710** women who had been examined by multiple fluoroscopy between 1930 and 1952. **The observed data, however, demonstrate with high statistical confidence, a reduction of the relative risk of breast cancer to 0.66 (P=0.05) at 15 cGy and 0.85 (P=0.32) at 25 cGy.** The second author, in his 1996 revision of this study, removed this highly significant contradiction of the LNT hypothesis by lumping all low-dose data into a single 1-49 cGy category. **The study actually predicts that a dose of 15 cGy would be associated with 7000 fewer deaths in these million women.** Lauriston S. Taylor, past president of the NCRP, consider application of LNT theory for calculations of collective dose as, "Deeply immoral uses of our scientific heritage."

49.7 METABOLIC AND RADIATION DNA DAMAGE CONTROL

During the past decade rapid advances in our knowledge of molecular biology and cell function enable us to understand why low-dose radiation is associated with positive health effects in contrast to the carcinogenic effect of high-dose radiation. Our understanding is based upon current, cellular molecular biology observations. Estimates are based on published data and recent personal communications.

- Two to three percent of all metabolized oxygen is converted to free radicals (reactive oxygen species (Sohal, R.S. and Weindruch, R. Oxidative stress, caloric restriction and aging. Science 1996; 273: 59-63), **10^{10} /cell/d, that produce about 10^6 DNA oxidative adducts/cell/d. These include about 0.5 double strand breaks/cell/d** (Pollycove, M. and Feinendegen, L. Quantification of human total and mis/ unrepaired DNA alterations: Intrinsic and radiation induced. Unpublished data). In addition, a relatively small number of metabolic DNA alterations are produced by DNA replication and thermal instability. **By comparison, 1 cGy low LET radiation produces 20 DNA oxidative adducts/cell that include an average of 0.4 double strand breaks/cell.**

- Over eons of time, as multicellular animals developed and metabolized **oxygen,** a complex DNA damage-control biosystems evolved. **The damage corresponding to 10^{10} free radicals/cell/day is largely prevented by antioxidants that scavenge approximately 99% of these free radicals. RMH Note**: All of the numbers referring DNA alterations/damages are estimations and do not necessarily agree with other estimates. Suffice it to say that exponential numbers of DNA oxidative alterations/ damages occur daily. The resultant ~10^6 DNA oxidative adducts/cell/d are reduced by enzymatic repair to about 10^2 mis/unrepaired DNA alterations/cell/d. apoptosis, differentiation, necrosis and the immune system remove approximately 99% of these mis/unrepaired DNA alterations so that an average of ~1 mutation/cell/d (possibly 2-3) accumulates during the lifetime of a stem cell to decrease DNA damage-control capability with associated aging and malignant growth. This remarkably efficient biosystem prevents precocious aging and malignancy unless impaired by genetic defects or damaged by high doses of radiation or other toxic agents. I have already advised you that this is not necessarily true.

- How much does background radiation add to the metabolic accumulation of mutations? **A much larger fraction of double strand breaks occurs in DNA oxidative adducts produced by radiation than in those produced by metabolism (2×10^{-2} vs. 5×10^{-7}).** The mis/unrepaired fraction of these double strand breaks is also much larger than that of other metabolic DNA oxidative adducts (~10^{-1} vs. 10^{-4}). Nevertheless, **the number of metabolic DNA oxidative adducts (~10^6/cell/d) is so much greater than the number of oxidative adducts from low LET background of 0.1 cSv/y (5×10^{-3}/cell/d), that an average of only ~10^{-7} radiation mutation/cell/d is added to ~1 metabolic mutation/ cell/d.**

49.8 RESPONSE TO LOW-DOSE RADIATION

The activity of DNA damage control biosystems is decreased by high-dose radiation, but adaptively responds with increased activity to low-dose radiation (e.g., <30 cGy) (Feinendegen, L.E., Loken, M.K., Booz, J., Muhlensiepen, H., Sondhaus, C.A. and Bond, V.P. Cellular mechanisms of protection and repair induced by radiation exposure and their consequences for cell system responses. Stem Cells 1995; 13(1): 7-20), (Feindendegen, L.E., Sondhaus, C.A., Bond, V.P. and Muhlensiepen, H. Radiation effects induced by low doses in complex tissue and their relation to cellular adaptive responses. Mutation Res 1996; 199-205), (Yamaoka, K. Increased SOD activities and decreased lipid peroxide in rat organs induced by low X-radiation. Free Rad Bio Med 1991; 11: 3-7), (Duke, R.C., Ojcius, D.M. and Young, J.D-E. Cell suicide in health and disease. Sci Am 1996; Dec 80-87).

The efficiency of this biosystem is increased by the adaptive responses to low-dose ionizing radiation. This is well documented in UNSCEAR, 1994: (United Nations Scientific Committee on the effects of Atomic Radiation. Sources and Effects of Ionizing Radiation. UNSCEAR 1994 Report to the General Assembly, with Scientific Annexes. New York, 1994; Annex B. Adaptive Response to Radiation in Cells and Organisms. 185-272).

"There is substantial evidence that the number of radiation-induced chromosomal aberrations and mutations can be reduced by a small prior conditioning dose in proliferating mammalian cells in vitro and in vivo.

"There is increasing evidence that cellular repair mechanisms are stimulated after radiation-induced damage...Whatever the mechanisms, they seem able to act not only on the lesions induced by ionizing radiation but also on at least a portion of the lesions induced by some other toxic agents.

"As to the biological plausibility of a radiation-induced adaptive response, it is recognized that the effectiveness of **DNA repair in mammalian cells is not absolute**...An important question, therefore, is to judge the balance between stimulated cellular repair and residual damage."

This statement applies not only to the mutations produced by radiation and other toxic agents, but also to the unmentioned enormous number of daily metabolic mutations. The operative effect of reducing metabolic mutations by the adaptive response of the damage-control biosystems to low-dose radiation is the critical factor, not reduction of the relatively negligible number of mutations produced by low-dose radiation.

Assuming a 20% increased efficiency of biosystems control in response to a ten-fold increase of annual background radiation from 0.1 cGy/y to 1 cGy/y, radiation mutations would indeed increase from 1×10^{-7}/cell/d to 8×10^{-7}/cell/d but metabolic mutations would decrease from ~1/cell/d to ~0.8/cell/d. "The balance between stimulated cellular repair and residual damage" is a decrease of mutations for an average of ~1 mutation/cell/d to ~0.8 mutation/cell/d."

UNSCEAR did not consider that the increase of radiation mutations is negligible compared to the operative effect of the adaptive response to low-dose radiation upon the high-background of metabolic mutations. **The biologic effect of radiation is not determined by the number of DNA mutations it creates, but by its effect on the biosystems that controls the relentless enormous burden of oxidative DNA damage**. High-dose radiation impairs this biosystems with consequent significant increase of metabolic mutations and corresponding risk **increments Low-dose radiation stimulates the DNA damage-control biosystems with consequent significant decrease of metabolic mutations and corresponding risk decrements.**

U.T.O.P.I.A.

This reduction of gene mutations in response to low-dose radiation provides a biological explanation of the statistically significant observations of mortality and cancer mortality risk decrements, and contradicts the biophysical understanding of the basic mechanisms upon which, ultimately, the NCRP's confidence in the LNT hypothesis is based.

49.9 CONCLUSION

I have included the data on low dose ratio hormesis for two reasons. First, I feel that there is a strong connection between low dose radiation exposure and the generation of RONS and excited states. We know that this is one of the major effects of ionizing radiation from countless past studies. Secondarily, I feel that this information and concept should be brought to the attention of more medical scientists.

My **Unified Theory** would predict that low dose radiation would generate more RONS/ excytomers, which would decrease cancer growths, decrease infections and increase the life span.   In fact, these are the things that radiation hormesis accomplishes. This is in direct contradistinction to the **Free Radi-Crap theory of aging and oxidative stress.**

50 OPINIONS OPPOSING THE HOWES SINGLET OXYGEN DELIVERY SYSTEM

To maintain intellectual integrity, I must present a summary of the literature which would oppose the therapeutic use of the Howes Singlet Oxygen Delivery system.

ARGUMENTS AGAINST USE OF EITHER HYDOGEN PEROXIDE OR SODIUM HYPOCHLORITE FOR TUMOR OR CANCER THERAPY

The American Cancer Society and the British Columbia Cancer Society have clearly stated their opposing positions, and the dangers, to hydrogen peroxide therapy and/or oxygen therapy. The opinions of tens of thousands of physicians and medical scientists of North America, which includes British Columbia, Canada and the United States of America, are summarized by excerpts from their publications as follows:

1. The British Columbia Cancer Agency and the American Cancer Society provide information on their website www.bccancer.bc.ca and www.cancer.org regarding hydrogen peroxide and its use in treatment as follows:

The "Summary" and "Professional Evaluation/Critique" sections of this Unconventional manual are cited directly from the medical literature, and are intended to help in the objective evaluation of alternative/complementary therapies.

Summary
"After studying the literature and other available information, the American Cancer Society has found no evidence that treatment with hydrogen peroxide or other 'hyperoxgenating' compounds is safe or results in objective benefit   in the treatment of cancer. Lacking such evidence, the American Cancer Society strongly urges individuals with cancer not to seek such treatment." (CA)

"Patients with cancer should not consider oxygen therapies as either alternative (first-line) or adjunct (complementary) therapies." (Cassileth)

"Oxygen therapy can destroy cells, including those of the blood-forming organs. Very high does can seriously damage health or even cause death." (Ontario)

Description/Source/Components

"Hydrogen peroxide is unstable and decomposes violently when in direct contact with tough surfaces or traces of organic or particulate matter. **Light, agitation, heating, or chemical substances like carbonates, proteins, chlorides, charcoal, and iron all accelerate the rate of hydrogen peroxide decomposition in solution.** One volume of 30% hydrogen peroxide solution will yield 100 volumes of oxygen gas when it decomposes." (Green)

50.1 PROFESSIONAL EVALUATION/CRITIQUE

"Hydrogen peroxide does participate in the bactericidal processes within activated phagocytic cells. But when it escapes from the cells into the adjacent extracellular space during the inflammatory process, it becomes a major contributor to the tissue damage seen in lung disease, malignancies, and hemolysis. The presence of pharmacological concentrations of hydrogen peroxide in the blood is clearly a double-edged sword which can easily cause as much harm as it can cause good." (Green)

"In 1988, the U.S. Postal Service issued Donsbach a cease and desist order to stop him from claiming that the hydrogen peroxide used orally or intravenously is effective against cancer or arthritis, or that it is fit for human consumption." (U.S. Congress)

"Researchers now understand that cancer cells' lower-than-normal respiration is due to the fact that tissue surrounding cancer cells receives less oxygen because it has fewer blood vessels feeding it. Oxygen therapies have not been found useful against cancer and are not used as mainstream cancer treatments." (Cassileth)

50.2 TOXICITY/RISKS

"A continuous infusion of peroxide that results in 0.01 volume per 100 ml blood can cause an arterial gas embolism [sudden blocking of an artery] and irreversible lung damage. That such adverse reactions do occur is clear from reports in the medical literature. These incidents include: oxygen gas emboli, necrosis [the sum of the morphological changes indicative of cell death], and gangrene following peroxide enemas or colonic lavage [washing out of the colon]; emphysema [accumulation of air in tissue or organs] following peroxide mouthwash or gargle; and ulcerative colitis [inflammation of the colon], gas embolism, and emphysema following deep wound irrigation. Peroxide ingestion results in respiratory arrest, seizures, gas embolism in the portal circulation, shock, and acute hemolysis [disruption of red blood cell membrane cause release of hemoglobin]. Stroke and multiple cerebral infarcts and venous embolism follow irrigation of anal fistula [one opening on the cutaneous surface of the anus] and irrigation of surgical wounds." (Green)

"Promoters of hydrogen peroxide tend to downplay its potential for harm….in fact, however, during the past three years, six children have been seriously poisoned and one died as a result of accidentally during the concentrated solution stored in their refrigerator. The product in the fatal case had been obtained by mail order as an alternative medicine. A near-fatal case of ingestion by an adult also has been reported." (CA)

"The present study clearly demonstrates that H_2O_2 acts as a carcinogen. Reactive oxygen intermediates have been reported to induce single-strand breaks in cellular DNA, oxidation of DNA bases, chromosomal aberrations, and DNA-protein cross-links." (Okamoto)

Hydrogen peroxide injections can have dangerous side effects. High blood levels of hydrogen peroxide create oxygen bubbles that can block blood flow and cause gangrene and death. Acute hemolytic crisis [destruction of blood cells] has also been reported following intravenous injection of hydrogen peroxide,. Women who are pregnant or breast-feeding should not use this method. (ACS)

In short, the American Cancer Society position on hydrogen peroxide, which it recommends to all physicians and patients, stated it best when they said:

"There is currently no scientific evidence that hydrogen peroxide therapy is effective for treating any of the conditions that have been claimed (which includes cancer and tumors)."

The medical establishment considers hydrogen peroxide therapy and/or oxygen therapy as non-therapeutic, illegal and possibly criminal.

References

American Cancer Society (1998). "Hydrogen Peroxide Treatment."
http://www.cancer.org/alt_therapy/hydrogenPeroxide.html
CA (Anonymous). "Questionable methods of cancer management hydrogen peroxide and other 'hyper oxygenation' therapies." CA: a Cancer Journal for Clinicians 1993 43:47-56.
Cassileth, B.R. Alternative medicine handbook: a complete reference guide to alternative and complementary therapies. New York. W.W. Norton & Co., 1998. 194-196.

Green, S. Oxygenation therapy: unproven treatments for cancer and AIDS. Sci Rev Alt Med 1998 1:6-12.

Okamoto M. et al. Transformation in vitro of a nontumorigenic rate urothelial cell line by hydrogen peroxide. Cancer Research 1996 56:4649-4653.

Ontario Breast Cancer Information Exchange Project. Guide to unconventional cancer therapies. 1st ed. Toronto: Ontario Breast Cancer Information Exchange Project, 1994 242-247.

U.S. Congress, Office of Technology Assessment. Unconventional cancer treatments. Washington, D.C.: U.S. Government Printing Office 1990 Sept:114

50.3 SELECTIVE REVIEW OF THE SCIENTIFIC LITERATURE OPPOSING THE USE OF HYDROGEN PEROXIDE

The following information was obtained from the **Chemical Summary for Hydrogen Peroxide,** CAS No. 7722-84-1, July 1995, 10 pages. At website http://circa.ornl.gov/documents/HydrogePeroixide.pdf. This summary is based on information retrieved from a systematic search limited to secondary sources (see appendix A). These sources include online databases, unpublished EPA information, government publications, review documents, and standard reference materials. No attempt has been made to verify information in these databases and secondary sources.

50.3.1 Acute Toxicity

Ingestion of large amounts of hydrogen peroxide causes chest and stomach pain, loss of consciousness, and motor disorders in humans and has caused mortality in experimental animals. Inhalation of high concentrations of vapor or mist causes irritation of nose and throat in humans. In appropriate solution, hydrogen peroxide is used in topical and dental gels.

1. <u>Humans</u> - In five persons who accidentally drank about 50 mL of a 33% hydrogen peroxide solution, symptoms included stomach and chest pain, retention of breath, foaming at the mouth, and loss of consciousness. Later, motor and sensory disorders, fever, microhemorrhages and moderate leucocytosis were noted. All recovered completely within 2-3 weeks (IARC 1985).

Inhalation of high concentrations of hydrogen peroxide vapor or mist may cause extreme irritation and inflammation of the nose and throat (ACGIH 1991).

Cases of rupture of the colon, inflammation of the anus or rectum, and ulcerative colitis have been reported following hydrogen peroxide enemas (IARC 1985).

A characteristic whitening of the skin occurs after topical application of hydrogen peroxide (1-30%), which is believed the result of avascularity of the skin produced by oxygen bubbles acting microembolically in the capillaries (IARC 1985).

Hydrogen peroxide as a topical gel is used to cleanse minor wounds or minor gum inflammation (HSDB 1995). Hydrogen peroxide concentrate is caustic and should not be tasted undiluted (HSDB 1995).

2. <u>Animals</u> - The intravenous LD50 of hydrogen peroxide in rats was reported to be 21 mg/kg (IARC 1985). The following percutaneous LD50s have been determined: rabbit, 630 mg/kg, rat, 700 to >7500 mg/kg (IARC 1985).

Rats receiving 2.5% hydrogen peroxide (equivalent to approximately 3.5 g/kg/da) in their drinking water died within 43 days (IARC 1985). (Further experimental details not supplied).

50.3.2 Subchronic/Chronic Effects

In experimental animals oral administration of hydrogen peroxide causes dental, liver, kidney, stomach and intestinal damage. Inhalation exposure of hydrogen peroxide caused skin irritation and sneezing in dogs, and high mortality in mice.

Animals - Dose-related growth retardation, induction of dental caries and pathological changes in the periodontium were observed in young male rats receiving 1.5% hydrogen peroxide as their drinking fluid (equivalent to approximately 2.1 g/kg/day) for 8 weeks (IARC 1985).

Effects observed in mice treated for 35 weeks with 0.15% hydrogen peroxide as their drinking fluid (equivalent to approximately 0.29 g/kg/day) included degeneration of hepatic and renal tubular epithelial tissues, necrosis, inflammation, irregularities of tissue structure of the stomach wall, and hypertrophy of the small intestine wall. Concentrations in excess of 1% (equivalent to approximately 1.9 g/kg/day) resulted in pronounced weight loss and death within two weeks (IARC 1985). In a sequential study of mice treated with 0.4% hydrogen peroxide in drinking water (equivalent to approximately 0.76 g/kg/day), gastric erosion was observed at 30 days and was present consistently throughout the 108 week study period (IARC 1985).

Dogs exposed 6 hours/day, 5 days/week for 6 months at an average vapor concentration of 7 ppm (9.73 mg/m3) of 90% hydrogen peroxide, developed skin irritation, sneezing, lacrimation, and bleaching of the hair. Autopsy disclosed pulmonary irritation and greatly thickened skin, but no hair follicle destruction. No significant changes in blood or urinary parameters were observed (ACGIH 1991).

Following eight 6-hour exposures to hydrogen peroxide at a concentration of 79 mg/m3 (56.88 ppm), 7/9 mice died (U.S. EPA 1988). Following exposure to hydrogen peroxide at 93 mg/m3, 6 hours/day, 5 days/week for 30 exposures , 1/10 rats died (U.S. EPA 1988).

50.3.3 Carcinogenicity

IARC has assigned an overall carcinogen city rating of 3 to hydrogen peroxide: no data in humans, limited data in laboratory animals. Gastric and duodenal lesions including adenomas, carcinomas, and adenocarcinomas have been observed in mice treated orally with hydrogen peroxide. Marked strain differences in the incidence of tumors have been observed. Papilloma development has been observed in mice treated by dermal application.

Animals - IARC has assigned an overall carcinogen city rating of 3 to hydrogen peroxide: limited data in laboratory animas (IARC 1987).

Groups of 98, 101, and 99 C57BL/6J mice of both sexes were given 0, 0.1, and 0.4% hydrogen peroxide (a solution of 30% for food additive use) in distilled water (approximately 60-250 mg/kg/day) as drinking water for 100 weeks. Tumors observed were as follows: control, 1 duodenal adenoma, 0.1%, 6 adenomas, 1 carcinoma of the duodenum; 0.4%, 2 adenomas, 5 carcinomas of the duodenum (p <0.05). Survival data were not given (IARC 1985).

Another group of 138 male and female C57BL/6N mice were treated with 0.4% hydrogen peroxide (a solution of 30% for food additive use) in distilled water (approximately 250 mg/kg/day) as drinking water, for up to 700 days with intermediate sequential groups sacrificed. 'Nodules' (hyperplastic lesions, adenomas and carcinomas) were found in the duodenum and stomach from 90 days until the end of the experiment. The lesions did not appear to increase in frequency over time, but atypical hyperplasia appeared late and 5% of the animals developed duodenal adenocarcinoma. No such lesions appeared in the controls (IARC 1985).

In other experiments, marked strain differences were observed in the development of gastric and duodenal 'nodules' in mice treated with 0.4% hydrogen peroxide (a solution of 30% for food additive use) in distilled water (approximately 250 mg/kg/day) as drinking water for 90 to 210 days (IARC 1985).

There was an inverse relationship between the incidence of duodenal 'nodules' (hyperplastic lesions, adenomas, carcinomas) and level of duodenal mucosal catalase activity in mice treated for 210 days with 0.4% hydrogen peroxide (approximately 250 mg/kg/day) in drinking water. Strains tested were: C3H/HeN, B6C3Fl, C57BL/6N and C3H/C b/s, with the following catalase activities: 5.3, 1.7, 0.7, and 0.4×10^{-4} k/mg protein, respectively. 'Nodule' incidences were 2/18, 7/22, 21/21, and 22/24 (IARC 1985).

Mice received twice weekly topical applications of 30% hydrogen peroxide diluted 1:1 in 0.2 mL acetone for 25 weeks; 3/57 had papillomas at that time. No squamous-cell carcinoma was found when animals were observed up to 50 weeks (IARC 1985).

CITED REFERENCES

IARC. 1985. International Agency for Research on Cancer. Hydrogen Peroxide. In: IARC Monographs on the Evaluation of Carcinogenic Risk of Chemicals to Humans: Allyl Compounds, Aldehydes, Epoxides and Peroxides, vol. 36. IARC, Lyon, pp. 285-314.

ACGIH. 1991. American Conference for governmental Industrial Hygienists, Inc. TLVs®. Documentation of the Threshold Limit Values and Biological Exposure Indices, 6th ed. ACGIH, Cincinnati, OH., p 782-783.

HSDB. 1995. Hazardous Substances Data Bank. MEDLARS Online Information Retrieval System, National Library of Medicine.

U.S. EPA. 1988. U.S. Environmental Protection Agency. Reportable Quantity Document for Hydrogen Peroxide. Office of Solid Waste and Emergency Response, Environmental Criteria and Assessment Office, U.S. EPA, Cincinnati, OH., 9 p.

IARC . 1987. International Agency for Research on Cancer. IARC Monographs on the Evaluation of Carcinogenic Risk of Chemicals to Man. Overall evaluations of carcinogenicity. An updating of Vols. 1 to 42. IARC, Lyon, p. 64.

50.3.4 Discussion

Oxygen has many reactive oxidizing forms, which are collectively referred to as reactive oxidative and nitrative species (RONS). However, they are also referred to by a wide variety of other names, such as: reactive oxygen metabolites, reactive oxygen intermediates, active oxygen species, reactive oxidizing species, etc. RONS is a term which includes all highly reactive, oxygen-containing molecules, including free radicals. The most prominent of the ROS are the superoxide anion radical (O_2^-), singlet oxygen ($^1O^*_2$), hydrogen peroxide (H_2O_2), hypochlorous acid (HOCl), nitric oxide (NO.), the peroxyl radical (ROO.), the hydroxyl radical (OH.), ozone (O_3), the alkoxyl radical (RO.) and the peroxynitrite radical (ONOO-). **These RONS are reported to play major causation roles in up to 100 human disease states,** including aging, cancer, dementia, arteriosclerosis, diabetes, arthritis, inflammation, ischemia-reperfusion injury and oxidative stress (Gutteridge, J. M. C. Free radicals in disease processes: A compilation of causes and consequences. Free Radical Res Commun 1993; 19: 141). The RONS are produced under physiological and pathophysiological conditions by what are considered pathobiochemical mechanisms. RONS and free radicals have been receiving scientific attention for decades and are increasingly attracting general public interest, which is best illustrated by a quote from an April 6, 1992 Time magazine article as follows:

"Free radicals are cellular renegades; they wreak havoc by damaging DNA, altering biochemical compounds, corroding cell membranes and killing cells outright. Such molecular mayhem, scientists increasingly believe, plays a major role in the developments of ailments like cancer, heart or lung disease and cataracts. Many researchers are convinced that the cumulative effects of free radicals also underlie the gradual deterioration that is the hallmark of aging in all individuals, healthy as well as sick."

This quote aptly illustrates the scientific and medical mindset of the time, which would have considered introduction of free radicals or RONS into tissue as clinical heresy. This attitude has persisted up to the present time throughout the scientific community. Additional RONS induced dysfunctions and/or diseases include cardiomyopathy, diabetes mellitus, porphyria, halogenated liver injury, adriamycin cardiotoxicity, segmental progeria disorders, cataractogenesis and multiple sclerosis (Halliwell, B., Gutteridge, J.M.C., Cross, C.E. Free radicals, antioxidants and human disease: Where are we now. J Lab Clin Med 1992; 119: 598-620). RONS are physiologically manufactured for the purpose of killing invading microorganisms, but they also inflict damage on nearby tissues, and are thought to be of pathogenic significance in a large number of diseases including, emphysema, acute respiratory syndrome, atherosclerosis, reperfusion injury, malignancy and rheumatoid arthritis. (Babior, B.M. Phagocytes and Oxidative Stress. Am J Med 2000; 109: 33-44). In short, free radical oxidative damage has been implicated in almost every major chronic disease.

In 1956, Denham Harman introduced the theoretical concept of oxidative stress, which has prevailed up to the present time, in which RONS total levels within a cell or organism exceeds the anti-oxidative capability of that cell or organism (Harman D. Aging: A theory based on free radical and radiation chemistry. J Gerontol 1956; 11: 298-300).

The introduction of exogenous sources of any of the RONS agents through inhalation, intravenous infusion or by direct tissue injection with reagents such as hydrogen peroxide or hypochlorous acid would have been considered to be harmful at the tissue sites closest to their introduction, with concomitant collateral damage to the area and to the overall health of the organism. Additionally, **it would have been even more deleterious to combine hydrogen peroxide and hypochlorous acid, which would have generated an even more harmful third RONS, namely, the highly reactive electronically excited singlet molecular oxygen ($^1O_2$).** Additionally, RONS, such as singlet oxygen, have very short half-lives and tend to react with the first molecule in their path such as fat (lipid), protein, DNA or sugar moieties. Attack by hydrogen peroxide, related to many disease states, has led to the identification of irreversibly damaged cellular components, including lipid-derived malondealdehyde, carbonyl group-containing proteins, 4-hydroxynonal-conjugated protein and 8-hydroxy-2'-deoxyguanosine derived from DNA (Teixeira, A. J., Ferreira, M.R., van Dijk, W.J., van de Werken, G. and de Jong., A.P. Analysis of 8-hydroxy-2'-deoxyguanosine in rat urine and liver DNA by stable isotope dilution gas chromatography/mass spectrometry. Anal Biochem 1995; 226: 307-319). Chain reactions can follow interactions between singlet oxygen with lipids and reactions with DNA can induce mutagenic changes. Superoxide and hydrogen peroxide, in the presence of ferrous or cuprous ion [the Fenton reaction, (Stadtman, E. R. Protein oxidation and aging. Science 1992; 257: 1220-1224)], both produce the highly reactive hydroxyl radical (OH.), which causes a multiplicity of modifications in DNA. Oxidative assault by (OH.) radical on the deoxyribose moiety will lead to the release of free bases from DNA, thus generating strand breaks with various sugar modifications and simple abasic (AP) sites. RONS produced AP sites are major DNA damage components in which DNA bases are lost. Additionally, it has been estimated that endogenous RONS-DNA interactions can result in about 200,000 base lesions per cell per day. Thus, **it would have been considered extremely deleterious, dangerous, and destructive to add additional RONS agents to living cells or systems, which would have increased their levels of oxidative stress.** In fact, the scientific and lay literature was, and still is, replete with articles pushing the wondrous benefits of daily consumption of multitudes of antioxidant agents and concoctions. Furthermore, because the mitochondrion is the primary site for the cell's oxidative metabolism and RONS production, mitochondria molecules (e.g., DNA, lipids, and proteins) are said to sustain the most free radical damage and is associated with several degenerative diseases including Parkinson's, Alzheimer's and Huntington's diseases. Human cancer cells over produce hydrogen peroxide (Szatrowski, T., and Nathan, C. Production of large amounts of hydrogen peroxide by human tumor cells. Cancer Res 1991; 51: 794-798). This observation may be causally linked to the cancer phenotype, in that low levels of hydrogen peroxide and superoxide stimulate cell growth (Burdon, R. Superoxide and hydrogen peroxide in relation to mammalian cell proliferation. Free Radic Biol Med 1995; 18: 775-794). **Again, scientific thinking was, and still is, that hydrogen peroxide is mutagenic and administration of additional quantities would have been, and are, contraindicated.** Investigators even raised cautions about the ingestion of commonplace hydrogen peroxide-containing substances, such as coffee, saying that coffee owes its direct mutagenicity to H_2O_2 formation (Stadler R.H., Turesky R.J., Muller, O., Markovic, J. and Leong-Morgenthaler, P.M. The inhibitory effects of coffee on radical-mediated oxidation and mutagenicity. Mutat Res 1994; 308(2): 177-190).

Pathological conditions such as hypercholesterolemia, atherosclerosis, hypertension, smoking and diabetes are associated with increased oxidative stress. Research evidence suggests that RONS can increase eNOS (endothelial nitric oxide synthase) expression and hydrogen peroxide is the mediator of the eNOS up-regulation (Lopez-Ongil, S., Hernandez-Perera, O., Navarro-Antolin, J., Perez de Lema, G., Rodriguez-Puyol, M., Lamas, S. and Rodrigueq-Puyol, D. Role of reactive oxygen species in the signaling cascade of cyclosporine a-mediated up-regulation of enos in vascular endothelial cells. Br J Pharmacol 1998; 124: 447-454), (Drummond, G. R., Cai, H., Davis, M.E., Ramasamy, S. and Harrison, D.G. Transcriptional and posttranscriptional regulation of endothelial nitric oxide synthase expression by hydrogen peroxide. Circ Res 2000; 86: 347-354). Hydrogen peroxide induces eNOS transcription by likely involving CaM kinas II and janus kinase 2 (Cai, H., Davis, M.E., Drummond, G.R. and Harrison, D.G. Induction of endothelial no synthase by hydrogen peroxide via a ca(2+)/calmodulin-dependent protein kinase ii/janus kinase 2-dependent pathway. Arterioscler Thromb Vasc Biol 2001; 21: 1571-1576). **Again, RONS, and more specifically hydrogen peroxide has been directly linked to the above pathological conditions, including aging, which would further contraindicate exogenous additions of peroxide to cells or organisms** (Halliwell, B. and Gutteridge, J.M. Role of free radicals and catalytic metal ions in human disease: An overview. Method Enzymol 1990; 186: 1-85).

The electron transport chain of mitochondria causes the univalent reduction of molecular oxygen to the superoxide anion radical (O_2^{-}), which can then enzymatically or spontaneously dismutate to hydrogen peroxide (H_2O_2) (Stadtman, E. R. Protein oxidation and aging. Science 1992; 257: 1220-1224). Hydrogen peroxide can also be generated by arachidonic acid metabolizing enzymes, xanthine oxidase, nitric oxide synthase, cytochrome P450 and in response to ultraviolet radiation. Further, hydrogen peroxide can be produced by a variety of extracellular stimuli including cytokines, neurotransmitters, peptide growth factors, hormones, and phorbol myristate acetate (PMA) (Krieger-Brauer, H. I. and Kather, H. The stimulus-sensitive H_2O_2-generating system present in human fat-cell plasma membranes is multireceptor-linked and under antagonistic control by hormones and cytokines. Biochem J 1995; 307: 1079-1088). **Over all, hydrogen peroxide has been, and still is, considered to be a dangerous molecule, as it relates to crucial intracellular functions** (Sahu, S. C. Oncogenes, oncogenesis, and oxygen radicals. Biomed Environ Sci 1990; 3: 183-201).

RONS and hydrogen peroxide have been implicated as causative agents in lung injury such as Acute Respiratory Distress Syndrome (ARDS) (alveolar damage), asthma (airway epithelial damage), chronic obstructive pulmonary disease COPD), and interstitial pulmonary fibrosis (Cross, C. E., van der Vliet, A., O'Neill, C.A. and Eiserich, J.P. Reactive oxygen species and the lung. Lancet 1994; 344: 930-933), (Jobsis, Q., Raatgeep, H.C., Hermans, P.W. and de Jongste, J.C. Hydrogen peroxide in exhaled air is increased in stable asthmatic children. Eur respir J 1997; 10: 519-521), (Worlitzsch, D., Herberth, G., Ulrich M. and Doring, G. Catalase, myeloperoxidase and hydrogen peroxide in cystic fibrosis. Eur Respir J 1998; 11: 377-383).

Apoptosis or programmed cell death is an orderly sequence in which cells destroy themselves or "commit suicide." RONS agents have been shown to induce apoptosis via different pathways and is initiated at "death receptors" that are members of the TNF-receptor (TNFR) family in the plasma membrane. Hydrogen peroxide-induced apoptosis appears to involve membrane death receptors by the induction of new protein expression and the Fas pathway (Yamakawa, H., Ito, Y., Naganawa, T., Banno, Y., Nakashima, S., Yoshimura, S., Sawada, M., Nishimura, Y., Nozawa, Y. and Sakai, N. Activation of caspase-9 and -3 during H2O2-induced apoptosis of PC12 cells independent of ceramide formation. Neurol Res 2000; 22: 556-564). Furthermore, it has been found that H_2O_2 inhibits the ability of 4 different chemotherapy drugs (VP-16, doxorubicin, cisplatin, and AraC) to induce apoptosis in human Burkitt lymphoma cells. H_2O_2 shifts the form of cell death from apoptosis to pyknosis/necrosis, which occurs after a significant delay compared with chemotherapy-induced apoptosis (Shacter, E., Williams, J.A., Hinson, R.M., Senturker S. and Lee Y.J. Oxidative stress interferes with cancer chemotherapy; inhibition of lymphoma cell apoptosis and phagocytosis. Blood 2000; 96(1): 307-313).

Another form of biological damage directly caused by hydrogen peroxide, and not O_2^{-} or OH., is with the lens of the eye in organ culture (Zigler, J.S., Jernigan, H.M., Jr., Garland, D. and Reddy, V.N. The effects of "oxygen radicals" generated in the medium on lenses in organ culture: inhibition of damage by chelated iron. Arch. Biochem. Biophys 1985; 241: 163-172). Additionally, studies have shown that human urothelial cells can be transformed to low grade neoplastic cells by H_2O_2 and suggest that H_2O_2 may be involved in the development of bladder cancer (Tamatani T., Hattori K., Nakashiro K., Hayashi, Y., Wu, S., Klumpp, D., Reddy, J.K. and Oyasu, R. Neoplastic conversion of human urothelial cells in vitro by overexpression of H_2O_2-generating peroxisomal fatty acyl CoA oxidase.

Int J Oncol 1999; 15(4): 743-749). Addition of hydrogen peroxide to cells in culture can lead to transition metal ion dependent radical mediated oxidative DNA damage. Hydrogen peroxide has even been found to activate HIV production. Investigators reported that H_2O_2 reacts with vanadate, which produces peroxides that have potent biological effects including the activation of the long terminal repeat (LTR) of human immunodeficiency virus type I (HIV-I) (Kazazi, F., Koehler, J.K. and Klebanoff, S.J. Activation of the HIV long terminal repeat and viral production by H_2O_2-vanadate. Free Radic Biol Med 1996; 20(6): 813-820).

50.3.5 Summary

RMH Note: Summarizing the effects of hydrogen peroxide on cells and organisms, for over half a century, H_2O_2 has been incorrectly and causally implicated in about 100 human disease conditions, which has been widely written about and discussed in the scientific, medical and lay literature. The alleged dangers of hydrogen peroxide have been, and are, well known.

The dangers of hydrogen peroxide are of such dire consequences that humans are well endowed with multiple lines of defense against H_2O_2 and RONS. Enzymes that rapidly break down hydrogen peroxide, such as catalase and glutathione peroxidase, are present in all cells and tissues. Furthermore, normal human serum contains high protective levels of catalase (Leff, J.A., Oppegard, M.A., Terada, L.S., McCarty, E.C. and Repine, J.E. Human serum catalase decreases endothelial cell injury from hydrogen peroxide. J Appl Physiol 1991; 71: 1903-1906). Hydrogen peroxide is widely regarded as a cytotoxic agent such that its levels must be minimized by the action of antioxidant defense enzymes. Thus, since cells have high levels of catalase and peroxidase, which act to immediately break down H_2O_2, it would seem unwise to attempt to accurately and quantitatively add exogenous hydrogen peroxide to serum, cells or tissue.

It is widely accepted that oxidants, such as RONS, derived from activated neutrophils and from endothelial cells can increase the permeability of endothelial monolayers in vivo and in vitro. Among these oxidants, H_2O_2 is thought to be perhaps the most important in microvascular injury, since changes in endothelial permeability often occur as a result of H_2O_2 exposure (Berman, R.S. and Martin, W. Arterial endothelial barrier dysfunction: actions of homocysteine and the hypoxanthine-xanthine oxidase free radical generating system. Br J Pharmacol 1993; 108: 920-926). The increased permeability produced by H_2O_2 is thought to require second messenger activation, e.g., increase cell calcium (Doan, T.N., Gentry, D.L., Taylor, A.A. and Elliott, S.J. Hydrogen peroxide activates agonist-sensitive Ca2+-flux pathways in canine venous endothelial cells. Biochem J 1994; 287: 209-215), and protein kinase C activity (Siflinger-Birnboim, A., Lum, H., Del Vecchio, P.J. and Malik, A.B. Involvement of Ca2+ in the peroxide-induced increase in endothelial permeability. Am J Physiol 1996; 270(14): L973-L978). H_2O_2 is also directly toxic to endothelial cells (Martin, W.J., II. Neutrophils kill pulmonary endothelial cells by a hydrogen-peroxide-dependent pathway: An in vitro model of neutrophil-mediated lung injury. Am Rev Respir Dis 1984; 130: 209-213), inhibits anion transport (Hinshaw, D.B., Burger, J.M., Delius, R.E., Hystop, P.A. and Omann, G.M. Inhibition of organic anion transport in endothelial cells by hydrogen peroxide. Arch Biochem Biophys 1992; 298: 464-470), simulates sodium-potassium pump activity (Meharg, J.V., McGowan-Jordan, J., Charles, A., Parmelee, J.T., Cutaia, M.V. and Rounds, S. Hydrogen peroxide stimulates sodium-potassium pump activity in cultured pulmonary arterial endothelial cells. Am J Physiol 1993; 265(9): L613-L621), and can lead to DNA damage (Imlay, J.A., Chin, S.M. and Linn, S. Toxic DNA damage by hydrogen peroxide through the Fenton reaction in vivo and in vitro. Science 1988; 240: 640-642).

50.4 OPPOSING THERAPEUTIC USE OF NAOCL

Hypochlorite; Hypochlorous Acid; Hypohalous Acid (Sodium Salt)

The following is an editorial statement from: Breaking News: Volume 6 Edition 1, January 2002 Edition.

Sodium hypochlorite (NaOCl), the active ingredient in chlorine bleach, is a chemical with more than its share of potential risks and negative characteristics, among them:

Toxicity. Chlorine bleach is highly toxic, corrosive if swallowed or inhaled. It is the source of more poison exposures than any other substance--over 60,000 incidents reported to poison control centers in 1999 alone (according to statistics from the American Association of Poison Control Centers, Toxic Exposure Surveillance System, www.aapcc.org). Of note, these statistics also indicate that ocular, dermal, and inhalation exposures, while less frequent than ingestion cases, tend to be more serious.

Chlorine concentrations of 30 parts per million (ppm) cause immediate chest pain, vomiting, and coughing; at 430 ppm, death occurs in 30 minutes; and exposures of 1000 ppm cause death in minutes (see U.S. EPA Air Toxic Website). In addition, it can combine with other wash room chemicals in hazardous ways: with certain substances, like ammonia or acids, it forms a toxic gas.

Generation of trihalomethanes (and other chlorination by products). In the presence of organic matter (tissue, serum, etc.), found in abundance on health care laundry textiles, chlorine forms harmful byproducts, including trihalomethanes (THMs), the most common class of chlorination by products (chloroform is a THM). Overexposure to trihalomethanes may increase the following risks to human health: liver, kidney, and central nervous system damage, miscarriages, neural tube effects, and cancer (esp. of the bladder, colon and rectum).

The U.S. EPA regulates trihalomethanes and soon will lower the allowable amounts in drinking water from 100 to 80 parts per billion (rule took effect for large water systems in Jan. 2002).

Sodium hypochlorite (NaOCl) which is commonly used as a household bleach is known to have adverse effects when ingested such as, mucosal irritation, corrosive activity and vomiting. Investigators have shown that 4% solutions of sodium hypochlorite with 0.5% sodium hydroxide given by the intragastric route to rats, produced damage to the lungs, the livers, and the kidneys. Also, erosive changes were present in the stomachs. Similar histopathological changes were observed when bleach was given by I.V. administration (Andiran, F., Tanyel, F.C., Ayhan, A. and Hicsonmez, A., Systemic harmful effects of ingestion of household bleaches. Drug Chem Toxico 1999; 22(3): 545-553).

Sodium hypochlorite (NaOCl), when added to water, dissolves to form hypochlorous acid. Hypochlorous acid (HOCl) is a **strong oxidizing and chlorinating species**, which is formed from hydrogen peroxide and chloride and has been implicated in lipid peroxidation by human phagocytic cells.

50.4.1 Myeloperoxidase

Hypochlorous acid is also formed by the enzymatic action of **myeloperoxidase (MPO),** which is considered to be of major importance in inflammatory processes such as arteriosclerosis. Catalytically active MPO is a component of human atherosclerosis tissue (Daugherty, A., Rateri, D.L., Dunn, J.L. and Heinecke, J.W. Myeloperoxidase, a catalyst for lipoprotein oxidation, is expressed in human atherosclerosis lesions. J Clin Invest 1994; 94: 437-444). The in vivo relevance of the MPO/H$_2$O$_2$/Cl- system damage has been demonstrated by the observation that HOCL epitopes of LDL have been detected in human atherosclerosis lesions using specific monoclonal antibodies (Hazell, L.J., Arnold, L., Flowers, D., Waeg, G., Malle, E. and Stocker, R.   Presence of hypochlorite-modified proteins in atherosclerotic lesions. J Clin Invest 1996; 97: 1535-1544). Investigators have also reported that reagent HOCl or HOCL generated by the MPO/H2O2/Cl- system can initiate peroxidation in lipoproteins and liposomes (Panasenko, O.M. The mechanism of the hypochlorite-induced lipid peroxidation. Biofactors 1997; 6: 181-190). Additionally, cholesterol chlorohydrin formation by reagent HOCl has been found in various cell types including erythrocytes, neutrophils and mammary carcinoma cells, which could mediate powerful biologic effects in the artery wall since other oxygenated sterols are cytotoxic and mutagenic and potent regulators of cholesterol homeostasis in cultured mammalian cells (Carr, A.C., van den Berg, J.J., and Winterbourn, C.C. Chlorination of cholesterol in cell membranes by hypochlorous acid. Arch Biochem Biophys 1996; 332: 63-69).

In the presence of chloride ions, the action of peroxidases, such as myeloperoxidase, on hydrogen peroxide produces hypochlorous acid (HOCl), which at even low molar concentration levels of 10-20 micromoles/liter acts to damage proteins on cell membranes and destroy their function (Cochrane, C.G. Cellular injury by oxidants. Am J Med 1991; 91(C): 23S-30S).

Sodium Hypochlorite and Hypochlorous Acid Toxicity

Sodium hypochlorite (NaOCl) is one of the most commonly used irrigating solutions in endodontic dental practice as an antibacterial and cleansing agent. Mehra and Clancy report the formation of a facial hematoma during endodontic therapy with the use of NaOCl. They report this intracanal medicament's potential toxicity (Hehra P., Clancy, C. and Wu, J. Formation of a facial hematoma during endodontic therapy. J Am Dent Assoc 2000; 131(1): 67-71).

In a study testing the cytotoxicity of liquid disinfectants, when investigators measured the integrity of cellular membrane, metabolic activity, or cell growth, they found that there is a several-hundredfold difference in the relative toxicity of various disinfecting substances. The concentration toxic in 50% of the cell population (TC(50)) that was found for each disinfectant was similar in a variety of cell lines from human, monkey, or mouse origin. Statistical analysis of TC(50)s suggests that liquid disinfecting agents could be classified in three main groups according to their relative toxicity, with (1) **mild** (TC(50)> 1mM, including phenol, **hydrogen peroxide**, and formaldehyde), (2) **moderate** (1mM>TC(50)>0.1mM, **sodium hypochlorite**), and (3) severe (TC(50)<0.1mM, glutaraldehyde, cupric ascorbate, and per acetic acid) toxicity. These data suggest a vast difference in the potential risk of various disinfectants and sterilants. The data presented in this study should help to define the relative toxic risk of different disinfecting substances to patients and healthcare personnel and assist in the selection of safer microbicidal formulations. (Sagripanti J.L. and Bonifacino A. Cytotoxicity of liquid disinfectants. Surg Infect (Larchmt) 2000; 1(1): 3-14).

HOCl has been implicated as a causative agent in rheumatoid arthritis and investigators have found that nitrite (NO(2)(-)) accumulation at chronically inflamed sites where both HOCl and nitric oxide (NO) are over produced may be cytoprotective against damage induced by HOCl (Whiteman, M., Rose, P., Siau, J.L and Halliwell, B. Nitrite-mediated protection against hypochlorous acid-induced chrondrocyte toxicity: A novel cytoprotective role of nitric oxide in the inflamed joint? 2003; 48(11): 3140-3150).

It is well known that **HOCl and H$_2$O$_2$ can hemolyze** human erythrocytes (RBC's) or kill monkey kidney cells in culture. Studies indicate that like peroxide, NaOCl also synergizes with membrane-perforating agents and with **a protease** to kill epithelial cells and further implicates such "cocktails" in cell injury or inflammation (Ginsburg, I., Sadovnic, M., Yedgar, S., Kohen, R. and Hibac, J. Hemolysis of human erythrocytes by hypochlorous acid is modulated by amino acids, antioxidants, membrane-perforating agents and by divalent metals. 2002; 36(6): 607-19).

Commercial 5% NaOCl can also produce structural and molecular alterations on the collagen and glycosaminogly-cans of mineralized and dematerialized dentin (Oyarzun, A., Cordero, A.M. and Whittle, M. Immunohistochemical evaluation of the effects of sodium hypochlorite on dentin collagen and glycosaminoglycans. 2002; 28(3): 152-156).

There have been studies on the therapeutic efficacy of the topical antiseptic sodium hypochlorite (NaOCl) for antibacterial activity and in parallel the cytotoxicity mechanisms by which hypochlorite and chloramines generated therefrom induce oxidative tissue damage, which further influences the wound-healing process. The early NaOCl-produced cytotoxic action on cultured fibroblasts was cell ATP depletion which occurred at 0.00005% (with FCS 2%) followed by dose-and time-dependent decreases, reaching levels below 5% of control values. Using the 3'-[phe-nyl amino-carbonyl)-3,4-tetrazolium]-bis(4-methoxy-6-nitro)benzene sulfuric acid metabolic assay to evaluate cell death, we observed that NaOCl concentrations greater than 0.05% provoked null fibroblast survival at all exposure times assayed. **Hypochlorous acid proved to exert a rapid inhibitory effect on DNA synthesis, consis-tent with its primary role in bacteria killing by phagocytes.** (Hidalgo, E., Bartolome, R. and Dominguez, C. Cytotoxicity mechanisms of sodium hypochlorite in cultured human dermal fibroblasts and its bactericidal ef-fectiveness. Chem Biol Interact 2002; 139(3): 265-282).

It has been suggested that the **primary target of hypochlorite must be sulfhydryl and amino groups in proteins** and that the lipid peroxidation may proceed as the secondary reaction, which is induced by radicals gen-erated from sulfenyl chlorides and chloramines.

Taurine has been shown to be an effective scavenger of hypochlorous acid (HOCl). The role of HOCl is well estab-lished in tissue damage associated with reperfusion injury mediated by neutrophils. The role of HOCl in CNS injury and inflammation reactions has not been well established. Myeloperoxidase activity is present in the CNS and it has been associated with ischemia injury. Studies now clearly show that taurine is an efficient scavenger of HOCl and can prevent neuronal damage caused by HOCl. Since myeloperoxidase expression in the CNS is increased by ischemia, one function of taurine released during an ischemia event may be to scavenge HOCl and provide neuro-protection (Kearns, S. and Dawson, R., Jr. Cytoprotective effect of taurine against hypochlorous acid toxicity to PC12 cells. Adv Exp Med Biol 2000; 483: 563-570).

-Addition of reagent HOCl (3-25 mm) did not induce mononuclear leukocytes with any DNA strand breaks (Mutation Research, 1992; 265: 255-261).

-HOCl and H_2O_2 were both used at physiologically relevant final concentrations of 12.5 μM, which was non-cytotoxic for human leucocytes according to eosin exclusion and lactate dehydrogenase release assays (Mutation Research, 1992; 265: 256).

-HOCl from PMNs auto activates collagenase that leads to breakdown of basement membranes.

51 SINGLET OXYGEN TOXICITY

The organic and biological chemistry of molecular oxygen is of extraordinary interest. Oxygen plays an important role in aging, damage to materials in the environment, cellular pathology (for example, the damage following stroke or heart attack) and many other areas. The details of the chemical reactions underlying these processes are poorly understood. The Foote group uses preparative, physical -organic and bioorganic methods to study the chemistry of molecular oxygen in photochemical and biological processes. Reactive intermediates include singlet oxygen ($^1O_2$, a metastable excited state of molecular oxygen) superoxide ion, and other oxygen species. (Chimin Sheau, Saeed Khan and Christopher S. Foote "Low-Temperature Photosensitized Oxidation of a Guanosine Derivative of an Imidazole Ring-Opened Product" (submitted to J Am Chem Soc), Murphy, S.T., Krasnovsky, A.A., Jr. and Foote, C.S. "High Efficiency of Singlet-Oxygen-Sensitized Delayed Fluorescence with Tetra-tert-butylphtalocyanine: A Potential singlet Oxygen Sensor" (submitted to J Am Chem Soc 1999).

Singlet oxygen is very toxic to organisms because it reacts with important biological molecules such as unsaturated lipids, utilizable amino acids, and nucleic acids, particularly guanosine derivatives of DNA. The resulting reactions cause destruction of membranes, enzyme inactivation, and mutations, all of which can lead to cell death. They are carrying out extensive studies of the reactions with biological target molecules and have characterized many of the primary products of these reactions. For example, photooxidation of guanosine derivatives produce endoperoxides that are stable only at low temperatures. This reaction is responsible for genetic damage caused by sensitizing molecules, light, and oxygen. (Ping Kang and Christopher S. Foote, Synthesis of a 13C, 15N Labeled Imidazole and Characterization of the 2;5-endoperoxide and its Decomposition, Tetrahedron Lett. accepted).

Dr. Christopher S. Foote summary at website: http://www.chem.ucla.edu/dept/Faculty/foote.html :

Oxygen-dependent photosensitized toxic effects are extremely common in nature. A particularly exciting application of this type of chemistry is the use of a photosensitizer, light, and oxygen to kill tumor cells selectively in humans. Studies of the mechanism and preparation of more effective sensitizers are in progress.

Robert J. Stackow and Robert Bernstein in an article entitled, "The chemistry of Visible Light," state the following:

Photodynamic Therapy

The reactivity of singlet oxygen in biological systems has been harnessed for beneficial purposes in a medical procedure known as photodynamic therapy (PDT). In this procedure photosensitizers are preferentially absorbed by tumor or cancer cells, rather than surrounding tissues. This is followed by irradiation of the tumor cells with visible light, causing singlet oxygen to be formed, hopefully killing the unwanted cells.

The advantage of PDT over other cancer therapies is its simplicity: It only requires a photosensitizer, oxygen and light. The difficulties associated with PDT are getting the photosensitizer to localize in the tumor cells and getting the light to the tumor cells containing the photosensitizer. For these reasons PDT is most successful on surface tumors such as skin cancers, certain cancers of the eye, and esophageal cancer, where application and irradiation of the areas are facile.

While the limitations associated with **PDT** may seem significant, alternative methods available for fighting these tumors are typically much harsher on the patient's overall health. This motivates researchers in the field of photodynamic therapy to widen the scope of its applicability.

Singlet Oxygen at UCLA

The future of PDT will involve finding or synthesizing photosensitizers that can work with red light. This is extremely desirable because out of the colors that make up white light, red light penetrates through the body's tissues the most easily. This phenomenon can be easily observed in a darkened room by holding a hand over a flashlight. The hand will glow red because the red light is able to pass all the way through the tissues. With photosensitizers which can work with red light, tumors which are internal, thus inaccessible to the current generation of photosensitizers, may become treatable with PDT.

In the research group of Professor Christopher S. Foote, in the Department of Chemistry and Biochemistry at UCLA, a major part of our research involves trying to utilize many of the concepts described here. In an effort to further our understanding of these processes, we are currently attempting to synthesize new and more potent photosensitizers with wider applicability for PDT, further elucidate the mechanisms by which they form singlet oxygen and other products, and continue investigations to determine how singlet oxygen reacts with different substrates.

Dr. Foote, the very man who, as early as 1964, had described the hydrogen peroxide reaction with sodium hypochlorite to produce excited singlet oxygen, is leading teams of scientists in attempts to find better photosensitizers to treat cancer with PDT. Four decades later, nowhere in the literature has Dr. Foote described or eluded to any attempt to use the simple peroxide/hypochlorite generation of singlet oxygen for the treatment of diseases such as cancer, arteriosclerosis, AIDS, etc. Yet, he and his team of investigators spend countless hours and dollars trying to chemically modify photosensitizers to better treat these diseases. Clearly, the elegance and simplicity of the Howes Method of Singlet Oxygen therapy has not occurred to any of them!

Additionally, Dr. Vincent DeVita, former Director of the National Cancer Institute, who is now the Chairman of Light Sciences Corporation www.lightsciences.com is currently studying and basing development on its extensive IP portfolio of 246 issued Patents covering a pipeline of photosensitizer drugs...in treating proliferate diseases. Evidently, my Singlet Oxygen Methods have not occurred to these astute and highly qualified investigators, who are spending millions of dollars to develop better photosensitizers to treat cancer. Furthermore, their literature and publications mention nothing whatsoever about the generation of singlet oxygen by the peroxide/hypochlorite system.

Studies have shown that tert-butyl hydroperoxide and methyl linoleate hydroperoxide **reacts with hypochlorite** to give peroxyl and/or alkoxyl radicals with little formation of $^1O_2$. In contrast to H_2O_2, **which gives $^1O_2$ exclusively** (Noguche, N., Nakada, A., Itoh, Y., Watanabe, A. and Niki, E. Formation of active oxygen species and lipid peroxidation induced by hypochlorite. Arch Biochem Biophys 2002; 392(2): 440-447).

51.1 GENERAL DISCUSSION

Other investigators have discussed the wide range of biochemical damage that is caused by the harmful singlet oxygen species in biological systems (Briviba, K., Klotz, L.O., Sies, H. Toxic and signaling effects of photochemically or chemically generated singlet oxygen in biological systems. Biol Chem 1997; 378(11): 1259-1265). The oxidative damage that results from singlet oxygen can have wide spread effects. **Proteins appear to quench about 80% of the singlet oxygen produced in cell membranes.** (Kanofsky, J.R. Quenching of singlet oxygen by human red cell ghosts. Photochem Photobiol 1991; 53: 93-99). The quenching leads to damage of the protein that can bring about membrane depolarization. (Specht, K. G. and M. A. J. Rodgers. Plasma membrane depolarization and calcium influx during cell injury by photodynamic action. Biochem Biophys Acta 1990; 1070: 60-68).

Singlet oxygen can damage bimolecules and thus exert toxicity (for reviews, see Sies, H. Biochemistry of oxidative stress. Angew Chem Int Ed. England 1986; 25: 1058-1071), (Piette, J. Biological consequences associated with DNA oxidation mediated by singlet oxygen. J Photochem Photobiol B Biol 1991; 11: 241-260), (Sies, H and Menck, C.F. Singlet oxygen induced DNA damage. Mutat Res 1992; 275: 367-375). **Damage to DNA consists primarily of the oxidation of guanine residues, mainly to 7-hydro-8-oxodeoxyguanosine** (Piette, 1991). Upon replication, this leads to G:C to T:A transversions and is part of the mutagenic action of singlet oxygen (Decuyper-Debergh, D., Piette, J. and van de Vorst, A. Singlet oxygen-induced mutations in M13 lacZ phage DNA EMBO J 1987; 6: 3155-3161), (Kouchakdigan, M., Bodepudi, V., Shibutani, S., Eisenberg, M., Johnson, F., Grollman, A. P. and Patel, D. J. NMR structural studies of the ionizing radiation adduct 7-hydro 8-oxodeoxyguanosine (8-oxo-7H-dG) opposite deoxyadenosine in a DNA duplex. 8-Oxo-7H-dG(syn)-dA(anti) alignment at lesion site. Biochemistry 1991; 30: 1403-1412), (Piette, J., Epe, B., Ballmaier, D., Roussyne, I., Briviba, K and Sies, H. DNA damage by peroxynitrite characterized with DNA repair enzymes. Nucleic Acids Res 1996; 24: 4105-4110). It has been hypothesized that singlet oxygen produced endogenously in Escherichia coli stationary phase cells is responsible for DNA damage and the high mutation rates found under these conditions (Bridges, B.A. and Timms, A. Effect of endogenous carotenoids and defective RpoS sigma factor on spontaneous mutation under starvation conditions in Escherichia coli: Evidence or the possible involvement of singlet oxygen. Mutat Res 1998; 403: 21-28). **7-Hydro-8-oxodeoxyguanosine is also formed in mitochondria DNA on treatment of human lung fibroblasts with methylene blue plus light.** (Anson, R.M., Croteau, D.L., Stierum, R.H., Filburn, C., Parsell, R. and Bohr, V.A. Homogenous repair of singlet oxygen-induced DNA damage in differentially transcribed regions and strands of human mitochondria DNA. Nucleic Acids Res 1998; 26: 662-668). Similarly, human lung WI-38 fibroblasts exposed to gas-phase singlet oxygen resulted in sister chromatid exchange (Eisenberg, W.C., Taylor K and Guerrero, R.R. Cytogenetic effects of singlet oxygen. J Photochem Photobiol B 1992; 16(3-4): 381-4).

Investigators have determined the deleterious effects of singlet oxygen ($^1O_2$), generated by thermal decomposition of the water-soluble endoperoxide 3,3'-(1,4-naphythylidene)dipropionate ($NDPO_2$), on plasmid DNA. Their findings indicate that $^1O_2$ can induce DNA lesions which are repaired by an error-prone process in prokaryotic and eukaryotic cells (Di Mascio, P, Menck, C.F., Nigro, R.G., Sarasin, A and Sies, H. Singlet molecular oxygen induced mutagenicity in a mammalian SV40-based shuttle vector Photochem Photobiol 1990; 51(3): 293-298).

Singlet oxygen ($^1O_2$) is a product of several biological processes and can be generated in photodynamic therapy, through a photosensitization type II mechanism. $^1O_2$ is able to interact with lipids, proteins and DNA, leading to cell killing and mutagenesis, and can be directly involved with degenerative processes such as cancer and aging. Investigators theorize that singlet oxygen interaction with cell membranes may generate secondary products that could react with DNA, leading to mutagenic lesions (Cavalcante A.K., Martinez, G.R., Di Mascio, P., Menck, C.F. and Agnez-Lima, L.F. Cytotoxicity and mutagenesis induced by singlet oxygen in wild type and DNA repair deficient Escherichia coli strains. DNA Repair (Amst) 2002; 1(12): 1051-1056).

Mutations of mitochondria (mtDNA) accumulate during normal aging. The most frequent mutation is a 4,977-base pair deletion also called the common deletion, which is increased in photoaged skin. Oxidative stress may play a major role in the generation of large scale mtDNA deletions. These studies provide evidence for the involvement of reactive oxygen species in the generation of aging-associated mtDNA lesions in human cells and indicate a previously unrecognized role of singlet oxygen in photoaging of human skin (Berneburg, M., Grether-Beck, S., Kurten, V., Ruzicka, T., Briviba, K., Sies, H. and Krutmann, J. Singlet oxygen mediates the UVA-induced generation of the photoaging-associated mitochondria common deletion. J Biol Chem 1999; 274(22): 15345-15349).

Studies on the oxyR gene, whose product regulates the expression of the enzymes and proteins that are needed for cellular protection against oxidative stress, suggests that **the oxyR regulon plays an important protective role in singlet oxygen-mediated cellular damage**, presumably through the protection of antioxidant enzymes (Kim, S.Y., Kim, E.J. and Park, J.W. Control of singlet oxygen-induced oxidative damage in Escherichia coli. J Biochem Mol Biol 2002; 35(4): 353-357).

Singlet oxygen is responsible for both the oxidative damage of biomolecules and its presence can lead to the activation of signal transduction pathways **Activation of the Fas pathway to apoptosis was initiated in human leukemia HL-60 cells by $^1O_2$** (Zhuang, S., Demirs, J.T. and Kochevar, I.E. Protein kinase C inhibits singlet oxygen-induced apoptosis by decreasing caspase-8 activation of the Fas-FasL pathway. J Surg Res 2001; 101: 183-189). **Singelt oxygen also initiated rapid apoptosis by a mechanism involving p38 activation.** (Zhuang, S., Demirs, J.T. and Kochevar, I.E. P38 mitogen-activated protein kinase mediates bid cleavage, mitochondria dysfunction and caspase-3 activation during apoptosis induced by singlet oxygen but not by hydrogen peroxide. J Biol Chem 2000; 275: 25939-25948).

Proteins comprise approximately 68% of the dry weight of cells and tissues and are therefore potentially major targets for oxidative damage and singlet oxygen generated by the transfer of energy to ground state (triplet) molecular oxygen by either protein-bound, or other, chromophores or other enzymes can bring about changes to both the side-chains and backbone of amino acids, peptides, and proteins. Such processes can result in the transmittal of damage to other biological targets and may play a significant role in bystander damage, or dark reactions, in systems where proteins are subjected to oxidation (Davies, M.J. Singlet oxygen-mediated damage to proteins and its consequences. Biochem Biophys Res Commun 2003; 305(3): 761-70).

Other investigators are trying to introduce singlet oxygen into cells or tissue by complex, free radical, multiple-step chemical reactions, or by utilizing anaerobic enzymes, endoperoxide decomposition, while still others are using the luciferin (luciferase) light-producing enzyme systems. Worldwide, countless others are busily changing chemical side group moieties on heme-containing proteins or manufacturing an enormous array of hematoporphyrin derivatives, in attempts to "overcome limitations and improve" their singlet oxygen delivery systems.

51.1.2 Summary

The Howes Singlet Oxygen Delivery System is a quantitative, highly reproducible, reliable, non-radicallic, single-step method, which is completely made of crucial physiological compounds (which are, in fact, present in steady state levels in all aerobic cells) and which breaks down into completely harmless and needed end products of saline (NaCl & H_2O) and ground state oxygen.

The prevailing prejudice against reactive oxygen species (RONS) is manifestly illustrated in the November 2003 issue of Readers Digest. In quoting Dr. Bruce Ames, a highly respected biochemist at University of California at Berkley, he states, "free radical oxidation doesn't just rise with aging--it causes it. The more that mitochondria 'leak' free radicals (i.e., oxygen radicals), the more those radicals end up damaging the mitochondria, which in turn leak even more free radicals." In bold print, the article states, "The ultimate irony: The thing we need most to live--oxygen--is what's

killing us." Statements such as this, which appear in both the lay press and in scientific publications, point out the currently accepted dogma which states that oxygen and its radicals are highly toxic, even lethal. I believe that the overall data shows that they are wrong.

**"Modern man arrives upon this earth hell-bent
and hard-wired for:
oxygen consumption, for RONS/excytomer (EMOD) production,
intellectual curiosity for fear of the unknown,
basic drives for pleasure and perpetuation of our unique double helix,
an ability to create, equaled by a propensity to destroy,
a self-cure system coupled with a homeostatic over-ride,
compensatory religiosity for our sinful ways,
a fight or flight reflex which opposes societal regulation,
and an assured face-to-face rendezvous with the Reaper."**

R.M. Howes, M.D., Ph.D.

8/24/04

52.0 EPIPHANY: PRINCIPLES OF UNIFICATION

In considering the incredible range of results seen with varying qualified laboratory investigators and in view of the diametrically opposed clinical results, seen with clinicians versus practitioners of alternative medicine, there is an eminent need for a view towards unification. With an overview and appreciation of the history of medicine, I have concluded that, at least the following principles are playing a key role in the production of such a non-uniform spectrum of results and contributing to the confusion and contradictions (both experimental and clinical) concerning oxygen metabolism:

1 **Ground state oxygen organismal, cellular and organelle levels in**
physiological living/breathing conditions, should be the basis for objective research studies, as opposed to over-emphasis of artifactual in vitro conditions. Without an adequate supply of ground state oxygen, our cells will not be able to generate adequate levels of RONS/excytomers.

2 **The non-linearity and multi-phasic nature of RONS/excytomers reactions.** Deficient levels "allow" development of pathogens, cancer and aging.
Normal levels maintain homeostasis.
High levels kill pathogens and cancer.

3 **The curious and amazing behavior of the electron.** I have written
in-depth about the effects of moving, adding or losing a singular electron within oxygen's orbitals and many other molecules. Keep in mind that it takes one quintillion electrons/sec. to power a light bulb. The same electrons, that flow from the hydro-electric turbines at the Hoover Dam, to power many Western cities, are the same entities which flow along the cytochromes of the electron transport chain to power our cells and thus, our lives. The same electrical force used for an electrocution is the same force which initiates heart beats and processes thought.

4 **The internal milieu,** as it specifically relates to the growth of pathogens and
cancer. Virchow, Lister and Bernard were acutely aware of this principle and I believe that it applies, in large part, to the specific cellular redox biochemical status and the integrity of the immune system.

5 **Natural variation of studied subjects:** male vs. female, old vs. young, fat
vs. thin, fed vs. fasted, known diets vs. ad lib diets, healthy vs. diseased, active vs. inactive, rat vs. mouse, dog vs. cat, organ vs. a different organ, tissue vs. a
different tissue cell type vs. a different cell type, etc.

6 **Differing methods of data evaluation.** Biometrics, statistical analysis,
epidemiological correlations, definitions of study groups included and excluded, differing levels of confidence and p values, etc. lead to difficulty in getting the true picture with many studies. Intentional over-usage of complex and arcane scientific lingo and terms only serves to impress the author, who hopes to shield himself (herself) from careful scrutiny of established and neophyte scientists. As Dr, Steele said, upon reading a draft of UTOPIA, "Some folks are overwhelmed by the exuberance of their own verbosity." Was that a compliment or an ins…?

7 **Dosis sola venenum facit**. Only **the dosage** makes the poison.

This helps explain the confusing data relating to so many pharmaceutical studies, dose-response curves and clinical trials. It also applies to the reactions of redox agents, whereby they can act as either an antioxidant or a pro-oxidant. Also, take into account the phenomenon of low dose activation and high dose inhibition. Multi-phasic dose-related reactions are not uncommon.

8 The almighty auto-pilot, whereby our mind and body is constantly acting

on its own to maintain a healthy state. I believe that this is perhaps one of the most overlooked of these principles by Western medicine. **Our entire constitutional make up is hard-wired for self-cure**, from the cellular components and organelles, to the entirety of the organism. When this system fails, in a normal aerobic organism, illness or disease is manifested. A state of good health is a manifestation of normalcy. The most illustrative case of the auto-pilot is during sleep and/or a comatose state.

9 The placebo effect, in which the studied agent serves as a "triggering mecha-

nism" for the activation of the body's self-cure system. The mystery of touch, rubbing, sugar pills, bread pills and injections of physiological saline will continue to confound clinical studies and therapeutic regimens.

10 Bias of investigators. Unquestionably, many of our "scientific" studies are

set up with "a point to prove," whether to further a reputation, to get FDA approval of a medication or to fulfill a grant objective. These studies are flawed before they even begin, because of a "pre-prejudicial" influence.

11 A lack of honesty and integrity. Unfortunately, profit motivates the pub-

lication of countless dishonest articles and the manufacture and dispersal of innumerable, ineffective nostrums, which are so readily available today. I dare say that there has never been a time in man's history, with more deceptive and ignominious quacks, charlatans and hucksters. Profit drives the healthcare industry, especially the pharmaceutical groups and the non-patentability, of a potential disease-fighting or life saving agents, should not preclude development of these products. I strongly advise all of you to perform due diligence in acquainting yourself with the medications that you are contemplating taking. More and more, I am seeing reports of harmful side effects of standard antibiotics, to fanciful cycloxygenase inhibitors, to TNF blockers, etc. Please be careful. Remember the lesson of medical history which teaches that man has frequently had the best healing results when there was no medical intervention. Certain pharmaceuticals are wonderful, but only if you really need them.

12 Relative to my **"cellular uncertainty principle,"** I believe that the cell is a

uni-verse contained within the macro-verse of the organism, just as the identifiable cosmological uni-verse is a component of the all-encompassing multi-verse. Just as Stephen Hawking believes that we can gain only limited knowledge of the universe, I believe that we have limits to our understanding of the living/breathing cell. The ultimate answer to many philosophical/scientific queries, as well as looming questions in physics, religion and string theory, may be that, **"Some things just are."** I believe that, although we may be capable of conceiving the staggering exponential happenings within the living/breathing cell, we may not be able to comprehend them. Concepts, such as invisible matter and dark energy are no more difficult to understand than the cellular cross-talk, which constantly occurs within our entire bodies, through flesh, blood and bone, many at about the speed of light. Even today, investigations are revealing that the cellular nucleus is not just a holding compartment for the genome, but is filled with complex biochemical reactions and complicated control mechanisms which were heretofore completely unanticipated.

13 Misleading epidemiological associations. The misinterpretation and mis

application of highly touted epidemiological associations are the equivalent of dragging a school of red herrings across the "truth trail" and thus, leading us astray in our pursuit and attempts to capture the "fox of knowledge." Countless quantities of time and mega-sums of money have been and are squandered chasing many of these meaningless tangents of distraction.

"Sham medicine" is, and will be, a thriving financial empire.

53 THE CRESCENDO AND GRAND FINALE: IT'S RAN-TASTIC!!

I have presented the data discussing the bactericidal, fungicidal, virucidal, parasiticidal and tumoricidal activity of RONS, especially hydrogen peroxide and singlet oxygen. I have proposed a unique delivery system for singlet oxygen, based on my laboratory and clinical data, which I now know will, at a minimum, kill squamous cell carcinoma in mice and basal cell carcinoma in man. I have pointed out, in box-car letters, the flaws with the free radical theory of aging and oxidative stress.

If you have studied this data, with an open mind, I believe that I have presented a compelling and convincing case to support my Unified Theory. Theoretically, my approach offers new hope for control and/or cure of cancer, AIDS, malaria, viral and bacterial infections and insights into the aging process.

I believe that, *what the ancients referred to as thymos or pneuma* and what I refer to as oxygen, carries a unique, life-sustaining quality, which is manifested by alterations of its electronic structure and that for the most part, the overall effects of these oxygen modifications (RONS/excytomers) are of crucial importance to the perpetuation of all aerobic life forms, inclusive of man. Further, I believe that the RONS/excytomers are a cardinal component of man's system of self-cure.

The benefits of oxygen far out weigh its alleged "cause-for-all-diseases-and-aging accusations."   In fact, it appears that the benefits of many of oxygen's modifications also have considerable salutary regulatory and signaling properties, which are in stark contrast to the past demonization of all of these reactive species.

In man's historical trek down the trail which leads from medical ignorance to scientific enlightenment, which rapidly proceeds to intellectual arrogance, there have been many wasteful digressions of disillusionment, only to arrive at illogical dead ends, thereby, squandering precious centuries of potential "times of discovery." A cursory review of medical history reveals that we are currently only stumbling out of the starting blocks, whilst attempting to trudge up the slippery slope of the learning curve for biochemical and biological truths. Impediments to man's progress have been in the form of political and religious demagoguery and out-and-out fear of knowledge.

I have shown you the secret maps of convergence, leading to oxygen's hidden treasures, buried deep within the living/breathing aerobic cell. I have pointed out the folly of the free radical theory of aging and oxidative stress and have repeatedly cautioned you to avoid the pitfalls of interpretations of epidemiological associations and the booby traps of in vitro studies.

I encourage all investigators to speak of truths, as they feel them in their hearts, even though doing so, may render them vulnerable to the possible vitriol of their critics, the termination of their funding, the rejection of their publications and/or banishment by their peers. Such are the lessons that have been and are presently being taught by our past and as was said by Michelangelo, "I am still learning."

Randolph M. Howes M.D., Ph.D.

AUTHOR AND SUBJECT INDEX:

Since this is an e-book, the author and subject index can be readily accessed by utilizing the "Find" feature.

To use this feature,
      left click on "Edit" to drop the menu.
      Left click on "Find" (Ctrl+F) (symbol is binoculars)

This will bring up the "Find and Replace window."
      In the rectangular space, which appears at "Find What,"
            type in "the name of the author desired" or "the subject of the search"

After filling in the desired search term, left click the "Find Next" box on the lower portion of the window.

The computer will take you to your requested search term for either an author or a specific word or subject.

NITRIC OXIDE: RADICAL THOUGHTS IN VEIN

It's a reactive gas, that can pass, within or to a cell
It's a radical notion, that this chemical potion, can keep us feeling well.
With pressures arterial, it's managerial, and makes hypertension subside
Relaxing smooth muscle, so a blood corpuscle has a less stressful ride.

From stroke prediction, to drug addiction, it seems to be every place
Intestinal motility, to learning ability, to the sunburn on your face.
With "NO" compunction, for your lung function, down to your appetite
It's in control, your mating pole, on your honeymoon night.

With too high levels, disease revels, from diabetes to stroke to arthritis
With levels too low, your penis won't grow, so we take Viagra inside us.
When a neutrophil, moves in for the kill, it appears to be the answer
There are rumors, it fights tumors, and may even kill cancer.

Take nitric oxide, add a superoxide, to produce peroxynitrite
Its power could have, and damage would have, made Nobel shout "Dynamite."
Proteins and DNA, and fats get out of its way, because of its harmful proclivity
Old peroxynitrite, causes molecular fright, because of its radical activity.

Cyclic GMP, may not be, the source of eternal youth
And biological norms, of three isoforms, won't show you divine truth.
But Robert, Ferid and Louis, have given to us, a discovery called sensational
They won the prize, and will save lives, from being observational.

So nitric oxide, has two sides, from pollutant to savior
It can be magic, or it can be tragic, it has a radical behavior.
It seems unbelievable, and inconceivable, that this is a miracle gas
If you disprove it, I'll behoove it, then I'll kiss your ... cheek.

A Tribute to Lou Ignarro, Nobel Laureate

Randolph M. Howes, M.D., PhD.
Copyright® 2001

DISCLOSURE AND DISCLAIMER

Made in United States
Orlando, FL
09 January 2025

57111044R00285